Periodontal Therapy

Clinical Approaches and Evidence of Success

Periodontal Therapy
Clinical Approaches and Evidence of Success
Volume 1

Edited by

Myron Nevins, DDS
Diplomate, American Board of Periodontology
Associate Clinical Professor of Periodontology
Harvard School of Dental Medicine
Boston, Massachusetts

Adjunct Professor
Department of Periodontics, School of Dentistry
University of North Carolina at Chapel Hill
Chapel Hill, North Carolina

Institute for Advanced Dental Studies
Swampscott, Massachusetts

James T. Mellonig, DDS, MS
Diplomate, American Board of Periodontology
Professor, Head Specialist Division and
Director Advanced Education Program
Department of Periodontics
The University of Texas Health Science Center at San Antonio
San Antonio, Texas

Associate Editor
Emil G. Cappetta, DMD
Diplomate, American Board of Periodontology
Clinical Professor
University of Medicine and Dentistry of New Jersey
Newark, New Jersey

Private Practice
Summit, New Jersey

Quintessence Publishing Co, Inc
Chicago, Berlin, London, Tokyo, Paris, Barcelona,
São Paulo, Moscow, Prague, and Warsaw

Library of Congress Cataloging-in-Publication Data

Periodontal therapy : clinical approaches and evidence of success /
   edited by Myron Nevins, James T. Mellonig.
       p.   cm.
   Includes bibliographical references and index.
   ISBN 0-86715-309-1
   1. Periodontal disease—Treatment. 2. Periodontal disease—
Atlases. I. Nevins, Myron. II. Mellonig, James T.
   [DNLM: 1. Periodontal Diseases—therapy. 2. Periodontal Diseases—
atlases.   WU 240 P4472 1998]
   RK361.P4614 1998
   617.6'3206—dc21
   DNLM/DLC
   for Library of Congress   97-42610
                                     CIP

quintessence
books

©1998 by Quintessence Publishing Co, Inc

Quintessence Publishing Co, Inc
551 North Kimberly Drive
Carol Stream, Illinois 60188

Editor: Betsy Solaro
Production: Michael Shanahan and Timothy M. Robbins
Cover design: Michael Shanahan

Printed in Japan

CONTENTS

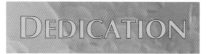

DEDICATION

This effort has been made possible by the patience and encouragement of my wife, soul mate, and best friend, Marcy, the wind beneath my wings. She and my sons, Michael and Marc, have understood and encouraged my fascination with periodontics, an occupation and an avocation.

—Ron Nevins

To my wife Karen, the love of my life and sage counsel, who allowed me, without any reservation, to pursue every goal in periodontics I dreamed possible and to my children, Tim, Amy, and Kim, who light up my life.

—Jim Mellonig

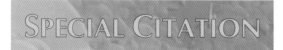

SPECIAL CITATION

Role models are an integral factor in the growth and maturity of every individual. We were fortunate to have Gerald M. Kramer and Gerald Bowers to guide and encourage our maturation, and we remain ever grateful for their efforts.

PREFACE

Every text is a reflection of its time. In this text, we have made every effort to identify contemporary periodontics, to examine the long-term results of periodontal treatment, and to base this treatment on the available evidence. We have been careful not to be overzealous in our effort to categorize periodontal therapy, but to allow for the mixing and matching of treatment regimens to suit the needs of the patient. We have, however, directed this text toward a definite goal of therapy, that of offering each patient the solution we would select for ourselves.

Contemporary periodontics is a reflection of the dedication, integrity, and imagination of the clinicians, educators, and researchers in the field. Early investigators followed diverse paths—many were educated in oral pathology or oral medicine—but by teaching and publishing their findings, they all shared a dedication to the pursuit of excellence. In truth, much progress resulted from the clash of ideas from diverse investigators, each committed to a single method.

Innovative investigators continued to reexamine the traditional beliefs and to ask impertinent questions. Many early studies were tainted with bias, and much time was to pass before improved scientific methods would emerge. Although bias can still rear its ugly head, a moment of reflection reveals that we still cannot clearly and precisely identify the etiology of adult periodontitis or understand refractory periodontitis. Yet we continue to hold in high esteem our teachers' teachers, today's role models, and their contribution to the body of knowledge that makes it possible for us to better serve our patients. Any health care professional restricted to treating chronic disease with no cure on the horizon must possess an ever-expanding armamentarium and a zest for challenge. The strength and spirit of our forefathers helps us move forward.

Our role models would look with respect upon recent developments in the field. Advances in periodontal regeneration diagnostics and osseointegration are a reflection of the cooperation and exchange of information of an international coterie of periodontists. Despite their different philosophies and approaches, periodontists have been able to congregate for World Workshops in Clinical Periodontics to scrutinize the available knowledge using a system designed to provide evidence-based findings. It is our hope that we are able to recognize meaningful evidence without losing sight of our end point goals. The field of periodontics remains a work in progress.

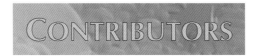

CONTRIBUTORS

John R. Bednar, DMD
Assistant Clinical Professor
Department of Orthodontics
Boston University School of Dental Medicine
Boston, Massachusetts

John F. Bruno, DDS, MS
Associate Clinical Professor
Department of Periodontology
Tufts University School of Dental Medicine
Boston, Massachusetts

Michael A. Brunsvold, DDS, MS
Diplomate, American Board of Periodontology
Associate Professor
Department of Periodontics
The University of Texas Health Science Center
  at San Antonio
San Antonio, Texas

Nicholas M. Dello Russo, DMD, MScD
Diplomate, American Board of Periodontology
Instructor in Periodontology
Harvard School of Dental Medicine

Private Practice
Boston, Massachusetts

Sergio De Paoli, DDS
Private Practice
Ancona, Italy

Institute for Advanced Dental Studies
Swampscott, Massachusetts

Gary S. Greenstein, DDS, MS
Diplomate, American Board of Periodontology
Clinical Professor of Periodontics
University of Medicine and Dentistry of New Jersey
Newark, New Jersey

Private Practice
Freehold, New Jersey

James J. Hanratty, DDS
Diplomate, American Board of Periodontology
Assistant Clinical Professor
Department of Periodontology
Tufts University School of Dental Medicine
Boston, Massachusetts

Institute for Advanced Dental Studies
Swampscott, Massachusetts

Perry R. Klokkevold, DDS, MS
Adjunct Associate Professor and Clinical Director
Section of Periodontics
University of California, Los Angeles
School of Dentistry
Center for the Health Sciences
Los Angeles, California

J. Gary Maynard, Jr., DDS
Diplomate, American Board of Periodontology
Clinical Professor of Periodontics
School of Dentistry, Medical College of Virginia
Virginia Commonwealth University
Richmond, Virginia

Howard T. McDonnell, DDS, MS
Diplomate, American Board of Periodontology
Faculty Director of Resident Education and Training
United States Air Force Periodontics Residency
Wilford Hall Medical Center
Lackland Air Force Base, Texas

Michael P. Mills, DMD, MS
Diplomate, American Board of Periodontology
Chairman and Program Director
United States Air Force Periodontics Residency
Wilford Hall Medical Center
Lackland Air Force Base, Texas

Kevin G. Murphy, DDS, MS
Diplomate, American Board of Periodontology
Private Practice
Baltimore, Maryland

Marc L. Nevins, DMD, MMSc
Clinical Instructor
Department of Periodontology
Harvard School of Dental Medicine
Boston, Massachusetts

Michael G. Newman, DDS
Diplomate, American Board of Periodontology
Adjunct Professor
Section of Periodontics
University of California, Los Angeles
School of Dentistry
Center for the Health Sciences
Los Angeles, California

Richard J. Oringer, DDS, DMSc
Assistant Professor
Department of Periodontics
State University of New York
Stonybrook, New York

Stefano Parma-Benfenati, MD, DDS, MScD
Department of Periodontology
University of Ferrara
Ferrara, Italy

Adriano Piatelli, MD, DDS
Professor and Chairman
Department of Oral Pathology
University of Chieti
Chieti, Italy

Ralph P. Pollack, DMD, MScD
Diplomate, American Board of Periodontology
Former Assistant Clinical Professor of Periodontology
Boston University School of Graduate Dentistry

Former Lecturer, Postgraduate Periodontics
Harvard University
Boston, Massachusetts

Gary M. Reiser, DDS
Diplomate, American Board of Periodontology
Assistant Clinical Professor
Department of Periodontology
Tufts University School of Dental Medicine
Boston, Massachusetts

Institute for Advanced Dental Studies
Swampscott, Massachusetts

Michael P. Rethman, DDS, MS
Diplomate, American Board of Periodontology
Chief Periodontist
Tripler Army Medical Center
Honolulu, Hawaii

Paul A. Ricchetti, DDS, MScD
Diplomate, American Board of Periodontology
Associate Clinical Professor of Periodontology
Case Western Reserve University School of Dentistry
Cleveland, Ohio

Private Practice
Mayfield Heights, Ohio

Louis F. Rose, DDS, MS
Diplomate, American Board of Periodontology
Professor of Surgery and Medicine
Allegheny University of the Health Sciences
Chief, Division of Dental Medicine and Surgery
Director of Implant Dentistry
Allegheny University Hospitals

Professor of Periodontics
University of Pennsylvania School of Dental Medicine
Philadelphia, Pennsylvania

Barbara J. Steinberg, DDS
Professor of Surgery and Medicine
Allegheny University of the Health Sciences
Assistant Director, Division of Dental Medicine and Surgery
Director, General Practice Residency
Allegheny University Hospitals

Clinical Associate Professor of Oral Medicine
University of Pennsylvania School of Dental Medicine
Philadelphia, Pennsylvania

Carlo Tinti, MD, DDS
Private Practice
Flero, Italy

Paolo Trisi, DDS
Department of Oral Pathology
University of Chieti
Chieti, Italy

Roger J. Wise, DDS
Diplomate, American Board of Periodontology
Lecturer, Harvard School of Dental Medicine
Department of Orthodontics
Boston, Massachusetts

Institute for Advanced Dental Studies
Swampscott, Massachusetts

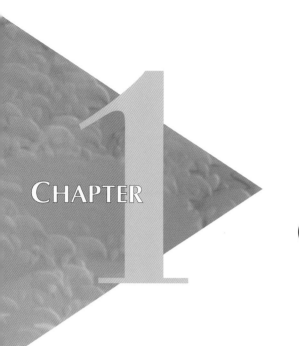

CHAPTER

Essentials of Periodontal Treatment Planning for Chronic Adult Periodontitis

Myron Nevins, DDS

edentulism: tooth loss
caries: decay

All periodontal therapeutic decisions must be predicated on preserving and improving the esthetic, phonetic, and functional dentition as perceived by both the therapist and the patient. Although it is impossible to circumvent the modifiers of physical health, patient behavior, financial capabilities, and performance variabilities as they pertain to treatment modalities, there must be an end-point goal of treatment that comes to fruition.

There were three major categories of problems facing public health dentistry in the early 1960s: edentulism, dental caries, and periodontal disease. The research of Brånemark and his colleagues[1-3] has resolved the issue of edentulism and poorly fitting dentures for those individuals willing and able to consider implant treatment. Fluoridation has reduced dental caries from an epidemic to a manageable clinical problem. Periodontal disease, however, continues to pose a threat. The bacterial etiology is now an accepted fact rather than a vague hypothesis, but the specific microorganisms responsible for chronic adult periodontitis have yet to be identified.[4-6] Commonly found patterns of disease appear to be the result of a combination of microorganisms acting in concert with a host's reduced capacity to resist disease.

The vast majority of patients that present to a periodontal practice suffer chronic adult periodontal disease.[7] Very few have truly refractory disease that does not respond appropriately to traditional treatment regimens. There is currently no profile of such patients that allows them to be identified before treatment begins, however, so they enter into the patient pool undetected. Other forms of the disease, such as juvenile periodontitis, are unusual, and thus the

application progress in their diagnosis and treatment is limited to a small patient population.

The purpose of this chapter is to share a perception of clinical treatment that has proven to be long lasting when the clinician and patient are committed to a well-organized, sincere periodontal maintenance program. The sequence of treatment and the accompanying organizational skills become essential in directing patient treatment. Unfortunately, there is a paucity of clinical studies that provide randomized controlled data that would truly affect evidence-based decision making for many therapies. Therefore, the basis of treatment planning that is suggested is a reflection of the author's experience with patient care melded with the clinical and research evidence that is available.[8-12]

Diagnosis

All patients should be committed to debridement treatment before a periodontal decision-making consultation[13,14] (Figs 1-1a and 1-1b). The time of consultation is thus conceived as an introduction to corrective treatments and a commitment to an ongoing maintenance of the result. The most important issue at consultation is the number and length of strategic clinical roots that can be retained and, if needed, restored to achieve a comfortable, functional, esthetic dentition.[15,16]

The *clinical root* is defined as that portion of the tooth root that is connected to the alveolar process by the periodontal ligament. The *clinical crown* comprises the remainder of the tooth structure.

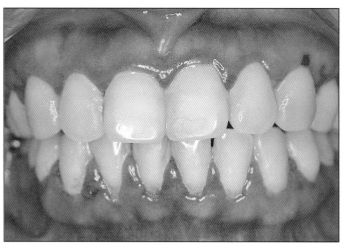

Fig 1-1a This patient has presented for treatment with inflamed red gingiva that is hyperplastic and bleeds easily on probing.

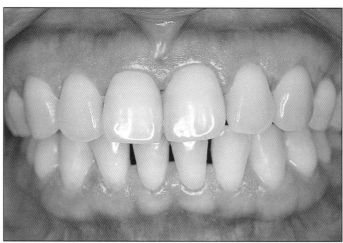

Fig 1-1b The form and color of the gingiva have returned to acceptable parameters. The tissue is pink and reduced in volume after debridement due to an improved state of cleanliness. It is at this time that the need for further periodontal treatment should be assessed.

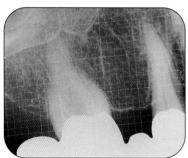

Fig 1-2a The two-dimensional radiograph provides accurate information as to the level of interproximal bone. It does not, however, reveal the loss of radicular attachment because of the buccolingual width of the tooth and the thin buccal plate of bone.

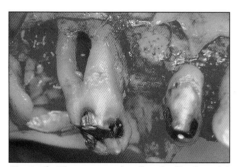

Fig 1-2b The same molar after the fixed partial denture has been removed. It is now that the three-dimensional loss is revealed.

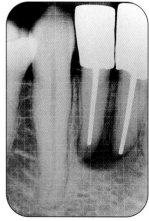

Fig 1-3a There are obvious problems relating to the periapical areas of the incisors. It is impossible to estimate the level of radicular bone on the canine. The two-dimensional radiograph is a reduction of the three-dimensional tooth and alveolar process.

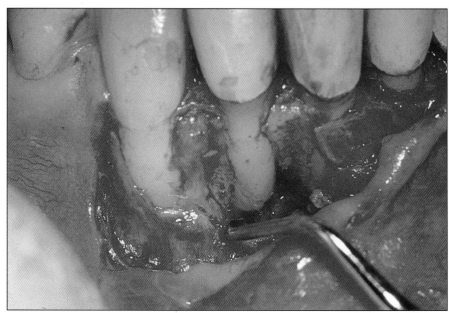

Fig 1-3b Flap reflection reveals that several millimeters of bone have been lost from the buccal surface of the canines and the lateral incisor. The buccal plate of bone is too thin to note the loss in the radiograph in Fig 1-3a.

Conventional periapical radiographs are two-dimensional reductions of three-dimensional teeth and their supporting alveolar process (Figs 1-2a and 1-2b). Interproximal and interradicular bone height are visible, but the radicular height of bone is difficult to ascertain because it is usually thin (Figs 1-3a and 1-3b). The loss of thicker palatal and lingual plates, described as a circumferential defect, is commonly observed[17] (Fig 1-4). These radiographs do identify the length of the clinical roots and provide significant information when they are made at the proper horizontal and vertical angles.

Phase I: Nonsurgical Treatment

All treatment of the periodontally compromised patient is divided into three phases. Phase I includes efforts to stop the problem from becoming worse, including the gathering of all pertinent diagnostic information; debridement treatment; analgesic endodontic therapy; adult tooth movement; and stabilization procedures. This nonsurgical therapy will provide the opportunity to realize the potential of a clean mouth. It will include supragingival and subgingival scaling with and without local anesthesia. A personalized education of the patient should be provided so that the patient can participate at home. The goal of phase I treatment is to contain the active disease.

Teeth in primary occlusal trauma should receive appropriate relief through selective grinding, orthodontic repositioning, or the use of a bite appliance. Teeth in secondary occlusal trauma should be considered for a form of permanent stabilization, such as intracoronal splinting or a provisional prosthesis. Orthodontic therapy is a valuable adjunct to this phase of treatment (see Fig 1-4). The end goal of phase I should be the conversion of dirty, mobile teeth to clean, stable teeth. It is also an appropriate time for strategic extractions to protect the remaining periodontium (Figs 1-5a to 1-5g).

Nonsurgical Periodontal Treatment

- Plaque control education
- Supragingival and subgingival scaling
- Root planing with local anesthesia
- Occlusal adjustment through selective grinding
- Provisional stabilization
- Endodontic therapy
- Adult tooth movement
- Reevaluation

The result of debridement should be pink, nonbleeding gingiva (see Fig 1-1b). This has led many to be misdirected to believe that pink tissue is synonymous with periodontal health, but it is only at this time that the clinician can

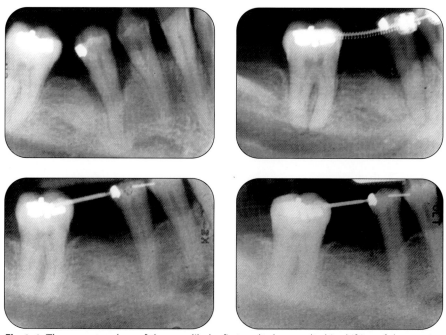

Fig 1-4 The premature loss of the mandibular first molar has resulted in drifting of the remaining posterior teeth. The second premolar demonstrates vertical osseous lesions on both proximal surfaces. Minor tooth movement has been utilized to reposition the teeth in their proper place. This was followed by placement of an autogenous bone graft and stabilization of the remaining teeth. The treatment plan called for the construction of a fixed partial denture to replace the missing first molar, but financial constraints have precluded this event. The radiographic series covers a period of 12 years.

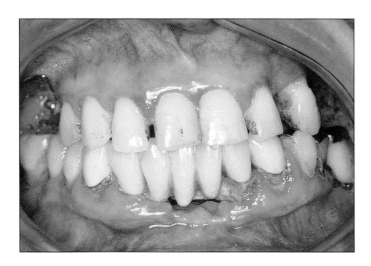

Fig 1-5a This patient has presented for the initial visit with advanced periodontal disease. There is an immediate indication for debridement therapy and the development of a treatment plan.

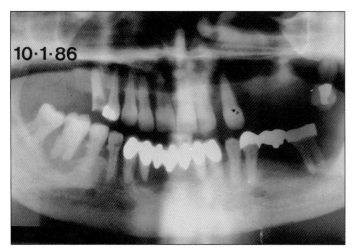

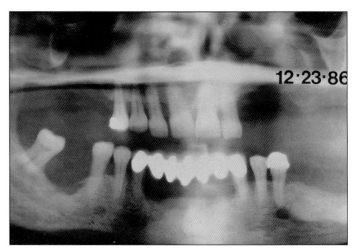

Fig 1-5b The original panoramic radiograph reveals the need to make decisions about several teeth. The mandibular right first molar should be extracted before there is any further damage to the supporting structures of the approximating teeth. The mandibular left molar and the maxillary left molar will be extracted immediately. The maxillary left canine has no bone support remaining and exhibits degree III mobility. The prognosis of the mandibular incisors is questionable, and the maxillary right second premolar will be eliminated because of bone loss, caries, and tooth position. It is necessary to stop the problem from getting worse. **Fig 1-5c** Panoramic radiograph taken after strategic extractions.

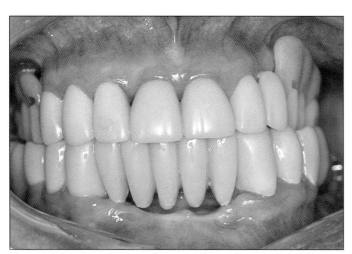

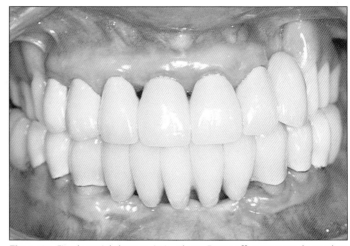

Fig 1-5d Provisionalization of the dentition after initial debridement treatment. The mandibular provisional prosthesis is fixed; the maxillary anterior provisional partial denture is fixed with a cantilevered left canine. The attachment for the partial denture is in this tooth.

Fig 1-5e Fixed partial denture is in place. Every effort was made to place the margins supragingivally when possible.

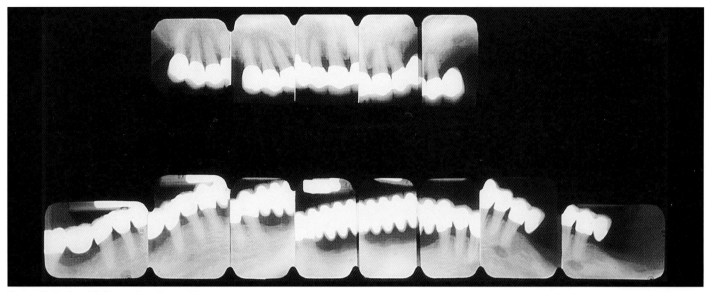

Fig 1-5f Updated full-mouth radiographic survey.

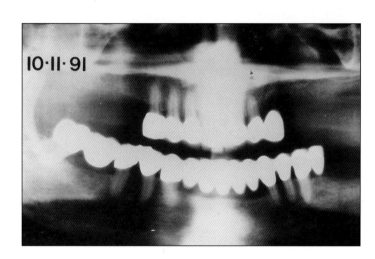

Fig 1-5g Panoramic radiograph taken 5 years after treatment with the fixed partial denture in place.

determine if the patient has the dexterity and desire to continue to phase II, the corrective part of treatment.

Phase II: Corrective Treatment

This phase of treatment addresses the deformities that result from preexisting periodontal disease. There are circumstances when orthodontic tooth movement occurs in phase II. Now it is time to consider the use of pocket elimination therapy and mucogingival surgery, the treatment of furcations on multirooted teeth, the use of periodontal regeneration procedures, and the placement of dental implants. Adjunctive treatment, such as endodontics for sectioned teeth and the construction of the permanent prosthesis, eventually conclude this phase of treatment.

Corrective Treatment

- Adult tooth movement
- Implant placement
- Periodontal surgery
- Endodontic therapy
- Reevaluation of the dentition and periodontium
- Finished restoration

---

maintenance & prevention

The third phase of treatment will protect the result that has been previously attained. It requires an ongoing commitment to diligence, an ever-increasing staff size, and, periodically, a significant enlargement of the treatment facility.[18]

It is important to provide a doctrine with some dogma that will pertain to all clinical treatments. It is also impossible to practice periodontics with "canal vision." Therefore, the dogma includes the following:

1. Use of debridement treatment
2. Maintenance of the result
3. Existence of interproximal embrasures
4. Recognition of the biologic width and its application to restorative dentistry
5. Placement of all margins of new restorations on sound tooth structure

Examination of a cross section of long-term results allows us to share a recipe for treatment that will be successful for most patients who present to a periodontist's office. The vast majority of these patients exhibit chronic adult periodontitis; a small number have rapidly progressive periodontitis, and there is minimal incidence of refractory disease. *Refractory periodontal disease* is defined as disease in multiple sites that continue to demonstrate attachment loss after appropriate therapy.[7] Therefore, most patients respond to appropriate periodontal treatment.

Appropriate treatment includes debridement, stabilization when necessary, pocket elimination, and maintenance therapy. Although many dentitions will also require orthodontics, pharmacologic agents, endodontics, and dental implants, the basic recipe for treatment will resolve the most common of all periodontal disease entities. This is not surprising because the etiology of chronic periodontitis is clearly bacterial.

Recipe for Treatment of Chronic Adult Periodontitis

- Debridement
- Stabilization
- Pocket elimination
- Maintenance therapy

Debridement

Debridement must be the first goal when the patient with adult chronic periodontitis is treated. If the patient does not demonstrate the skills and the desire to achieve this goal, it is difficult to justify the administration of more sophisticated treatment. Pink, nonbleeding gingiva will result from the professional's and patient's participation in a program to achieve a clean mouth, but pink gingiva is not necessarily synonymous with periodontal health (Figs 1-6a and 1-6b).

It is at this time that periodontal probing procedures are most important because the periodontist must now decide if surgical treatment is indicated. Each area of the dentition must be individually evaluated to determine whether the patient and the hygienist can possibly provide a blanket of control without further treatment.

Stabilization

The issue of stabilization for loose teeth can only be addressed on a basis of clinical observation because there have been no long-term studies that provide direct evidence that would be applicable to a specific patient.[19] If the patient's chief complaint is mobile teeth and an inability to masticate properly, stabilization is best performed early in treatment. These procedures are indicated for teeth that demonstrate at least a degree II mobility and have insufficient clinical roots to realistically anticipate an end result of stable teeth without mechanical intervention (Figs 1-7a to 1-7e). There is little or no value attached to stabilizing teeth based solely on the anticipation that they later will become mobile as a result of treatment.

Primary occlusal trauma describes teeth with significant clinical roots for which clinical stability is anticipated as a result of corrective treatment[15] (Figs 1-1, 1-7b, and 1-7d).

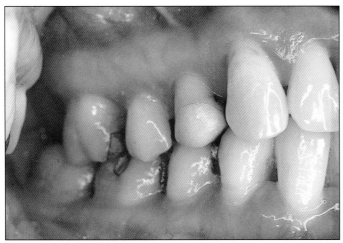

Fig 1-6a Results of debridement therapy. The tissues are pink and the patient is demonstrating a willingness to cooperate.

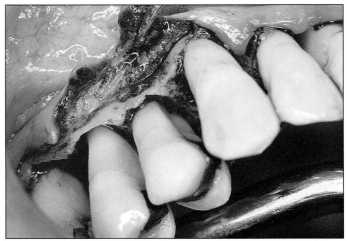

Fig 1-6b It is decided to open the tissues and eliminate granulation tissue that would not be accessible without flaps. A resective procedure would have provided no opportunity to treat the osseous lesions. It is also obvious that the pink tissue in Fig 1-6a is not synonymous with periodontal health.

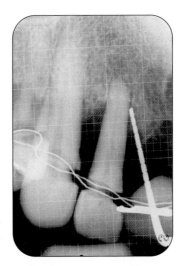

Fig I-7a The lateral incisor has been stabilized as one step in an effort to eliminate the maxillary partial denture. This tooth would never be stable because it has an inadequate clinical root.

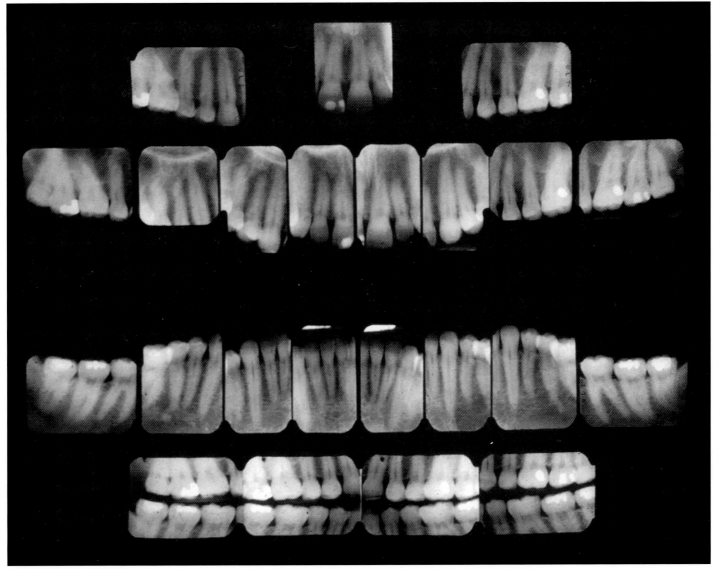

Fig I-7b This radiographic survey reveals long clinical roots and therefore allows an optimistic periodontal prognosis.

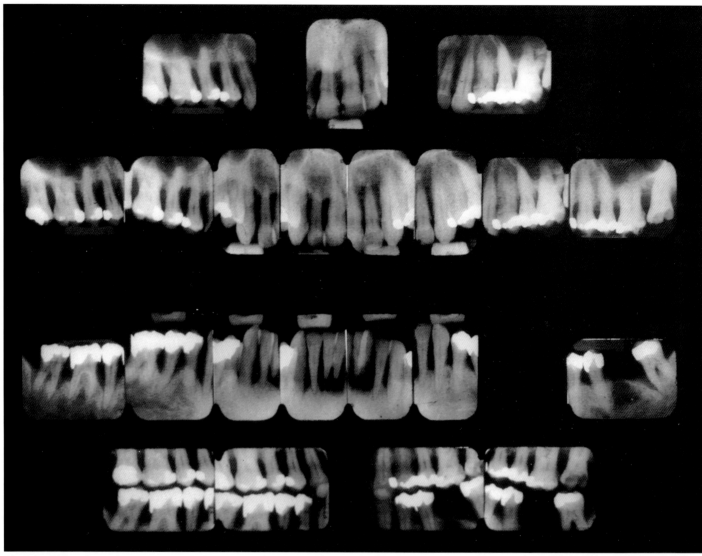

Fig 1-7c This radiographic survey reveals short clinical roots and advanced periodontal disease. The prognosis for this dentition is questionable.

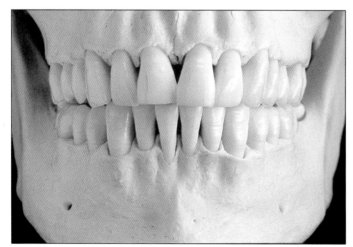

Fig 1-7d In this intact dentition, the roots are covered by alveolar bone to within 1 mm of the cementoenamel junction. The mandibular right central incisor demonstrates root structure not encompassed by bone because of the position of the tooth.

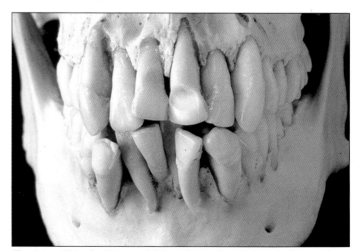

Fig 1-7e This dentition exhibits advanced periodontal disease, long clinical crowns, and short clinical roots. The prognosis of this dentition is questionable.

Secondary occlusal trauma describes teeth with insufficient clinical roots that will not be stable, regardless of the execution of clinical treatment[15] (Figs 1-7a, 1-7c, and 1-7e).

Pocket Elimination

The geographic position of a pocket may influence the treatment decision. A 5-mm probing depth from the cemento-enamel junction in the area of a furcation on a molar will mandate treatment in the form of pocket elimination,[20] whereas the same depth between the maxillary central incisors would strongly indicate the need for nonsurgical treatment. Clinical research has demonstrated that it is difficult or impossible to predictably remove the accretions on a root surface in a pocket that is deeper than 4 mm.[21,22] Human histologic evidence demonstrates that the pink interdental papilla resulting from root debridement, with or without chemotherapy, has not necessarily returned to a histologic state of health[23] (Figs 1-8a and 1-8b). Ulcerated epithelium, significant round-cell infiltrate, and a disorientation of the connective tissue complex of the gingival corium are still present. The clinician is thus faced with three possibilities for a probing depth of more than 4 mm:

1. Maintenance as is
2. Reduction by subtraction
3. Reduction by addition

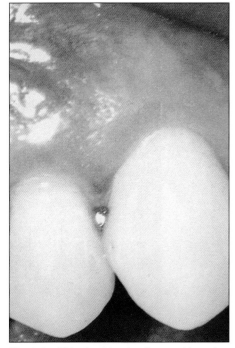

Fig 1-8a This dentition has been subjected to root planing to resolve periodontal inflammatory disease. The papilla is now pink and does not bleed with probing. It is possible that deep cleaning procedures can reverse the damage to the soft tissue papilla, but is this periodontal health? (From Dragoo.[23])

Fig 1-8b The block section of the two teeth shown in Fig 1-8a demonstrates disorientation of the gingival papilla with deep hyperplasia. There is severe infiltration of inflammatory cells and disorganization of the connective tissue corium. Alveolar crest (AC), junctional epithelium (JE), cementum (CE), inflammatory infiltrate (I), proliferating epithelial strands (RP), sulcular epithelium (SE). (From Dragoo.[23])

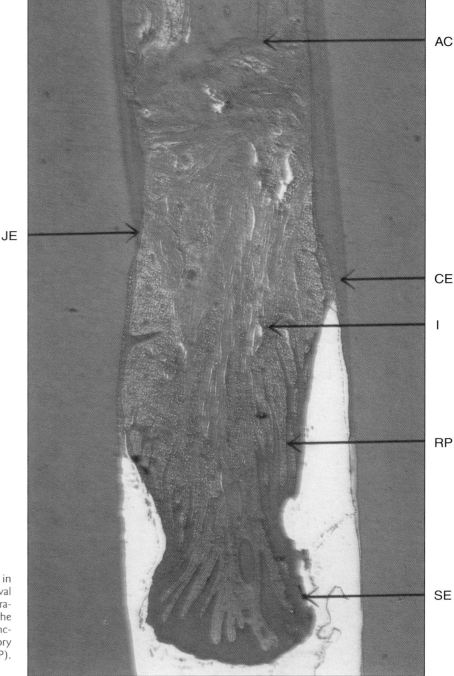

1st Premolar   Canine

The periodontist is expected to select the treatment modality that will provide the further retention of attachment apparatus for the longest period of time.[10] After the result of nonsurgical treatment is established, it is important to address the question of predictability. The selection of periodontal regeneration is always preferable (Figs 1-9a to 1-9e), but is not the best solution for shallow bone defects, and some teeth with deep infrabony lesions may be best suited for extraction (Fig 1-10).

Osseous lesions have been comfortably compartmentalized as consisting of one-, two-, and three-wall defects.[24] The novice, therefore, collates the radiographic and clinical evidence, expecting to find a pure form of lesion. The reality is that almost all bone deformities of the periodontium are a combination of the three types and might be better described as being *confined* or *not confined* (Fig 1-9c). The predictability of treatment will be predicated on the number of osseous walls present. Although there is substantial evidence recording the successful regenerative treatment of advanced osseous defects,[25–33] it is reasonable to assume that the one-wall portion of a deep defect should be treated by ostectomy and that the two- and three-wall portions should be treated by periodontal regeneration techniques.[34] The important issue is that both addition and subtraction result in the resolution of the periodontal pocket and present an area that is cleansable by both the patient and the dental hygienist.[35]

Some clinicians claim that the result of debridement therapy should be observed and a worsening of the problem should be documented before surgical correction is considered. This is very difficult to accomplish in a mobile society with multidisciplinary treatment that has to be coordinated. It is dependent on unusual compliance by the patient and diligence from the referring dentist, a rare combination. It is therefore important to conclude the decision-making process and treat the patient before there is unplanned procrastination and further destruction of the periodontium (Fig 1-11).

It is important to establish the goals of ostectomy treatment.[35,36] The interproximal bone must be flat from mesial to distal and from buccal to lingual. The interproximal bone should be occlusal or at approximately the same level as the radicular bone (Figs 1-12a and 1-12b). The opposite, described as *reverse architecture*, will result in continued soft tissue pocketing.[37] The correction of such discrepancies by ostectomy is exercised only after careful analysis. Deep lesions are not candidates, because ostectomy would depreciate the prognosis of relatively healthy neighboring teeth (see Fig 1-9a). There is also a limit as to how much bone can be realistically removed in cases of secondary occlusal trauma, and compromise may be introduced if regeneration is not an option (Fig 1-12c). The goal of parabolic architecture will be influenced by the size of the embrasure, because it is more difficult to control soft tissue growth in narrow interproximal sites.[38,39]

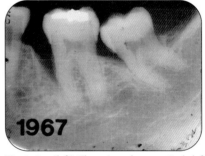
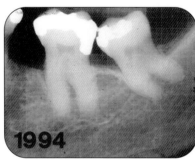
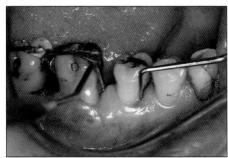

Fig 1-9a *(left)* There is a deep vertical defect on the mesial surface of the second molar. Osseous resection is not the preferred treatment because significant bone would be reduced from the distal surface of the premolar. *(right)* This tooth has been treated with an autogenous bone graft. After 27 years, the lesion appears well treated and the tooth is very serviceable to the patient.

Fig 1-9b Deep periodontal pockets remain after debridement therapy. It is unnecessary to stabilize these teeth because the mobility is slight.

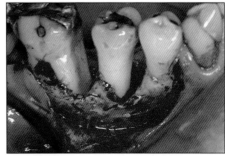
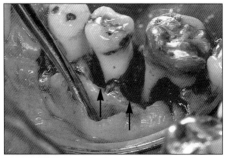
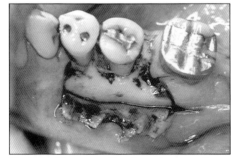

Fig 1-9c Buccal and lingual flaps have been elevated, and the granulation tissue has been removed. Note the remaining deep, uncontained periodontal pockets, consisting of one and two walls.

Fig 1-9d The reflection of the lingual flap reveals the extent of the bone loss on the lingual surface *(arrows)*.

Fig 1-9e Eleven months after autogenous bone grafting, there is almost a complete regeneration of the lost supporting bone.

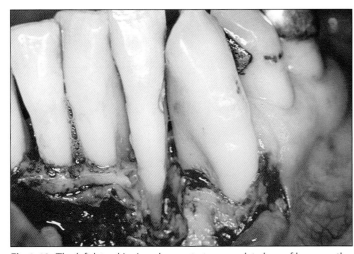

Fig 1-10 The left lateral incisor demonstrates complete loss of bone on the buccal and distal surfaces. It is important to reach a conclusive decision before more bone is lost on the mesial surface of the canine. The prognosis for regeneration is not good, because even if the bone could be restored to the level of approximating bone, the tooth would still have a guarded prognosis. Therefore, this tooth should be extracted.

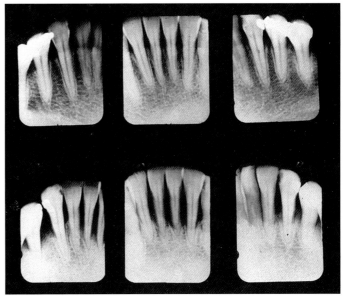

Fig 1-11 The top row of radiographs demonstrates the situation at initial presentation of the patient. This patient decided not to follow through with corrective procedures, even though there was crestal loss of bone in several areas. She was informed that this was a measure of her susceptibility to her own microbiota. The patient's interpretation was that the bleeding had stopped and that therefore her dentition was healthy. The bottom row of radiographs shows the same patient's dentition, 10 years later. The clinical roots are greatly reduced, and the prognosis for the dentition has changed from favorable to questionable.

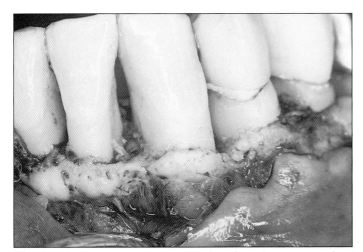

Fig 1-12a In the reverse osseous architecture, bone is more coronal on the buccal surface than it is interproximally. The defects are shallow and lend themselves to osseous correction.

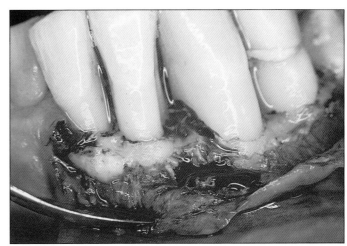

Fig 1-12b The bone morphology has been corrected to create a positive architecture.

Fig 1-12c Long clinical crowns usually mean short clinical roots. Note the large embrasure between the canine and first premolar and the small embrasure between the two premolars. It is necessary to limit bone resection for these teeth because the clinical roots are short.

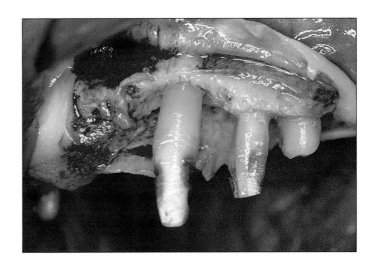

Case Reports

It is necessary to observe the results of debridement, stabilization (where necessary), and pocket elimination that are committed to long-term maintenance to appreciate the validity of the proposed recipe for success. The following four case studies have been selected to demonstrate the success of such treatment.

Case 1

In the first patient, a mandibular dentition articulates with a maxillary denture. The original radiographic survey demonstrated appreciable interproximal loss of bone between all of the remaining teeth (Figs 1-13a and 1-13b). The second molars were extracted by the referring dentist, but the other teeth all exhibit clinical stability or minimal

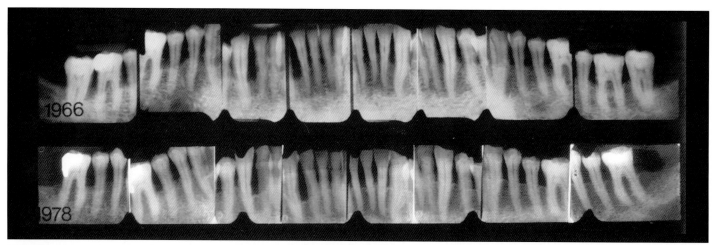

Fig 1-13a *(top row)* In 1966, the patient presented with 14 mandibular teeth. There was interproximal pocketing in all areas and obvious loss of bone. The second molars were extracted at that time by the referring dentist. *(bottom row)* In 1978, the clinical roots of the 12 surviving teeth exhibit the same length they did 12 years earlier; therefore, there has been no further loss of bone. This patient was treated with pocket reduction therapy following debridement treatment. The periodontal maintenance schedule has a periodicity of 3 months.

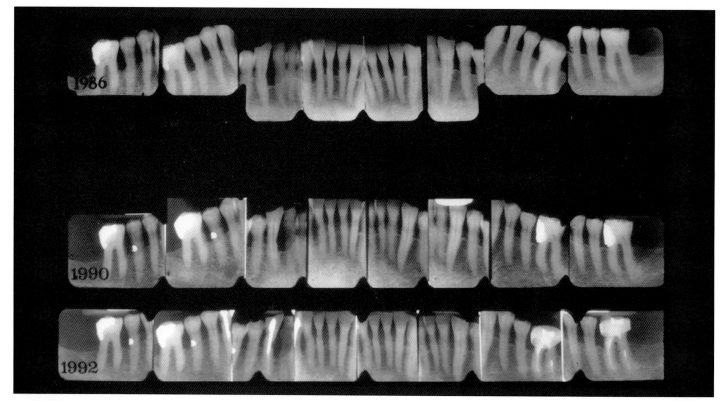

Fig 1-13b Continued history of the patient in Fig 1-13a. There has been no further loss of bone in *(top row)* 1978, *(middle row)* 1990, or *(bottom row)* 1994. This case has now been followed for 28 years. It demonstrates that pocket elimination therapy is efficacious, especially when the patient is compliant. The restoration of the left first molar is inadequate, and the prognosis of this tooth is now questionable.

mobility. Treatment, consisting of pocket reduction therapy by ostectomy and apically repositioned flaps, was provided in 1966, and the result is documented until 1994. There has been no further surgical treatment, loss of teeth, or loss of interproximal bone to date.

This case demonstrates that periodontal disease can be attenuated and does not worsen as a natural phenomenon. This patient has not failed to attend a maintenance visit, with a periodicity of 3 months, in 29 years, and his desire to keep his teeth is evidenced in a better-than-average performance of oral hygiene measures.

Case 2

The second case is that of a 38-year-old woman with a complete maxillary denture and a mandibular dentition of 10 teeth. Her chief complaint involved the mobility of her teeth, which inhibited mastication. Phase I of therapy included debridement and stabilization to change a mobile, dirty dentition to a stable, clean dentition. Phase II treatment included mucogingival surgery to enlarge the buccal vestibule and thus enhance the patient's ability to clean. It also included the use of autogenous bone from the

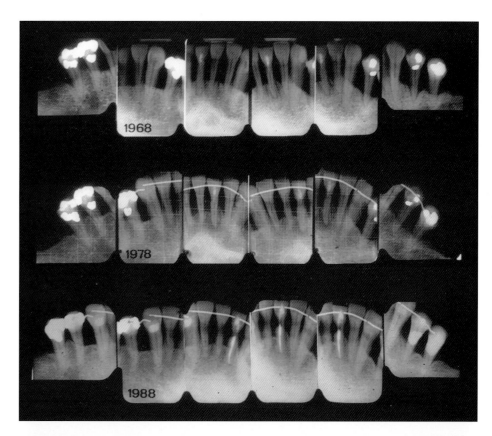

Fig 1-14a *(top row)* This patient presented with 10 mandibular teeth, all of which demonstrated significant loss of supporting structure (1968). *(center row)* The mobile, dirty teeth have been treated by debridement and stabilization. *(bottom row)* Twenty years later, the 10 teeth are still present and there is at least as much bone as there was initially. Osseous resection is not the correct treatment for teeth with minimal clinical roots, so every effort was made to regenerate lost periodontium. The donor source of the bone grafting was the edentulous maxilla.

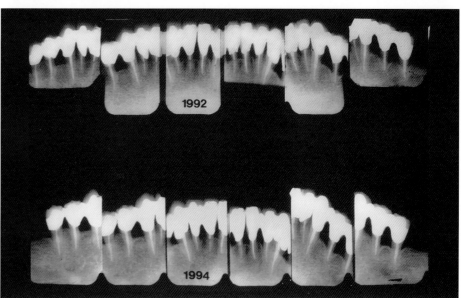

Fig 1-14b This case has been followed for 26 years. It was necessary in 1988 to commit the patient to restorative dentistry.

edentulous maxilla to resolve vertical lesions that could not be treated by ostectomy because of the small clinical roots.

This case study demonstrates the preservation of these 10 teeth, after 20 years of observation, with at least the quantity of bone initially present (Fig 1-14a). The teeth were then committed to a complete-coverage prosthesis with the final observation of 28 years (Fig 1-14b). This patient has continued with a periodontal maintenance program with compliance similar to that of the patient in case 1.

Case 3

The third case is limited to the mandibular anterior teeth. The recipe of debridement, stabilization, pocket elimination, and maintenance has resulted in long-term maintenance of the remaining teeth and their periodontium (Fig 1-15a). This patient is an example of unusual compliance, as evidenced by the lack of dental plaque at the time of her appointment for professional debridement (Fig 1-15b). She clearly understands the relationship of bacterial plaque

to further loss of periodontium and is motivated to avoid further problems.

Case 4

The fourth patient presented with advanced periodontal destruction throughout the dentition. The maxillary arch was treated definitively with a periodontal prosthesis, but financial limitations resulted in staged treatment for the mandible. The observation of the lingual surface of the mandibular incisors identified the mandibular partial denture as an etiologic factor that had to be immediately eliminated (Figs 1-16a and 1-16b). The first direction of treatment was the application of debridement and stabilization procedures, which, together with the elimination of the removable partial denture, resulted in pink tissue with little or no attached gingiva for the right incisors (Fig 1-16c). A lingual gingival graft was performed to protect the remaining periodontium and provide a fiber-apparatus barrier against further inflammatory disease (Figs 1-16d and 1-16e).

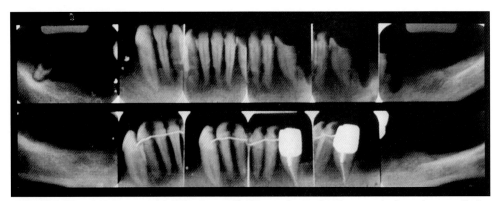

Fig 1-15a This patient presented with six mandibular anterior teeth. The root tip from the mandibular molar was extracted. The recipe of treatment included debridement, stabilization, pocket elimination, and maintenance. The mobile incisors were stabilized with an A splint rather than a partial denture. This eliminates any possibility that the partial denture will come in contact with the gingiva.

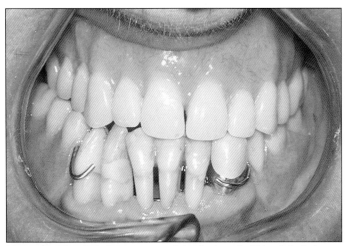

Fig 1-15b The clinical appearance of the final result. This clinical photograph was taken at a maintenance visit *before* the cleaning procedure. The patient obviously understands the importance of debridement and the danger of plaque.

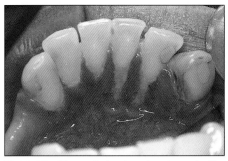

Fig 1-16a The periodontium has been badly damaged by a combination of events. The damage on the lingual surface of the incisors has been caused by a removable partial denture. Note the difference between the color of the tissue surrounding the teeth and that of the tissue of the edentulous ridge.

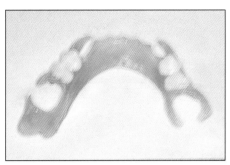

Fig 1-16b Removable partial denture that must be eliminated.

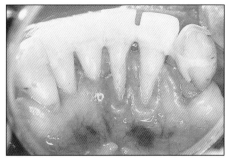

Fig 1-16c Observation of the lingual surface after debridement and stabilization treatment reveals that the dirty, mobile teeth are now clean, stable teeth. Figure 1-16a indicates that there is little potential for a collagen fiber apparatus that would be strong enough to resist inflammatory periodontal disease on the lingual surface of these teeth.

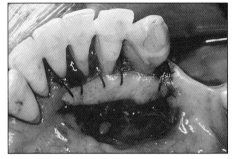

Fig 1-16d A free gingival graft is placed to provide a better barrier against inflammatory disease.

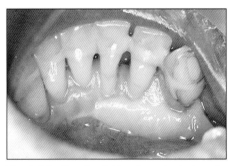

Fig 1-16e Result of the free gingival graft procedure.

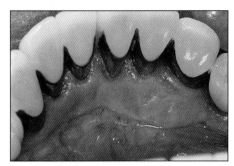

Fig 1-16f Twenty years later, this barrier remains effective.

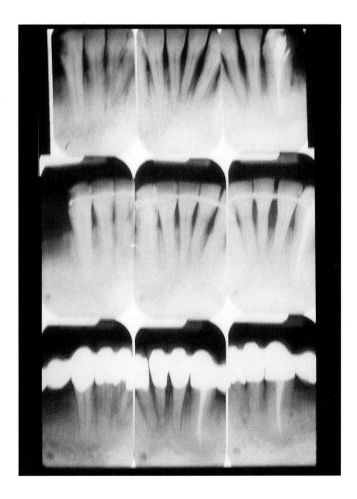

Fig 1-16g *(top row)* Note the apparent loss of interproximal bone in the original radiographic survey. *(middle row)* Obvious improvement after debridement and stabilization. This observation is probably influenced by the elimination of the active inflammatory lesions. *(bottom row)* Radiographs made 22 years after treatment.

The patient continues to participate in the maintenance of these teeth, and a permanent prosthesis has been constructed. It is worth noting that, 10 years after construction of the permanent prosthesis, the patient continues to struggle with plaque control (Figs 1-16f and 1-16g). It is a foolish mistake for the periodontist to be deluded into thinking that all patients will be paragons of oral cleanliness. People are creatures of habit and it is unlikely that the average patient will participate perfectly in a periodontal maintenance program.

Phase III: Maintenance Therapy

Phase III is that part of treatment designed to preserve the results accomplished in phase II. It demands an ever-increasing number of staff and a physical plant that can absorb the necessary growth of a practice.[18,40] It is impossible to consider providing this service for every patient treated in a periodontal practice because of numerical limitations, referral patterns, and the availability of staff to accomplish the goals on a timely basis (see Chapter 26).

Occupational difficulties, marital problems, and behavioral issues with children challenge patients' compliance. The difficulty encountered by people who attempt to stop smoking or continually fail to maintain weight loss with dieting is also evidenced in the lack of compliance with dental hygiene.[41,42] In spite of this, the recognition of a patient who is susceptible to periodontal disease demands the availability of a serious maintenance program.[18]

Septic Versus Aseptic Lesions

It is necessary to distinguish between a septic and an aseptic periodontal lesion. The vast majority of lesions encountered are septic (bacterial), and the aseptic problem is usually related to tooth malpositioning or mobility resulting from occlusal trauma. A radiograph identifying periodontal health will reveal a flat interdental crest of bone that is parallel to a projected line connecting adjacent cementoenamel junctions[43] (Figs 1-17a to 1-17c). The crest should be approximately 1 mm apical to this line to provide space for the transeptal fibers that attach to the cervical cementum of adjacent teeth as Sharpey's fibers.

Malpositioning

Malpositioned teeth frequently demonstrate uneven osseous crests (Figs 1-18a to 1-18d). If no superimposed inflammatory defect is present, the level of the crest will be

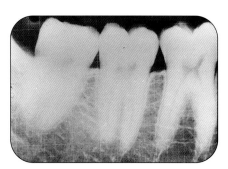

Fig 1-17a This radiograph demonstrates the preferred position for the alveolar crest in health. The interproximal bone between the proximal surfaces of two adjacent teeth is parallel to an imaginary line connecting the cementoenamel junctions. It is positioned 1 mm apical to the cementoenamel junctions, leaving room for the insertion of the transeptal fibers.

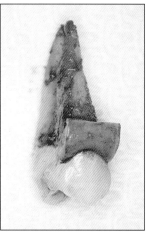

Fig 1-17b Extracted premolar with a collar of gingival tissue still attached.

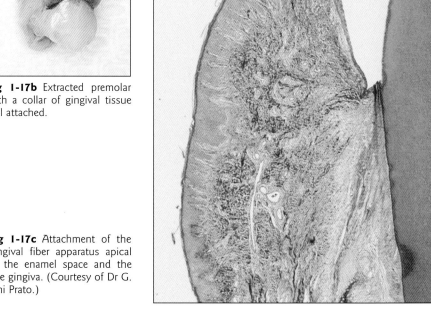

Fig 1-17c Attachment of the gingival fiber apparatus apical to the enamel space and the free gingiva. (Courtesy of Dr G. Pini Prato.)

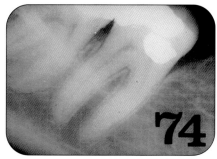

Fig 1-18a The mandibular first molar is missing, and the mandibular second molar is tilted mesially. This creates an uneven alveolar crest that will be parallel to the line connecting the two adjacent cementoenamel junctions.

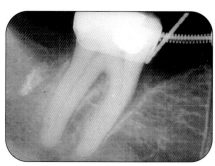

Fig 1-18b The periodontal probe does not extend apically beyond the cementoenamel junction, indicating that the connective tissue attachment to the tooth is intact. Removal of the orthodontic appliance should result in correction of the periodontal lesion.

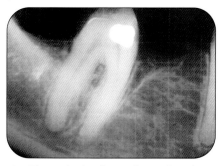

Fig 1-18c The orthodontic appliance has been eliminated, and a provisional fixed partial denture placed to stabilize the tooth. There is an excellent clinical root and the furcation is intact. In a short period, the apparent osseous deformity is replaced by radiographic evidence of the healing of the periodontium.

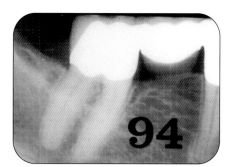

Fig 1-18d A fixed partial denture has been placed, and a radiograph taken after 17 years reveals an intact periodontium and no evidence of the earlier osseous deformity caused by orthodontic treatment.

Fig 1-18e Histologic observation of a tooth during orthodontic movement. The supracrestal fiber attachment and the epithelium are intact on the surface of the cementum and enamel, respectively. The osseous crest is undergoing a remodeling process, and the blood vessels in the periodontal ligament are engorged. This is similar to Fig 1-18b. The alveolar crest is disturbed, but the soft tissue attachment to the tooth is intact, so that the area is aseptic and the osseous radiographic changes will be reversible.

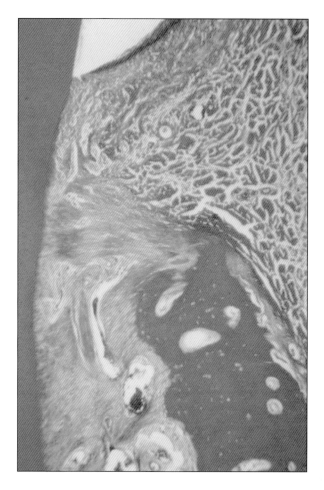

parallel to a line connecting approximating cementoenamel junctions in a radiograph. The correction of the position of the tooth will correct the radiographic osseous deformity, but a radiograph made during orthodontic tooth movement can be disarming unless amplified by a periodontal probe. An inability to probe is evidence that the connective fiber apparatus is intact (see Fig 1-18b). This means that the area is aseptic and the elimination of the etiology will result in the resolution of the osseous deformity without surgery. Periodontal surgery probably would be destructive, because it would establish communication between the oral cavity and the aseptic bone defect of the noninflammatory lesion.

Occlusal Trauma

The concept that occlusal trauma results in a periodontal pocket was proven fallacious by the research of Cohen[44] and Cohen et al.[45] The previously accepted hypothesis that a heavy occlusion results in stenosis of the gingival vasculature cannot be supported, because the gingival vasculature remains patent in teeth with high restorations in the monkey model (Fig 1-19). This defused the concept that a periodontal pocket is the result of diminished circulation, caused by occlusal trauma.

It is common for the mandibular molar that is tipped mesially to be in trauma. The correction of this occlusal problem will resolve the radiographic bone discrepancy in a nonsurgical fashion, if correction takes place before an inflammatory lesion is superimposed on the discrepancy[46,47] (Figs 1-20a and 1-20b).

Mandibular Incisor Recession

Although once thought to be related to occlusal trauma, most recession on mandibular incisors can be related to a discrepancy between the buccolingual dimension of the tooth and the buccolingual width of the alveolar process. When the tooth is too large there is an absence of buccal plate, and an inflammatory lesion results in gingival recession (see Chapter 18). This is especially true when there is a limited buccal vestibule. The resolution of this problem is found in mucogingival surgery (Figs 1-21a and 1-21b). Even in the presence of incisal wear, long-term observation of such treatment demonstrates the validity of this approach.[21]

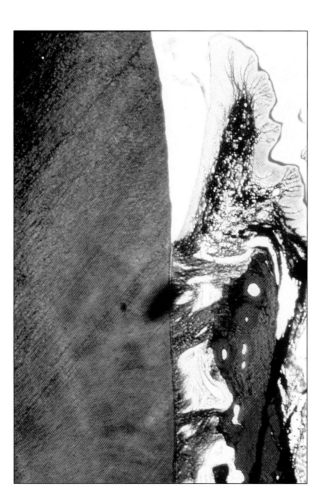

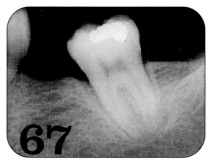

Fig 1-19 This canine tooth has been placed in supraocclusion to test the hypothesis that a tooth in occlusal trauma would experience a breakdown of the periodontal soft tissues because of stenosis of the blood vasculature of the gingival papilla. Indian ink infusion into the carotid artery, immediately postmortem, demonstrates that the vasculature of the gingival papilla is patent. It is also an opportunity to observe that little or no vasculature extends into the epithelium.

Fig 1-20a The mandibular molar is tipped mesially and in occlusal trauma (1967). The periodontal ligament on the mesial surface is widened, but the discrepancy cannot be probed.

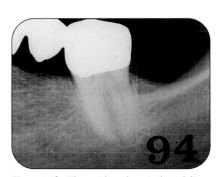

Fig 1-20b The widened periodontal ligament was eliminated by the construction of the fixed partial denture. This radiograph, from 1994, demonstrates that the problem has been corrected and remained corrected over a period of 27 years.

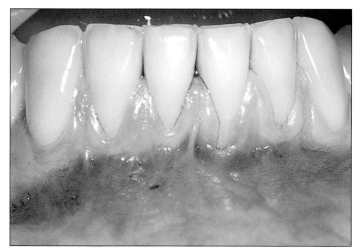

Fig 1-21a The mandibular incisors demonstrate gingival recession to the level of the shallow vestibule. Note the incisal wear that has occurred.

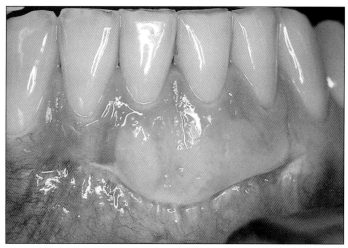

Fig 1-21b One year after a gingival graft has been placed, there is a deepened vestibule and the incisor roots are completely covered with gingiva. There is minimal probing. No occlusal therapy has been performed; therefore, the occlusion can be absolved as an etiologic factor in the gingival recession.

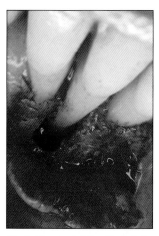 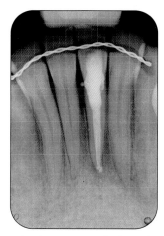 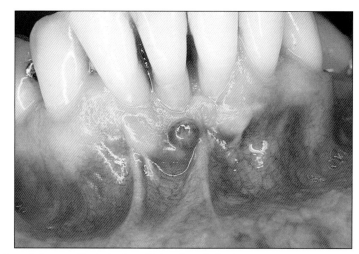

Fig 1-22a to 1-22c An infrabony pocket is present on the buccal surface of the mandibular incisor. Although endodontic treatment has been performed, the fistula continues on the buccal surface of the central incisor.

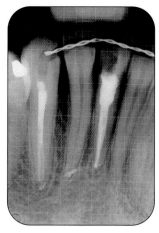 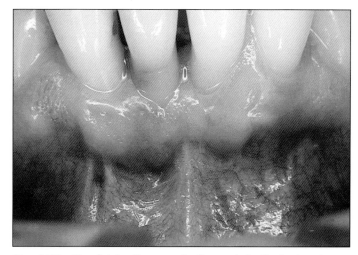

Fig 1-22d Pulp testing demonstrated that the mandibular right canine was nonvital. After endodontic therapy was performed for this tooth, the fistula disappeared. Note the track of cement leading from the canine to the apical area of the central incisor. This is probably the line of drainage of the periapical lesion on the canine.

Fig 1-22e The fistula disappeared after endodontic treatment was performed on the canine.

Pulpal Problems

The presence of an infrabony pocket on the buccal surface of a mandibular incisor is rare (Figs 1-22a to 1-22e), so it is necessary to consider pulpal etiology, especially if operative dentistry was recently performed.

Treatment of Multirooted Teeth

All problems for single-rooted teeth become more complicated in multirooted teeth. The geographic placement of these teeth presents special difficulties for the arrival at an exact diagnosis, the performance of corrective treatment, and the maintenance of the results. It is necessary to consider the following issues:

1. State of repair of the tooth
2. Periodontal pocketing and loss of attachment
3. Furcation invasion
4. Presence or absence of embrasures
5. Mobility
6. Root form
7. Length of the edentulous span
8. Tooth position
9. Occlusion

These issues are addressed in Chapters 13 and 14.

Goals of Treatment

Even the most advanced cases of periodontal disease can be successfully treated with the aforementioned recipe for treatment. It is critical that untreatable teeth be identified at the outset of treatment and not committed to treatment regimens that will be discouraging to both the clinician and the patient[48] (Figs 1-23a to 1-23h). It is essential to use non-surgical therapies before a commitment is made to surgical treatment, because they are usually reversible and allow the selection of appropriate treatments for specific patients. The corrective treatment must be definitive and achieve an end goal that can be maintained by the patient and the health care professional.

The patient must be continually observed over significant periods of time with the mind set toward control rather than cure because there is never a moment when the patient who has demonstrated severe susceptibility will not be considered a potential periodontal patient. However, it is necessary to accomplish a treatment plan that does not require continual corrective treatment. The goal for all patients is to reach a plateau where the case is easily maintained by the patient and hygienist; circumstances that preclude costly treatment frequently change and may allow the introduction of prosthetics or implants many years after the original thrust of treatment. It is necessary to preserve the remaining teeth and periodontium so that this can be accomplished.

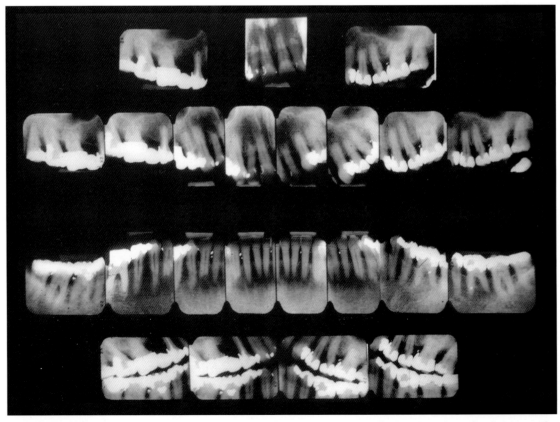

Fig 1-23a A full-mouth radiographic survey (1970) reveals severe periodontal disease throughout the dentition. The patient's finances are limited, and the prognosis for the maxillary molars is poor.

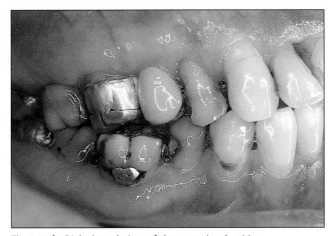

Fig 1-23b Right lateral view of the posterior dentition.

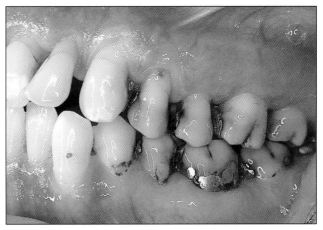

Fig 1-23c Left lateral view of the posterior dentition.

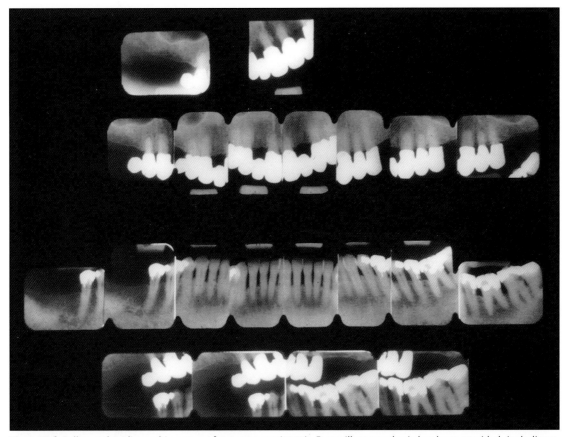

Fig 1-23d Full-mouth radiographic survey after treatment (1972). A maxillary prosthesis has been provided, including a second premolar cantilever on the right side. (Courtesy of Dr. H.M. Skurow.)

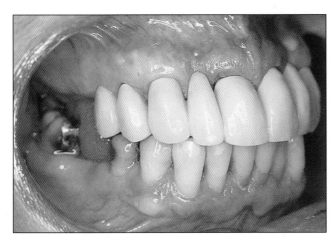

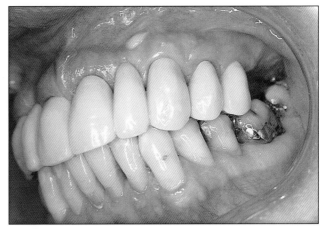

Figs 1-23e and 1-23f Lateral views at the conclusion of treatment. Note that the dentition ends as a premolar occlusion.

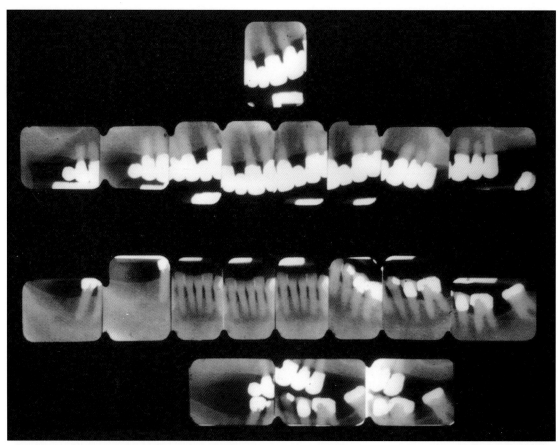

Fig 1-23g Full-mouth radiographic survey, 17 years after treatment (1987).

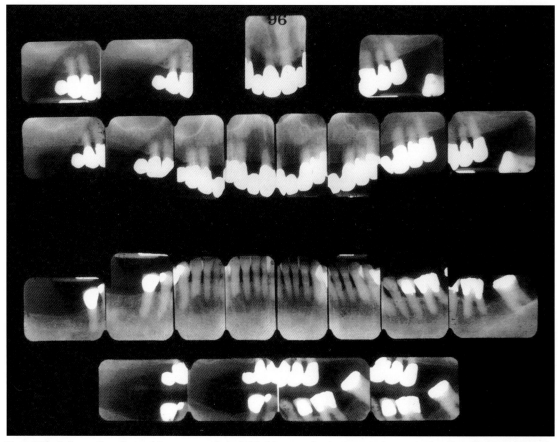

Fig 1-23h Full-mouth radiographic survey made in 1996, 26 years after treatment, demonstrating that all abutment teeth are still in place.

Premolar Occlusion

An abbreviated dentition is a practical end goal but is best selected after there is an opportunity to test the patient's response.[16] The biologic trial restoration (provisional fixed partial denture) provides the patient with an opportunity to decide if he or she is satisfied with the esthetics and masticatory function. It is best to allow the patient to use the provisional prosthesis before his or her answers are measured.

The construction of a premolar occlusion with or without a single cantilever has served many patients successfully for long periods of time.[17] This information is pertinent for both the natural dentition and implant-supported dentitions when the treatment direction is initiated for the periodontally compromised patient.[49,50]

The periodontium should and can outperform the prosthesis. When this happens, it is possible to replace the prosthesis with minimal periodontal correction (Figs 1-24a to 1-24h). The barometer of success of such treatment is a traditional radiographic survey. If treatment results in the preservation of the selected abutment teeth and the supporting bone, a new prosthesis is constructed that should continue in a satisfactory fashion for the patient.

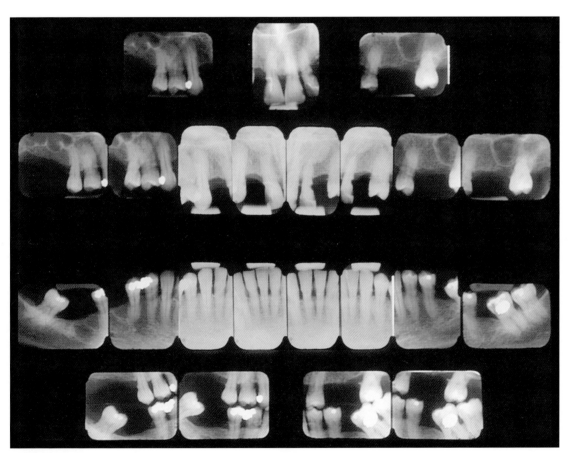

Fig 1-24a Original full-mouth radiographic survey, made in 1968.

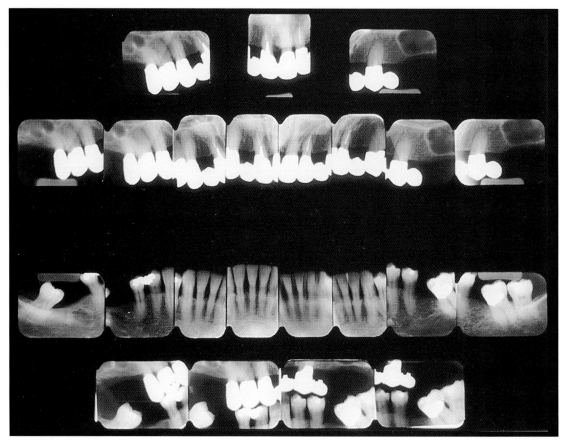

Fig 1-24b Radiographic survey after treatment in 1969.

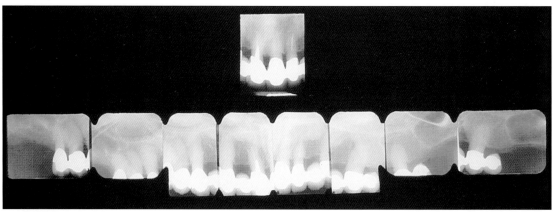

Fig 1-24c Radiographic survey made in 1980.

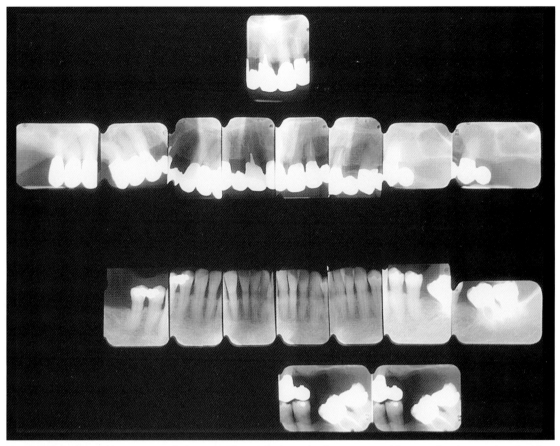

Fig 1-24d Radiographic survey made in 1994. The original prosthesis, constructed in 1968, has been replaced with a new ceramometal prosthesis. There is a premolar occlusion on the right side and a premolar occlusion on the left side that includes a cantilevered second premolar.

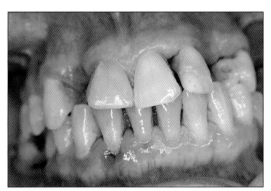

Fig 1-24e When the patient originally presented, the maxillary left canine, second premolar, and molars were missing or untreatable. It was immediately evident that any fixed prosthesis would have limited support on the left side.

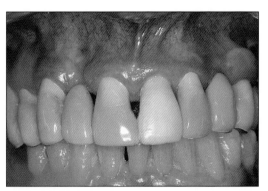

Fig 1-24f The original prosthesis needed to be replaced for esthetic reasons. There is no necessity to correct any periodontal problems because there is no pocketing or mucogingival problem after 24 years.

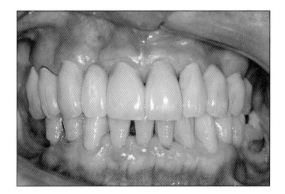

Fig 1-24g New prosthesis is in place. If the number of teeth and the bone levels are the same, an existing prosthesis can be replaced by a new prosthesis. This is only possible if treatment has preserved the periodontium for the abutment teeth. (Courtesy of Dr. H.M. Skurow.)

References

1. Brånemark P-I, Breine U, Adell R, Hansson BO. Osseointegrated implants in the treatment of the edentulous jaw: Experience from a 10-year period. Scand J Plast Reconstr Surg 1977;11(suppl 16).

2. Brånemark P-I, Zarb GA, Albrektsson T (eds). Tissue-Integrated Prostheses: Osseointegration in Clinical Dentistry. Chicago: Quintessence, 1985.

3. Adell R, Lekholm U, Rockler B, Brånemark P-I. A 15-year study of osseointegrated implants in the treatment of the edentulous jaw. Int J Oral Surg 1981;6:387–416.

4. Löe H, Theilade E, Jensen SB. Experimental gingivitis in man. J Periodontol 1965;36:177–187.

5. Page RC, Schroeder HE. Pathogenesis of inflammatory periodontal disease. A summary of current work. Lab Invest 1976;33:235–249.

6. Slots J, Moenho D, Langebaek J, Frandsen A. Microbiota of gingivitis in man. Scand J Dent Res 1978;86:174–181.

7. Caton J. Periodontal diagnosis and diagnostic aids. In: Nevins M, Becker W, Kornman K (eds). Proceedings of the World Workshop in Clinical Periodontics. Chicago: American Academy of Periodontology, 1989:I-1–I-32.

8. Lindhe J, Nyman S. The effect of plaque control and surgical pocket elimination on the establishment and maintenance of periodontal health. A longitudinal study of periodontal therapy of advanced disease. J Clin Periodontol 1975;2:67–79.

9. Lindhe J, Westfelt E, Nyman S, Socransky SS, Heijl L, Bratthall G. Healing following surgical/non-surgical treatment of periodontal disease. J Clin Periodontol 1982;9:115–128.

10. Lindhe J, Westfelt E, Nyman S. Socransky SS, Haffajee AD. Long-term effect of surgical/non-surgical treatment of periodontal disease. J Clin Periodontol 1984;11:448–458.

11. Olsen CT, Ammons WF, von Belle G. A longitudinal study comparing apically respositioned flaps with and without osseous surgery. Int J Periodont Rest Dent 1985;5(4):11–33.

12. Isidor F, Karring T. Long term effect of surgical and non-surgical periodontal treatment: A 5-year clinical study. J Periodont Res 1986;21:462–472.

13. Claffey N, Nyland K, Kiger R, Garrett S, Engelburg J. Diagnostic predictability of scores of plaque, bleeding, suppuration and probing depth for probing attachment loss. J Clin Periodontol 1990;17: 108–114.

14. Baderstein A, Nilveus R, Engelburg J. Scores of plaque, bleeding, suppuration and probing depth to predict probing attachment loss. J Clin Periodontol 1990;17:102–107.

15. Amsterdam M, Abrams L. In: Goldman H, Schlugar S, Fox L, Cohen DW (eds). Periodontal Therapy. St Louis: Mosby, 1964:762–799.

16. Skurow H, Nevins M. The rationale of the preperiodontal provisional biologic trial restoration. Int J Periodont Rest Dent 1988;8(1):9–29.

17. Prichard JF. Interpretation of radiographs in periodontics. Int J Periodont Rest Dent 1983;3(1):9–39.

18. Nevins M. Long-term periodontal maintenance in private practice. J Clin Periodontol 1996;23:273–277.

19. Waerhaug J. Justification for splinting in periodontal therapy. J Prosthet Dent 1969;22:201–208.

20. Wang H, Burgett F, Shyr Y, Ramfjord S. The influence of molar furcation involvement and mobility on future clinical periodontal attachment loss. J Periodontol 1994;65:25–29.

21. Waerhaug J. Healing of the dento-epithelial junction following subgingival plaque control. II: As observed on extracted teeth. J Periodontol 1978;49:119.

22. Stambaugh RV, Dragoo MR, Smith DM, Carasali L. The limits of subgingival scaling. Int J Periodont Rest Dent 1981;1(5):31–42.

23. Dragoo MR, Grant DA, Gulverg D, Stambaugh R. Experimental periodontal treatment in humans. I: Subgingival root planing with and without chlorhexidine gluconate rinses. Int J Periodont Rest Dent 1984;4(3):9–30.

24. Goldman HM, Cohen DW. The infrabony pocket: Classification and treatment. J Periodontol 1958;29:272–291.

25. Machtei EE, Schallhorn RG. Successful regeneration of mandibular class II furcation defects: An evidence-based treatment approach. Int J Periodont Rest Dent 1995;15:146–167.

26. Nyman S, Lindhe J, Karring T, Rylander H. New attachment following surgical treatment of human periodontal disease. J Clin Periodontol 1982;9:290–296.

27. Cortellini P, Bowers GM. Periodontal regeneration of intrabony defects: An evidence-based treatment approach. Int J Periodont Rest Dent 1995;15:128–145.

28. Gottlow J, Nyman S, Lindhe J, Karring T, Wennström J. New attachment formation in the human periodontium by guided tissue regeneration. Case reports. J Clin Periodontol 1986;13:604–616.

29. Schallhorn RG, McClain PK. Combined osseous composite grafting, root conditioning and guided tissue regeneration. Int J Periodont Rest Dent 1988;8(4):8–31.

30. McClain PK, Schallhorn RG. Long-term assessment of combined osseous composite grafting, root conditioning and guided tissue regeneration. Int J Periodont Rest Dent 1993;13:9–27.

31. Mellonig JT. Decalcified freeze-dried bone allograft as an implant material in human periodontal defects. Int J Periodont Rest Dent 1984;4(6):41–55.

32. Becker W, Becker BE. Treatment of mandibular 3-wall intrabony defects by flap debridement and expanded polytetra-fluorethylene barrier membranes. Long-term evaluation of 32 patients. J Periodontol 1993;64:1138–1144.

33. Bowers GM, Chadroff B, Carnevale R, Mellonig J, Corio R, Emerson J, et al. Histologic evaluation of new attachment apparatus formation in humans. Part III. J Periodontol 1989;60:683–693.

34. Ochsenbein C. Combined approach to the management of intrabony defects. Int J Periodont Rest Dent 1995;15:329–343.

35. Kramer G. The case for ostectomy—A time-tested therapeutic modality in selected periodontitis sites. Int J Periodont Rest Dent 1995;15:229–237.

36. Ochsenbein C. A primer for osseous surgery. Int J Periodont Rest Dent 1986;6(1):8–47.

37. Schlugar S. Osseous resection: A basic principle in periodontal surgery. Oral Surg Oral Med Oral Pathol 1949;2:316–325.

38. Nevins M. Interproximal periodontal disease: The embrasure as an etiologic factor. Int J Periodont Rest Dent 1982;2(6):9–27.

39. Kramer GM. A consideration of root proximity. Int J Periodont Rest Dent 1987;7(6)9–34.

40. Becker W, Becker B, Berg L. Periodontal treatment without maintenance: A retrospective study in 44 patients. J Periodontol 1984; 55:505–509.

41. Wilson TG, Glover ME, Schoen J, Baust C, Jacobs T. Compliance with maintenance therapy in a private periodontal practice. J Periodontol 1984;55:468–473.

42. Wilson TG, Kornman KS, Newman MG. Advances in Periodontics: Supportive Periodontal Treatment for Patients with Inflammatory Periodontal Diseases. Chicago: Quintessence, 1992:195–203.

43. Ritchey B, Orban B. The crests of the interdental alveolar septa. J Periodontol 1953;24:75.

44. Cohen DW. Changes in the attachment apparatus in occlusal trauma. Alpha Omegan 1951;45:20.

45. Cohen DW, Keller G, Feder M, Livingston E. Effects of excessive occlusal forces in the gingival blood supply. J Dent Res 1960;39:677.

46. Brown IS. Effect of orthodontic therapy on periodontal defects. J Periodontol 1969;40:577.

47. Wise RJ, Kramer GM. Predetermination of osseous changes associated with uprighting tipped molars by probing. Int J Periodont Rest Dent 1983;3(1):69–81.

48. Yulzari J. Strategic extraction in periodontal prosthesis. Int J Periodont Rest Dent 1982;2(6):51.

49. Strub JR, Lintner H, Marinello CP. Rehabilitation of partially edentulous patients using cantilever bridges: A retrospective study. Int J Periodont Rest Dent 1989;9:365–376.

50. Kayser AF. A shortened dental arch: A therapeutic concept in reduced dentitions and certain high risk groups. Int J Periodont Rest Dent 1989;9:427–450.

CHAPTER 2

The Interdental Embrasure and Interproximal Periodontal Disease

Myron Nevins, DDS

The damage resulting from inflammatory periodontal disease can be ascertained by observation of the radicular and interproximal periodontium.[1] Radicular changes are more visible and are frequently recognized by the patient and the dental health team, whereas interproximal disease is usually silent and asymptomatic, so that it, like other chronic diseases, is overlooked. The most routine dental procedures have the potential to disrupt the integrity of the protecting soft tissues, thus creating a pathway for the inflammatory lesion and the resultant loss of bone[2] (Figs 2-1a and 2-1b).

Periodontally compromised patients demonstrate the loss of interproximal interradicular bone on dental radiographs.[3] The elimination of periodontal pockets and the refinement of interproximal dental restorations to create an environment that is easily cleansed are critical to the success of treatment to preserve the remaining bony housing for the teeth.[4,5]

Interdental Soft Tissue Anatomy

The gingival unit acts as the physical barrier to the septic lesion at the interface of oral bacterial activity and the sterility of the underlying crest of bone.[6,7] The soft tissues that protect the bony housing include the transseptal fibers, which immediately cover the crest and attach into the cementum on the proximal surfaces of adjacent teeth in the form of Sharpey's fibers. The junctional epithelium is found occlusal to the fiber apparatus and the gingival sulcus, which is surrounded by the free gingiva. Direct evidence links the etiology of the septic lesion to bacterial plaque and the resulting inflammatory lesion.[8–10] The exogenous and endogenous reactions clearly are capable of destroying the attachment apparatus and resulting in a diminished periodontal prognosis.

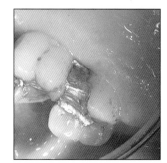

Fig 2-1a The interproximal embrasure is completely occluded by an overhanging alloy restoration. The pink gingiva gives no indication of the interproximal disease.

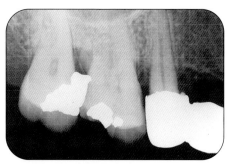

Fig 2-1b The radiograph reveals the correlation between the overhanging alloy and the loss of interdental bone. Note the apparent invasion of the distal furcation on the first molar.

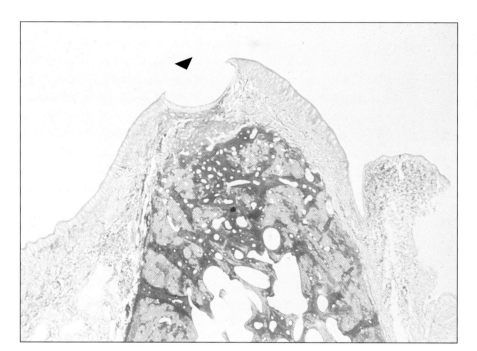

Fig 2-2 Histologic section of an interproximal space. The interdental bone is convex or flat. Note the interdental col under the contact point. This concavity is lined with a very thin, cuboidal epithelium of four or five cell layers in thickness. The intact connective tissue interspersed between the bone and the epithelium represents transseptal fibers.

In the absence of inflammation, there is no direct evidence that excessive occlusal force will result in the permanent loss of the alveolus[11] (see Chapter 8). Because most patients react to minimally high occlusal restorations, stronger forces loaded in a vertical axis would exhaust a patient's tolerance and he or she would seek relief.

The interdental col is described as a concavity of soft tissue connecting the buccal and lingual or palatal peaks of gingiva under the contact point of two teeth when the soft tissue papilla totally fills the interproximal space.[12] The buccal and lingual papillae are covered with stratified squamous epithelia, but this concavity, or col, is covered with epithelia of only a few cell layers in thickness. The method with which the weaker epithelia blends with the oral epithelia is unclear, but it is reasonable to assume that this interface of epithelia, together with the col lining, may be a weak link in the soft tissue protection of the underlying osseous crest. This line of reasoning could lead to the speculation that any interproximal dental procedure has the potential to be an iatrogenic factor.

The anatomic soft tissue col is not mimicked in the underlying crest of bone, which displays a flat or convex form in a state of health (Fig 2-2). There is no col or soft tissue concavity when the papilla does not fill the interproximal space, that is, after therapy has been performed to eliminate a periodontal pocket or when a diastema occurs between teeth.

Disruption of the Soft Tissue Barrier

There are many dental procedures that must be performed even if they result in minor disruption of the soft tissue papilla. A routine example is the restoration of molar interproximal caries in the adolescent dentition in the presence of altered passive eruption. Most people have sufficient innate resistance to periodontal disease to withstand minor injuries without exhibiting measurable detrimental results. However, it is impossible to determine who has a predilection for periodontal disease; therefore, it is important to routinely perform meticulous dentistry for interproximal restorations[13,14] (Fig 2-3).

It is necessary to program interproximal accessibility into all prostheses. The so-called temporary restoration used in standard operative procedures is no exception; if the provisional restoration prevents cleansing of the area, an inflammatory lesion will result.[15] Properly constructed provisional crowns can mask superficial evidence of periodontal problems and should be removed to allow a complete clinical examination (Figs 2-4a and 2-4b). It is possible that the previous tooth preparation and crown margin extended significantly subgingivally and that periodontal surgery is necessary to expose adequate clinical crown to finish a margin.

It is wrong to permanently cement a new restoration in the absence of periodontal health. A red, ulcerative interproximal papilla is indicative of a loss of epithelium and an open wound; histologic observation reveals round-cell infiltration and almost total disruption of the connective tissue fiber apparatus (Figs 2-5a to 2-5c). It is unlikely that such an interdental papilla can protect the integrity of the underlying bony septa or that the papilla will revert spontaneously to health after the delivery of the final restoration.

The alveolar housing for the roots of anterior teeth is narrower than that for posterior teeth (Figs 2-6a and 2-6b) and may exhibit a crest limited to facial and lingual lamina dura with little or no cancellous bone interspersed between the two cortical plates.[16] The disruption of the soft tissue barrier in these regions will probably result in a horizontal loss of interproximal bone. The buccolingual dimension of

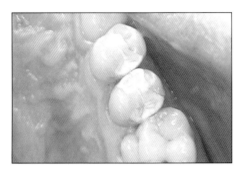

Fig 2-3 All dental restorations should be carved to emulate the original tooth structure. There should be firm contact points between restorations and the natural surfaces of adjacent teeth.

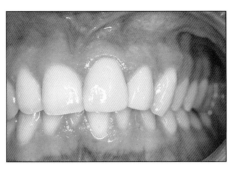

Fig 2-4a Provisional crowns for the maxillary left central and lateral incisors are in place. The gingiva appears to be pink and healthy. However, the referring dentist indicated that he is unable to resolve the underlying problems nonsurgically.

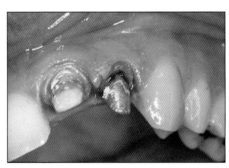

Fig 2-4b It is necessary to remove the provisional crowns to correctly assay the need for periodontal correction. The interdental papilla continues to be red, indicating a lack of epithelium. This problem has not been corrected by the new provisional crowns or the patient's efforts to cleanse. An additional problem is that the previous tooth preparations, for the crowns that failed, extended too far subgingivally. It would be impossible to correct the tooth preparations without extending significantly subgingivally. Therefore, surgery must be performed to expose additional tooth structure.

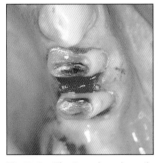

Fig 2-5a The interdental papilla between the premolars is red and inflamed at the time of insertion of the permanent fixed partial denture. Periodontal surgery had been performed in preparation for the restorative dentistry.

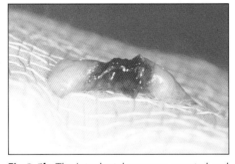

Fig 2-5b The interdental area was resected and submitted as a biopsy specimen. Note the pink interdental papilla joined by a red mass of tissue.

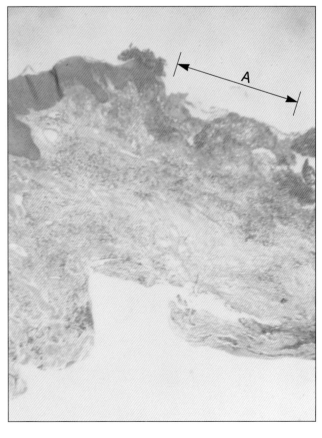

Fig 2-5c The histologic section of the resected tissue demonstrates an interruption of the epithelium and ulceration corresponding to the red area (A). The connective tissue corium is completely disrupted and heavily infiltrated with inflammatory cells. It is hard to imagine that this connective tissue could be reorganized simply by the cementation of a permanent fixed partial denture. It is important that the epithelium, the first line of body defense, be intact when the prosthesis is cemented and that the underlying connective tissues be well organized to protect the underlying bone.

the interproximal bone is larger as the alveolar process widens to accommodate the larger-rooted posterior teeth (Fig 2-6c). The destruction of the soft tissue barrier will be more likely to result in bone loss with a vertical component because of the distance between the two cortical plates and the space therein, occupied by cancellous bone.

Interproximal Osseous Lesions

The most frequently noted osseous lesion occurs when there is loss of bone under the contact point, but minimal bone damage at the line angles of the teeth, that is, the shallow interproximal bone crater[17] (Fig 2-7a). Periodontal treatment must prevent the reinitiation of this lesion after periodontal corrective therapy has been accomplished.[18] The three possible treatment modalities for an interproximal pocket are maintenance, reduction by subtraction, or reduction by regeneration. Each situation will have to be treated with special care, but an intrabony pocket demands a specific decision. The shallow crater is usually best treated by ostectomy,

whereas the deeper intrabony pockets should be treated by regeneration or a combination of regeneration and ostectomy.[19–21] The loss of interproximal bone should not be allowed to continue to the point that it becomes necessary to extract the tooth (Fig 2-7b).

A limited anterior embrasure may be more tolerable than a limited posterior embrasure (see Figs 2-6a and 2-6b). The buccolingual distance to be cleansed is smaller and the demand for dexterity is more reasonable. With the transition from the unrestored to the restored dentition, the complexity of decisions changes dramatically. The retention of one or more mandibular incisors may not offer an appreciable benefit to the total supporting apparatus of the arch and may provide insurmountable difficulties to the interproximal restoration (Figs 2-8a and 2-8b). The lack of an embrasure will disturb the integrity of the soft tissue attachment and offer little or no chance to provide the patient with adequate access for cleansing the prosthesis. The recognition of this problem may lead the clinician to remove one incisor and to reposition the remaining incisors orthodontically to provide cleansable embrasures (Figs 2-9a and 2-9b).

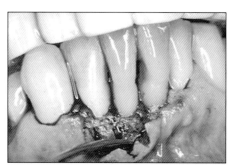

Fig 2-6a The embrasures between the mandibular incisors are small. There is some possibility that the patient will be able to floss between these teeth because they are in the anterior portion of the mouth and they are single rooted.

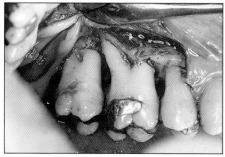

Fig 2-6b The interproximal embrasure between maxillary molars is frequently impossible to cleanse. The distobuccal root of the first molar diverges toward the mesiobuccal root of the second molar, resulting in an embrasure that narrows as it extends apically. Because the furcation of the maxillary first molar is located approximately 4 mm apical to the cementoenamel junction, it is likely that there is a loss of bone between the distal and palatal roots of this tooth. This will make it impossible for the patient or the hygienist to keep this area free of plaque. The solution may be the resection of the distobuccal root.

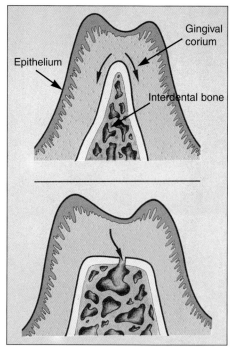

Fig 2-6c The alveolar housing is much wider buccolingually in the posterior part of the mouth because it must accommodate the larger root structures. The wider interdental area posteriorly is more prone to intrabony pockets.

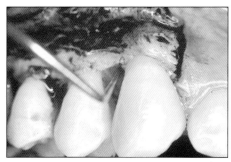

Fig 2-7a The interdental crater between the maxillary canine and first premolar is shallow, and the prospects for regeneration are not good. This type of defect is best treated by ostectomy and osteoplasty. It is important to isolate osseous lesions at the time of surgery so that specific treatment decisions can be rendered.

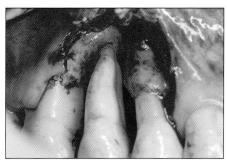

Fig 2-7b It is too late to treat this tooth with periodontal regenerative techniques. It is very important that the tooth be removed before there is any further damage to the supporting structure of the adjacent teeth.

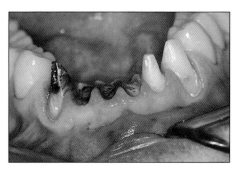

Fig 2-8a The mandibular central incisors and right lateral incisor have no clinical crown. The root proximity is a perceived difficulty when completing a cleansable prosthesis.

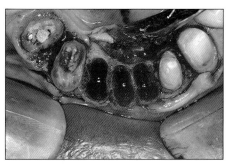

Fig 2-8b The postextraction clinical observation reveals very thin interdental septa of bone. It would have been very difficult to construct approximating restorative margins that would be cleansable; therefore the teeth were removed.

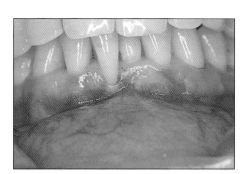

Fig 2-9a The mandibular incisors are crowded and difficult to cleanse (1970).

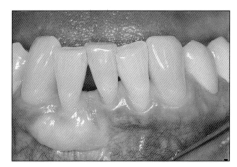

Fig 2-9b The prominent right central incisor was extracted, and the other teeth were repositioned. After 26 years, the patient continues to exhibit periodontal health and embrasures that can be kept clean.

Maxillary Anterior Dentition

The maxillary anterior sextant offers an interesting dichotomy of thought. Although long-term health demands attention to pocketing, the esthetic needs of the patient frequently demand compromise (Figs 2-10 and 2-11). The replaced flap or the Widman flap offers an immediate solution, in that the flap is placed in an attractive position,[22] but the technique[10,11] is unlikely to reestablish an attachment to the tooth and tends to perpetuate pocketing.[23] This places the patient at risk for continued deterioration of the interdental crest, unless he or she is that rare example of absolute periodontal compliance.

Even then, a more definitive treatment result is preferred before a final prosthesis is fabricated. If the bone lesion is vertical and treatable by a regeneration procedure, the esthetics will be preserved. Pocket reduction via subtraction is of limited value, unless all the maxillary anterior teeth are included in a prosthesis that will redesign the embrasures and establish a somewhat uniform size of the teeth (Figs 2-12a to 2-12f). Sometimes the best answer may be to eliminate a specific tooth or all incisors to reach a conclusion that correlates periodontal health and fine esthetics (Figs 2-13 and 2-14).

Some embrasures are limited in the coronal area but offer the possibility to be opened because the roots diverge apical to the cementoenamel junction. It is necessary to gain access to the seam of the root and the alveolar process via flap surgery and then to reduce the excess tooth structure to open the embrasure (Figs 2-15a to 2-15e). This does not suggest that roots that are parallel can be reduced to create an artificial subgingival embrasure. This would result in poor marginal adaptation of the prosthesis because the discrepancy would be filled with granulation tissue (Figs 2-16 to 2-18).

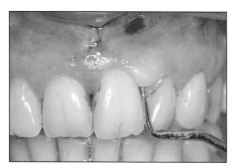

Fig 2-10a There is an 8-mm interdental pocket between the maxillary central and lateral incisors. The periodicity of periodontal abscesses is approximately 6 weeks.

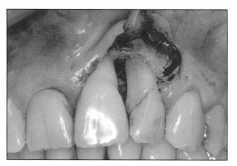

Fig 2-10b Periodontal flaps are elevated to reveal the root surfaces, which have been root planed and demonstrate significant loss of supporting bone. It is impossible to position the buccal flap at the crestal bone, and therefore it is necessary to determine the position arbitrarily.

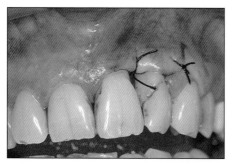

Fig 2-10c The flap is sutured in place at a level that will help preserve reasonable esthetics. There is no correlation between the level of the osseous crest and flap placement.

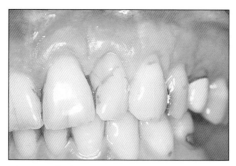

Fig 2-10d The patient presents with a periodontal abscess again, 16 weeks after periodontal surgery. The abscess will necessitate administration of local anesthesia and root planing, supplemented by antibiotic therapy. Financial limitations preclude a definitive treatment plan and necessitate pocket maintenance. However, this would be an unacceptable end goal if a prosthesis were to be introduced in this region.

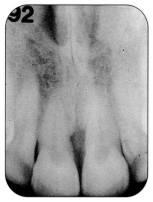 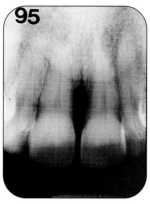

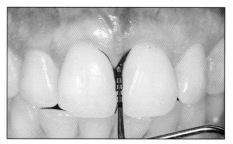

Fig 2-11a The radiographs demonstrate the loss of the septum between the maxillary central incisors. *(left)* The area was treated surgically in 1992. *(right)* The patient has continued to be under periodontal supervision (1995).

Fig 2-11b There is an interdental probing of 9 mm between the maxillary central incisors. It is very important to stop the loss of bone.

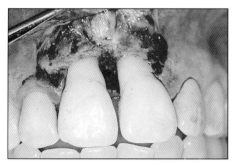

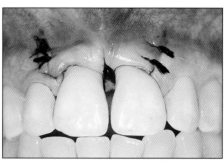

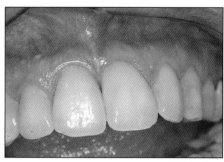

Fig 2-11c Periodontal flaps have been elevated, revealing significant loss of supporting bone for both teeth. It will be difficult to decide where to place the flap when suturing.

Fig 2-11d It is necessary to compromise and place the flap more coronally than the level of the alveolar process. Even the compromise will result in the loss of the papilla between the central incisors.

Fig 2-11e After the area has healed, composite has been added interproximally to encourage the regrowth of the papilla. The patient has no difficulty using a floss threader to debride the area. A procedure such as this requires an exceptional effort by the restorative dentist and the patient. (Courtesy of Dr. John Machell.)

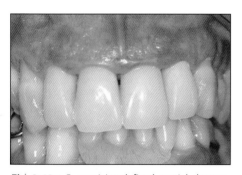

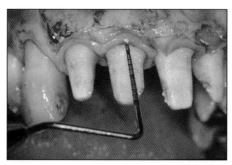

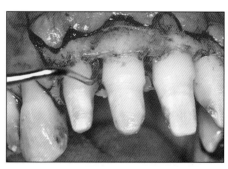

Fig 2-12a A provisional fixed partial denture has replaced existing crowns. There is deep interproximal pocketing that must be corrected before the final prosthesis is constructed.

Fig 2-12b The buccal flap has been elevated, but the pocketed collar of tissue remains. It will be necessary to remove this tissue entirely to visualize the osseous deformities that exist.

Fig 2-12c Only with the provisional prosthesis removed and the buccal and palatal flaps elevated can all the granulation tissue be removed. This procedure provides an opportunity to eliminate the interdental craters by addition or subtraction, as is necessary. In this instance, the shallow interdental craters will be resolved by ramping the bone toward the palate.

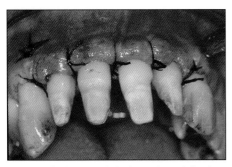

Fig 2-12d The partial-thickness buccal flap has been repositioned at the osseous crest. This enables the tissue to heal and the elements of the biologic width to fill in as dictated by the location of the teeth in the alveolar process.

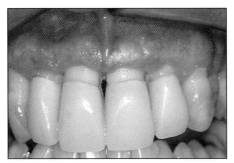

Fig 2-12e The gingiva has demonstrated some creeping attachment during this period of time. The distance from the gingiva to the final line of the tooth preparation is much less than in Fig 2-12d, the immediately postoperative view of the surgery. It is important to allow time (6 to 8 weeks) to pass before the final prosthesis is constructed, so that the gingiva can achieve its desired level. This differential in tissue height can be attributed to the development of the entities of the biologic width.

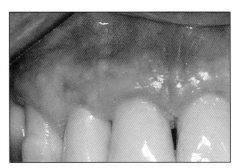

Fig 2-12f The permanent restorations are in place.

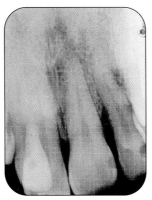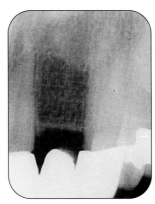

Fig 2-13a *(left)* The preoperative radiograph demonstrates an interdental crater between the left central and lateral incisors. *(right)* The postoperative radiograph, taken 17 years later, demonstrates complete healing of the extraction socket.

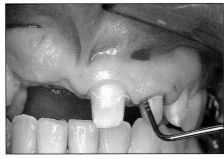

Fig 2-13b Although the gingival tissue is pink and nonbleeding, there is a deep bone defect on the mesial surface of the left lateral incisor. The original treatment plan called for extraction of this tooth, but the restorative dentist decided to retain it in the provisional bridge.

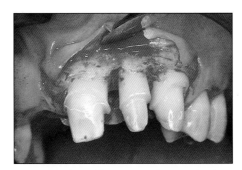

Fig 2-13c Flap reflection reveals excessive loss of supporting bone in the area between the central and lateral incisors. Use of osseous resection to achieve parabolic architecture is contraindicated because the teeth would be too long. The lesion is too shallow for predictable regeneration; in addition, regeneration procedures would delay the final restoration for some months to determine if further surgery is necessary. The lateral incisor is a nonstrategic tooth.

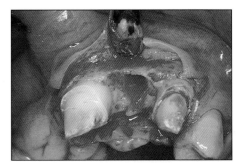

Fig 2-13d The lateral incisor has been extracted; this provides an opportunity to see the interdental crater on the distal surface of the central incisor. The need to develop parabolic architecture is avoided, and the bone can be ramped to the palate without creating a solution with a difficult esthetic component. The lateral incisor is not strategic and does not provide significant support to the proposed final prosthesis.

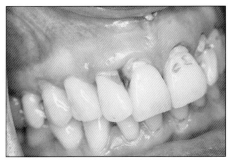

Fig 2-14a There is a deep interdental crater between the maxillary right central and lateral incisors. The lateral incisor is rotated, creating a very narrow embrasure between the two teeth. (Courtesy of Dr. H.M. Skurow.)

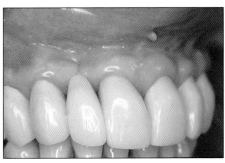

Fig 2-14b The lateral incisor has been removed and replaced with a pontic as part of the final prosthesis.

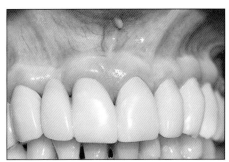

Fig 2-14c The patient has been able to clean the interproximal areas of this fixed prosthesis for an extended period (14 years). There is no gingival recession from any crown margins.

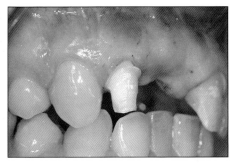

Fig 2-15a There is a very limited potential for an embrasure between the lateral incisor and canine. In an effort to avoid a problem of marginal fit, an extended shoulder preparation has been created.

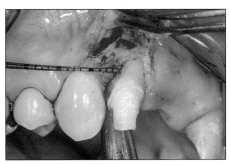

Fig 2-15b A buccal flap has been reflected. It reveals the potential to enlarge the embrasure because of the divergence of the roots. There is a distal triangle of clinical crown that can be reduced with tooth preparation.

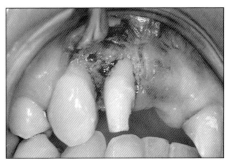

Fig 2-15c The embrasure has been opened by tooth preparation.

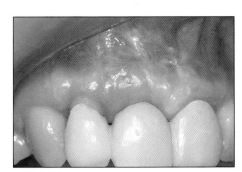

Fig 2-15d The provisional prosthesis is in place, and healing is observed.

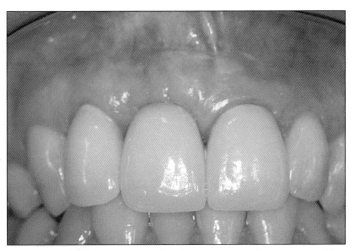

Fig 2-15e The final restoration has been constructed. (Courtesy of Dr. John Machell.)

Maxillary Posterior Dentition

All embrasures that are bordered by roots with concavities are precarious because proximal osseous defects are commonplace, especially on the mesial surface of the maxillary first premolars (see Fig 2-7a). The proximal concavity makes the construction of a cleansable restoration difficult and also challenges the patient's dexterity. Interestingly, this is the area frequently selected as the site for precision attachments to interlock fixed restorations. Such treatment reduces the patient's capacity to cleanse by reducing the size of the embrasure.

Perhaps the most difficult decision involves the interproximal space between the maxillary first and second molars (Fig 2-19). The wider teeth result in a larger buccolingual distance that is difficult to cleanse, and an intraradicular periodontium that is quite susceptible. It is important to address limited embrasures as a part of the initial treatment plan and to resolve all periodontal problems before the teeth are restored. It may be that one molar has an excellent prognosis and one a poor prognosis, in which case a strategic extraction would be in order. When both teeth have a good prognosis and an inadequate interproximal embrasure, and the treatment plan calls for complete-coverage restora-

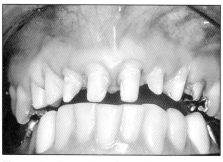

Fig 2-16a A provisional prosthesis has been removed and there appear to be adequate embrasures. The restorative dentist reports that he is unable to find the end of the finish line of the tooth preparations.

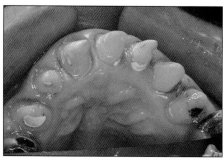

Fig 2-16b The occlusal view also reveals apparent embrasures. These teeth were crowned to correct crowding. This is a poor decision because it will be very difficult to create cleansable embrasures.

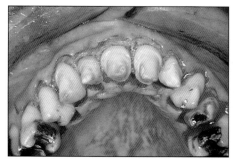

Fig 2-16c Buccal and palatal flaps have been elevated, revealing the apical extension of the original tooth preparations and the lack of embrasures between the prepared teeth. It is not plausible to use tooth preparation to open embrasures, if there is no space between the two adjacent roots (compare Figs 2-15b and 2-15c).

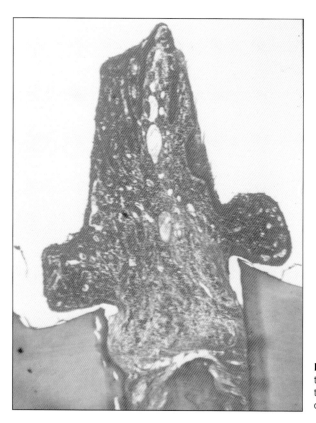

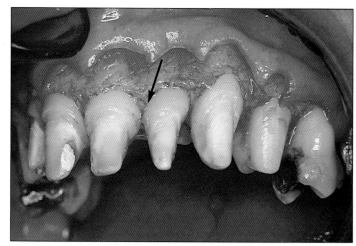

Fig 2-18 A buccal view reveals no potential for an embrasure between the left incisors *(arrow)*.

Fig 2-17 A human histologic section demonstrating what might be anticipated when the permanent fixed partial denture was cemented in Fig 2-16b. Soft tissue would cover the finish lines and interfere with proper seating of the prosthesis. The soft tissues are composed of disorganized granulation tissue.

tions, the preferable treatment would be the utilization of orthodontics to create an embrasure (Figs 2-20a and 2-20b).

If orthodontic treatment is not in order, the embrasure can be opened by removing a root from one or both of the molars[24–27] (Figs 2-21a to 2-21d and 2-22). This would pose the choice of which root to remove—the distobuccal root of

the first molar or the mesiobuccal root of the second molar. In the absence of furcation involvement, it is necessary to consider the root anatomy of these teeth. The distobuccal root of the first molar is round, and the distal furcation is found about midway between the distobuccal and distopalatal line angles (Figs 2-23a and 2-23b). The

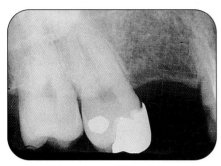

Fig 2-19 The radiograph reveals that there is no potential for an embrasure. It is possible for these teeth to remain in a state of periodontal health when no restoration is attempted, but it is not possible to prepare these teeth and fit interdental margins and still provide a cleansable embrasure for a patient.

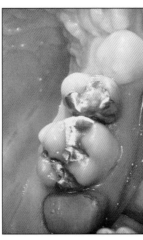

Fig 2-20a The patient has lost the permanent crown for the maxillary second molar, which has drifted mesially to contact the first molar.

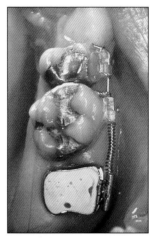

Fig 2-20b Minor tooth movement has been introduced to recreate an embrasure between the first and second molars.

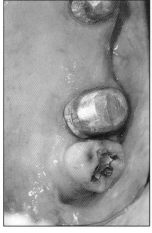

Fig 2-21a A telescopic retainer is in place in preparation for the delivery of a final fixed prosthesis. There is no embrasure, and the interproximal probing depth is 8 mm.

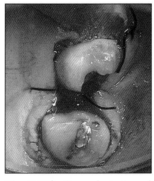

Fig 2-21b A much improved embrasure has been created by preparing both teeth and removing the distobuccal root of the first molar.

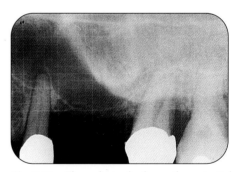

Fig 2-21c The radiograph shows the potential for an embrasure if both teeth were prepared. The approximating roots deviate from each other. There has been extensive loss of interproximal bone, and the distal furcation has lost bone.

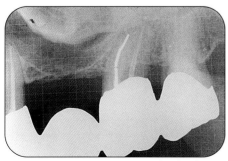

Fig 2-21d The postsurgical radiograph shows the finished prosthesis in place. Note the embrasure.

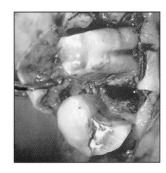

Fig 2-22 A mesial root has been removed to relieve a difficult embrasure between the molars. The bone is intact between the distal and palatal roots, and the patient will be able to clean this area with direct cleaning.

mesiobuccal root of the second molar is generally flat and oblong, and the mesial furcation is approximately two thirds the distance to the palate.

Thus, the removal of the mesiobuccal root of the second molar resolves a tight embrasure more significantly than does the removal of the distobuccal root of the first molar. In addition, it will probably be easier to educate the patient about direct-approach cleansing of this awkward restoration than it will be to teach back-action cleansing techniques for the restoration of a first molar without a distal root. Endodontic failure is possible, and most patients would prefer to preserve the first molar.

It is difficult to initiate the conversation and the chain of events that must ensue when a root resection is proposed solely to open an embrasure, but it does not require many failures to recognize the importance of this decision. The perpetuation of a narrow embrasure with the construction of a permanent prosthesis has the potential to severely limit the periodontal prognosis. Premature failure is discouraging to both the patient and the dental team and must be kept at a minimum (Figs 2-24a to 2-24c).

There is some opportunity to enhance the interproximal space by employing tooth preparation when the flaps are reflected during the surgical intervention. This will be determined by the direction of the roots as they proceed apically, and is only applicable if they are divergent from each other and offer a larger embrasure if the teeth are prepared (see Figs 2-21c and 2-21d).

Periodontal disease and/or caries frequently dictate the decision as to which root should be extracted in the restoration of teeth afflicted with advanced periodontal disease. The resultant embrasure should first be tested in a provisional restoration before final restorations are constructed (Figs 2-25a to 2-25c). It is imperative that the periodontist, the restorative dentist, and the laboratory technician share the same goals.

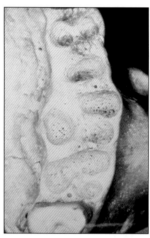

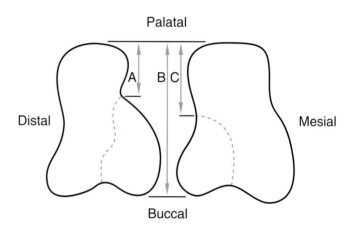

Fig 2-23a The placement of the maxillary posterior quadrant in the alveolus. The furcation on the mesial aspect of the molars is about two thirds the distance to the palate because of the oblong shape of the mesial root. Of particular interest is the interproximal space between the two molars, where the distal furca is about midway from the palate to the buccal.

Fig 2-23b The position of the distal furcation on the first molar and the mesial furcation on the second molar. If everything else is equal, the removal of the mesial root on the second molar will provide more embrasure space between these two difficult teeth. The distance from the palatal surface of the maxillary molar to the mesial furcation (*A*); the total buccopalatal width of the interdental space between 2 maxillary molars (*B*); the distance from the palatal surface of the maxillary molar to the distal furcation (*C*).

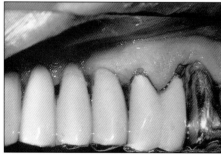

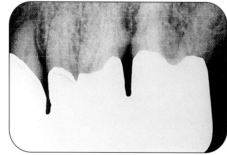

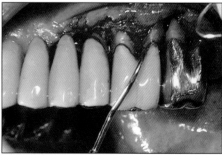

Fig 2-24a The embrasure between the maxillary molars is limited.

Fig 2-24b Six years after completion of the prosthesis, the approximating roots of the molars are almost contacting each other. This limits the prosthetic restorations and the patient's ability to clean this very difficult area. There is a radiolucency apical to the convergence of the roots.

Fig 2-24c The surgical procedure performed at the time of the radiograph reveals extreme loss of the interproximal bone. This failure supports the decision to remove and open an embrasure before a prosthesis is constructed.

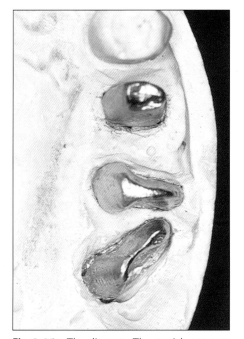

Fig 2-25a The die cast. The mesial root was removed from the maxillary first molar because of caries. The distal root was removed from the maxillary second molar because of periodontal disease. The root concavities and the small embrasure between the molars dictate the need to test the possibility of controlling plaque and periodontal disease before completion of the finished prosthesis.

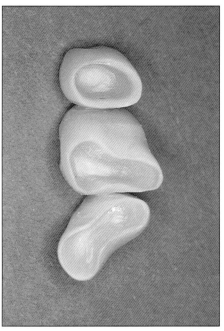

Fig 2-25b *(cervical view)* The patient will use this provisional restoration as a trial restoration.

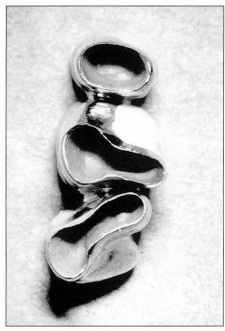

Fig 2-25c The permanent prosthesis is a reproduction of the provisional restoration.

Mandibular Molars

The restoration of mandibular molars offers similar complexities relative to difficult access for both the dentist and the patient. These are frequently amplified by premature loss of the first molar and the mesial drifting of the second and third molars. When the second and third molar tilt mesially, the contact points slip and the embrasure is narrowed. The ensuing restoration of one or both of these teeth will jeopardize the size of the interdental embrasure. The solution to the tilted mandibular molar is the correction of the tooth position for both mandibular molars, or the extraction of one and the orthodontic uprighting of the molar that remains.[27,28] This is usually accomplished before periodontal surgery.

The Soft Tissue Barrier and Periodontal Health

If a periodontal state of health is established interproximally before construction of the final restoration, and if that state of health is not disturbed during the construction of the restoration and exists on the day the restoration is delivered to the patient, it is reasonable to anticipate the existence of an intact soft tissue interproximal papilla that will protect the integrity of the underlying bone. This would necessitate that there be no damage to the interproximal papilla during tooth preparation, impression taking, try-in, and final cementation. This hypothesis depends on a conception of intracrevicular or supragingival marginal placement that will not challenge the integrity of the attachment of supracrestal fibers into the cementum of adjacent teeth.[29,30] It is important to avoid detaching the connective tissue attachment to the tooth. Because neither the sulcus nor the junctional epithelium is vascularized, any bleeding that occurs during the performance of restorative dentistry will be a result of damaging the connective tissue.

An intact soft tissue attachment at the conclusion of corrective treatment is imperative to long-term periodontal health. For predictable success, this intact soft tissue attachment must be supplemented with a maintenance program of logical periodicity carried out in a compliant patient.[31,32,33]

Further damage and continued bone loss will be contingent on future destruction of the soft tissue protectorate. It is to this end that all patients must be educated to cleanse interproximally with some instrument other than a toothbrush. Not every person can master dental floss or tape, and interproximal brushes are preferable for cleansing root concavities and splinted teeth.

References

1. Nevins M. Interproximal periodontal disease—the embrasure as an etiologic factor. Int J Periodont Rest Dent 1982;2(6):9–27.

2. Kramer GM. A consideration of root proximity. Int J Periodont Rest Dent 1987;7(6):9–34.

3. Prichard JF. Interpretation of radiographs in periodontics. Int J Periodont Rest Dent 1983;3(1):9–39.

4. Lindhe J, Nyman S. The effect of plaque control and surgical pocket elimination on the establishment and maintenance of periodontal health. A longitudinal study of periodontal therapy of advanced disease. J Clin Periodontol 1975;2:67–79.

5. Townsend Olsen C, Ammons WF, Van Belle C. A longitudinal study comparing apically repositioned flaps with and without osseous surgery. Int J Periodont Rest Dent 1985;5(4):11–33.

6. Goldman HM. Histologic topographic changes of inflammatory origin in the gingival fibers. J Periodontol 1952;23:104.

7. Goldman HM. The relationship of the epithelial attachment to the adjacent fibers of the periodontal membrane. J Dent Res 1944;23:177.

8. Löe H, Theilade E, Jensen SB. Experimental gingivitis in man. J Periodontol 1965;36:177–187.

9. Page RC, Schroeder HE. Pathogenesis of inflammatory periodontal disease. A summary of current work. Lab Invest 1976;33:235–249.

10. Slots J, Moenho D, Langebaek J, Frandsen A. Microbiota of gingivitis in man. Scand J Dent Res 1978;86:174–181.

11. Keller GJ, Cohen DW. India ink and perfusion of the vascular plexus of oral tissues. Oral Surg Oral Med Oral Pathol 1955;8:539.

12. Cohen B. Morphological factors in the pathogenesis of periodontal disease. Br Dent J 1959;107:31.

13. Maynard JG Jr., Wilson RD. Physiologic dimensions of the periodontium fundamental to successful restorative dentistry. J Periodontol 1979;50:170–174.

14. Lytle JD, Skurow HM. The interproximal embrasure. Dent Clin North Am 1971;15:641.

15. Skurow HM, Nevins M. The rationale of the preperiodontal provisional biologic trial restoration. Int J Periodont Rest Dent 1988;8(1):9–29.

16. Gher ME, Vernino AR. Root anatomy: a local factor in inflammatory periodontal disease. Int J Periodont Rest Dent 1981;1(5):53–63.

17. Bahat O, Glover ME, Ammons WF, Kegel W, Selipsky H. The influence of soft tissue on interdental bone height after flap curettage. I. A study involving six patients. Int J Periodont Rest Dent 1984;4(2):9–25.

18. Jenkins W, Wragg P, Gilmour W. Formation of interdental soft tissue defects after surgical treatment of periodontitis. J Periodontol 1990;61:564–570.

19. Selvig RA, Rersten BG, Wikesjö UME. Surgical treatment of intrabony periodontal defects using expanded polytetrafluoroethylene barrier membranes: Influence of defect configuration on healing response. J Periodontol 1993;64:730–733.

20. Kramer GM. The case for ostectomy—a time tested therapeutic modality in selected periodontitis sites. Int J Periodont Rest Dent 1995;15:229–237.

21. Ochsenbein C. Combined approach to the management of intrabony defects. Int J Periodont Rest Dent 1995;15:329–343.

22. Ramfjord S. Present status of the modified Widman flap procedure. J Periodontol 1977;48:558.

23. Bahat O, Glover ME, Ammons WF. The influence of soft tissue on interdental bone height after flap curettage. II. Histologic findings after six months. Int J Periodont Rest Dent 1984;4(2):25–31.

24. Klavan B. Clinical observation following root amputation in maxillary molar teeth. J Periodontol 1975;46:1–5.

25. Langer B, Stein SD, Wagenberg B. An evaluation of root resections. A ten year study. J Periodontol 1981;52:719–722.

26. Carnevale G, Di Febo G, Fuzzi M. A retrospective analysis of the perio-prosthetic aspect of teeth re-prepared during periodontal surgery. J Clin Periodontol 1990;17:313–316.

27. Carnevale G, Pontorieno R, Hürzeler M. Management of furcation involvement. Periodontics 2000 1995;9:69–89.

28. Brown IS. Effect of orthodontic therapy on periodontal defects. J Periodontol 1969;40:577.

29. Wise RJ, Kramer GM. Predetermination of osseous changes associated with uprighting tipped molars by probing. Int J Periodont Rest Dent 1983;3(1):69–81.

30. Wilson RD, Maynard JG. The relationship of restorative dentistry to periodontics. In: Prichard JF (ed). The Diagnosis and Treatment of Periodontal Disease in General Dental Practice. Philadelphia: Saunders, 1979, ch 28.

31. Nevins M, Skurow HM. The intracrevicular restorative margin, the biologic width and the maintenance of the gingival margin. Int J Periodont Rest Dent 1984;4(3):31–50.

32. Becker W, Becker B, Berg L. Periodontal treatment without maintenance: a retrospective study in 44 patients. J Periodontol 1984;55:505–509.

33. Wilson TG, Shannon H, Temple R. The results of efforts to improve compliance with supportive periodontal treatment in a private practice. J Periodontol 1993;64:311–314.

CHAPTER 3

A Long-Term Maintenance Program

Myron Nevins, DDS
Richard J. Oringer, DDS, DMSc
Marc L. Nevins, DMD, MMSc

The premise of periodontics is to retain the natural dentition in a state of health and function (Figs 3-1a to 3-1m). The goal of active periodontal therapy is to create a stable environment that can be maintained by a partnership of patient self-care and timely professional visits. This professional treatment, better termed *supportive* *periodontal therapy* (SPT), is actually an extension of active treatment and is meant to maintain the results of corrective therapy. Although it is not possible to accurately identify patients who will experience further attachment loss, it is well accepted that microbial plaque is the main etiologic agent for periodontal disease. Therefore, the main objective

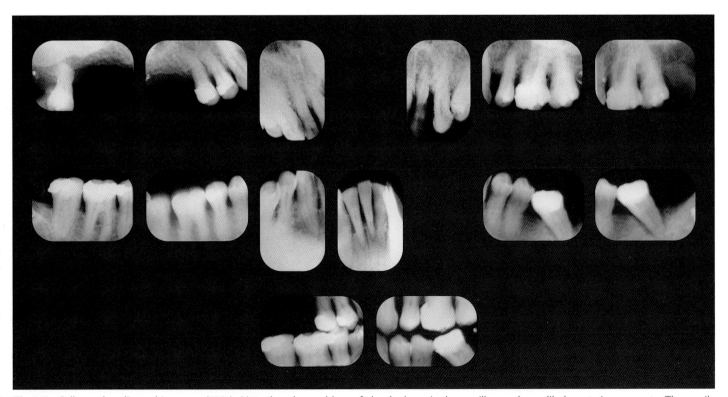

Fig 3-1a Full-mouth radiographic survey (1951). Note the advanced loss of alveolar bone in the maxillary and mandibular anterior segments. The maxillary right second molar, maxillary left first molar, and mandibular left second molar have been lost.

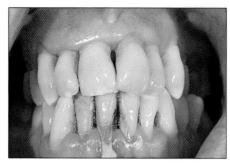

Fig 3-1b The clinical presentation in 1951 reveals advanced adult periodontitis.

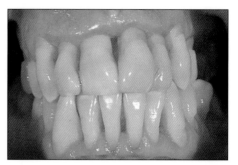

Fig 3-1c Periodontal surgical treatment has been completed (1951). (Courtesy of Dr. G.M. Kramer.)

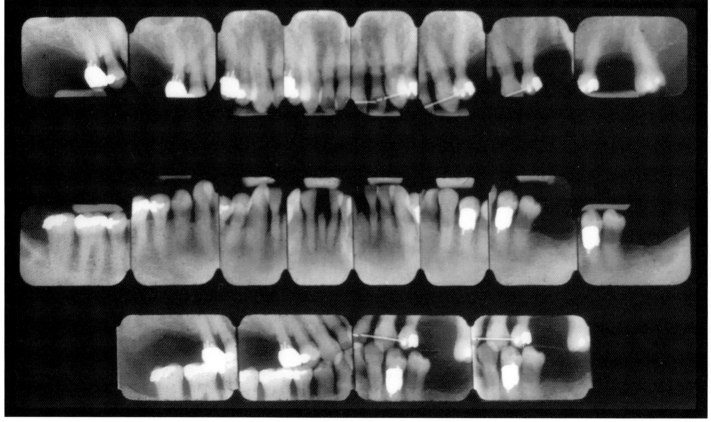

Fig 3-1d Full-mouth radiographic survey (1970). The mandibular central incisor is fractured at the gingiva.

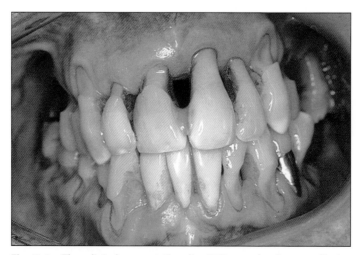

Fig 3-1e The clinical presentation in 1970 reveals the mandibular provisional fixed partial denture replacing the lost incisor.

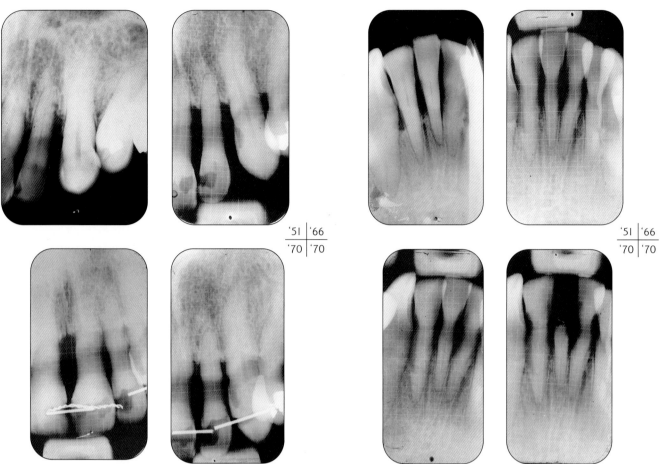

Fig 3-1f Bone loss is attenuated after corrective periodontal surgery. Intracoronal splints have been placed after orthodontic retraction of the maxillary incisors.

Fig 3-1g There has been no progressive periodontal disease, but the central incisor has fractured as a result of aggressive oral hygiene and scaling and root planing.

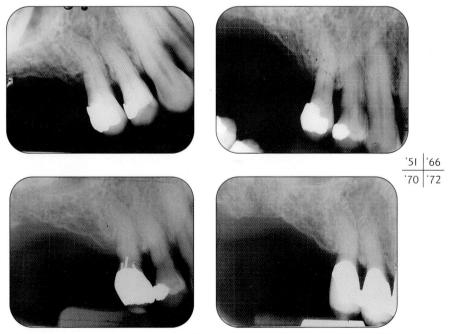

Fig 3-1h After treatment of active disease, the patient has been successfully maintained with premolar occlusion.

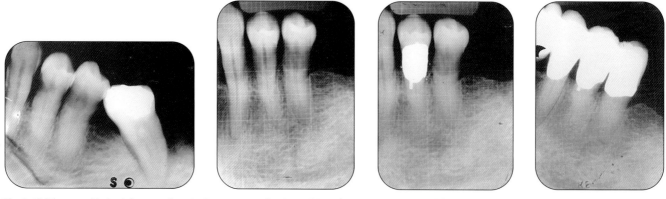

Fig 3-1i The mandibular left second molar is present at the time of initial treatment (1951). *(left to right)* 1951, 1966, 1970, 1972.

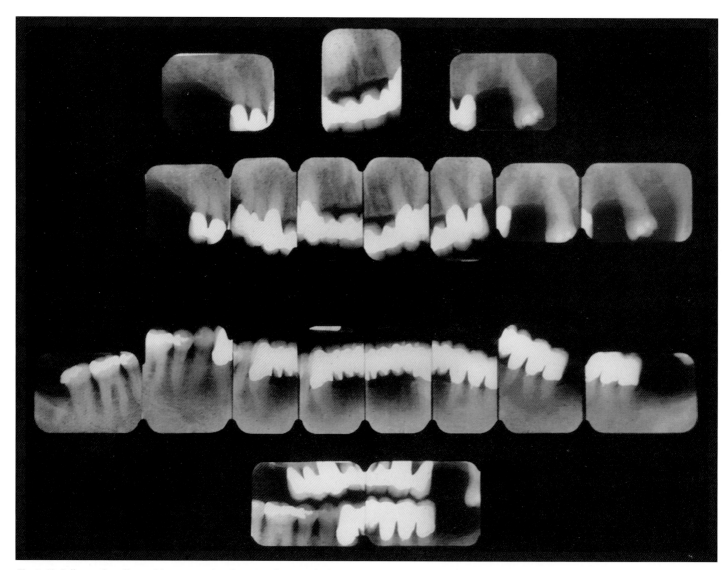

Fig 3-1j Full-mouth radiographic survey taken in 1972 after prosthetic reconstruction.

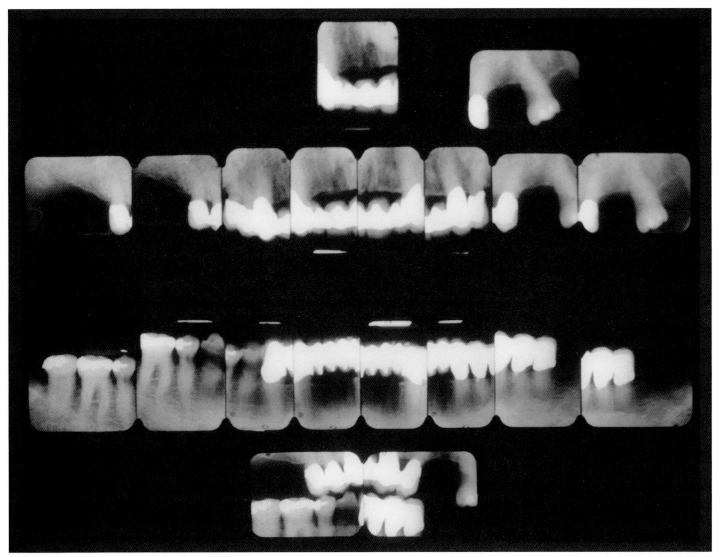

Fig 3-1k Full-mouth radiographs taken in 1993 reveal maintenance of alveolar bone and the marginal integrity of the prostheses. There has been no additional tooth loss over 40 years. Note the lack of supereruption of the maxillary left and mandibular right second molars, which are without functional antagonists.

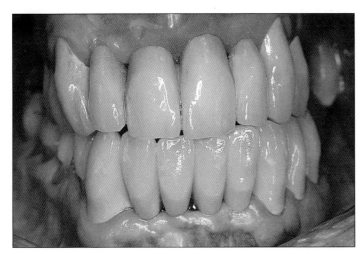

Fig 3-1l Clinical view in 1972 after cementation of the porcelain-fused-to-metal prosthesis. (Courtesy of Dr. H.M. Skurow.)

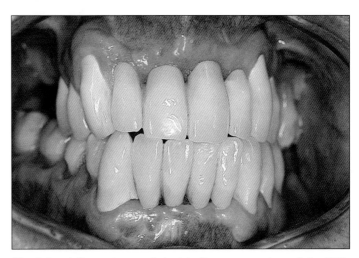

Fig 3-1m Inflammatory periodontal disease was stopped in 1951. Prosthetic reconstruction was completed in 1972 to correct compromised esthetics. The esthetics of the prosthesis is maintained in 1993, after 21 years in function.

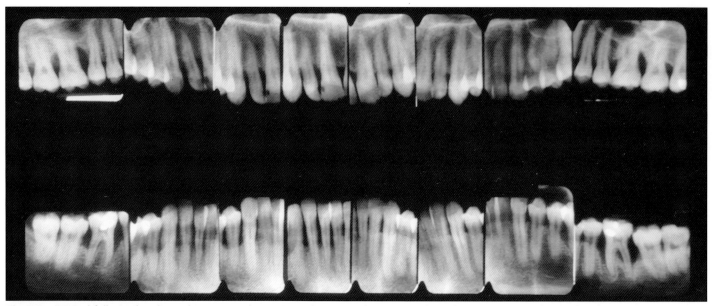

Fig 3-2a Original full-mouth radiographic survey, taken in December 1970. There is overt loss of osseous support for the four first molar areas and in the incisor regions.

of SPT is to reduce the patient's risk of active periodontal destruction by nonspecifically lowering bacterial levels, usually with mechanical instrumentation.[1]

It is important to recognize that patients present with various levels of disease, and different patients will require different approaches to maintenance therapy. The concept of individualizing maintenance therapy for each patient as well as the factors to consider will be discussed. Factors to be addressed include the appropriate goals of active therapy, the length and periodicity of visits, the individual who should provide treatment, the patient's behavior, the size of the office, and economic pressures.

Controlling Periodontal Disease

Individuals with a history of periodontal disease are susceptible to future loss of attachment.[2] First it is necessary to address the available evidence on how to best control periodontal disease. All would agree that the goal of periodontal health is better served by shallow sulci than by pathologically deepened pockets, but many continue to debate whether shallow sulci are an achievable goal of corrective treatment.[3] There is evidence that long-term pocket elimination therapy can be successful in patients with advanced periodontal disease who demonstrate optimal plaque control.[4–6] These studies establish the maintenance periodicity to be 3 to 6 months, very similar to the schedule followed by most private practices.

The clinical advantages of a plaque-free mouth have been further established by Rosling et al,[7] but the data are difficult to replicate in private practice, because in their subjects home care was augmented by a professional debridement every 2 weeks. Various treatment modalities have been shown to have equally poor results in the absence of plaque control.[8] The search for realistic treatment regimens that have been shown to halt future breakdown has made it clear that treatment provided during active therapy is the cornerstone of successful maintenance therapy (Figs 3-2a to 3-2e). Because the recall intervals will be dependent on the abilities of both the patient and the hygienist to debride the dentition, it is necessary to recognize the level of disease and consider appropriate treatment so that maintenance therapy can become a realistic possibility.

Once a periodontal patient, always a periodontal patient? Perhaps not, but there is little reason to suspect that it is possible to decrease patient susceptibility beyond making plaque control more accessible. How should the long-term success of periodontal treatment be evaluated? A review of the literature indicates that factors to consider include tooth loss, radiographic bone loss, loss of clinical attachment, interradicular loss of bone for multirooted teeth, mobility, and perhaps the periodicity of symptoms.[9–11] Other factors might include esthetics, phonetics, comfort, and a general feeling of well-being. As we consider our perception of this complicated issue, radiographic comparisons appear to offer a secure objective assessment. Ultimately, the outcome of periodontal treatment can be addressed by quantifying tooth loss.[10–12]

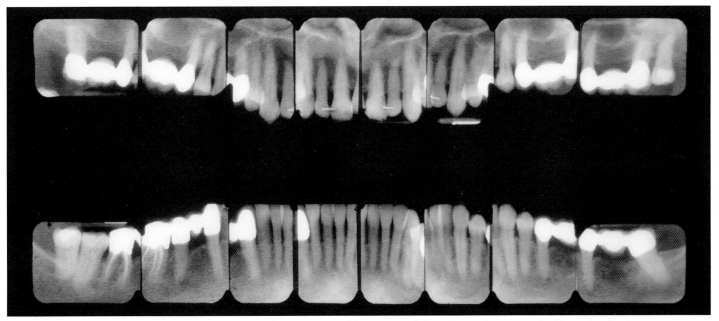

Fig 3-2b Full-mouth radiographic series, taken in 1994, showing successful treatment of the patient, who presented with postlocalized juvenile periodontitis. The maxillary anterior teeth were stabilized after completion of orthodontic therapy. There has been no further tooth loss since extractions during active therapy in 1970.

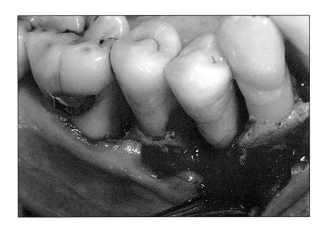

Fig 3-2c A mucoperiosteal flap has been reflected in the mandibular right quadrant to reveal the osseous lesions on the mesial surface of the first molar and both proximal surfaces of the first premolar. The lesion on the mesial surface of the first molar had been decorticated to promote regeneration. An autogenous bone graft was used.

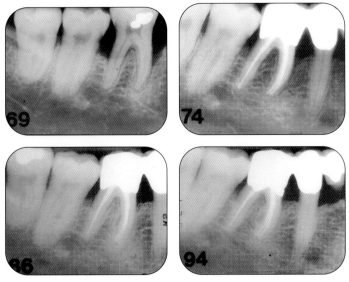

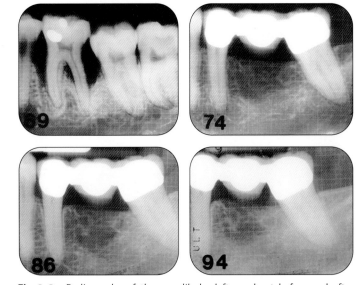

Fig 3-2d Periapical radiographs of the mandibular right quadrant reveal that successful treatment in 1970 has been maintained for more than 24 years. The first premolar was extracted because it had deep, uncontained proximal lesions and a clinical mobility of degree III.

'69	'74
'86	'94

Fig 3-2e Radiographs of the mandibular left quadrant before and after removal of the mandibular left first molar. There is obvious repair of the saddle area, along with protection of the osseous septa of the abutment teeth. The bone under the pontic has not been resorbed over time.

'69	'74
'86	'94

More advanced disease results in deeper pockets, intra-bony defects, furcation involvement, and mobile teeth and is frequently complicated by restorative needs (Figs 3-3a to 3-3e).[10,11] It requires a different therapeutic approach. How can the patient be expected to care for such problems, and what are the limitations of a maintenance visit? There are very few patients in any practice that fit into the plaque-free category, and thus it is necessary to consider the conscientious individuals who populate private practice maintenance programs.[7,13]

Periodontists are limited to controlling rather than curing the disease process. When there is improvement of the periodontal environment, plaque control can be readily accomplished at timely professional visits and by the patient during intervals between treatments.[14] Most patients are more compliant with a toothbrush than with any form of interdental debridement.[15] Therefore, most tooth-threatening periodontal problems are interdental, specifically the areas that are most difficult to cleanse. Angular osseous crests have been demonstrated to be a predictor of further loss of the periodontium.[16] The interproximal pocket greater than 5 mm allows three treatment approaches: maintenance, reduction by subtraction, and reduction by addition. The nonsurgical approach avoids the risk of phonetic and esthetic compromise in the maxillary anterior sextant, but it is less effective in areas that are more difficult for

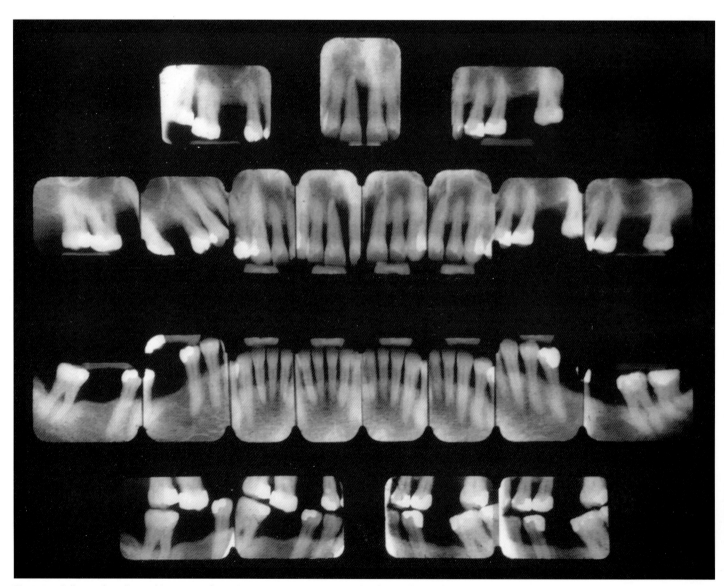

Fig 3-3a Full-mouth radiographic survey of a patient presenting in 1969 with advanced periodontal disease. Note the bone loss approaching the apex of the maxillary right central incisor.

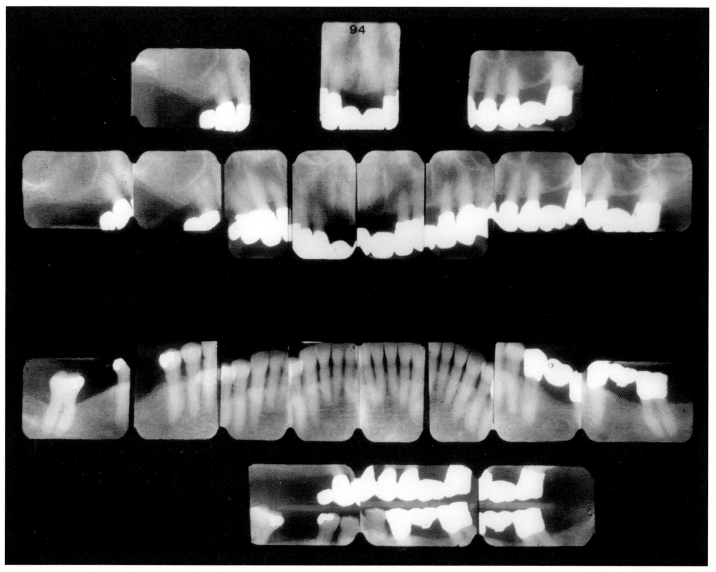

Fig 3-3b Radiographs taken in 1994 show that disease has not progressed after periodontal-prosthetic treatment. The maxillary right cantilever was used to resolve esthetic difficulties.

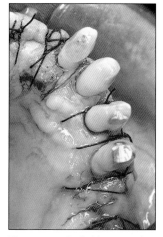

Fig 3-3c Definitive pocket elimination surgery is performed after provisionalization. The flap margins are placed at the osseous crest.

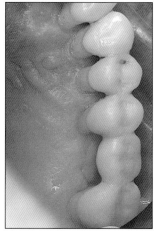

Fig 3-3d Healed surgical result prior to completion of the prosthesis.

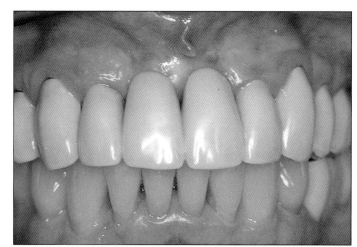

Fig 3-3e Final prosthesis in place.

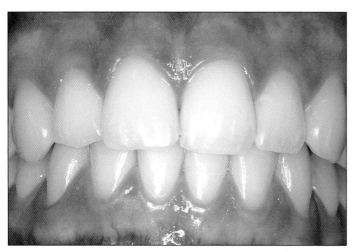

Fig 3-4 Normal-length teeth with interdental papillae intact. Probing depths are minimal, and there are no multirooted teeth with furcation problems. Professional debridement exercises will consume less time in this dentition than in the dentition in Figure 3-5.

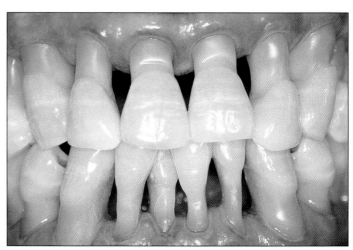

Fig 3-5 The anterior view of this dentition reveals elongated clinical crowns with old fixed restorations in place. It will take an experienced dental hygienist a full hour to fulfill the 3-month maintenance needs of this patient.

the patient and hygienist to debride.[17] There is common agreement as to the efficacy of nonsurgical treatment for the treatment of gingivitis and for some cases of mild periodontitis, because the disturbance of the periodontal environment is usually minimal.[18–21]

Components of SPT

Periodic comprehensive clinical periodontal and radiographic examinations are necessary to document attachment levels and crestal bone levels, which are the gold standard for longitudinal assessment of successful periodontal therapy. Full-mouth radiographic surveys made at respectable time intervals identify bone changes and are also necessary to screen for caries, pulpal pathosis, and other lesions. It is the responsibility of the periodontist monitoring patients in a recall system to identify carious lesions, faulty margins, and occlusal discrepancies.

Plaque control and oral hygiene evaluation should be completed at each supportive periodontal visit. No specific hygiene program appears to be superior, but repeated instruction at each visit is important for patients to maintain optimal oral home care.[22] The dentist and dental hygienist must clinically examine the periodontium before beginning instrumentation. It is important to explore all

surfaces of the teeth to determine where scaling and root planing are needed.

The exploratory stroke can be accomplished with a sharp curette (or an explorer) and is followed by a working stroke on those surfaces where tactile roughness is detected. Sites with calculus and minimal pocket depth should be scaled, whereas sites with significant pocket depth and calculus will require scaling and root planing. These deeper sites may require local anesthetic to facilitate patient comfort during root planing. Scaling and root planing are followed by tooth polishing with a rubber cup and pumice or with air abrasive. The length of time needed to accomplish these tasks varies with the length of exposed tooth structure, pocket depths, furcation involvement, and the proficiency of oral home care (Figs 3-4 and 3-5).

Factors Affecting the SPT Program

Periodontal maintenance (SPT) may be the critical factor when disease stabilization is evaluated over a significant time frame.[23,24] This message has been handed down from generation to generation of periodontists as gospel, but the problems associated with such a statement are far from resolved.[21,25] The variables that need to be addressed in a maintenance system in private practice include corrective

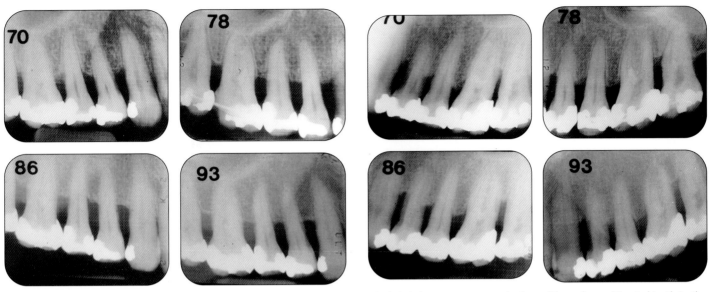

Fig 3-6a Resective therapy has been successfully maintained over a 23-year period. It is important to stop the loss of bone for multirooted teeth in the maxillary posterior quadrants before furcation involvement becomes a factor.

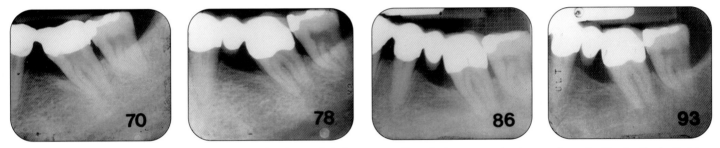

Fig 3-6b The mandibular left quadrant has been treated with periodontal surgery, and prosthetic treatment has been performed without orthodontic intervention. Pontic space has been created by tooth preparation. This improved access has facilitated oral home care by the patient.

therapeutic decisions, staff availability, patient behavior, the size of the treatment facility, and economic pressures (insurance benefits and the prevailing dental community). The periodicity and length of maintenance visits indicate that considerable effort is needed to effectively accomplish the goal of providing a valuable maintenance program for periodontal patients.

Physical Health Factors

The maintenance visit provides the practitioner the opportunity to obtain interim medical and dental histories. Patients may visit dentists and not physicians, so the dentist may identify pathoses such as hypertension, diabetes (through accurate history), dermatologic disorders in the head and neck region, and lesions intraorally (see Chapter 5). In addition, the dentist may provide information on smoking cessation, which can improve long-term outcomes for periodontal conditions.[26] The efficacy of procedures such as guided tissue regeneration are compromised by smoking and absence of plaque control.[27] Osseointegrated implants have also been shown to be less successful among smokers, and patients must be informed that smoking is a risk factor against successful treatment.[28]

Interradicular Bone Loss (Furcations)

In most cases of advanced disease, there is involvement of multirooted teeth with interradicular loss of bone (Figs 3-6a and 3-6b).[10] Both class II and class III furcations present difficult cleansing problems to the hygienist, the patient, and, specifically, the restorative dentist (Fig 3-7).[17] The technique of root resection has proven efficacious on long-term evaluation and reduces some of the most challenging areas to cleanse (Figs 3-8 and 3-9)(see Chapters 13 and 14).[29] Although the periodontal regenerative armamentarium has been expanded through contemporary developments, it only addresses a limited percentage of periodontal defects.[30–36] Recently, Pontoriero and Lindhe[37] reported that guided tissue regeneration therapy provided no gains in probing attachment and bone levels for interproximal maxillary class II or mandibular class III furcations. The gains of regenerative therapies have been demonstrated to be at risk if maintenance is inadequate.[27]

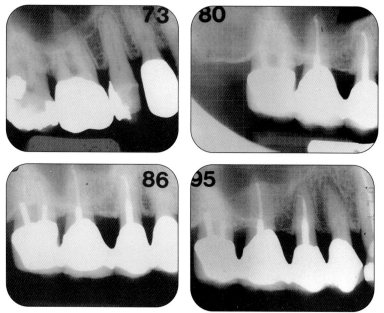

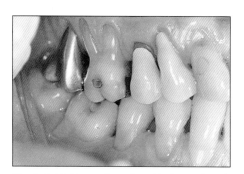

Fig 3-7 Multirooted teeth with long clinical crowns and furcation involvement. The patient and hygienist alike are challenged to maintain a plaque-free environment.

Fig 3-8 Advanced periodontal disease with maxillary furcation involvement has been successfully treated with resective therapy, including root amputation for the first molar. Definitive treatment of the furcation problem has resulted in periodontal stability over time.

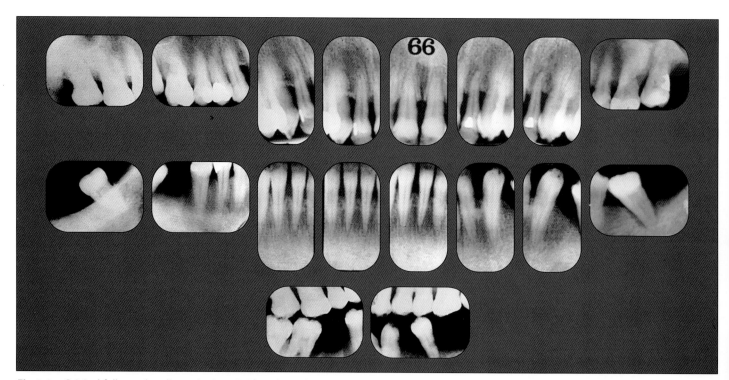

Fig 3-9a Original full-mouth radiographs (1966). There is moderate-to-severe bone loss, including a severe lesion on the mandibular right molar, which was treated with an autogenous bone graft in 1996.

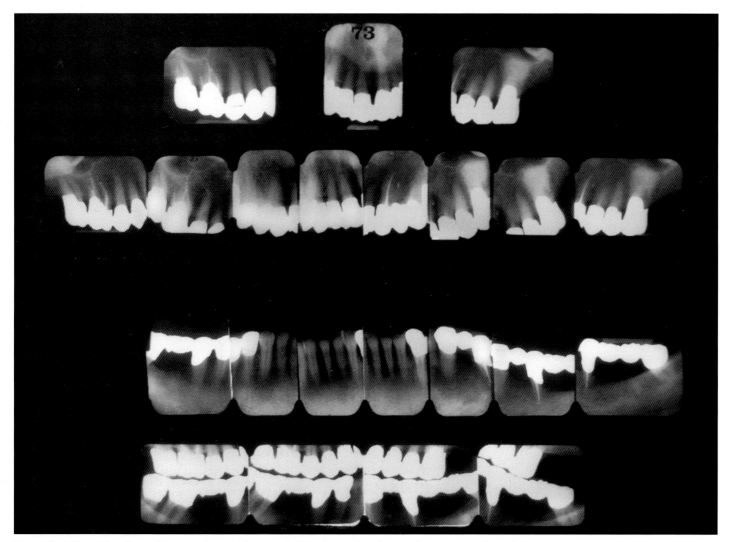

Fig 3-9b Full-mouth radiographic series (1973) after completion of periodontal surgical treatment and prosthetic restoration.

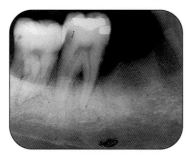

Fig 3-9c The molar has both an infrabony mesial defect and furcation involvement. This defect was treated with an autogenous bone graft.

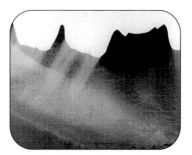

Fig 3-9d The defect has been successfully resolved, and the molar is able to serve as an abutment for the fixed partial denture.

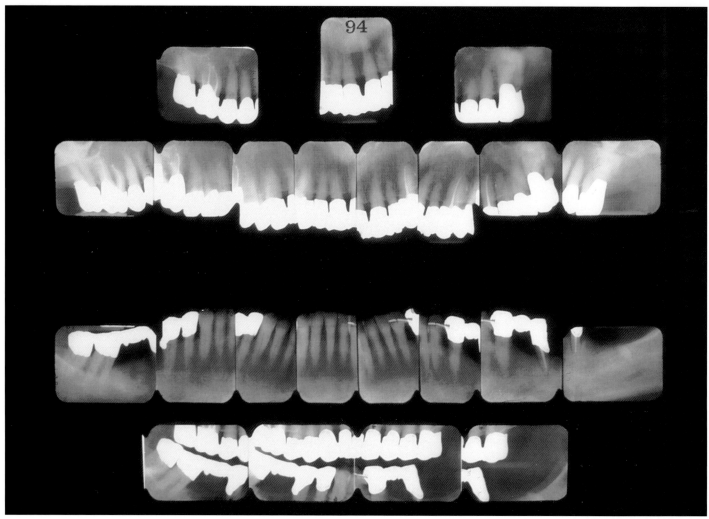

Fig 3-9e Full-mouth radiographs (1994). The bone graft has been maintained after 29 years. The original maxillary prosthesis is still in function. The mandibular left second molar has been lost.

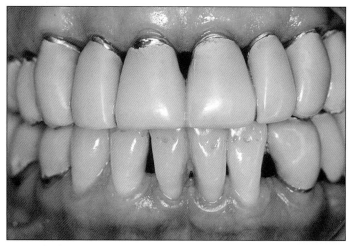

Fig 3-9f After 29 years, the original fixed prosthesis is in place. Although there has been some loss of acrylic resin, there is minimal recession at the gingival margin. This clinical photograph was taken prior to a maintenance visit. The exceptional oral home care of the patient is evident.

Refractory Disease

The periodontal disease of a very small percentage of the patient population in every practice is refractory; these patients will require more frequent visits and present recurrent problems, regardless of the treatment provided (Fig 3-10).[1-4] There is no specific bacterial profile or diagnostic method available to identify those patients who will not respond to traditional therapy.[38] In patients suspected to have refractory disease, a medical examination, including hematologic screening to determine adequate immune function, may be beneficial.[39] As these patients are identified, they will require specific maintenance regimens. Once again, the determining factor will be the ability to maintain a plaque-free environment, because the progressive destruction will not occur in the absence of microorganisms.[40]

A patient with refractory periodontitis who refuses repetitive surgical treatment and has areas with recurrent pocketing may require shorter maintenance intervals, often from 6 to 8 weeks. In addition, microbial testing and adjunctive antibiotic therapy might be indicated for the treatment of patients who demonstrate an enhanced suspectibility to

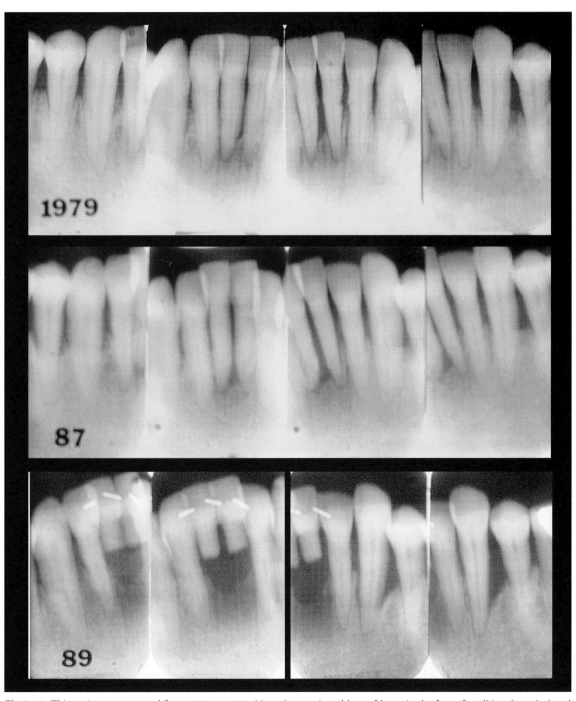

Fig 3-10 This patient was treated from 1979 to 1989. Note the continued loss of bone in the face of traditional surgical and nonsurgical periodontal treatment.

periodontal pathogens.[41] It is important to examine these patients frequently, both clinically and radiographically, to monitor attachment levels and crestal bone heights. It is also important to continually inform the patient of current diagnosis and prognosis at recall examinations to prepare the patient for future needs, which may include dental implants.

Availability of Auxiliary Personnel

The limited availability of auxiliary personnel to participate in debridement activities affects the availability of SPT. Debridement is usually performed by the dental hygienist or the dentist; the standard time for a maintenance visit is 1 hour. Teeth with long clinical crowns and exposed furcation areas and fixed restorative dentistry require a longer commitment of time to achieve the same result as less compromised problems. The 1-hour visit includes the time required to prepare the dental operatory to meet contemporary sterilization standards; to welcome the patient and examine the oral cavity; to check for caries; to chart periodontal problems; to enhance oral hygiene techniques; and to dismiss the patient and arrange the next visit[42]—and this is in addition to complete debridement of the dentition.

This process must be carried out for approximately eight patients each day. Even a utopian office setting requires patients to have a periodontium with few complications if these goals are to be met. Each time a pocket of greater than 5 mm or a furcation is encountered, the likelihood of controlling disease decreases because of the difficulty of completely removing debris from the root surface.[21,25,43,44] If the dentist offers these services without a hygienist, the role can quickly preclude corrective dentistry.

Laws in many geographic locations restrict the number of dental hygienists that can be employed in one office. Some countries have inadequate training facilities and others have no training facilities to produce hygienists. A small number do not allow hygienists to participate in patient treatment. Many countries have a dentist-to-patient ratio that excludes the possibility of definitive periodontal care.[45–47] All of the above circumstances mandate more definitive end points of active periodontal treatment, because recall visits with a reasonable periodicity are unlikely.

A full-time hygienist works five 8-hour days. This schedule, of course, differs in every office, but, for the sake of argument, approximately 1,900 hours per year are available for treatment by the hygienist. This means that only 500 patients can be seen by one hygienist in a periodontal recall practice with an average periodicity of 3 months. Even this availability suffers if the hygienist makes radiographs, spends time reinforcing the patients' method of debride-

ment, and participates in multiple-visit root planing as a part of initial preparation. Contrast this with the number of patients that accumulate over a 10-year time frame if a periodontist sees just 10 new patients a month, or 120 patients a year. Even the loss of some patients as a result of a change of location, death, or disenchantment with the service provided cannot solve the equation.[48]

As a practice matures, it becomes necessary to employ multiple hygienists, even if only to offer SPT to individuals with a seriously compromised periodontium. Concomitant to this development is the need to increase the administrative staff to arrange appointments and attend to billing and third-party considerations. It also requires a larger physical plant and results in a major commitment to proper patient maintenance.[48]

Patient Compliance

Historical data provided by the few studies that exist prepare clinicians for disappointment with compliance in the periodontal maintenance system.[49–52] Research has also established that surgically treated individuals on a maintenance program seriously outperform those who do not participate.[12] It is well established that some individuals will survive with the most sketchy maintenance and others will struggle with the best care, but it is not possible to identify accurately the problematic cases in advance with contemporary methods of diagnosis.[39,53,54]

All of this is further complicated by the behavioral characteristics encountered in the patient population. Most people are creatures of habit; a supreme effort must be expended to create new habits, but it requires relatively little to offset them. Financial or occupational instability, divorce proceedings, and coping with the errant behavior of children are common events. Any one of these factors is enough to challenge an individual's dedication to periodontal maintenance.

Outside Forces

Successful maintenance treatment is further threatened by the Solomonistic idea that patients should be shared by the periodontist and referring dentist.[22] Both situations offer inherent limitations because there are gaps in performance, different time frames are offered to the patient, and it is difficult to arrange appointments with patients. In truth, many patients relapse unnecessarily. Third parties (the insurance industry), with inadequate knowledge of disease control and a compelling interest only in finances, too frequently interfere unconscionably by suggesting to patients that an extended time frame between visits is acceptable.

Conclusion

The sum total of the variables that challenge an effective maintenance system support the argument for effective, definite periodontal treatment. The goals of therapy should bear in mind the burden of maintaining the result attained by treatment and the challenges that are commonplace in contemporary society. Although definitive treatment in itself is far from a panacea, it does make it easier for both the compliant patient and the health professional charged with accomplishing debridement at the professional level to help control the circumstances that lead to inflammatory periodontal diseases.

References

1. Wilson TG, Glover ME, Schown J, Baust C, Jacobs T. Compliance: a review of the literature with possible applications to periodontics. J Periodontol 1987;58:706–714.

2. Grbic JT, Lamster IB, Celenti RS, Fine JB. Risk indicators for future clinical attachment loss in adult periodontitis: Patient variables. J Periodontol 1991;62:322–329.

3. Kieser JB. Nonsurgical periodontal therapy. In: Lang NP, Karring T (eds). Proceedings of the 1st European Workshop on Periodontology. London: Quintessence, 1994:131–158.

4. Lindhe J, Nyman S. The effect of plaque control and surgical pocket elimination on the establishment and maintenance of periodontal health. A longitudinal study of periodontal therapy of advanced disease. J Clin Periodontol 1975;2:67–79.

5. Lindhe J, Westfelt E, Nyman S, Socransky SS, Haffajee AD. Long-term effect of surgical/nonsurgical treatment of periodontal disease. J Clin Periodontol 1984;11:448–458.

6. Olsen CT, Ammons WF, von Belle G. A longitudinal study comparing apically repositioned flaps with and without osseous surgery. Int J Periodont Rest Dent 1985;5(4):11–33.

7. Rosling B, Nyman S, Lindhe J, Jern B. The healing potential of the periodontal tissues following different techniques of periodontal surgery in plaque-free dentitions: a two-year clinical study. J Clin Periodontol 1976;3:233–250.

8. Nyman S, Lindhe J, Rosling B. Periodontal surgery in plaque-infected dentitions. J Clin Periodontol 1977;4:240–249.

9. Marshall-Day CD, Stephano RG, Quigley LF. Periodontal disease: prevalence and incidence. J Periodontol 1977;4:185–203.

10. Hirschfild L, Wasserman B. A long-term survey of tooth loss in 600 treated periodontal patients. J Periodontol 1978;49:225–237.

11. McFall WT. Tooth loss in 100 treated patients with periodontal disease: a long-term study. J Periodontol 1982;53:539–549.

12. Becker W, Becker B, Berg L. Periodontal treatment without maintenance: a retrospective study in 44 patients. J Periodontol 1984;55:505–509.

13. Kennedy JE, Bird W, Palcanis K, Dorfman H. A longitudinal evaluation of varying widths of attached gingiva. J Clin Periodontol 1985;12:667–675.

14. McFall WT. Supportive treatment. In: Nevins M, Becker W, Kornman K (eds). Proceedings of the World Workshop in Clinical Periodontics. Chicago: American Academy of Periodontology, 1989:IX-1–IX-28.

15. Ciancio SG. Non-surgical periodontal treatment. In: Nevins M, Becker W, Kornman K (eds). Proceedings of the World Workshop in Clinical Periodontics. Chicago: American Academy of Periodontology, 1989:II-1–II-20.

16. Papapanou PN, Wennström JL. The angular bony defect as indicator of further alveolar bone loss. J Clin Periodontol 1991;18:317–322.

17. Nordland P, Garrett S, Kiger R, Vanooteghem R, Hutchens LH, Egelberg J. The effect of plaque control and root debridement in molar teeth. J Clin Periodontol 1987;14:231–236.

18. Löe H, Theilade E, Jensen SB. Experimental gingivitis in man. J Periodontol 1965;36:177–187.

19. Ramfjord SP, Knowles JW, Nissle RR, Burgett F, Shick RA. Results following three modalities of periodontal therapy. J Periodontol 1975;46:522–526.

20. Listgarten MA, Slots J, Novotny A, et al. Incidence of periodontitis recurrence in treated patients with and without cultivable Actinobacillus actinomycetemcomitans, Prevotella intermedia, and Porphyromonas gingivalis: a prospective study. J Periodontol 1991;62:377–386.

21. Claffey N, Nyland K, Kiger R, Garrett S, Egelberg J. Diagnostic predictability of scores of plaque, bleeding, suppuration and probing depth for probing attachment loss. J Clin Periodontol 1990;17:108–114.

22. Axilsson P, Lindhe J. Effect of controlled oral hygiene procedures on caries and periodontal disease in adults: results after six years. J Clin Periodontol 1981;8:239–248.

23. Axelsson P, Lindhe J. The significance of maintenance care in the treatment of periodontal disease. J Clin Periodontol 1981;8:281–294.

24. Wilson TG. Supportive periodontal treatment for patients with inflammatory periodontal diseases. In: Wilson TG, Kornman KS, Newman MG (eds). Advances in Periodontics. Chicago: Quintessence, 1992:195–203.

25. Baderstein A, Nilveus R, Egelberg J. Scores of plaque, bleeding suppuration and probing depth to predict probing attachment loss. J Clin Periodontol 1990;17:102–107.

26. Ah MKB, Johnson GK, Kaldahl WB, Patil KD, Kalkwarf KL. The effect of smoking on the response to periodontal treatment. J Clin Periodontol 1994;21:91–97.

27. Cortellini P, Pini Prato G, Tonetti M. Periodontal regeneration of human infrabony defects. V. Effect of oral hygiene on long-term stability. J Clin Periodontol 1994;21:606–610.

28. Bain C, Moy P. The association between the failure of dental implants and cigarette smoking. Int J Oral Maxillofac Implants 1993;8:609–615.

29. Carnevale G, DiFebo G, Tonelli MP, Marin C, Fuzzi M. A retrospective analysis of the periodontal-prosthetic treatment of molars with interradicular lesions. Int J Periodont Rest Dent 1991;11:189–205.

30. Nyman S, Lindhe J, Karring T, Rylander H. New attachment following surgical treatment of human periodontal disease. J Clin Periodontol 1982;9:290–296.

31. Gottlow J, Nyman S, Lindhe J, Karring T, Wennström J. New attachment formation in the human periodontium by guided tissue regeneration: case reports. J Clin Periodontol 1986;9:290–296.

32. Schallhorn R, McLain P. Combined osseous composite grafting, root conditioning and guided tissue regeneration. Int J Periodont Rest Dent 1988;8:9–32.

33. Bowers GM, Chadroff B, Carnevale R, et al. Histologic evaluation of new attachment apparatus formation in humans. Part III. J Periodontol 1989;60:683–693.

34. McLain PK, Schallhorn RG. Long-term assessment of combined osseous composite grafting: root conditioning and guided tissue regeneration. Int J Periodont Rest Dent 1993;13:9–28.

35. Cortellini P, Bowers GM. Periodontal regeneration of intrabony defects. Int J Periodont Rest Dent 1995;15(2):128–145.

36. Machtei EE, Schallhorn RG. Successful regeneration of mandibular class II furcation defects. Int J Periodont Rest Dent 1995;15:146–167.

37. Pontoriero R, Lindhe J. Guided tissue regeneration in the treatment of degree II furcations in maxillary molars. J Clin Periodontol 1995;22: 756–763.

38. Attstrom R, van der Velden U. Consensus report of session I. In: Lang NP, Karring T (eds). Proceedings of the 1st European Workshop on Periodontology. London: Quintessence, 1994:120–126.

39. Adams DF. Diagnosis and treatment of refractory periodontitis. Curr Opin Dent Curr Sci 1992;2:33–38.

40. Socransky SS, Haffajee AD. Evidence of bacterial etiology: a historical perspective. Periodontology 2000 1994;5:7–25.

41. Rams TE, Slots J. Antibiotics in periodontal therapy: an update. Compend Contin Educ Dent 1992;12:1130–1145.

42. Schallhorn R, Snider LE. Periodontal maintenance therapy. J Am Dent Assoc 1981;103:227.

43. Waerhaug J. Healing of the dento-epithelial junction following subgingival plaque control II: As observed on extracted teeth. J Am Dent Assoc 1978;49:9–29.

44. Stambaugh RV, Dragoo M, Smith D, Carasali L. The limits of subgingival scaling. Int J Periodont Rest Dent 1981;1:31–41.

45. Baskar PK. Current status of periodontal treatment in India. J NZ Soc Periodontol Asian Pacific Suppl 1994;1:18–19.

46. Cao C. The present status of periodontal treatment in China. J NZ Soc Periodontol Asian Pacific Suppl 1994;1:9–10.

47. Vongsurasit T. The current status of periodontal treatment in Thailand. J NZ Soc Periodontol Asian Pacific Suppl 1994;1:11–12.

48. Nevins M. Long-term maintenance in private practice. J Clin Periodontol 1996;23:273–277.

49. Wilson TG, Glover ME, Schoen J, Baust C, Jacobs T. Compliance with maintenance therapy in a private periodontal practice. J Periodontol 1984;55:468–473.

50. Mendoza AR, Newcomb GM, Nixon KC. Compliance with supportive periodontal therapy. J Periodontol 1991;62:731–736.

51. Checchi L, Pellicioni GA, Galto MRA, Kelescian L. Patient compliance with maintenance therapy in an Italian periodontal practice. J Clin Periodontol 1994;21:309–312.

52. Demetriou N, Tsami-Pandi A, Parashis A. Compliance with supportive periodontal treatment in private periodontal practice: a 4-year retrospective study. J Periodontol 1995;66:145–149.

53. Greenstein G. Advances in periodontal disease diagnosis. Int J Periodont Rest Dent 1990;10:351–375.

54. Wilton JMA, Johnson NW, Curtis MA, et al. Specific antibody responses to subgingival plaque bacteria as aids to the diagnosis and prognosis of destructive periodontitis. J Clin Periodontol 1991;18:1–15.

Diagnosing Destructive Periodontal Diseases

Gary S. Greenstein, DDS, MS
Michael P. Rethman, DDS, MS

During the last decade, clinical trials provided data that dictated that established dogma regarding the etiology and pathogenesis of periodontal diseases be modified. Historically, it was believed that tissue inflammation, once it was initiated by bacteria, would slowly and continuously increase in severity if left untreated.[1] Therefore, it seemed logical to conclude that detection of putative periodontal pathogens or clinical signs of disease indicated that definitive periodontal therapy was needed. However, longitudinal studies have demonstrated that these premises were often misleading.

Currently, the following concepts are considered valid:

1. Gingivitis frequently does not proceed to periodontitis.[2]
2. Disease progression may be episodic or continuous.[3,4]
3. The rate of deterioration may be fast or slow.[5]
4. Patients with periodontitis harbor both active and nonactive pockets.[6]
5. Only a small percentage of pockets in a patient with periodontitis will typically demonstrate loss of clinical attachment within 1 or 2 years.[7–10]
6. Detection of putative pathogens may[11,12] or may not be associated with future disease progression.[13–15]

The realization that sites with inflamed bleeding pockets do not necessarily reflect current or future disease progression underscored the need for reinterpretation of clinical parameters and spurred development of additional diagnostic tests. Consequently, these advances raised questions as to why, when, and where additional testing is needed beyond appraisal of clinical signs of disease. This chapter provides an overview of available diagnostic methods. Furthermore, it addresses principles of diagnostic testing and the therapeutic implications of utilizing an information base that fluctuates as the threshold for progressive periodontitis is changed.

Defining Periodontal Disease

Link Between Etiology and Clinical Signs of Disease

Periodontitis (adult, juvenile, refractory, etc) causes destruction of the specialized tissues that provide support for the dentition. These diseases should be considered infections of the periodontium, because there are bacterial etiologies and immune responses.[12] However, individuals who are colonized by putative pathogens are not necessarily infected or diseased. Therefore, it is important to differentiate among these terms:[16]

1. *Colonization* refers to the multiplication of microbes without a tissue or immune response.
2. The term *infection* connotes that colonization has occurred and has been accompanied by an immune response (cellular or humoral).
3. The term *disease* indicates that an infection has caused detectable, but not necessarily irreversible, damage to the host.[16] Disease is a rare consequence of infection; however, infection is often a necessary basis for disease.

More than 500 bacterial species have been detected in the oral cavity; however, only 10 to 20 are frequently associated with the presence of disease.[17] The precise interactions among bacteria and with the host that permit commensal organisms to be pathogenic or allow exogenous bacteria to colonize are not fully understood. Similarly, there are no data regarding the size of an inoculum needed to initiate disease.[18] Ultimately, complex interactions in an ecological niche or habitat determine if an organism will induce disease. In other words, modification of the microenvironment must occur and the host must be unable to adequately respond to the bacterial challenge at a particular time and site before potentially pathogenic organisms can cause harm.[16,18]

With regard to the origins of putative pathogens, there are conflicting opinions as to whether certain bacteria are exogenous (foreign) or endogenous (normal) inhabitants of the oral cavity. Organisms such as *Porphyromonas gingivalis* and *Actinobacillus actinomycetemcomitans* (*Aa*) are considered exogenous by some investigators for the following reasons:[19]

1. Their detection is frequently associated with the presence of disease.
2. They are not cultured from the majority of healthy subjects.
3. These organisms are often associated with a large antibody response that is atypical for endogenous organisms.
4. They can usually be eliminated from the oral cavity.

In contrast, several lines of evidence suggest that *P gingivalis* and *Aa* may be endogenous and participate in opportunistic infections:

1. Many individuals are colonized by these organisms without manifesting signs of periodontal disease.[14,18,20-26]
2. Some periodontally healthy patients may have low levels of antibodies reactive with *P gingivalis* and *Aa*.[27]
3. There is evidence to indicate that these putative pathogens are genetically heterogeneous and consist of many clonal types, a finding consistent with endogenous organisms.[18,28-31]

In general, the data support the concept that periodontal diseases are opportunistic infections. However, it is unresolved whether all pathogens are endogenous or if some, such as *Aa*, are exogenous. Regardless of their origin, for disease to occur it appears that the mere presence of pathogens is not as critical as the host response. Therefore, it can be concluded that periodontal supportive therapy and good oral hygiene habits are important to ensure that subgingival putative pathogens remain below a certain pathogenic threshold.

Types of Periodontal Disease

There are different types of periodontal diseases. *Gingivitis* is the most prevalent and is characterized by redness, bleeding on probing, and an inflammatory infiltrate in the connective tissue. Traditionally, it was believed that untreated gingivitis eventually converted to periodontitis. This dogma has been refuted, and it is now recognized that gingivitis infrequently proceeds to progressive periodontitis.[2] However, gingivitis usually precedes, and is often associated with, progressive periodontitis. Therefore, if *periodontitis* is thought of as an apically progressing inflammatory lesion of the connective tissue, immediately adjacent to teeth or implants, then it is reasonable to conclude that elimination of all signs of inflammation should remain a primary objective of periodontal therapy.

There are different types of progressive periodontitis, all of which are characterized by loss of connective tissue and alveolar bone:[32]

1. *Adult periodontitis* is the most prevalent form and usually affects individuals older than 35 years of age.
2. *Early-onset periodontitis* is found in three forms:
   a. *Prepubertal* (localized and generalized) affects the primary dentition.
   b. *Juvenile* (localized and generalized) occurs around puberty.
   c. *Rapidly progressive* usually occurs in patients 20 to 30 years old.
3. *Periodontitis associated with systemic diseases.*
4. *Necrotizing ulcerative periodontitis.*
5. *Refractory periodontitis* is associated with patients who do not respond to conventional therapy.

Although periodontal diseases are infections, the type of periodontitis cannot be differentiated by microbiologic or immunologic techniques. In general, characterization of different types of periodontitis is based on the age of onset, clinical and radiographic findings, underlying health, and the response to therapy. Furthermore, because their etiologies remain poorly understood, it may be difficult to refer to a specific type of periodontitis.

Periodontitis as a Syndrome

Periodontal diseases have been referred to as a "periodontal destructive syndrome."[33] The term *syndrome* is used to label a pattern of morbid signs and symptoms whose etiologies are not fully understood.[33] This concept was supported by research by Moore et al.[6] They microbiologically monitored 20 patients who lost 2 mm of clinical attachment and found distinct differences in the microflora at healthy and diseased sites. However, they detected no differences in the percent or type of bacteria at active and inactive sites. This finding underscored that the triggering mechanisms that upset the host-parasite balance remain unknown.

In general, the term *periodontal destructive syndrome* appears to be a more accurate label for periodontal afflictions than *periodontitis* or *periodontal disease(s)* for the following reasons:

1. The terms *periodontitis* and *periodontal disease(s)* can be misleading, because they imply that the multifactorial etiologies of this syndrome are understood and that predictable periodontal therapies have been defined.

2. The label *syndrome* can be used more clearly to refer to different sites within a dentition, where disease progression may occur as a result of a variety of microbes.

3. The term *syndrome* can be used more clearly to denote that periodontal afflictions are a series of infections that occur at different rates and irregular time intervals.

Therefore, *periodontal disease syndrome* may be a better term to collectively describe different types of periodontitis, because it underscores that many issues associated with the etiology, pathogenesis, and therapy of periodontal disease(s) remain unclear.

Effect of Gold Standards on the Information Base

Rationale for Selecting a Gold Standard[34]

Absolute proof that periodontal disease progression occurred is provided by histologic assessment of connective tissue attachment or alveolar bone loss. However, it is impractical to collect biopsy material at sequential time points. Therefore, surrogate parameters have to be used. Currently, to assess progressive periodontitis, only loss of alveolar bone and clinical attachment can be objectively measured.[35] Thus, in the context of periodontal diagnosis, the term *gold standard* is sometimes used to refer to clinical or radiographic measures of disease progression (loss of probing attachment or alveolar bone).[35] The former is usually employed in longitudinal clinical trials to avoid the biohazards associated with radiographs.[5]

To compensate for errors associated with probing, different amounts of probing attachment loss (eg, 0.4, 1, 2, or 3 mm) have been used as thresholds for progressive periodontitis.[5] Problems inherent in manual periodontal probing can be reduced by using stents and electronic pressure-sensitive probes. However, the variable most confounding to probing measurements during a clinical evaluation is gingival status. The extent of the gingival inflammatory infiltrate can affect probing measurements. When the tissue is heavily infiltrated, the probe may penetrate through the junctional epithelium and up to 1 mm into connective tissue even though there is no histologic loss of connective tissue attachment.[36] Therefore, it is not possible to precisely define an absolute amount of probing attachment loss that can be used as a universal measure for disease progression.

Actually, measurement conditions in individual offices and longitudinal trials will determine the amount of attachment loss that must occur for a site to be declared actively deteriorating. Factors that affect selection of disease thresholds include the probing force, the type of probe used, and the standard deviation of replicated probing assessments.

Thus, there is no established gold standard for clinical assessment of progressive periodontitis. Rather, certain defined rules are used to establish thresholds that represent reasonably unbiased assessments of disease activity.[35,37]

Prevalence of Periodontal Diseases

Table 4-1 lists investigations that have addressed the prevalence of adult periodontitis.[38–41] However, there is variation in the results because these studies used a variety of populations and standards to detect the presence of disease.[38–41]

Table 4-1 Prevalence of periodontitis*

Study	Location	n[†]	Prevalence[‡]	Criterion[§]
Brown et al[38]	USA (workers)	15,132	12.8%	CAL: 5 mm
Horning et al[39]	USA (military)	1,984	14.2%	PD: 5 to 7 mm
Miyazki et al[40]	50 countries	—	5–20%	PD: 6 mm
Pilot and Miyazki[41]	Europe	38,274	5–15%	PD: 6 mm; CAL: 4 mm

 * From Greenstein.[37] Reprinted with permission.
 † Number of patients evaluated.
 ‡ Percentage of patients with periodontitis.
 § Criterion for disease detection at one site or more per patient: CAL = clinical attachment loss; PD = probing depth.

For instance, in the study by Brown et al,[38] when a 5-mm loss of clinical attachment was used as the standard, 12.8% of assessed individuals were found to have lost clinical attachment at one or more sites. However, if a 3-mm threshold (25% of a length of a root) was employed, then 44% of the population was considered affected.[38]

Other factors that may contribute to underestimation of disease prevalence are the use of survey teeth and measurements performed at line angles instead of interproximally.[42–44] Overall, the data, which indicated 5% to 20% of the assessed individuals manifest periodontitis, probably underestimated the prevalence of periodontitis in the general population.

Incidence of Disease Progression

Table 4-2 includes studies that have addressed the incidence of disease progression in patients with untreated periodontitis.[4,7–10] The results of these investigations indicated the following:

1. The incidence of breakdown is limited, infrequent, and may be episodic.
2. About 40% to 90% (a mean of 58%) of individuals with periodontitis manifest disease progression in at least one site within 6 to 24 months.
3. From 0.99% to 29% of the sites will deteriorate. However, when a high criterion (2.5 mm) was used to define progression, disease detection was low (0.99%).[7] Contrastingly, if a low threshold (0.4 mm) was used, then disease incidence was high (29%).[24] Obviously, threshold selection affects data interpretation. If the high and low figures are eliminated, it appears that 5% to 10% of the infected sites demonstrate disease progression.

4. Around 20% of all patients exhibit 60% of all sites that deteriorate.

It can be concluded that a small percentage of individuals are at great risk and manifest the majority of sites that deteriorate. Accordingly, identification of these individuals has become a focus of research.

Patterns of Disease Progression

Socransky et al[1] described several models of disease progression that may occur in different patients or sites within the same patient: the continuous, random burst, and asynchronous multiple burst theories. Most traditional periodontal therapy is based on the continuous theory, which assumes disease progression is slow, continuous, and progressive. However, there are problems with this concept. For example, epidemiologic studies do not assess the rate at which lesions progress, and they cannot differentiate between new sites that are developing and old sites that are becoming worse. Therefore, this type of investigation cannot be used to clarify patterns of disease progression. Furthermore, sometimes clinical attachment loss is too fast or too slow to conform with this model. A large number of lesions also do not seem to change at all, and sometimes disease progression is brought under control.

To compensate for shortcomings of the continuous model, Goodson et al[3] proposed the random burst hypothesis, which theorizes that there are sudden bursts of disease activity followed by periods of remission and even repair. However, it was not proposed that disease activity was random with respect to location or cause. Therefore, Zimmerman[45] suggested that this model be called the *episodic burst theory*. Furthermore, Zimmerman[45] proposed

Table 4-2 Disease progression in patients with periodontitis*

| Study | n[†] | No. of sites[‡] | T[§] | Criterion[‖] | Deterioration (%) | |
					Patients[¶]	Sites[#]
Grbic et al[7]	75	11,466	6 mo	2.5 mm	41.3	0.99
Deas et al[8]	21	2,094	9 mo	2 mm	90.0	6.1
Persson and Page[9]	25	200	24 mo	2 mm	40.0	10.7
Halazonetis et al[10]	55	24,720	5–12 mo	1.75 mm	42.0	5.0
Jeffcoat and Reddy[4]	30	—	6 mo	0.4 mm	77.0	29.0

* From Greenstein.[37] Reprinted with permission.
† Number of patients monitored.
‡ Number of sites monitored.
§ Evaluation period (in months).
‖ Disease activity threshold.
¶ Percentage of patients deteriorating in at least one site.
# Percentage of sites deteriorating.

that the asynchronous multiple burst model, which refers to breakdown occurring during specific periods (eg, puberty), be called the *synchronous burst hypothesis.*

The lack of clarity with regard to which models of disease progression usually occur was recently underscored by Jeffcoat and Reddy.[4] They monitored adult periodontitis for 6 months and assessed the prevalence of clinical attachment loss using various thresholds (0.4 to 2.4 mm). When a 0.4-mm threshold was employed, 76% of the sites broke down in a linear fashion and only 12% deteriorated in bursts of disease activity. The finding that a linear pattern of disease progression was more common when a small threshold was employed corroborates the contention that, when high thresholds are used, the more subtle changes are not detected.

It is apparent that standards used to assess disease progression can affect the interpretation of disease progression patterns. In general, periodontal diseases can be thought of as a series of infections whose patterns of progression may vary depending on the host response. Therefore, it is not possible to predict the pattern of disease progression at any particular site.

Understanding Diagnostic Testing

Decision Matrices

Many diagnostic tests are being developed to detect or predict disease progression. To determine the capabilities of each test, a clinical threshold must be selected that denotes the presence of disease. In Table 4-3, disease is considered present when there is 2 mm or more loss of clinical attachment;

disease is not present if the loss is less than 2 mm. Thresholds are also used for diagnostic tests undergoing evaluation so that a positive or negative result can be reported.

A comparison of the positive or negative test results with the presence or absence of progressive periodontitis will generate four outcomes, seen in the decision matrix (see Table 4-3): true positive, false positive, false negative, and true negative.[46,47] These data can then be used to calculate characteristics of diagnostic tests: diagnostic specificity, sensitivity, and positive and negative predictive values.

Sensitivity, Specificity, and Predictive Values

Sensitivity refers to the percentage of times a test is positive when (in the case of periodontal diseases) progressive periodontitis is present. *Specificity* indicates the percentage of times a test is negative when progressive periodontitis is absent. These values are calculated in subpopulations in which researchers already know if patients are diseased or healthy. Therefore, sensitivity and specificity values are of little help to clinicians who are assessing patients. Clinicians may find this information helpful when selecting a test, but it will not provide information with regard to diagnostic accuracy in a clinical situation where there is a mixed population (healthy and diseased individuals).

To know how often a test will forecast a correct diagnosis in a mixed population, therapists need to be apprised of the positive and negative predictive values for a test. A positive predictive value indicates the percentage of time a positive test correctly predicts progressive periodontitis, and a negative predictive value indicates how often a negative test confirms health (see Table 4-3).

Unfortunately, predictive values are affected by the prevalence of disease in a population. Therefore, in a typical general practice, the negative (ie, healthy) predictive

Table 4-3 Decision matrix*

Diagnostic test	Disease present (CAL > 2 mm)	Disease absent (CAL < 2 mm)
Positive	a True positive	b False positive
Negative	c False negative	d True negative

*From Greenstein.[37] Reprinted with permission.

Sensitivity = a/a + c.
Specificity = d/b + d.
Positive predictive value = a/a + b.
Negative predictive value = d/c + d.
CAL = clinical attachment loss.

value of a diagnostic test would be higher than in a periodontal practice, because the general practice has fewer patients at risk. Conversely, this means that in a typical periodontal practice, a positive test result is more likely to be accurate than in a general practice. These phenomena suggest that diagnostic test thresholds that are set should be based on the type of dental practice environment. An example of how prevalence affects positive predictive values is illustrated in a later section that discusses aspartate aminotransferase (see p. 70).

Effect of Disease Thresholds on Diagnostic Test Characteristics

Selection of disease thresholds that impact sensitivity, specificity, and positive and negative predictive values are determined by several factors.[34] If it is decided that the test should be very sensitive, so that all individuals with disease or disease progression are detected, then a low cutoff point is chosen. This will provide high sensitivity and high positive predictive values, but it will be associated with an increased occurrence of false-positive results (low specificity and low negative predictive values). This may be desirable when screening for a serious or life-threatening disease, because disease detection is critical and confirmation can be attained by subsequent tests.

Contrastingly, confirmation testing requires strict or high thresholds to limit the number of false-positive results. The test is now more specific (high specificity and high negative predictive values), but less sensitive. This type of testing is needed to ensure that expensive or risky therapy is not mistakenly undertaken.

Thus, thresholds for diagnostic tests in clinical practice are dictated by several factors. These include the mortality and morbidity of the disease process, the time necessary to perform the test, the monetary cost, and the consequences of overtreatment and/or undertreatment.

Risk Assessment

It is no longer appropriate to consider all people at equivalent risk of developing different types of periodontitis.[48–53] Therefore, many investigators are trying to clarify which risk markers are associated with increased risk of developing periodontal diseases. In general, risk markers can be classified as risk indicators or risk factors. *Risk indicators* are variables that are not necessarily etiologic for periodontitis (eg, pockets), whereas *risk factors* are thought to be causal (eg, bacteria).[49]

Over the years, numerous risk markers have been proposed for periodontal diseases. Currently, there is substantial evidence to indicate that the following factors predispose individuals to the development of periodontitis: smoking,[52] diabetes,[50] neutrophil defects,[51] and elevated levels of some subgingival microbes.[49] These risk markers and others are undergoing intensive research. Nevertheless, periodontal diseases have multiple risk factors. Therefore, it should not be expected that one risk factor will consistently be associated with the development of disease, and it should not be expected that elimination of one risk factor will completely eliminate the risk of developing disease.[48]

Risk factors are addressed either prospectively or retrospectively, and the direction of these assessments will determine the type of calculations needed.[53] In prospective studies (eg, controlled clinical trials), risk factors are identified prior to the development of disease. In these studies, relative risk, which is a ratio of the risk of developing disease in individuals exposed to a risk factor to the risk in the unexposed group, is frequently reported to characterize the strength of an association between a risk factor and disease development. In contrast, odds ratios are frequently used in retrospective studies to provide information concerning risk of developing disease, because the incidence rate is not available.[53]

Generally, the following scheme provides a guideline for interpreting the strength of odds ratios and relative risk: 1 = no association; 2 = likelihood of an association, 3 = strong association; and 4 = very strong association.[49]

Interpretation of Traditional Clinical Parameters and New Technologies for Diagnostic Assessments

Physical Alterations

Probing Depths

Clinical probing depth measurements are an integral part of a periodontal examination. However, 1-mm fluctuations are within acceptable probing discrepancy (eg, the standard deviation for replicate probing assessments is 0.82 mm).[54] Therefore, clinicians utilizing manual probing should seek out alterations of 2 mm or greater in probing depths or clinical attachment levels. A change of 2 mm can be interpreted to indicate that clinical attachment loss occurred with a relatively high degree of confidence.[55–57] If an electronic pressure-sensitive probe that provides greater precision (ability to measure accurately) and reproducibility of measurements is used, a smaller threshold can be employed. Nevertheless, results must be interpreted cautiously when low thresholds (eg, 0.4 mm) are employed because probe penetration can vary depending on tissue inflammation.

A single probing depth measurement can delineate locations that are difficult to maintain and can identify sites with advanced attachment loss, but at any specific time does not

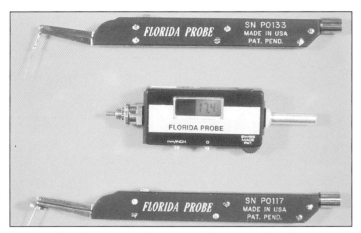

Fig 4-1a The Florida Probe (Florida Probe Co, Gainesville, FL) is an accurate pressure-sensitive device used to measure probing depth. Two models are available; *(top)* the regular probe and *(bottom)* the disc probe. (From Greenstein.[37] Reprinted with permission.)

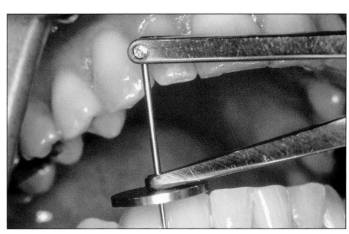

Fig 4-1b The disc probe facilitates recording of relative clinical attachment levels. It uses the occlusal surface as a fixed reference point to the base of the pocket. (From Greenstein.[37] Reprinted with permission.)

reflect progressive periodontitis. For example, the presence of moderate probing depths (4 to 6 mm) is a poor predictor of disease progression.[55,56,58] Deep probing depths also do not necessarily predict imminent deterioration; however, 21% to 44% of sites greater than or equal to 7 mm, when monitored for 1.5-mm changes for more than 2 years, experienced progressive periodontitis.[55,56,58] Furthermore, when these areas were monitored for 3.5 and 5 years the percentage of deteriorating sites increased to 50%.[59,60] It can be concluded that deep probing depths and advanced clinical attachment loss are risk indicators that merit careful monitoring.

Recession or coronal migration of the gingiva can interfere with the ability of replicate probing assessments to detect progressive periodontitis. To avoid these confounding occurrences, measurements of clinical attachment level can be recorded. However, this task is laborious, requires patience, and can take 10 minutes per quadrant. Therefore, these data are infrequently scored during routine patient management. Furthermore, it can be contended that recession and coronal gingival migration are not routinely associated with progressive periodontitis.[61–63] Nevertheless, it would be beneficial to measure clinical attachment levels at problematic sites to ensure objective monitoring. In general, clinicians must appraise the pros and cons of each recording technique depending on the status and dental history of individual sites and patients.

Pressure-sensitive probes increase the precision and reproducibility of probing measurements[64] (Figs 4-1a and 4-1b). Clinicians desiring these benefits can utilize automated devices, which also can provide electronic data storage.[64] However, these devices require more time to use, are costly, and can be uncomfortable, and the use of small thresholds to detect disease progression may increase false-positive findings. Furthermore, despite greater precision,

the reproducibility of the data is not necessarily better unless multiple probing assessments are performed.[65] Therefore, use of pressure-sensitive probes during routine patient management provides advantages and disadvantages. Although their use is not essential, individual clinicians will need to decide if these devices provide more accurate measurements and allow better record keeping in their practice settings.

Bleeding After Probing

Bleeding after probing is indicative of an inflammatory lesion in the connective tissue subjacent to the junctional epithelium.[66] In areas inaccessible to visual inspection (eg, the base of pockets), the presence or absence of bleeding provides an objective diagnostic sign that can be easily monitored and used to evaluate periodontal status. Bleeding assessments can be standardized by using a pressure-sensitive probe; however, forces greater than 25 g may induce bleeding at healthy sites.[67]

Bleeding after probing cannot be used to differentiate among gingivitis, stable periodontitis, and progressive periodontitis lesions.[53,56,59,60] In general, bleeding assessments are poor predictors of future disease progression. However, investigators indicated that 47% of the 7-mm probing depths that bled[55] and 30% of sites that consistently bled on probing[68] experienced clinical attachment loss during a 2-year observation period.[55]

Gingival tissues that bleed or do not bleed exhibit specific histologic differences. Furthermore, although bleeding may not be a good positive predictor of clinical attachment loss, its absence is an excellent negative predictor of future attachment loss.[69] Therefore, absence of bleeding on probing is desirable and suggests low risk of further breakdown.

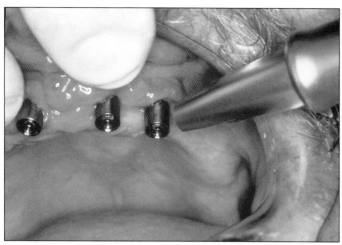

Fig 4-2a The Periotest (Bioresearch, Milwaukee, WI) can be used to precisely assess tooth mobility or the firmness of implants. (From Greenstein.[37] Reprinted with permission.)

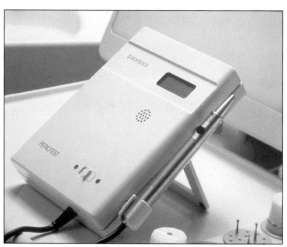

Fig 4-2b Periotest data are recorded visibly and audibly by the instrument console, which is located on the bracket table. (From Greenstein.[37] Reprinted with permission.)

Hypermobility

Tooth mobility can result from usual masticatory stress on a healthy, but reduced, periodontium (previously diseased) or from excessive forces placed on an anatomically uncompromised periodontium (normal and healthy). The degree of mobility will depend on the direction and magnitude of displacing forces acting on the dentition. This response will be modified by periodontal status (normal versus reduced or inflamed versus noninflamed).[70]

The relationship between disease progression and hypermobility in humans has not been clarified.[71] Occlusal trauma induced in squirrel monkeys with periodontitis did not accelerate attachment loss but did result in some irreversible interproximal bone loss. In contrast, occlusal trauma in beagle dogs exacerbated attachment loss.[70] Regardless of which concept is correct, current information dictates that eradication of inflammation is critical and reduction of tooth mobility is secondary.[72] However, posttreatment clinical results have been better in patients in whom occlusal adjustment was performed prior to periodontal therapy than in unadjusted controls.[73]

After therapy, teeth with reduced periodontia may demonstrate increased but stable mobility patterns. This reflects accommodation to occlusal forces. Loose teeth are not more susceptible to plaque-induced infections, do not precipitate a shift of gingivitis to periodontitis, and often do not need to be splinted.[71,72] However, increasing mobility reflects ongoing remodeling of the periodontium and dictates the need for interceptive therapy.

An instrument that can assess mobility has become commercially available (Figs 4-2a and 4-2b).[74] The device contains an electronically driven tapping head that percusses the tooth on the buccal aspect. The handpiece contains a microcomputer that records the time it takes the periodontium to return the tooth to its original position, thereby reflecting periodontal status. A baseline score indicating mobility does not necessarily reflect progressive periodontitis. However, an increasing or decreasing value may reflect a change in periodontal status.

Amount of Keratinized Gingiva

Traditionally, it was assumed that several millimeters of keratinized tissue were needed to maintain gingival health; however, this concept has been modified.[75–79] Investigators have demonstrated that gingival tissues can remain healthy with less than 1 mm of keratinized or attached gingiva,[75] and there was no correlation between the amount of recession and the width of attached gingiva.[76] Furthermore, narrow and wide zones of keratinized tissue are equally prone to developing clinical and histologic signs of inflammation.[77] Therefore, sites with minimal keratinized tissue must be assessed in light of recent data, and it should not be assumed that a band of keratinized tissue is essential to maintain periodontal health.[75–79]

On the other hand, there are indications for augmentation of keratinized attached gingiva at specific sites when one or more of the following conditions is noted: chronic inflammation, continued recession, root sensitivity, and esthetic disfigurations.[75] Enhancement of attached keratinized gingiva prior to placement of subgingival crown margins has also been advocated, because subgingival restorations are associated with an increased inflammatory response.[78]

Radiographic Assessments

Conventional Radiographs

Conventional radiographs do not indicate if bone loss is progressing or stable. Therefore, replicate assessments need to be performed on standardized radiographs to detect bone resorption. In general, radiographs underestimate disease activity.[80–82] For example, intact cortical plates obscure medullary bone loss, and 30% of crestal bone can be resorbed before it is detected on radiographs.[80] Furthermore, prior to radiographic detection of bone loss, 4 mm of clinical attachment can be lost.[81] Conventional radiographs also are usually not accurate for comparing the density of bone before and after therapy.[82]

The white line observed at the crest of the alveolar bone, referred to as the *crestal lamina dura*, is frequently assessed by clinicians. Its absence has been interpreted to indicate the presence of periodontitis. However, several studies that investigated the relationships between lamina dura and clinical parameters of disease have reported that this interpretation is inconsistent with objective data.[83,84] In contrast, the presence of crestal lamina dura may be a predictor of continued health.[85] Thus, conventional radiographs are not sensitive indicators of progressive periodontitis.

Subtraction Radiography

In this method, geometrically and densitometrically standardized pairs of radiographs, taken at different times, are compared using computer techniques. These images are more sensitive for detecting alveolar changes than are conventional radiographs.[86] Additionally, examiners can more accurately and quickly identify osseous lesions with subtraction radiography.[87,88]

Subtraction radiography has become commercially available. However, the relationship between attachment loss and changes in osseous density is unclear.[8] Furthermore, because bone densitometer measurements are highly sensitive indicators of change, and attachment loss of 2 mm is a highly specific indicator of disease progression, it may be unrealistic to expect a simple and direct correlation between the two techniques.

Despite the superior sensitivity of subtraction radiographs, their routine use in patients is not advisable, because continuous monitoring of patients with radiographs (eg, every 3 months) could create a problem regarding radiation hygiene.

Bacteriologic Evaluations

Correlations between specific organisms and disease progression can serve as a biologic basis for increased usage of microbiologic testing, despite technical and conceptual problems encountered during bacteriologic assays.[89]

Bacterial assessments can be used to assess for organisms that may precipitate disease progression, to monitor recall intervals, to determine effects of therapy and most importantly, to direct antibiotic therapy.

Bacterial Cultures

Culturing is the reference method for determining the microbial composition of plaque samples. It enables identification of major plaque components and permits in vitro evaluation of sensitivity to antimicrobial agents. Culturing has proven especially valuable for patients who do not respond to conventional treatment. Slots et al[90] reported that one third of refractory sites harbored yeast, enteric rods, or pseudomonads.

Bacteriologic testing laboratories provide guidelines to indicate whether the level of putative pathogens present is of low, moderate, or great risk to the patient.[91] However, these guidelines are arbitrary because there is a lack of substantial information to indicate that detection of alleged pathogens can predict future disease activity.[13,14] One recent prospective study concluded that the presence of putative pathogens could be used to predict disease progression (2-mm loss of clinical attachment) at only 20% of the sites.[13] It was concluded that their absence was a better predictor of no further attachment loss than their presence was of disease progression.[13]

In conclusion, bacterial assessments are not efficient for predicting disease progression. However, they can direct antibiotic therapy, and detection of putative pathogens dictates careful monitoring.[11]

Phase and Dark-Field Microscopic Monitoring

Bacterial morphotypes (shapes) can be identified with phase or dark-field microscopic evaluation; however, this type of assessment does not facilitate species identification. Numerous studies have indicated that diseased sites are usually associated with decreased coccoid cells and increased numbers of motile forms, especially spirochetes.[92–94] Comprehensive studies have found that spirochetal assessments failed to predict the following: recurrence of disease, onset of gingivitis, and progressive loss of clinical attachment at individual sites.[92–94] Furthermore, some pathogens seen in juvenile periodontitis (*A actinomycetecomitans*) or adult gingivitis (*P gingivalis* and *Prevotella intermedia*) are neither spirochetal or motile. Therefore, they would be undetected by phase or dark-field microscopy. Overall, the variations related to microscopic monitoring impede its use as a reliable diagnostic test.

DNA Probes

Deoxyribonucleic acid (DNA) probes identify specific sequences of nucleic acids that are unique to each individual bacterial species, thereby permitting detection of organisms. This technique is more sensitive than culturing, can

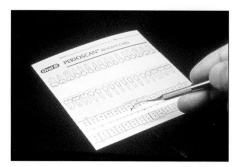

Fig 4-3a BANASCAN (formerly called Perioscan) is a test for anaerobic organisms (Walter J. Loesche, University of Michigan, Ann Arbor, MI). Plaque is collected with a curette from specific sites and placed on a card that is numbered to correspond to teeth in the arch. (From Greenstein.[37] Reprinted with permission.)

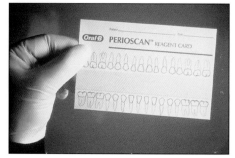

Fig 4-3b The card is folded on itself, which brings the enzyme into contact with the plaque samples. During incubation, an enzymatic reaction results in a blue hue on sites where an anaerobic infection is present. At present, this test is not commercially available in the United States. (From Greenstein.[37] Reprinted with permission.)

detect a minimum of 10^3 microbes, and is not dependent on maintaining viable cells.[95,96] At present, commercially available testing is limited to assessing for six microbes (*P gingivalis, P intermedia, A actinomycetemcomitans, Eikenella corrodens, Campylobacter rectus, Fusobacterium nucleatum*). The results are categorized as fewer than 10^3 organisms (low risk), 10^3 to 10^4 organisms (moderate risk), and greater than 10^5 organisms (high risk). These are guidelines and should be used in conjunction with other clinical assessments because individuals may not manifest pathosis at these levels. However, if elevated levels of putative pathogens are detected, it is advisable to initiate therapy to reduce or eliminate these bacteria, because they present a potential risk.

In general, similar to culturing, DNA probes may be most useful for assessing areas not responding to therapy, for monitoring patients with *Aa*-associated juvenile periodontitis, and for evaluating therapeutic efficacy.

Enzymatic Tests

Enzymatic detection of several anaerobes can be accomplished based on the ability of *P gingivalis, Treponema denticola,* and *Bacteroides forsythus* to produce an enzyme that hydrolyzes a trypsinlike substrate, N-benzoyl-DL-arginine-2 napthylamide (BANA). This assay induces a color reaction with a dye indicative of the presence of one or more of the above organisms (Figs 4-3a and 4-3b).[97] The ability of the test to identify *T denticola* and *P gingivalis* was confirmed by immunologic assays (ELISA)[98–101] and DNA probes.[99] In one clinical trial, it was reported that, after initial therapy, BANA-positive sites lost significantly more attachment in the following year than did teeth that tested BANA negative.[100] The BANA test also was utilized to identify patients with anaerobic infections, which were treated with metronidazole.[101] This assay provides a rapid chairside test (15 minutes) to detect anaerobic infections. However,

it is limited to those organisms already mentioned and, similar to culturing, their detection is not necessarily indicative of disease status.

Recently, a test kit that provides rapid assessment for the presence of *A actinomycetemcomitans, P intermedia,* and *P gingivalis* was developed. A 5-minute, user-friendly, enzyme immunoassay is used to detect specific surface antigens for the bacteria. The test visually differentiates and semiquantitates antigens for these organisms.[102,103] However, similar to results of other microbiologic tests, the results must be interpreted in conjunction with other clinical parameters.

Host Responses

Temperature Evaluations

Utilization of changes in temperature at specific sites and within patients has been explored as a diagnostic tool to detect inflammatory changes associated with periodontal disease (Figs 4-4a and 4-4b).[104–107] Several studies have indicated that higher temperatures are associated with inflammation.[104–107] However, nonsignificant correlations were determined between the patients' mean subgingival temperatures and clinical parameters.[105] Furthermore, when the predictive capacity (assessed retrospectively) of temperature was assessed longitudinally, it was only able to predict 3.9% of the sites that would deteriorate (2 mm) during the subsequent 2 months.[106] In contrast, 96% of the sites with increased temperatures did not break down.

Temperature assessments predicted clinical attachment loss better than did other clinical parameters at specific sites during a brief study.[106] However, the high percentage of sites that did not deteriorate and the confounding correlation between probing depths and temperature readings suggest that longer studies are needed to evaluate the utility of temperature assessments.

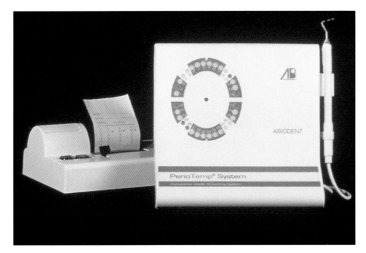

Fig 4-4a The Periotemp (Abiodent, Danvers, MA) assesses temperature changes. The console indicates green for cool, red for hot, and amber when the recorded temperature is between cool and hot. (From Greenstein.[37] Reprinted with permission.)

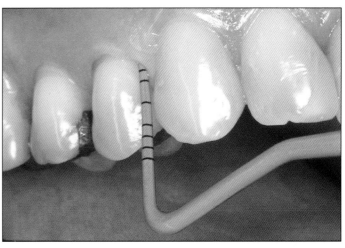

Fig 4-4b The temperature probe is inserted into a pocket to determine if the site is warmer than normal. (From Greenstein.[37] Reprinted with permission.)

With regard to individual subjects, the data suggested that mean sulcular temperature elevations may help identify subjects who are prone to additional attachment loss.[104,106,107] However, it needs to be determined whether subjects with higher temperature are at greater risk of deterioration or whether subjects with widespread disease have higher subgingival temperatures. Therefore, before temperature assessments are integrated into periodontal evaluations, additional data are needed to determine whether such measurements can identify individuals at risk of disease progression.

Immunologic Tests

Immunologic tests rely on antigen-antibody reactions. These assays can be used to identify specific plaque bacteria and to determine serum antibody levels to pathogens. Detection of microbes is usually accomplished by exposing antigens to fluorescein-labeled antibodies. This is a rapid test, but time consuming when used quantitatively.[108] The need for species-specific reagents and an immunofluorescent microscope probably limits its use in typical dental environments.

Immunologic assays may become more important as the need for microbiologic determinations becomes more precise. For instance, immunologic tests are needed to differentiate between the three serotypes of *A actinomycetemcomitans*. Because not all *Aa* serotypes produce leukotoxin, it is possible that serotype identification may be necessary to accurately determine the pathogenic potential of organisms.[109]

Host response to periodontal infections often includes production of antibodies. Enzyme-linked immunosorbent assays (ELISA) are frequently used to monitor antibody levels because they are very sensitive tests.[110] However, not all patients infected with putative pathogens demonstrate elevated antibody levels.

Recently, a screening test that detects antibodies to five suspected periodontal pathogens was developed. This sensitive immunodot assay uses a small amount of blood obtained from a finger stick. Because this test can detect immune phenomena that may occur prior to clinical attachment loss, it theoretically has the ability to identify patients at risk of developing disease progression. However, additional testing is needed to clarify what percentage of patients with increased antibody titers will develop signs of disease and after what duration.

The data must also be interpreted in light of the following considerations: Detection of antibodies does not reveal if the level of immunoglobulin is increasing or decreasing or if the individual is a carrier of putative pathogens.[110] Furthermore, specific levels of antibodies have not been clearly related to episodes of disease progression, and the test does not direct therapy to a specific site. Such a test has high scientific merit, but its clinical utility still needs to be defined.

Immunologic testing has also been used to detect neutrophil dysfunctions that are associated with various forms of periodontitis: prepubertal, juvenile, rapidly progressive, and refractory.[111] Nevertheless, this knowledge has not altered therapy, and, despite successful treatment, neutrophil impairments persist.[112,113] At present, there is no simple, rapid, chairside capability to assess neutrophil defects and it is unknown if detection of these defects can be used to predict disease progression.

Biochemical Evaluations

In the past, analysis of gingival crevicular fluid (GCF) provided little help in predicting progressive periodontitis. Recently, several constituents of gingival crevicular fluid were noted as possible predictors of disease progression: prostaglandins E$_2$,[114] beta-glucuronidase,[115] and interleukin.[116] However, detection of these host-produced biochemical markers of an inflammatory process requires extensive laboratory analysis, and currently no tests are available for integration into daily practice.

Collagenase, a neutral protease, is another GCF component undergoing research as a marker of inflammation. Compared with healthy sites, locations with gingivitis or periodontitis had higher levels of collagenase.[117,118] A chairside test to detect neutral protease levels (collagenase is the main neutral protease) was developed (Figs 4-5a to 4-5c).[119,120] However, there are no data showing a relationship between the level of collagenase and progressive periodontitis, and the test cannot differentiate between gingivitis and periodontitis. It also remains unclear if the amount of collagenase reflects disease progression or just pocket depth. At present, the test does not appear to provide more information than can be obtained by using traditional clinical assessments.

In patients with periodontitis, investigators also detected increased elastase levels, a neutral protease released by polymorphonuclear leukocytes.[121,122] Cross-sectional data have indicated that total elastase levels are higher at sites demonstrating attachment loss (enzyme levels 2.82 versus 2.03) and bone loss (enzyme levels 2.32 versus 2.01).[123] If 1-mm attachment loss and bone loss (5% change in radiodensity) were analyzed jointly, the elastase test provided an 82% sensitivity and 66% specificity. However, predictive values were not provided, and there was no clarification as to the relevance of a 5% change in osseous density to clinical attachment levels. Furthermore, no data have clarified what elastase levels are associated with gingivitis or deep inactive pockets or the ability of elastase levels to predict future clinical attachment loss.

The most comprehensively studied enzyme associated with periodontal disease is aspartate aminotransferase (AST) (Figs 4-6a and 4-6b). Increased levels of AST are detected in dogs with ligature-induced periodontitis,[124] in

Figs 4-5a to 4-5c Periocheck (Pro-Dentec, Batesville, AR) assesses for collagenase in the gingival crevicular fluid. (From Greenstein.[37] Reprinted with permission.)

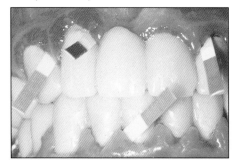

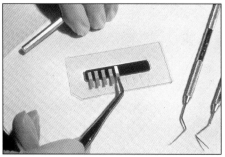

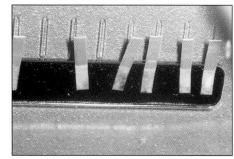

Fig 4-5a Filter strips are placed within the gingival sulcus.

Fig 4-5b The used filter strips are placed on collagen gel.

Fig 4-5c During incubation, the filter strips absorb a blue dye released by the gel. The amount of color on the strips is then compared to a colormetric chart to determine the amount of collegenase present. This test is FDA approved.

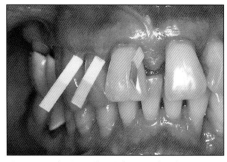

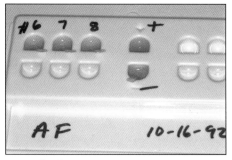

Fig 4-6a Periogard (Colgate-Palmolive, Piscataway, NJ) is a test for AST. Filter strips are placed at the orifice of the sulcus to collect gingival crevicular fluid (teeth 6, 7, and 8). (From Greenstein.[37] Reprinted with permission.)

Fig 4-6b The test results are negative because the color reaction in the individual wells of the plastic tray that correspond to teeth 6, 7, and 8 are similar to the negative control (marked [−] in the center of the plastic tray). At present, this test is not commercially available in the United States. (From Greenstein.[37] Reprinted with permission.)

humans with experimental gingivitis,[125] and in patients with periodontitis.[126] High levels of AST are also found at sites losing 2 mm of clinical attachment.[127–129] The precise temporal relationship between progressive periodontitis and the amount of AST in gingival crevicular fluid is unclear. In general, the data support the idea that detection of high levels of AST reflects periodontal pathosis. However, variations in AST levels have been observed between groups of active and inactive diseased sites and those with high and low Gingival Index scores.[126,127,129]

Recently, it was demonstrated that if an AST level of 800 μIU (international units) is used as a threshold, this test demonstrates a 0.93 sensitivity and a 0.68 specificity for detecting 2-mm loss of clinical attachment.[9] However, predictive values are 0.73, 0.50, and 0.20 when the prevalence of disease is 50%, 25%, and 10% in the treated population. This means that, when 25% of the assessed population is afflicted, the test will signal a correct diagnosis 50% of the time. At present, there are insufficient data to conclude that AST detection is indicative of ongoing or pending loss of clinical attachment.

Strategies for Diagnostic Testing[130]

Rationale for Testing

To promote optimal therapeutic decisions, diagnostic testing can be used to increase diagnostic certainty. Diagnostic testing is used to confirm or reject diagnostic hypotheses, to obtain prognostic data, to screen for hidden disease, and to reassure the patient and clinician. After a diagnosis is made, further testing can aid in the selection of antibiotics, the monitoring of patients, and the determination of therapeutic end points.

Determinants for Test Utilization

The initial decision to perform testing should be based on clinical findings and the dental and medical history. When a patient presents with a healthy periodontium (ie, no redness, bleeding, or purulence; minimal probing depths; and little or no clinical attachment loss), it is usually not necessary to confirm these clinical observations with diagnostic tests. However, there are exceptions: For example, if a child presents with juvenile periodontitis, microbiologic testing of an apparently healthy sibling is advisable.

If signs of disease are present, it is usually unnecessary to verify the patient's condition with nontraditional diagnostic testing. First, periodontal status is assessed and a treatment plan is developed. If the planned therapy is effective and has low risk, as does most periodontal therapy, then some

uncertainty about disease progression can be tolerated. Therefore, the need and expense of many tests can be avoided.

In general, the response to conventional therapy is the major determinant for further diagnostic testing in patients with periodontitis. However, there are some situations in which microbial testing may be of benefit prior to therapy, despite the obvious presence of disease. These include unusual types of periodontitis (eg, juvenile and prepubertal), systemically ill individuals, and patients taking long-term antibiotics.

If patients are responding to therapy, additional testing is probably unnecessary. However, when disease is refractory to conventional treatment, it may be useful to use other assessments to help direct therapy. For these patients, culturing and antibiotic sensitivity testing may have great utility, because they can guide antimicrobial therapy to control or eliminate elevated levels of putative pathogens.

Superfluous Testing

The potential exists for clinicians to engage in unnecessary diagnostic testing. Overreliance on testing may result from the pursuit of diagnostic certainty, malpractice concerns, patient requests, and/or professional peer pressure. Therefore, strategies must be developed to avoid the pursuit of diagnostic certainty beyond that required to delineate appropriate therapy.

In general, once diagnostic uncertainty is reduced, patients with adult periodontitis should be advised that additional testing techniques are available but probably will not alter the proposed treatment plan. Regardless, some patients may still desire additional diagnostic testing to convince themselves that the diagnosis is correct. This may increase patient acceptance of therapy, but it also may stimulate unnecessary or excessive evaluations. Similarly, peer pressure among clinicians to use tests to confirm the presence of disease can also result in superfluous testing.

Malpractice occurs when clinicians fail to meet the standard of care for diagnosis and treatment of periodontal diseases. At present, it is the author's opinion that most novel diagnostic tests have not provided crucial information for the diagnosis of adult periodontitis. Therefore, their utilization is unlikely to be considered a legal standard of care.

However, in patients with unique forms of periodontitis (eg, juvenile periodontitis), and especially in patients not responding to conventional therapy, tests such as culturing and antibiotic sensitivity testing are being used quite frequently, a critical step toward becoming a legal standard. The legal standard of care is continually redefined by case law. Therefore, some tests that affect clinical decision making, increase diagnostic certainty, and improve patient management may eventually become standards of care and will have to be integrated into the diagnostic armamentarium.

Conclusion

Diagnostic data must be interpreted in light of current concepts regarding the etiology and pathogenesis of periodontal diseases. Traditional clinical assessments will usually detect inflammatory lesions and direct clinicians to areas requiring therapy and possible additional testing. Although there are ample data to indicate that not all inflamed sites will deteriorate, the data strongly suggest that sites kept consistently free of inflammation will not lose clinical attachment. Therefore, in light of the morbidity associated with undertreatment and the inability to predict which inflamed sites are resistant or susceptible, elimination of all signs of inflammation remains an important clinical goal for the management of periodontal diseases.

The response to therapy is a major determinant of the need for supplemental evaluations. Additional testing may also be beneficial at certain sites or for individual patients when there is diagnostic uncertainty regarding the absence of presence of disease or when the medical or dental history suggests that a patient is at risk of developing periodontitis. Furthermore, supplemental testing becomes critical when therapy fails to improve and stabilize periodontal status. In these situations, microbiologic assessments and drug sensitivity testing are advantageous.

Currently, no one clinical or laboratory test can provide definitive diagnostic or prognostic information. Therefore, a combination of traditional and new clinical assessment methods can, in some cases, provide the most complete information for treatment planning.

Note: The opinions expressed herein are those of the authors and should not be construed to be those of the government of the United States.

References

1. Socransky SS, Haffajee AD, Goodson JM, Lindhe J. New concepts of destructive periodontal disease. J Clin Periodontol 1984;11:21–32.

2. Listgarten MA, Schifter CC, Laster L. 3-year longitudinal study of the periodontal status of an adult population with gingivitis. J Clin Periodontol 1985;12:225–238.

3. Goodson JM, Tanner ACR, Haffajee AD, Sornberger GC, Socransky SS. Patterns of progression and regression of advanced destructive periodontal disease. J Clin Periodontol 1982;9:472–481.

4. Jeffcoat MK, Reddy MS. Progression of probing attachment loss in adult periodontitis. J Periodontol 1991;62:185–189.

5. Greenstein G, Caton J. Periodontal disease activity: A critical assessment. J Periodontol 1990;61:543–552.

6. Moore WEC, Moore LH, Ranney RR, Smibert RM, et al. The microflora of periodontal sites showing active destructive progression. J Clin Periodontol 1991;18:729–739.

7. Grbic JR, Lamster IB, Celenti RS, Fine JB. Risk indicators for future clinical attachment loss in adult periodontitis. Patient variables. J Periodontol 1991;62:322–329.

8. Deas D, Pasquali L, Yuan CH, Kornman KS. The relationship between probing attachment loss and computerized radiographic analysis in monitoring progression of periodontitis. J Periodontol 1991;62:135–141.

9. Persson GR, Page RC. Diagnostic characteristics of crevicular fluid aspartate aminotransferase (AST) levels associated with periodontal disease activity. J Clin Periodontol 1992;19:43–48.

10. Halazonetis TD, Haffajee AD, Socransky SS. Relationship of clinical parameters to attachment loss in subjects with destructive periodontal diseases. J Clin Periodontol 1989;16:563–568.

11. Socransky SS, Haffajee AD. Implications of periodontal microbiology for the treatment of periodontal infections. Compend Contin Educ Dent 1994; suppl 18:S684–S693.

12. Socransky SS, Haffajee AD. Effect of therapy on periodontal infections. J Periodontol 1993;64:754–759.

13. Wennström JL, Dahlen C, Svensson J, Nyman S. *Actinobacillus actinomycetemcomitans, Bacteroides gingivalis* and *Bacteroides intermedius*: Predictors of attachment loss? Oral Microbiol Immunol 1987;2:158–163.

14. Listgarten MA, Slots J, Nowotny AH, et al. Incidence of periodontitis recurrence in treated patients with and without *Actinobacillus actinomycetemcomitans, Prevotella intermedia*, and *Porphyromonas gingivalis*. A prospective study. J Periodontol 1991;62:377–386.

15. MacFarlane TW, Jenkins WM, Gilmour WH, McCourtie J, McKenzie D. Longitudinal study of untreated periodontitis. II. Microbiological findings. J Clin Periodontol 1988;15:331–337.

16. Evans AS. Epidemiological concepts. In: Evans AS, Brachmen PL (eds). Bacterial Infections of Humans: Epidemiology and Control. New York: Plenum, 1991:3–58.

17. Moore WEC, Moore LVH. The bacteria of periodontal diseases. Periodontology 2000 1994;5:66–77.

18. Loos BG, Dyer DW, Genco RJ, Selander RK, Dickenson DP. Natural history and epidemiology. In: Shah HN (ed). Biology of the Species *Porphyromonas gingivalis*. Boca Raton, FL: CRC Press, 1993:1–31.

19. Genco RJ, Zambon JJ, Christersson LA. The origin of periodontal infections. Adv Dent Res 1988;2:245–259.

20. Zambon JJ, Christersson LA, Slots J. *Actinobacillus actinomycetemcomitans* in human periodontal disease. Prevalence in patient groups and distribution of biotypes and serotypes within families. J Periodontol 1983;54:707–711.

21. Slots J, Reynolds HS, Genco RJ. *Actinobacillus actinomycetemcomitans* in human periodontal disease: A cross sectional microbiologic investigation. Infect Immun 1980;29:1013–1020.

22. Asikainen S, Jousimies-Somer H, Kanervo A, Saxen L. *Actinobacillus actinomycetemcomitans* and clinical periodontal status in Finnish juvenile periodontitis patients. J Periodontol 1986;57:91–93.

23. Petit MDA, van Steenbergen TJM, Timmerman MF, de Graff J, van der Velden U. Prevalence of periodontitis and suspected periodontal pathogens in families of adult periodontitis patients. J Clin Periodontol 1994;21:76–85.

24. van Steenbergen TJM, Petit MDA, Scholte LHM, van der Velden U, de Graff J. Transmission of *Porphyromonas gingivalis* between spouses. J Clin Periodontol 1993;20:340–345.

25. Preus HR, Zambon JJ, Dunford RG, Genco RJ. The distribution and transmission of *Actinobacillus actinomycetemcomitans* in families with established adult periodontitis. J Periodontol 1994;65:2–7.

26. Alaluusua S, Asikainen S, Lai CH. Intrafamilial transmission of *Actinobacillus actinomycetemcomitans*. J Periodontol 1991;62:207–210.

27. Zafiropoulos GGK, Flores-de-Jacoby L, Hungurer KD, Nicengard RG. Humoral antibody responses in periodontal disease. J Periodontol 1992;63:80–86.

28. Caugant DA, Selander RK, Olsen I. Differentiation between *Actinobacillus (Haemophilus) actinomycetemcomitans, Haemophilus aphrophilus* and *Haemophilus paraphrophilus* by multilocus enzyme electrophoresis. J Gen Microbiol 1990;136:2135–2141.

29. Killian M, Theilade E, Poulsen K. Population structure of *Actinobacillus actinomycetemcomitans* [abstract 1]. J Dent Res 1994;73:940.

30. Loos BG, Mayrand D, Genco RJ, Dickinson DP. Genetic heterogeneity of *Porphyromonas (Bacteroides) gingivalis* by Genomic DNA fingerprinting. J Dent Res 1990;69:1488–1493.

31. Loos BG, Dyer DW, Whittam TS, Selander RK. Genetic structure of populations of *Porphyromonas gingivalis* associated with periodontitis and other oral infections. Infect Immunol 1993;61:204–212.

32. Caton J. Periodontal diagnosis and diagnostic aids. In: Nevins M, Becker W, Kornman K (eds). Proceedings of the World Workshop in Clinical Periodontics. Chicago: American Academy of Periodontology 1989:I-1–I-12.

33. Rethman M. Periodontal terminology [letter]. J Periodontol 1993;64:83.

34. Greenstein G, Lamster I. Understanding diagnostic testing and risk assessment for periodontal diseases. J Periodontol 1995;66:659–666.

35. Goodson JM. Selection of suitable indicators of periodontitis. In: Bader J (ed). Risk Assessment in Dentistry. Chapel Hill, NC: University of North Carolina, 1989:69–74.

36. Listgarten MA. Periodontal probing: What does it mean? J Clin Periodontol 1980;7:165–176.

37. Greenstein G. Assessment of periodontal disease activity: Diagnostic and therapeutic implications. In: Periodontal Disease Management. Chicago: American Academy of Periodontology, 1993;185–210.

38. Brown LJ, Oliver RC, Löe H. Periodontal status of US employed adults 1985–1986. J Am Dent Assoc 1990;121:226–235.

39. Horning GM, Hatch CL, Lutskus JL. The prevalence of periodontitis in a military treatment population. J Am Dent Assoc 1990;121:616–622.

40. Miyazki H, Pilot T, Leclercq MH, Barnes DE. Profiles of permanent conditions in adults measured by CPITN. Int Dent J 1991;41:74–80.

41. Pilot T, Miyazki H. Periodontal conditions in Europe. J Clin Periodontol 1991;18:353–357.

42. Persson GR. The effects of line-angle measurements on prevalence estimates of periodontal diseases. J Periodont Res 1991;26:527–529.

43. Rams TE, Oler J, Listgarten MA, Slots J. Utility of Ramjford index teeth to assess periodontal disease progression in longitudinal studies. J Clin Periodontol 1993;20:147–150.

44. Ainamo J, Ainamo A. Partial indicies as indicators of the severity and prevalence of periodontal disease. Int Dent J 1985;35:322–326.

45. Zimmerman SO. Discussion: Attachment level changes in destructive periodontal diseases. J Periodontol 1986;13:473–475.

46. Greenstein G, Lamster I. Understanding diagnostic testing for periodontal diseases. J Periodontol 1995;66:659–666.

47. Department of Clinical Epidemiology and Biostatistics. McMaster University Health Sciences Center. How to read clinical journals. II. To learn about a diagnostic test. Can Med Assoc J 1981;124:703–710.

48. Beck JD. Methods of assessing risk for periodontitis and developing multifactorial models. J Periodontol 1994;65:468–478.

49. Wolff LF, Gunnar D, Aeppli D. Bacteria as risk markers for periodontitis. J Periodontol 1994;65:498–510.

50. Oliver RC, Tervonen T. Diabetes—A risk factor for periodontitis in adults? J Periodontol 1994;65:530–538.

51. Hart TC, Shapira L, Van Dyke TE. Neutrophil defects as risk factors for periodontal diseases. J Periodontol 1994;65:521–529.

52. Bergstrom J, Preber H. Tobacco use as a risk factor. J Periodontol 1994;65:545–550.

53. Riegelman RK, Hirsch RP. Studying a Study and Testing a Test. How to Read the Medical Literature, ed 2. Boston: Little, Brown and Loe, 1989:127–175.

54. Haffajee AD, Socransky SS, Goodson JM. Comparison of different data analyses for detecting changes in attachment level. J Clin Periodontol 1983;10:298–310.

55. Vanooteghem R, Hutchen LH, Garret S, et al. Bleeding on probing and probing depth as indicators of the response to plaque control and root debridement. J Clin Periodontol 1987;14:226-230.

56. Badersten A, Nilveus R, Egelberg J. Effect of nonsurgical therapy. VII. Bleeding, suppuration and probing depths in sites with probing attachment loss. J Clin Periodontol 1985;12:432–440.

57. Gunsolley JC, Best AM. Changes in attachment level. J Periodontol 1988;59:450–456.

58. Nordland P, Garret S, Kiger R, et al. The effect of plaque control and root debridement in molar teeth. J Clin Periodontol 1987;14:231–236.

59. Claffey N, Nylund K, Kiger R, et al. Diagnostic predictability of scores of plaque, bleeding, suppuration and probing depth for probing attachment loss. 3½ years of observation following initial periodontal therapy. J Clin Periodontol 1990;17:108–114.

60. Badersten A, Nilveus R, Egelberg J. Scores of plaque, bleeding, suppuration and probing depth to predict probing attachment loss. 5 years of observation following nonsurgical periodontal therapy. J Clin Periodontol 1990;17:102–107.

61. Lindhe J, Okamoto H, Yoneyama T, et al. Periodontal loser sites in untreated adult subjects. J Clin Periodontol 1989;16:671–678.

62. Badersten A, Nilveus R, Egelberg J. Effect of nonsurgical therapy. II. Severely advanced periodontitis. J Clin Periodontol 1984;11:63–76.

63. Gorman NJ. Prevalence and etiology of gingival recession. J Periodontol 1967;38:316–322.

64. Magnusson I, Fuller W, Heins P, et al. Correlation between electronic and visual reading of pocket depths with a new developed constant probe force. J Clin Periodontol 1988;15:180–184.

65. Osborn J, Stoltenberg J, Huso B, et al. Comparison of measurement variability using a standard and constant force periodontal probe. J Periodontol 1990;61:497–503.

66. Greenstein G, Caton JG, Polson AM. Histologic characteristics associated with bleeding after probing and visual signs of inflammation. J Periodontol 1981;52:420–425.

67. Lang NP, Nyman S, Senn C, Joss A. Bleeding on probing as it relates to probing pressure and gingival health. J Clin Periodontol 1991;18:257–261.

68. Lang NP, Orsanic T, Gusberti FA, Siegrist BE. Bleeding upon probing. A predictor for the progression of periodontal stability. J Clin Periodontol 1986;13:590-596.

69. Lang NP, Adler R, Joss A, Nyman S. Absence of bleeding upon probing. An indicator of periodontal stability. J Clin Periodontol 1990;17:714–721.

70. Polson AM. The relative importance of plaque and occlusion in periodontal disease. J Clin Periodontol 1986;13:923–927.

71. Greenstein G, Polson AM. Understanding tooth mobility. Compend Contin Educ Dent 1988;9:327–337.

72. Polson AM, Kantor ME, Zander HE. Periodontal repair after reduction of inflammation. J Periodont Res 1979;14:520–525.

73. Burgett FG, Ramfjord SP, Nissle RR, Morrison EC, Charbeneau TD, Caffesse RG. A randomized trial of occlusal adjustment in the treatment of periodontitis patients. J Clin Periodontol 1992;19:381–387.

74. Olive J, Aparico C. The Periotest method as a measure of osseointegrated oral implant stability. Int J Oral Max Implants 1990; 5:390–400.

75. Hall WB. Gingival augmentation/mucogingival surgery. In: Nevins M, Becker W, Kornman K (eds). Proceedings of the World Workshop in Clinical Periodontics. Chicago: American Academy of Periodontology, 1989;VII-1–VII-21.

76. Tenenbaum H. A clinical study comparing the width of attached gingiva and the prevalence of gingiva recession. J Clin Periodontol 1982;9:86–92.

77. Freedman AL, Salkin LM, Stein MD, Green K. A 10 year longitudinal study of untreated mucogingival defects. J Periodontol 1992; 63:71–72.

78. Maynard JG, Wilson RD. Diagnosis and management of mucogingival problems in children. Dent Clin North Am 1980;24:683–704.

79. Dorfman H, Kennedy J, Bird W. Longitudinal evaluation of free autogenous gingival grafts. J Clin Periodontol 1980;7:316–324.

80. Ortman L, McHenry K, Hausmann E. Relationship between alveolar bone measured by 125/absorptiometry with analysis of subtraction radiographs. J Periodontol 1982;53:311–314.

81. Goodson JM, Haffajee AD, Socransky S. The relationship between attachment level loss and alveolar bone loss. J Clin Periodontol 1984;11:348–359.

82. Hausmann E. A contemporary perspective on techniques for the clinical assessment of alveolar bone. J Periodontol 1990;61:149–156.

83. Greenstein G, Polson AM, Iker H, Meitner S. Associations between crestal lamina dura and periodontal status. J Periodontol 1981;52:362–366.

84. Ainamo J, Tammisalo EH. Comparison of radiographic and clinical signs of early periodontal disease. Scand J Dent Res 1973;81:548–552.

85. Rams TE, Listgarten MA, Slots J. Utility of radiographic crestal alveolar lamina dura for predicting periodontitis disease-activity. J Clin Periodontol 1994;21:571–576.

86. Jeffcoat MK, Reddy MS, Webber RL, et al. Extraoral control of geometry for digital subtraction radiography. J Dent Res 1987;22:396–402.

87. Rethman M, Ruttiman U, O'Neal R, et al. Diagnosis of bone lesions by subtraction radiography. J Periodontol 1985;56:324–329.

88. Grondahl K, Grondahl HG, Wennström J, Heijl L. Examiner agreement in estimating changes in periodontal bone from conventional and subtraction radiographs. J Clin Periodontol 1987;14:74–79.

89. Socransky SS, Haffajee AD, Smith GL, et al. Difficulties encountered in the search for etiologic agents of destructive periodontal diseases. J Clin Periodontol 1987;14:588–598.

90. Slots J, Rams TE, Listgarten MA. Yeasts, enteric rods and pseudomonads in the subgingival flora of severe adult periodontitis. Oral Microbiol Immunol 1988;3:47–52.

91. Bragd L, Danlen G, Wilkstrom M, Slots J. The capacity of Actinobacillus actinomycetemcomitans, Bacteroides gingivalis and Bacteroides intermedius to indicate progressive periodontitis: A retrospective study. J Clin Periodontol 1987;14:95–99.

92. Evian CL, Rosenberg ES, Listgarten MA. Bacterial variability within diseased periodontal sites. J Periodontol 1982,53:595–598.

93. Listgarten MA, Schifter CC, Sullivan P, Rosenberg ES. Failure of a treated microbial assay to reliably predict disease recurrence in a treated periodontitis population receiving regularly scheduled prophylaxes. J Clin Periodontol 1986;13:768–773.

94. Listgarten MA, Levin S, Schifter CC, et al. Comparative differential dark-filled microscopy of subgingival bacteria from tooth surfaces with recent evidence of recurring periodontitis and from nonaffected surfaces. J Periodontol 1984;55:398–401.

95. French CK, Savitt ED, Simon SL, et al. DNA probe detection of periodontal pathogens. Oral Microbiol Immunol 1986;1:58–62.

96. Loesche WJ, Lopatin DE, Stall J, et al. Comparison of various detection methods for periodontopathic bacteria: Can culture be considered the primary reference standard? J Clin Microbiol 1992;30:418–426.

97. Loesche WJ. The identification of bacteria associated with periodontal disease and dental caries by enzymatic methods. Oral Microbiol Immunol 1986;1:65–70.

98. Loesche WJ, Bretz WA, Lopatin DE, et al. Multicenter clinical evaluation of a chairside method for detecting certain periodontopathic bacteria in periodontal disease. J Periodontol 1990;61:189–196.

99. Loesche WJ, Lopatin DE, Giordana J, et al. Comparison of the benzoyl-DL-arginine napthylamide (BANA) test, DNA probes, and immunologic reagents for ability to detect anaerobic periodontal infections due to Porphyromonas gingivalis, Treponema denticola, and Bacteroides forsythus. J Clin Microbiol 1992;30:427–433.

100. Loesche WJ, Giordana J, Hujoel PP. The utility of the BANA test for monitoring anaerobic infections due to spirochetes (Treponema denticola) in periodontal disease. J Dent Res 1990;69:1696–1702.

101. Loesche WJ, Schmidt BA, Morrison R. Effect of metronidazole on periodontal treatment needs. J Periodontol 1991;62:247–257.

102. Contestable P, Abrams C, Boyer B, Grogan E, Snyder B. A rapid immunoassay for the simultaneous detection of multiple suspected periopathogens [abstract C-302]. Abstracts of the General Meeting of the American Society of Microbiology 1991:392.

103. Corona-Howard H, Reynolds HS, Ryerson CC, Zambon JJ, Genco RG, Snyder B. Analytical performance of Evalusite Periodontal Test and comparison to culture [abstract 1181]. J Dent Res 1994;73:249.

104. Kung RTV, Ochs B, Goodson M. Temperature as a periodontal diagnostic. J Clin Periodontol 1990;17:557–563.

105. Haffajee AD, Socransky SS, Goodson JM. Subgingival temperature. I. Relation to baseline clinical parameters. J Clin Periodontol 1992;19:409–416.

106. Haffajee AD, Socransky SS, Goodson JM. Subgingival temperature. II. Relation to future periodontal attachment loss. J Clin Periodontol 1992;19:409–416.

107. Fedi PF, Killoy WJ. Temperature differences at sites in health and disease. J Periodontol 1992;63:24–27.

108. Zambon JJ, Bochachi V, Genco RJ. Immunological assays for putative periodontal pathogens. Oral Microbiol Immunol 1986;1:39–44.

109. Ebersole JL, Frey DE, Taubman MA, et al. Serologic identification of oral bacteroides ssp by enzyme linked immunosorbent assay. J Clin Microbiol 1984;19:639–644.

110. Wilton JMA, Johnson NW, Curtin MA, et al. Specific antibody responses to subgingival plaque bacteria as aids to the diagnosis and prognosis of destructive periodontitis. J Clin Periodontol 1991; 18:1–15.

111. Altman LC, Page GE, Vandersteen LI, et al. Abnormalities of leukocyte chemotaxis in patients with various forms of periodontitis. J Periodont Res 1985;20:553–563.

112. Van Dyke TE, Levine MJ, Genco RJ. Periodontol diseases and neutrophil abnormalities. In: Genco RJ, Mergenhagen SE (eds). Host-Parasite Interactions in Periodontal Diseases. Washington DC: American Society of Microbiology, 1982:235–245.

113. Page RC, Beatty P, Waldrop TC. Molecular basis for the functional abnormality in neutrophils from patients with generalized prepubertal periodontitis. J Periodont Res 1987;22:182–183.

114. Offenbacher S, Odle BM, Van Dyke TE. The use of crevicular fluid prostaglandin E2 levels as a predictor of periodontal attachment loss. J Periodont Res 1986;21:101–112.

115. Lamster TB, Oshrain RL, Harper DS, et al. Enzyme activity in crevicular fluid for detection and prediction of clinical attachment loss in patients with chronic adult periodontitis. J Periodontol 1988;59:516–523.

116. Stashenko P, Fujiyoshi P, Offenbacher MS, et al. Levels of interleukin-1B in tissue from sites of active periodontal disease. J Clin Periodontol 1991;18:548–554.

117. Larivee J, Sokek J, Ferrier JM. Collagenase and collagenase inhibitor activities in crevicular fluid of patients receiving treatment for localized juvenile periodontitis. J Periodont Res 1986;21:702–714.

118. Hakkarainen K, Uitto VJ, Ainamo J. Collagenase activity and protein content of sulcular fluid after scaling and occlusal adjustment of teeth with deep periodontal pockets. J Peridont Res 1988;23:204–210.

119. Bowers JE, Howley CE, Romberg E. A clinical test for proteolytic enzymes in gingival crevicular fluid. Comparison with periodontal probing depth and bleeding upon probing. Int J Periodont Rest Dent 1991;11:411–422.

120. Bowers JE, Zahradnik RT. Evaluation of a chairside gingival protease test for use in periodontal diagnosis. J Clin Dent 1989;1:106–109.

121. Cox SW, Eley BM. Detection of cathepsin B- and L, elastase-tryptase-trypsin-, and dipeptidyl peptidase IV-like activities in crevicular fluid from gingivitis and periodontitis patients with peptidyl derivatives of 7-amino-4-trifluoromethyl coumarin. J Periodont Res 1989;24:353–361.

122. Cox SW, Eley BM. Cathepsin B/L-, elastase-, trypsin- and dipeptidyl peptidase IV-like activities in gingival crevicular fluid. A comparison of patients. J Clin Periodontol 1992;19:333–339.

123. Palcanis KG, Larjava IK, Wells BR, et al. Elastase as an indicator of periodontal disease prognosis. J Periodontol 1991;63:237–242.

124. Chambers DA, Crawford JM, Mukherjee S, Cohen RL. Aspartate aminotransferase increase in crevicular fluid during experimental periodontitis in dogs. J Periodontol 1984;55:526–530.

125. Persson GR, DeRouen T, Page RC. Relationship between levels of aspartate aminotransferase in gingival crevicular fluid and gingival inflammation. J Periodont Res 1990;25:17–24.

126. Persson GR, DeRouen T, Page RC. Relationship between gingival crevicular fluid levels of aspartate aminotransferase and active tissue destruction in treated chronic periodontitis patients. J Periodont Res 1990;25:81–87.

127. Chambers DA, Imrey PB, Cohen RI. A longitudinal study of aspartate aminotransferase in human crevicular fluid. J Periodont Res 1991;26:65–74.

128. Page RC. Host response tests for diagnosing periodontal disease. J Periodontol 1992;63:356–366.

129. Imrey PB, Crawford JMM, Cohen RI, et al. A cross sectional analysis of aspartate aminotransferase in human gingival crevicular fluid. J Periodont Res 1991;26:75–84.

130. Greenstein G, Caton J. Commentary on periodontal diagnostic testing [guest editorial]. J Periodontol 1995;66:531–535.

131. Greenstein G. Diagnosis of periodontal diseases. Compend Contin Educ Dent 1994;15:750–801.

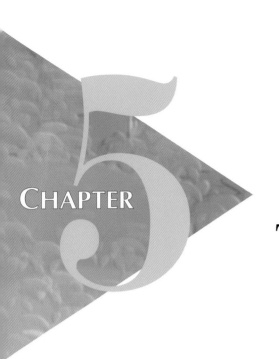

CHAPTER 5

Systemic Complications That Influence the Successful Treatment of Adult Periodontitis

Louis F. Rose, DDS, MD
Barbara J. Steinberg, DDS

Geriatric and medically compromised patients comprise a rapidly growing segment of the population, one whose medical, physical, and psychosocial problems may complicate dental treatment. Elderly or medically compromised patients frequently take one or more medications, such as steroids, anticoagulants, and immunosuppressive agents. Sophisticated surgical manipulation and medical intervention have made possible the ambulatory status of people with cardiovascular, endocrine, and regenerative disease, conditions that just a few years ago would have meant confinement or death. These facts, together with the increasing public awareness of dental health, easily explain the increase in the number of elderly and chronically ill patients occupying the reception areas of today's dentists.

The relationship of general health status and systemic disorders to periodontal disease has been studied extensively. With few exceptions, it is more accurate to consider systemic diseases to be contributing factors in the pathogenesis of periodontal disease rather than primary etiologic factors. Clinical observations alone are not sufficient to identify the systemic disease that may be contributing to the periodontal manifestations. If an alteration in general health is suspected to be a factor in the etiology of periodontal disease, it can only be confirmed by supplementing the clinical observations and dental history with a comprehensive medical history and, if indicated, a consultation with a physician.

Considering the increased likelihood of medical emergencies in this compromised population, it is the responsibility of every practicing periodontist to identify any patient who may be a potential medical risk. This chapter will discuss common systemic conditions, their effect on the periodontal tissues, and the subsequent management of the patient.

Genetic Risk Factors for Periodontal Disease

Periodontal diseases more than likely differ with respect to microbial etiology, host response, and progression of clinical disease. Although there are various types of periodontal diseases, they share the common characteristic of complex host–parasite interactions. The association of periodontal destruction with systemic disease, whether acquired or innate, underlies the importance of the host in maintaining periodontal health. The onset and progression of disease reflects the balance between homeostasis and destruction of the periodontal tissues.

Recent studies suggest that host susceptibility factors play an important role in high-risk patients, and that genetic control may be contributing to this risk.[1]

Evidence for genetic control of risk factors for some forms of periodontal disease comes from three major sources[1]:

1. The consistent association of periodontitis with certain genetically transmitted traits
2. Twin studies of adult-onset forms of periodontitis
3. Genetic studies of early-onset forms of periodontitis

Periodontal disease can no longer be thought of as a prevalent condition for which all people are at equal risk if they fail to practice good oral hygiene. It appears that microbial and host factors are important to disease susceptibility; neither, independently, seems sufficient to account for all forms of periodontal disease. Because periodontal diseases are more than likely diverse in etiology, any thought of a universal host risk factor is probably inappropriate. However, genetic studies of homogeneous forms of periodontal disease may serve as valuable model systems with which to explore the role of potential host susceptibility factors.

Periodontal Complications and Neutrophil Abnormalities

Neutrophils (also referred to as *polymorphonuclear leukocytes* [PMNs]) are the most abundant type of leukocytes present in the peripheral blood of humans, constituting approximately 40% to 70% of the total circulating leukocytes. The importance of these cells in combating infectious diseases is demonstrated through the increased susceptibility to recurrent bacterial infections observed in patients with defective neutrophil production or function.[2] As the primary circulating phagocytic cells, neutrophils play a key role in host defense against extracellular bacteria, especially pyogenic bacteria. They also play a role in the acute phase of inflammatory reactions.

Patients with neutrophil defects, which are either quantitative (neutropenia) or qualitative (adherence, chemotaxis, and microbicidal activity), often suffer from oral mucosal ulcerations, gingivitis, and/or periodontitis. Severe oral disease occurs with both primary and secondary neutrophil abnormalities. The primary neutrophil disorders characterized by severe periodontal disease include neutropenia (chronic or cyclic), leukocyte adhesion deficiency (LAD), Chédiak-Higashi syndrome, and drug-induced agranulocytosis. Neutrophil abnormalities that occur secondary to underlying systemic disease and that are also associated with severe periodontal disease include insulin-dependent (type I) and non–insulin-dependent (type II) diabetes; Papillon-Lefèvre syndrome; Down's syndrome; hyperimmunoglobulinemia E–recurrent infection syndrome (HIE), or Job's syndrome; inflammatory bowel disease (Crohn's disease); preleukemic syndrome; acquired immunodeficiency syndrome (AIDS); and acute myeloid leukemia.

Evidence that the neutrophil is a key protective cell against periodontal infection supports the concept that impaired neutrophil function is a risk factor for the development of periodontal disease.[2] Other factors that increase the risk of periodontal disease include smoking, drugs that depress neutrophils transiently (eg, corticosteroids), nutritional deficiencies in which neutrophils are suppressed

(especially in severe cases of protein calorie malnutrition), and severe bacterial infections with endotoxemia. Stress has also been implicated as a risk factor in certain forms of periodontal disease, such as acute necrotizing ulcerative gingivitis (ANUG). This may occur in two ways: *(1)* indirectly by changing behavior, resulting in poor oral hygiene; and *(2)* directly by suppressing host resistance through immunomodulators, such as adrenocorticosteroids, which are produced during stress.

Neutrophils function as a double-edged sword; although they are primarily protective, they also can act as proinflammatory cells capable of causing significant tissue destruction. Thus, neutrophil disorders that are either primary or secondary to systemic disease are frequently associated with severe periodontal disease. Therefore, neutrophil dysfunction is a risk factor for periodontitis, most likely lowering the host's resistance to periodontal pathogens.

Diabetes Mellitus

Historical Associations Between Periodontal Disease and Diabetes

Although earlier studies regarding the relationship between diabetes and the prevalence and severity of periodontal disease have been equivocal, more recent and comprehensive studies have now clearly proven that diabetes increases the risk of both severe periodontitis and the incidence of periodontal disease progression by approximately 2- to 3-fold[3,4] (Fig 5-1). The presence of pathogens, as well as dysfunction of neutrophils and host response, increased production of inflammatory mediators, and connective tissue alterations all contribute to the severity of periodontal disease. Many of the host response traits that increase susceptibility to periodontitis in otherwise healthy individuals are exaggerated in diabetic patients, who suffer from metabolic and vascular basement membrane changes that may also affect the periodontal tissues and flora.

Effect of Diabetes on Periodontal Flora

Several studies have focused on whether the oral flora in diabetic patients is different from that of nondiabetic patients. One study found bacterial patterns in the diseased sites of diabetic patients to be similar to those of healthy adults with periodontal disease. These sites commonly harbored *Porphyromonas gingivalis* and *Prevotella intermedia* in proportions similar to those in nondiabetic patients with adult periodontitis.[5] Other authors have reported higher levels of specific microorganisms, such as *Actinobacillus actinomycetemcomitans* and *Capnocytophaga*.[6] Zambon et al[7]

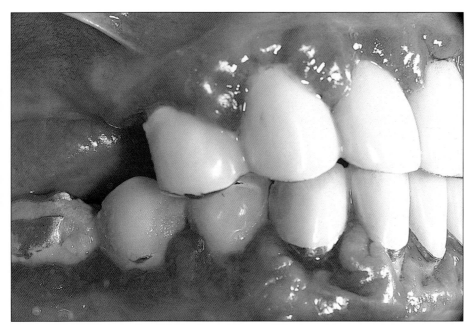

Fig 5-1 Severe periodontal disease in the diabetic patient.

studied the subgingival flora in a group of patients with non–insulin-dependent diabetes mellitus. The most frequently isolated microorganisms were *P intermedia,* followed by *Campylobacter rectus* and *P gingivalis.* The proportion of *P gingivalis* was reported to be higher in non–insulin-dependent diabetes mellitus patients with periodontitis. It is conceivable that, in the diabetic patient, the abnormal host defense mechanisms in addition to the hyperglycemic state can lead to the growth of a specific group of organisms.

Impaired Neutrophil Function

Neutrophil dysfunction usually leads to increased susceptibility to periodontitis.[8,9] Defects in chemotaxis and phagocytosis have all been reported in diabetic patients. Also, the severity of periodontal disease may be due to altered neutrophil chemotaxis in patients with diabetes or it may be a marker of a basic defect in neutrophil function. Other studies have noted impairment in neutrophil phagocytosis in patients with poorly controlled diabetes.[10]

Excessive Inflammatory Response

Insulin-dependent diabetes mellitus is associated with a specific loss of pancreatic beta cells, most likely due to an autoimmune reaction. This autoimmune trait is thought to be associated with genes linked to the HLA-DR3, HLA-DR4, and HLA-DRQ regions.[11,12] It is interesting to note that HLA-associated alleles in the same region have also been associated with severe forms of progressive periodontal disease.[13] Further research in this area can prove beneficial.

Collagen Turnover Defects

Both a marked decrease in collagen production and impairments in collagen degradation have also been reported in diabetic patients. The decrease in periodontal tissue collagen levels is thought to be a specific phenomenon in diabetes. Impaired collagen synthesis, as well as the defects in cellular response to tissue injury, can cause the delayed wound healing seen in patients with diabetes.

Impaired Wound Healing

Poor wound healing is a common problem in diabetic patients. This is characterized by a decrease in the quantity of wound collagen and lowered wound tensile strength. This alteration in wound healing has been attributed in part to nonenzymatic glycosylation of collagen and other wound proteins during periods of hyperglycemia and is thought to be highly correlated to blood glucose concentration.[14] Also, platelet-derived growth factor, epidermal growth factor, and transforming growth factor–β are thought to be limited at the wound site of the diabetic patient,[15] which may contribute to poor wound healing. In addition, wound collagenase activity has been shown to be increased in diabetic patients.[16]

Response to Periodontal Therapy

The literature is replete with articles discussing the effect of control of diabetes on periodontal status and the effects of periodontal therapy on glycemic levels.[17,18] Control of diabetes affects the host response and the environment for the growth of certain microorganisms and can thus affect the severity of periodontal disease.[19] It has been reported that patients with long-term poorly controlled diabetes have more proximal loss of attachment and bone under similar plaque conditions than patients without diabetes.[20] Also, it has been noted that rapid periodontal breakdown is not related to the diabetes per se but rather to the level of hyperglycemia.[21]

Studies support the fact that most patients with controlled diabetes respond well to conventional periodontal treatment.[22] Because diabetic patients may be more prone to infections, adjunct prophylaxis may be necessary if surgical therapy is considered. Because host response defects are considered to be part of the etiology in certain types of periodontal disease, antibiotics may improve the host response and reduce the number of pathogenic microorganisms. Presently there are no guidelines suggesting the use of antibiotics in diabetic patients and no studies indicating the contribution of antibiotics to the therapeutic outcome. It is strictly based on the practitioner's clinical judgment. The recommended dental treatment must consider the diabetic status of the patient, eg, controlled or uncontrolled, the diabetic complication, and the degree of periodontal disease.

Female Hormonal Alterations

Influence of Hormonal Alterations on the Periodontium in Women

Hormones exert a significant influence on body physiology throughout life. Women, in particular, experience hormonal variation under both physiologic and nonphysiologic conditions, such as hormonal therapy or the use of oral contraceptives. This section focuses on the influence of hormones on the periodontal tissues.

Puberty and Menstruation

During puberty, the production of sex hormones increases to a level that remains relatively constant throughout the normal reproductive period of women. Microbial alterations have been noted during puberty; these can be attributed to changes in the environment caused by the gingival tissue response to the higher concentration of sex hormones. In particular, some gram-negative anaerobes, such as *Prevotella intermedia*, have the ability to substitute estrogen and progesterone for menadione (vitamin K) as an essential growth factor.[23] Another gram-negative bacteria, *Capnocytophaga* species, increases as well, and this genus has been implicated in the increased bleeding tendency observed during puberty.[24]

Most periodontally healthy women experience few significant periodontal consequences as a result of hormonal changes at puberty or during menstruation. However, it has been reported that women with gingivitis experience exaggerated inflammation, reflected by an increased amount of gingival exudate, during menstruation; controls with healthy gingiva remain unaffected.[25] Thus, proper evaluation with appropriate treatment is suggested for compromised or susceptible individuals who otherwise require periodontal care.

Pregnancy

The hormonal changes that occur during pregnancy include elevations of both progesterone and estrogen. It has been noted that alterations in maternal susceptibility to infection in early gestation result from changes in the immune system. The periodontium is one of several tissue compartments that is potentially affected.[26] The oral pathologic conditions include gingivitis, pregnancy granuloma, periodontitis, and dental caries.

Pregnancy Gingivitis

Pregnancy gingivitis is a descriptive term for gingivitis occurring during pregnancy. Epidemiologic studies of pregnancy gingivitis show a prevalence ranging from 35%[27] to 100%.[28] The pattern of pregnancy gingivitis seems to follow the hormonal cycle. It initially increases with rising levels of gonadotropin, is maintained from the fourth to eighth months of gestation (with rising levels of estrogen and progesterone), and then decreases in the last month of pregnancy with the abrupt drop in hormone secretion.[29] It has been noted that, during pregnancy, increased levels of progesterone and estrogen parallel gingival inflammation and the concentration of *P intermedia*.[30]

The change in the subgingival environment more than likely is caused by an accumulation of active progesterone, whose metabolism is reduced during pregnancy,[31] and the ability of *P intermedia* to substitute vitamin K, which is an essential growth factor,[32] with progesterone and estrogen. Looking at the clinical presentation of pregnant women, Raber-Durlacher et al[33] noted that the periodontal pocket bleeding index was higher during pregnancy than it was 6 months postpartum. In addition, O'Neill[34] demonstrated that progesterone causes an increase in vascular permeability, polymorphonuclear leukocytes, and prostaglandin E2 in the gingival sulcus. Taken together, the immunosuppressive influence of progesterone, the increased levels of active progesterone in the gingiva, and the microbial shift toward increased proportions of *P intermedia* can exacerbate the gingival response to microbial plaque in pregnant women.

Although a significant proportion of pregnant women suffer from pregnancy gingivitis, this condition is both self-limiting and transient. Gingival tissues usually return to their original healthy state postpartum, when estrogen and progesterone levels reach baseline values. The ratio of anaerobic to aerobic microorganisms increases during the second trimester. This is followed by a reversal of these parameters in the third trimester. Women who are susceptible or have a preexisting gingival condition should seek treatment to prevent extension of the inflammatory process into deeper structures of the periodontium, which can lead to periodontitis.

Pregnancy Granuloma

Pregnancy granuloma is also known as *pregnancy tumor* and *epulis gravidarum*. However, pregnancy granuloma is the preferred term because its histologic presentation is similar to that of pyogenic granuloma.[35] The lesion has a predilection for the maxilla and, in particular, the anterior vestibular aspect. It usually presents as fiery red, pedunculated soft interdental tissue and is often covered with small fibrin spots. The lesions undergo rapid growth initially but are rarely larger than 2 cm (Fig 5-2). Pregnancy granulomas bleed readily if disturbed and demonstrate a tendency to recur following incomplete removal.[36] If left untreated, the lesion will either regress or develop into a residual fibrous mass postpartum.

Surgical removal is usually performed after parturition. However, if the lesion causes functional problems or appears to have deleterious effects on the adjacent periodontium, it can be safely removed under local anesthesia during a normal pregnancy, preferably during the second trimester.

Management of Pregnant Women

The pregnant woman requires special consideration when dental care is needed. During pregnancy, physical changes include increases in cardiac output, red cell mass, respiratory vital capacity, oxygen consumption, and respiratory rate.

As the fetus continues to grow, the mother's bladder and abdominal vessels are impinged on and the diaphragm is displaced upward, reducing respiratory volume.

The safety of the developing fetus is of concern; therefore treatment must be planned when the fetus is least affected. Because organogenesis occurs mainly in the first trimester, most developmental defects take place during this time. Although emergency dental treatment can be accomplished any time during pregnancy, the second trimester is considered the best time to render treatment because organogenesis is complete and the mother is not as uncomfortable as during the first and third trimesters.

Most medication appears to cross the placental barrier. Fetal exposure to compounds through the ingestion by the mother is the second most common cause of teratogenesis.[37] Central nervous system depression can occur with use of narcotics, and spontaneous abortions have been reported following administration of nitrous oxide. Additionally, use of tetracycline, vancomycin, and streptomycin should be avoided because they may cause staining of teeth (4 to 9 months, gestation) and may have ototoxic and nephrotoxic effects on the fetus. Erythromycin, penicillin, and cephalosporins are considered safe, but consultation with the patient's obstetrician is recommended before any drug is prescribed.

Radiographic exposure to the fetus is eliminated if the proper technique and equipment are used.[33]

Contraceptives

Hormonal contraceptives are based on the use of gestational hormones to induce a hormonal condition that simulates a state of pregnancy to prevent ovulation. A number of studies[38] have shown contraceptives to have various effects on gingival tissue. El-Ashiry et al[39] found an increase in clinically assessed inflammation in women using oral contraceptives, and Lindhe and Bjorn[40] observed an increased

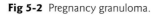

Fig 5-2 Pregnancy granuloma.

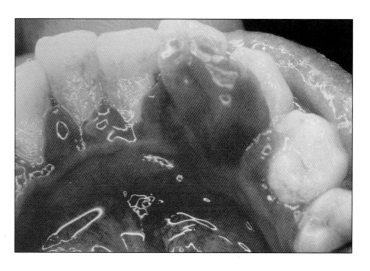

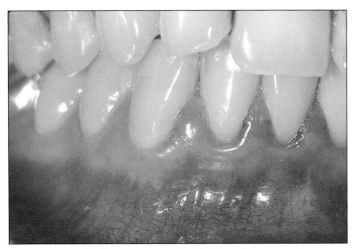

Fig 5-3 Gingival inflammation associated with oral contraceptives.

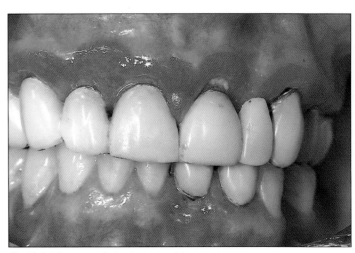

Fig 5-4 Menopausal gingivostomatitis.

amount of gingival exudate following months of regular use of oral contraceptives. In addition, women using oral contraceptives have a higher mean gingival inflammatory index than do control subjects who are not using contraceptives.[41] However, Knight and Wade[42] did not find any significant differences in Plaque Index and Gingival Index scores or more loss of attachment.

These results suggest that prolonged use of oral contraceptives may detrimentally affect the periodontium (Fig 5-3). More studies are required to determine the underlying mechanisms involved with these findings.

Menopause and Postmenopause

A number of investigators have linked menopause with some periodontal conditions (Fig 5-4). Moschil et al[43] demonstrated that women with functional disorders of the ovaries experienced more severe periodontal disorders and have mandibles with less mineral density than do healthy women with normally functioning ovaries. Moschil et al[43] suggested a potential correlation linking ovarian dysfunction, which could parallel menopause, and lowered bone density of the mandible with an increased incidence of periodontal disease. Groen et al[44] found that the incidence of periodontitis correlates with signs of generalized osteoporosis. But a positive cause-effect relationship between tooth loss from periodontitis and osteoporosis has yet to be demonstrated.

These results show that, although osteoporosis in women is not an etiologic factor in periodontitis, it may affect the severity of the disease in preexisting periodontitis. Women on hormonal replacement therapy experience problems similar to those of oral contraceptive users. Thus, menopausal and postmenopausal women in good gingival health cannot be considered to be at increased risk of periodontal disease.

Cardiovascular Disease

Periodontal Considerations and Management

Epidemiologic studies indicate that many individuals with cardiovascular disease either have periodontal disease or are edentulous. A Finnish group has evidence that, after conventional risk factors for stroke and heart attacks have been accounted for, there still remains a significant relationship between periodontal disease and cardiovascular disease.[45,46] A preliminary analysis of an investigation of the interrelationship of medical and dental health by Loesche[47] suggests that there is a statistical association between edentulousness and cardiovascular disease Loesche[47] suggested that these associations could be coincidental, reflecting a lifestyle of personal neglect, which predisposes to both heart disease and dental disease. He also noted that it is possible that missing teeth and periodontal disease are additional risk factors for heart disease by predisposing the individual to chronic low-grade infection.[47]

Cardiovascular disease affects approximately 43 million people in the United States today.[48] In fact, cardiovascular disorders comprise the highest percentage of serious diseases in the population of this country.[49] Addressing these problems in dentistry primarily involves focusing attention in two areas:

1. The prevention of bacterial endocarditis or endarteritis in patients susceptible to these infections
2. Dental management of the cardiac patient with ischemic heart disease, angina, myocardial infarction, and systemic hypertension[50]

Ischemic Heart Disease

There are two types of angina that the dental practitioner must recognize and treat should they occur in the dental office; stable angina and unstable angina. Stable angina is chest pain that results from a predictable amount of exertion and responds to rest or nitroglycerin. Patients with stable angina may receive dental care in short, minimally stressful morning appointments. Profound local anesthesia is highly recommended to prevent large amounts of endogenous epinephrine from being released in response to pain. The maximum allowed dose of epinephrine is 0.04 mg per appointment for a patient with stable angina. This converts to two cartridges of 1:100,000 epinephrine (0.02 mg of 1:100,000 epinephrine). Premedication with oral sedation, eg, tranquilizers, and nitrous oxide may be indicated.

Unstable angina is chest pain that occurs at rest or after variable amounts of exertion. It represents a significant change in the patient's anginal pattern (ie, new associated symptoms, a change in nitroglycerin response, or a new pain radiation pattern). It does not always respond to nitroglycerin. Patients with unstable angina should receive only emergency or minimal dental care and only after consultation with a physician. The hospital may be the most appropriate environment to provide dental treatment for these patients.

Myocardial Infarction

Myocardial infarction occurs when narrowed atherosclerotic coronary arteries become acutely occluded by a thrombus, leading ultimately to necrosis of the portion of the heart muscle supplied by that artery. The patient generally reports crushing, substernal pain, which frequently radiates to the neck, jaw, or left arm. The pain may be accompanied by shortness of breath, anxiety, nausea, and diaphoresis. The highest risk of death occurs during the first 12 hours, when the risk of ventricular fibrillation is highest.[51] Patients who have sustained a myocardial infarction within the last 6 months are at increased risk of an additional infarction.

Consequently, only minimal treatment for acute dental problems is advised within 6 months of an infarction and that only after consultation with the patient's physician. Elective dental care can usually be provided after 6 months have elapsed following a myocardial infarction. Consultation with the patient's physician is recommended. If no problems are noted, the dentist may proceed with treatment, employing those principles used when caring for the patient with a cardiac disorder, eg, angina. These principles include morning appointments, profound local anesthesia, as well as oral or inhalation sedation, if needed, and close monitoring of the patient's vital signs.

Valvular Heart Disease

The patient with valvular heart disease faces three basic risks: heart failure, hemodynamically significant arrhythmia, and infective endocarditis. The main concern of the periodontist when treating these patients is the possibility of endocarditis. Dental procedures involving manipulation of soft tissue that result in bleeding can produce a transient bacteremia. Bloodborne bacteria may lodge on damaged and abnormal heart valves, in the endocardium, or in the endothelium near congenital anatomic defects, resulting in bacterial endocarditis or endarteritis. It is not possible to predict which patients will develop this infection or which particular procedure will be responsible.[52]

Certain cardiac conditions are more often associated with endocarditis than others. The American Heart Association (AHA) in June 1997 stratified cardiac conditions into high, moderate, and negligible risk categories based on potential outcome if endocarditis develops.[52] Prophylaxis is recommended for individuals in the high and moderate risk categories and not recommended for those in the negligible risk group (Table 5-1).

Mitral valve prolapse (MVP) and the need for prophylaxis has always been a source of controversy. In the new guidelines an algorithm was developed to define more clearly when prophylaxis is recommended for patients with this condition (Fig 5-5).

Antibiotic prophylaxis for at-risk patients is recommended for dental and oral procedures likely to cause bacteremia (Table 5-2).

If a series of dental procedures is required, it may be prudent to observe an interval of 9 to 14 days between procedures to reduce the potential for the emergence of resistant strains of organisms.[52] The recommended standard prophylactic regimens for all dental, oral, and upper respiratory tract procedures are noted in Table 5-3. Some individuals may not be candidates to receive the standard prophylactic regimen. For individuals who are unable to take oral medications, a parenteral medication may be necessary. Table 5-3 also presents the regimens recommended by the AHA.

In addition, the AHA recommends antiseptic mouth rinses applied immediately prior to dental procedures to reduce the incidence or magnitude of bacteremia. Agents include chlorhexidine gluconate and povidone-iodine. At-risk patients can be given 15 mL of chlorhexidine via gentle oral rinsing for about 30 seconds prior to dental treatment; gingival irrigation is not recommended.

Individuals who take oral penicillin for secondary prevention of rheumatic fever or for other purposes may have viridans streptococci in their oral cavities that are relatively resistant to penicillin, amoxicillin, or ampicillin. In such cases, the physician or dentist should select clindamycin,

Table 5-1   Cardiac conditions associated with endocarditis[52]

Endocarditis prophylaxis recommended

High-risk category

Prosthetic cardiac valves, including bioprosthetic and homograft valves
Previous bacterial endocarditis
Complex cyanotic congenital heart disease (eg, single ventricle states, transposition of the great arteries, tetralogy of Fallot)
Surgically constructed systemic pulmonary shunts or conduits

Moderate-risk category

Most other congenital cardiac malformations (other than above and below)
Acquired valvar dysfunction (eg, rheumatic heart disease)
Hypertrophic cardiomyopathy
Mitral valve prolapse with valvar regurgitation and/or thickened leaflets

Endocarditis prophylaxis not recommended

Negligible-risk category
(no greater risk than the general population)

Isolated secundum atrial septal defect
Surgical repair of atrial septal defect, ventricular septal defect, or patent ductus arteriosus (without residua beyond 6 months)
Previous coronary artery bypass graft surgery
Mitral valve prolapse without valvar regurgitation
Physiologic, functional, or innocent heart murmurs
Previous Kawasaki disease without valvar dysfunction
Previous rheumatic fever without valvar dysfunction
Cardiac pacemakers (intravascular and epicardial) and implanted defibrillators

(From Dajani AS, et al.[52] Reprinted with permission.)

Table 5-2   Dental procedures and endocarditis prophylaxis[52]

Endocarditis prophylaxis recommended*

Dental extractions
Periodontal procedures including surgery, scaling and root planing, probing, and recall maintenance
Dental implant placement and reimplantation of avulsed teeth
Endodontic (root canal) instrumentation or surgery only beyond the apex
Subgingival placement of antibiotic fibers or strips
Initial placement of orthodontic bands but not brackets
Intraligamentary local anesthetic injections
Prophylactic cleaning of teeth or implants where bleeding is anticipated

Endocarditis prophylaxis not recommended

Restorative dentistry[†] (operative and prosthodontic) with or without retraction cord[‡]
Local anesthetic injections (nonintraligamentary)
Intracanal endodontic treatment; post placement and buildup
Placement of rubber dams
Postoperative suture removal
Placement of removable prosthodontic or orthodontic appliances
Taking of oral impressions
Fluoride treatments
Taking of oral radiographs
Orthodontic appliance adjustment
Shedding of primary teeth

* Prophylaxis is recommended for patients with high- and moderate-risk cardiac conditions.
† This includes restoration of decayed teeth (filling cavities) and replacement of missing teeth.
‡ Clinical judgment may indicate antibiotic use in selected circumstances that may create significant bleeding.

(From Dajani AS, et al.[52] Reprinted with permission.)

Table 5-3 Prophylactic regimens for dental, oral, respiratory tract, or esophageal procedures[52]

Situation	Agent	Regimen*
Standard general prophylaxis	Amoxicillin	Adults: 2.0 g; children: 50 mg/kg orally 1 hour before procedure
Unable to take oral medications	Ampicillin	Adults: 2.0 g intramuscularly (IM) or intravenously (IV); children: 50 mg/kg IM or IV within 30 minutes before procedure
Allergic to penicillin	Clindamycin	Adults: 600 mg; children: 20 mg/kg orally 1 hour before procedure
	or	
	Cephalexin[†] or cefadroxil[†]	Adults: 2.0 g; children: 50 mg/kg orally 1 hour before procedure
	or	
	Azithromycin or clarithromycin	Adults: 500 mg; children: 15 mg/kg orally 1 hour before procedure
Allergic to penicillin and unable to take oral medications	Clindamycin	Adults: 600 mg; children: 20 mg/kg IV within 30 minutes before procedure
	or	
	Cefazolin[†]	Adults: 1.0 g; children: 25 mg/kg IM or IV within 30 minutes before procedure

* Total children's dose should not exceed adult dose.
† Cephalosporins should not be used in individuals with immediate-type hypersensitivity reaction (urticaria, angioedema, or ana-
phylaxis) to penicillins.

(From Dajani AS, et al.[52] Reprinted with permission.)

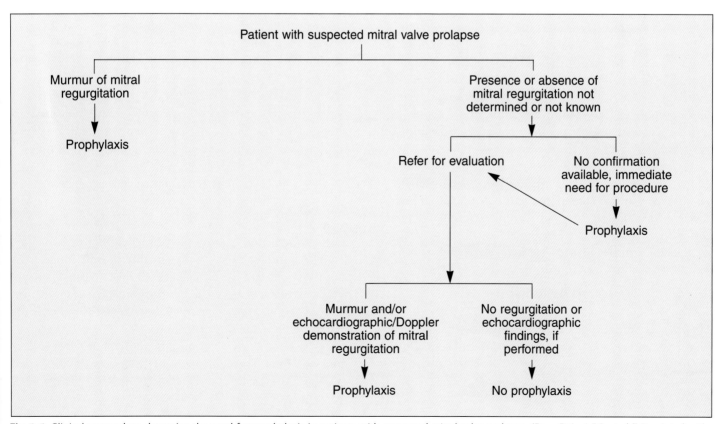

Fig 5-5 Clinical approach to determine the need for prophylaxis in patients with suspected mitral valve prolapse. (From Dajani AS, et al.[52] Reprinted with permission.)

azithromycin, or clarithromycin for endocarditis. Because of possible cross-resistance with the cephalosporins, this class of antibiotics should be avoided.

Individual judgments may have to be made for patients who do not fit established guidelines set forth by the AHA. Infectious disease or cardiology consultation should be obtained as indicated for patients who require multiple, prolonged, or unusual regimens of prophylactic antibiotic coverage. It has been accepted that adequate antibiotic prophylaxis does not preclude infective endocarditis; it only minimizes risks.

Anticoagulation Therapy

Patients with prosthetic valves, thromboembolic phenomena, or other flow disturbances are often therapeutically anticoagulated. Coumarin preparations, eg, warfarin (Coumadin), are the agents currently used for outpatient anticoagulation. The most common therapeutic dose of anticoagulant increases the patient's prothrombin time to twice that of normal clotting time.[53] The range of one and a half to two times the normal clotting time is considered within the range of safety to perform dental procedures likely to cause bleeding. Local measures to achieve hemostasis, including the use of Gelfoam, Surgicel, collagen, direct pressure, and primary closure, should also be taken.

When contemplating procedures likely to cause bleeding, it is appropriate for the dentist to communicate with the physician and request that dosage adjustments be made to keep the prothrombin time between one and a half and two times the control. This adjustment may need to be initiated two to three days prior to the procedure. Frequently, it is necessary to assess prothrombin time the morning of the dental appointment. After dental treatment, the patient should be advised to resume taking the anticoagulant as soon as possible (usually the day of the procedure). Because of the prolonged half-life of Coumadin, initial wound healing will be well under way before the prothrombin time again increases beyond the safe treatment range.

When local hemostatic measures fail in the anticoagulated patient, pharmacologic manipulation becomes necessary.[54] If the anticoagulated patient can tolerate a wait of several hours or more, vitamin K administration will reverse the effect of Coumadin. More urgent situations may require a transfusion of fresh-frozen plasma.

Hypertension

Systemic hypertension, defined as an elevation of arterial blood pressure, is a cardiovascular disorder that affects 10% to 15% of adults. The prevalence of hypertensive heart disease increases sharply with age. Elderly people with blood pressure readings of 140/90 mm Hg or less have a longer life expectancy than do others in their age group with higher blood pressure.[53]

The blood pressure of patients previously identified to have hypertension should be taken at each visit. Elective dental treatment for the patient with uncontrolled hypertension should be as conservative as possible. There are no contraindications to providing dental care for the patient with well-controlled hypertension. Complications and side effects of drugs used to treat hypertension include postural hypotension, mental confusion, depression, drowsiness, and xerostomia.

The use of epinephrine in combination with local anesthetics is not contraindicated in the hypertensive patient unless the systolic blood pressure is higher than 200 mm Hg and/or the diastolic is higher than 115 mm Hg.[55,56] Small amounts of epinephrine, 0.04 mg per appointment (approximately two cartridges containing 1:100,000), are recommended, compared to a maximum of 0.2 mg in a healthy 150-lb adult male (eight 1.8-mL cartridges of 1:100,000 and five and a half 1.8-mL cartridges of 1:50,000).[56] Profound anesthesia is indicated to prevent large amounts of endogenous epinephrine from being released in response to pain. Adequate aspiration is critical to prevent intravascular injection.[57] The use of a vasopressor to control local bleeding and the use of gingival retraction cord with vasopressors are contraindicated. Psychosedation techniques and oral and inhalation sedation, eg, tranquilizers and nitrous oxide, may be useful in treating this group of patients. Caution must be exercised, however, in the use of nitrous oxide for outpatient conscious sedation because hypoxia may produce startling increases in arterial blood pressure with calamitous results.

If general anesthetic agents are indicated, there is the risk for hypotension. Because of this risk, it is not recommended that general anesthetics be used on an outpatient basis in patients with significant hypertensive disease. Medical consultation and care in a hospital setting may be indicated.

Pacemakers

Pacemakers are often placed in patients who have frequent attacks of syncope or episodes of tachycardia or bradycardia. The pulse rate and rhythm quality of individuals with pacemakers should be assessed at each dental visit. There are two basic types of pacemakers: temporary, or transvenous, pacemakers and permanent pacemakers, of which the demand-type is the most common.

If a patient with a temporary transvenous pacemaker requires dental treatment, consultation with the physician concerning the need for antibiotic prophylaxis may be advised. Premedication prophylaxis is not necessary for permanent-type pacemakers, but the demand type of pacemakers are most sensitive to external electromagnetic forces, including pulp testers, ultrasonic scalers and electrosurgery units, and microwave ovens. This was a problem with older pacemakers, which were unipolar and poorly insulated. The new pacemakers are bipolar and better insulated, so that the small amount of electromagnetic radiation generated by dental equipment poses little threat to pacemaker function.[58]

Transplant Therapy

The dentist should participate in the treatment planning for patients about to undergo elective heart transplantation. Active and potential sources of infection should be eliminated, and necessary dental care should be accomplished, whenever possible, before the transplant. Patients who receive a heart transplant on an emergency basis and who have existing dental infection should be given antibiotics before and after the transplant. The decision as to which antibiotic to use is usually determined by the cardiothoracic surgeon with input from the dental practitioner.

Following the heart transplantation, recipients are maintained on immunosuppressive drugs for life. The intent of this immunosuppression is to blunt host rejection of the graft by suppressing T helper cells. These drugs may include cyclosporine, corticosteroids, antilymphocyte globulin, azathioprine, or a combination of these medications. All of the immunosuppressive agents may mask early manifestations of oral infection. Oral mucosal lesions suggestive of herpes simplex, candidiasis, or other fungal infections should be evaluated by cytologic examination, culture, and/or biopsy when indicated. These infections may lead to severe or disseminated disease in immunosuppressed patients and must be detected early so that antimicrobial therapy can be instituted.

Prophylactic antibiotics are recommended for all dental procedures likely to cause a bacteremia in patients taking immunosuppressive drugs. In addition, application of chlorhexidine to the surgical site may reduce the incidence of bacteremia.[52] In patients taking cyclosporine, the incidence of gingival hyperplasia exists. Cyclosporine-induced gingival hyperplasia is estimated to affect 30% of posttransplantation patients, and its rate of development is more rapid than is phenytoin-induced hyperplasia.[58] For patients taking adrenal-suppressive doses of corticosteroids, supplementations of steroids may be necessary prior to "stressful" dental procedures.

Hematologic Disorders

Acute Leukemias

Acute leukemias are cancers of the blood-forming organs, causing marrow failure and infiltration of various organs and tissues by blast cells. Once the leukemic process has been initiated, there is a progressive expansion of the leukemic population, especially stem cells.

Intraoral Signs and Symptoms

Intraoral signs and symptoms of leukemia are related to the severity of the deficiency of the mature normal white blood cells, red blood cells, and platelets. Other oral signs are caused by infiltration of leukemic cells into the oral tissues and side effects of chemotherapeutic drugs used to treat the disease.

It has been reported that there are oral lesions in more than 80% of patients with acute monocytic leukemia, in 40% of patients with acute myeloid leukemia, and in more than 20% of those with lymphoid leukemia.[59]

Acute leukemia frequently causes a massive infiltration of leukemic cells into the gingival tissues (Fig 5-6). The gingiva appears to have lost its normal contour and texture. It is hyperplastic, edematous, and bluish red, with blunting of the interdental papillae. Varying degrees of gingival inflammation, ulceration, and necrosis have been noted.[60–62]

Oral mucosal ulcers are common in patients with leukemia. These lesions may result from bacterial invasion caused by severe leukopenia or from mucosal atrophy caused by the direct effect of the chemotherapeutic drugs on the epithelial cells. Trauma from a dental prosthesis or teeth may result in large, secondarily infected ulcers that progress to facial cellulitis and septicemia.

Treatment

The oral complications that occur during leukemia may cause considerable difficulty for the patient. Toxemia, septicemia, gingival hemorrhage, marked discomfort and pain, and loss of appetite are a few of the complications that may arise. During the acute phase of the disease, only those procedures that are necessary to alleviate the pain, discomfort, and hemorrhaging should be performed.

On the other hand, during a period of remission every attempt should be made to achieve a state of periodontal health. The treatment should be conservative, consisting of the removal of all local irritants and instruction in good plaque control techniques. Treatment procedures involving long periods of time should be avoided.

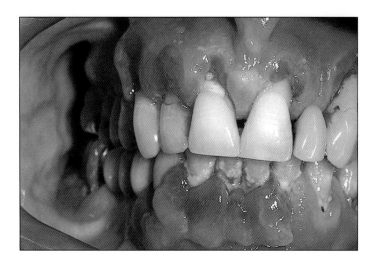

Fig 5-6 Oral manifestations of acute leukemia.

Thrombocytopenia

Severe gingival bleeding resulting from thrombocytopenia can often be managed successfully with localized treatment. The use of an absorbable gelatin sponge with topical thrombin or placement of microfibrillar collagen is often sufficient. Some authors have reported successful management of gingival bleeding with oral rinses of antifibrinolytic agents.[59] If these measures are not successful in stopping blood flow from an oral site, platelet transfusions may be necessary.

Two major types of thrombocytopenia purpura have been described. Primary (idiopathic) thrombocytopenic purpura is of unknown etiology. This is a relatively common form of the disease and occurs at any age. Secondary thrombocytopenia is due to a known etiologic factor, such as chemicals or drugs.

Oral Manifestations

The oral manifestations of thrombocytopenia may represent the initial signs of the disease. *Purpura*, the most common oral sign, is defined as any escape of blood into subcutaneous and/or submucosal tissues and includes petechiae and ecchymoses, which are often seen on the tongue, lips, and occlusal line of the buccal mucosa secondary to minor trauma. Purpura may be differentiated from vascular lesions by direct application of pressure on the area. These lesions will not blanch; they may be induced on the palate from the suction created by a complete denture. Other oral signs include spontaneous gingival hemorrhage and prolonged bleeding following trauma, toothbrushing, extractions, or periodontal therapy. Similar purpuric lesions are found on the skin. The patient may have a positive history of epistaxis, hematuria, melena, and increased menstrual bleeding.

Gingival biopsy is helpful in the diagnosis of thrombotic thrombocytopenic purpura because the gingiva is readily accessible, highly vascular, and amenable to hemostasis.

Treatment

Spontaneous gingival bleeding can usually be managed by oxidizing mouthwashes, but platelet transfusions may be required to stop the bleeding. Good oral hygiene and conservative periodontal therapy will help to remove plaque and calculus, which potentiate the bleeding. Accidental trauma can be avoided by replacing ill-fitting prostheses and removing all orthodontic appliances. These patients should be cautioned not to sleep with any removable prosthesis in place.

Emergency care during severe thrombocytopenic episodes consists of endodontic therapy, and when indicated, the administration of antibiotics and nonsalicylate analgesics. A stab incision and drainage may be performed, but blunt dissection of an abscessed area is to be avoided. Definitive dental treatment should be delayed until normal platelet function returns. Platelet levels greater than 50,000 mm³ are desired before dental treatment, and further transfusions are given as needed postoperatively to maintain hemostasis.

Block injections are to be avoided if the platelet count is below 30,000 mm³ because of the possibility of hematoma formation and airway obstruction. Infiltration anesthesia is used instead. Aspirin-containing analgesics are contraindicated because they may potentiate bleeding. Any drug that has previously induced a thrombocytopenic episode should not be used. Frequently, these patients are treated with steroids, which may further complicate dental treatment.

Hemophilia

Classic hemophilia (hemophilia A) is an inherited deficiency of functional factor VIII; the associated bleeding tendency is proportional to the severity of the deficiency. It is the most common inherited disorder of coagulation and is associated with serious and often apparently spontaneous bleeding. Individuals with mild hemophilia (5% to 25% of normal levels of factor VIII) *may* have little or no increase in bleeding and escape detection for years, whereas those with hemophilia of intermediate severity (factor VIII levels that are 1% to 4% of normal) usually have no spontaneous bleeding but may have bleeding with surgery or trauma.

Clinical Manifestations

The clinical manifestations of hemophilia A are directly related to the level of factor VIII. Hemarthroses are common clinical problems. In decreasing order of frequency, they involve the knee, ankle, hip, elbow, wrist, and shoulder. There is often a history of preceding trauma or stress, but this may be relatively minor. Classic hemophilia is treated by intravenous infusion of normal human factor VIII, in the form of cryoprecipitate or lyophilized concentrate. A plasma factor VIII level of higher than 30% must be achieved to halt bleeding.

Oral Manifestations

Episodic, prolonged bleeding, either spontaneous or traumatic, is the most common oral presentation. Bleeding from the nose, mouth, and lips may be severe. Hemarthroses, which may lead to ankylosis and erosion of the temporomandibular joint surface, are incapacitating and painful.

Treatment

Dental management should be directed toward prevention. Good oral hygiene will aid in the reduction of gingival bleeding. Oral prophylaxis can generally be accomplished without factor replacement. Bleeding caused by supragingival ultrasonic scaling or rubber cup prophylaxis is controlled by the platelets. However, deep scaling can cause serious hemorrhage in patients who have not had factor replacement.

Hematomas can be prevented by taking care during placement of radiographic film, when using high-speed vacuum and saliva ejectors, and in all oral tissue management. Foam rubber–tipped or gauze-padded instruments can minimize hematoma formation.

The administration of local anesthesia is a major concern in dental treatment. Dissecting hematomas, airway obstruction, and death are known complications of block anesthesia in hemophiliac patients. Injections should not be given unless the patient has a plasma factor VIII level of 50% or greater.

Periodontal surgery should be performed only if the anticipated therapeutic benefits outweigh the possibility of severe postoperative complications. No factor replacement is needed for probing and careful supragingival scaling. Replacement is necessary preceding deep scaling, curettage, and surgery. The objective of periodontal therapy in hemophiliac patients is to control gingival inflammation to an extent that allows the patient to perform oral hygiene and allows the therapist to perform maintenance and instrumentation with minimal fear of bleeding problems.

Surgical treatment has often been avoided because of the potential for continued bleeding. Before any surgery, complete coagulation studies, factor levels, and red cell types should be obtained. The patient should be tested for inhibitors, and replacement therapy should be available. Chemical cautery or electrosurgery should be avoided because of the possibility of tissue necrosis and secondary bleeding, and aspirin-containing analgesics should not be prescribed. All hemophiliac patients should be tested for hepatitis and human immunodeficiency virus (HIV) because of the quantity of blood products and transfusions they have received. Dental treatment is maximized while the patient is receiving replacement therapy. Therefore, the number of visits to achieve the desired results should be minimized.

Osteoporosis

Osteoporosis is a metabolic bone disorder and the most common cause of osteopenia in the elderly. It represents a disease state of skeletal metabolism in which the rate of bone matrix formation is depressed and is thus unable to compensate for the excessive resorption. Ossification is normal, but there is inadequate matrix to ossify.

Dental Considerations

The mandible, in addition to the long bones and vertebrae, may exhibit changes related to generalized osteoporosis. Although most patients with osteoporosis do not suffer from an underlying systemic disease, certain disease states cause a decrease in mineral density that may become apparent in the mandible and alveolar bone. For this reason, changes in the mandible and alveolar bone can be an important means of recognizing systemic diseases.

Osteoporosis of the mandible is usually manifested by a decrease in trabeculation. However, a decrease in mineral content of 30% to 50% is required before diminished bone density becomes apparent on dental radiographs. It has been shown that the densities of the mandible and radius are similarly affected by age; both show a comparable decrease in mineral density with increasing age.[63,64] Periodic, routine dental radiographs provide a means to compare density changes in the mandible over a period of time.

Acquired Immunodefiency Syndrome

Oral manifestations are very common early signs of symptomatic HIV infection, and more than 95% of AIDS patients will have oral changes during the course of their illness.[65] A comprehensive examination of the head, neck, and oral cavity for all patients can be very helpful in locating and monitoring orofacial conditions that are sometimes associated with HIV infection. Because orofacial manifestations of HIV infections are treatable, dental consultation should be sought promptly when these conditions develop. Oral infection can become life threatening in the severely immunocompromised patient.

For the purposes of this discussion, emphasis will be placed on HIV-associated periodontal lesions. However, some of the aforementioned oral problems may affect the gingiva as well (Kaposi's sarcoma, herpetic lesions, etc).

Periodontal Lesions Associated With HIV

Types

Unique forms of periodontal disease have been discovered in individuals infected with human immunodeficiency virus. Intraoral lesions may in fact be one of the first signs of HIV infection. Although the frequency of HIV-associated periodontal disease appears to be less than was previously thought, many researchers agree that an important factor influencing the prevalence of unique periodontal disease in the HIV population is the degree of immunodeficiency.[66]

The pathogenesis of HIV-associated periodontal diseases remains unclear but may be the result of a specific microflora and/or alterations in the host response.[66] Periodontal disease associated with HIV infection shows more severe signs and symptoms, responds less to standard periodontal therapy, progresses rapidly, and may be associated with a greater degree of tissue loss, bone exposure, and sequestration than conventional periodontal disease.

Both HIV gingivitis (HIV-G), presently called *linear gingival erythema* (LGE), and HIV periodontitis (HIV-P), now called *necrotizing ulcerative periodontitis* (NUP), have microbiologic profiles similar to that of conventional adult periodontitis, although these lesions are quite different clinically.[66]

Clinical Characteristics of Linear Gingival Erythema (Formerly HIV Gingivitis)

- Erythematous linear banding, usually 2 mm wide
- Diffuse petechial redness
- Minimal response to therapy
- Subtle lesion that may go unnoticed by an untrained examiner
- Early indicator of HIV infection
- Not associated with low T4-cell counts

Clinical Characteristics of Necrotizing Ulcerative Periodontitis

- Severe, deep pain
- Spontaneous gingival bleeding
- Extensive soft tissue necrosis
- Severe loss of periodontal attachment
- Rapid onset and progression
- Exposed osseous tissues
- Associated with low T4-cell counts

In addition to LGE and NUP, acute necrotizing ulcerative gingivitis has been associated with HIV infection. Differentiating between ANUG and NUP can be difficult. Both ANUG and NUP may, in some patients, progress to necrotizing stomatitis, which is characterized by extensive soft tissue necrosis, exposure of bone, and sequestration of dead bone fragments. Necrotizing stomatitis represents the most severe form of periodontal infection associated with HIV and is one of the more serious oral infections of HIV disease; in fact, it can be life threatening.

Treatment

Patients infected with HIV can safely receive dental care. The timing or extent of the treatment plan may need to be modified according to the patient's immunologic and hematologic status and general medical condition. Appropriate emergency treatment should be rendered and pain should be relieved in all stages of the disease.

Before periodontal treatment is initiated in the patient with HIV, it is prudent to consult with the patient's physician to establish the patient's current status. If severe thrombocytopenia is present, platelet replacement may be needed before surgical procedures are performed. Also, it must be determined if prophylactic antibiotics are needed to protect the patient with severe immune suppression from postoperative infection. Antibiotic prophylaxis before dental treatment is *not* indicated solely because of the patient's HIV-positive status. The decision to use prophylactic antibiotics depends on the concomitant medical condition, the procedure to be performed, and the patient's degree of immunodeficiency.

The rapidly progressive nature and severity of necrotizing ulcerative periodontitis requires early aggressive debridement of the local etiologic factors. Intrasulcular lavage with 10% povidone-iodine solution during debridement is suggested. Systemic broad-spectrum antibiotics should rarely be prescribed because of the potential for fungal overgrowth. Metronidazole, 250 mg, four times daily for 3 to 5 days, has been demonstrated to be effective during the acute treatment phase and to minimize fungal overgrowth.[67] If clinical signs and laboratory evidence of fungus are present, use of appropriate antifungal therapy is recommended.

With effective initial debridement and the use of suggested adjunctive chemotherapeutic agents, rapid resolution of even severe NUP lesions should be obtained. Good oral hygiene practices must be employed. Two or 3 days after the initial treatment, follow-up debridement, scaling, and root planing should be performed. Long-term management of periodontal health may be achieved but may require more frequent recall visits, excellent home care, and the use of a chemotherapeutic mouth rinse. Chlorhexidine (0.12%) mouthrinse, used twice daily, appears to be effective in long-term management of HIV-associated periodontal disease.[67]

Pharmacologic Considerations

Phenytoin

Gingival overgrowth occurs in about half of all individuals who ingest phenytoin on a chronic regimen as their sole antiepileptic medication. However, the prevalence of gingival overgrowth is much higher than it is when phenytoin is taken in combination with other antiepileptic agents. Both sexes and all races are susceptible to phenytoin-induced gingival overgrowth. Teenagers and young adults to about 30 years of age are affected more frequently than are middle-aged or elderly persons. The anterior labial surfaces of the maxillary and mandibular gingiva are most commonly and severely affected.

The earliest clinical signs of gingival change, soreness and tenderness, may occur 2 to 3 weeks after phenytoin therapy is started. Gingival overgrowth often becomes clinically apparent during the first 6 to 9 months of therapy, as interdental papillae overgrow and extrude, forming firm, mobile, triangular tissue masses. These increase in magnitude during the ensuing 1 to 2 years and may fuse mesially and distally and form a continuous curtain of overgrown marginal gingiva; maximum size is usually achieved within that time.[68]

Some disagreement exists as to the relationship between drug dosage and the severity of overgrowth. But the majority of studies do not support a statistically valid connection.[69]

Treatment of gingival enlargement may involve replacing phenytoin with an alternative drug, eg, carbamizipine or sodium valproate, in consultation with the patients physician. Conservative periodontal therapy, including frequent professional prophylaxis and a rigorous oral hygiene regimen, is recommended because the preponderance of evidence suggests that meticulous plaque control will prevent or significantly decrease the severity of the hyperplasia.[69] Surgical reduction of the hyperplastic tissue may be necessary if there is interference with function or appearance. Recurrence of overgrowth should be expected within 1 to 2 years, particularly in individuals under the age of 25 years, if the phenytoin regimen is continued.[70] If oral hygiene is poor, the recurrence of overgrowth may occur even sooner.

Cyclosporine

Cyclosporine has been used in the United States since 1984 for prevention of rejection phenomena following solid organ and bone marrow transplantation. Clinical trials currently ongoing in the United States may lead to approval by the US Food and Drug Administration for greatly expanded use of cyclosporine in the near future. Because of its effectiveness in so many disorders, it has been estimated that more than 1 billion persons worldwide will be taking cyclosporine in the next decade.

Cyclosporine exerts its effects by selective suppression of specific subpopulations of T lymphocytes, interfering with production of lymphokines and interleukins 1 and 2.[70]

The gingival lesions associated with cyclosporine are often clinically and histologically indistinguishable from those elicited by phenytoin. The clinical course is also similar, in that the lesions generally originate in the interdental area; all segments of the dental arch may be affected.

Calcium Channel Blockers

Nifedipine (Procardia) is a substituted dihydrophyridine used widely since 1978 in the treatment of angina pectoris and postmyocardia syndrome. It has been reported to induce gingival overgrowth in patients with heart disease. The gingival lesions elicited by nifedipine in humans are clinically similar to those elicited by phenytoin and cyclosporine. All segments of the dentition are susceptible to dihydropyridine-induced overgrowth, but the anterior facial aspects are most frequently and severely affected (Fig 5-7). Secondary inflammatory manifestations are common because oral hygiene is compromised by the excess tissue. The histopathologic picture is one of thickened epithelia that exhibit elongation of epithelial rete; the preponderance of redundant tissue is composed of connective tissue with abundant fibroblasts. Extracellular ground substance also appears to be in excess.

Clinical experience suggests that establishment of excellent plaque control and regular scaling and root planing will aid in preventing and moderating nifedipine overgrowth.

Verapamil hydrochloride (Calan) is another commonly prescribed calcium antagonist. Although structurally similar to nifedipine, it has not been associated with gingival overgrowth.

Cancer Chemotherapeutic Agents

Control of malignancies by chemotherapeutic agents has emerged in recent years as the primary treatment or as an adjunct to surgery and radiation. The actions of these drugs produce toxic effects on the body, both directly at the cellular level and indirectly by myeloimmunosuppression of the hematopoietic and lymphoid tissues.

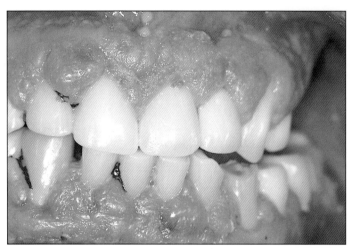

Fig 5-7 Gingival hyperplasia secondary to the use of calcium channel blockers.

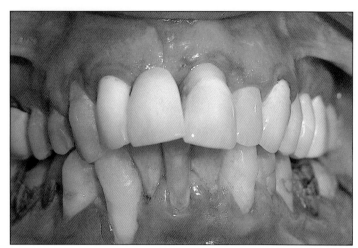

Fig 5-8 Acute periodontal infection in a patient on myelosuppressive chemotherapy.

Effects on the Periodontium

The diseased periodontium is a potential source of acute systemic infection in patients receiving myelosuppressive chemotherapy.[71,72] Acute periodontal infections in patients undergoing chemotherapy can occur in a setting of preexistent chronic periodontal diseases[72,73] (Fig 5-8). The exacerbation of preexisting periodontal disease is associated with elevated levels of periodontopathic organisms during episodes of granulocytopenia.[74]

Evaluation of Patients on Chemotherapeutic Agents

The periodontist should be aware of the emotional and physical needs of the patient and should know and understand the changes in the overall health of the patient. As a specialist, the periodontist should know the changes in the periodontium that chemotherapy may cause. The patient should have comprehensive clinical and radiographic regional examinations, with particular emphasis on those sites known to cause problems during chemotherapy, eg, infected or unrestorable teeth, ill-fitting prostheses, and sites affected by periodontal disease.

The examination must be done with full knowledge of the patient's hematologic parameters. Complications may arise if the therapy is aggressive and blood values are dangerously low. The absolute granulocyte count should be greater than $1,000/mm^3$ and the platelet count greater than $100,000 \ mm^3$ before any non-urgent dental procedures are undertaken. Prothrombin time should also be considered.[75]

Treatment of Patients on Chemotherapeutic Agents

Ideally, oral sources of bacteremia, eg, periodontal disease, hopeless teeth, pericoronal flaps, and periapical pathosis, should be eliminated prior to the onset of chemotherapy. If an emergent dental problem arises during chemotherapy

and significant deficiencies are noted in the blood cell count, a transfusion of blood components and broad-spectrum parenteral antibiotic prophylaxis must be considered before treatment. If the patient is scheduled to receive blood component transfusions as part of the supportive regimen, the emergent dental problem can usually be treated palliatively, and definitive dental treatment can be scheduled immediately following the transfusion.

Only the minimum necessary dental intervention should be provided to control acute dental problems occurring during active phases of myelosuppression secondary to chemotherapy. Review of the patient's hematologic profile and consultation with the physician responsible for the patient's care are mandatory.

After chemotherapy has been completed, definitive dental care may be provided for the patient. Consultation and coordination with the oncologist are mandatory. Again, the patient's hematologic status and the need for antibiotic prophylaxis should be considered.

Frequent recalls, management of symptoms, and aggressive preventive intervention should be part of the medical and dental treatment of patients receiving chemotherapy. Prescription of 0.12% chlorhexidine mouthrinse to reduce fungal and bacterial overgrowth is suggested.

If the gingival tissue bleeds easily or the granulocyte count is low, toothbrushing should be discontinued, and the teeth should be cleansed with moist gauze wrapped around the finger. Commercial mouthwashes dry the tissue, and their use should be avoided. Removable prostheses should not be worn while the patient is sleeping or at any time if they cause irritation to the tissue. Denture-soaking solutions should be changed daily.

Topical analgesics may be prescribed to provide relief from painful mucositis or ulceration. Viscous lidocaine 2%, lidocaine ointment 5%, dyclonine 1%, and diphenhydramine 0.5% mixed with milk of magnesia suspension, Kaopectate,

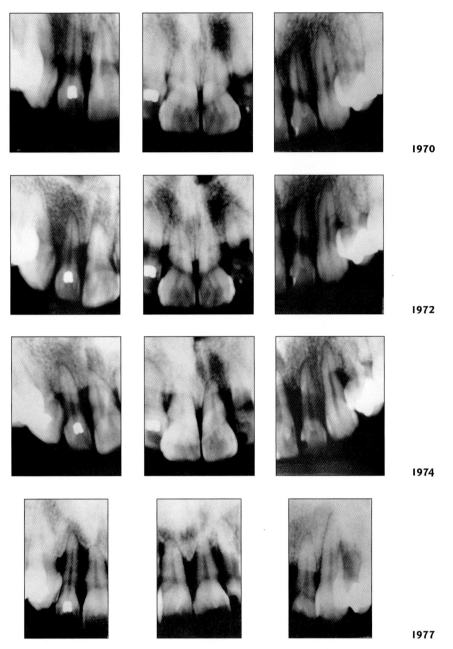

1970

1972

1974

1977

Fig 5-9 Effects of stress on the periodontium over 7 years.

or other topical analgesics can be applied ad lib to areas of painful mucositis or ulceration. In severe cases, use of topical cocaine or parenteral narcotics may be necessary.

Stress

There are many forms of stress, such as trauma, drug intoxication, and muscular fatigue, that may compromise the health of an individual. The systemic reactions that affect the body generally produce an interrelated nonspecific tissue change resulting from continued exposure to stress; these changes have been termed the *general adaptation syn-* *drome*. Thus, the adaptive mechanisms of the body in response to stress may reduce disease.

Relationship to Periodontal Disease

Resorption of alveolar bone, epithelial sloughing, degeneration of the periodontal ligament, reduced osteoblastic activity,[76] the formation of periodontal pockets,[77] and delayed wound healing of connective tissue and bone[78] have all been associated with stress (Fig 5-9).

Acute necrotizing ulcerative gingivitis is the periodontal disease reported to have a significant relationship to stress (Fig 5-10). Investigators have also suggested that emotional

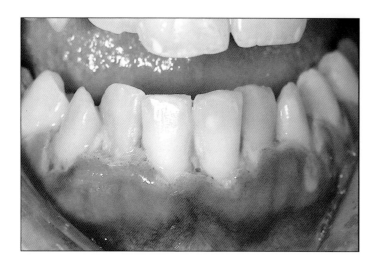

Fig 5-10 Acute necrotizing ulcerative gingivitis.

stress may affect the gingiva directly or indirectly. The direct route involves overt habits that may include poor oral hygiene, poor dietary habits, and smoking. Stress may alter the resistance of the periodontium to infection by acting on the autonomic nervous system and the endocrine system to affect such factors as circulating antibodies and gingival circulation. It has been hypothesized that the constriction of blood vessels that results from continual severe emotional upset may be a complicating or causative factor in the pathogenesis of periodontal disease. Constant vasoconstriction could result in a lack of oxygen and nutrients to the periodontal tissues.[79]

Researchers have noted a relationship between stress and the microbial flora associated with periodontal disease. The identified specific bacteria that were considered to be pathogenic for ANUG and implicated *Porphyromonus (Bacteroides) intermedius* as a significant bacterial entity in ANUG. Increased clinical steroid levels associated with stress may also be a precipitating factor. By weakening host inflammatory response, and by inducing ischemia in the gingiva, bacterial invasion may be enhanced. Corticosteroids may be an important nutritional factor of *P intermedius*, thus providing the organisms with a selective nutrient advantage, with subsequent overgrowth and increased inflammatory response.[80]

It has also been suggested that elevated levels of cortisol may produce alterations in the immune system.[81] These alterations may account for the decreased chemotactic and phagocytic response of polymorphonuclear leukocytes.

Treatment

In severely stressed patients, periodontal therapy is frequently dictated by the dentist's ability to communicate and motivate the patient. The dentist should consider referral of the patient to a psychiatrist or clinical psychologist for additional therapy if necessary. This may significantly enhance the result of periodontal treatment.

Cigarette Smoking and Periodontal Disease

Cigarette smoking is a risk factor for many diseases, and recent evidence indicates that it adversely affects periodontal health. A number of epidemiologic studies have shown strong associations between smoking and the prevalence and severity of periodontitis. There are data suggesting that smoking causes defects in neutrophil function, impairs serum antibody responses to periodontal pathogens, and potentially diminishes gingival fibroblast function.[82]

Periodontitis is less prevalent and less severe in former smokers than in current smokers, providing evidence that smoking cessation is beneficial. Smoking influences the response to treatment; smokers predominate among patients with refractory periodontitis that is resistant to conventional treatment. A patient's smoking history is a useful clinical predictor of future disease activity. During the last decade, a number of studies have reported strong associations between cigarette smoking and alveolar bone loss, tooth loss, and the prevalence and severity of periodontitis. Data suggest that the effect of smoking is direct and not caused by poor oral hygiene and increased dental plaque.[82]

There is evidence that cigarette smoking exerts both systemic and local effects. The reports that smokers with periodontitis have less gingival bleeding and inflammation than

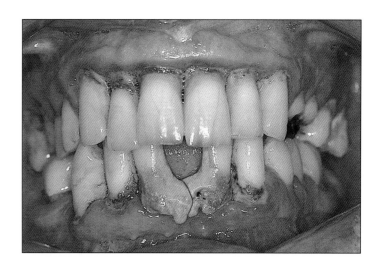

Fig 5-11 Gingiva associated with a heavy smoker.

nonsmokers support the hypothesis that smoking exerts local effects. Tobacco smoke contains cytotoxic and vasoactive substances, including nicotine, which can mediate the local effects. In addition, the pattern of pocketing in smokers differs from that in people who have never smoked. Smokers have proportionately more periodontal pocketing in the anterior segments of their dentition than those who have never smoked, a finding suggestive of local effects.

The documented systemic effects of cigarette smoking include inhibition of peripheral blood and oral neutrophil function, reduced antibody production, and alteration of peripheral blood immunoregulatory T–cell subset ratios. In addition, smoking is known to be associated with a reduction of skeletal bone mineral content. Studies suggest that the increased susceptibility of smokers is not related to the proliferation of a selected or an unusual bacterial species.[82]

Clinical Characteristics of Smokers

Smokers often present at a young age (20 to 30 years) with relatively severe and widespread periodontal disease, in which the gingival margins do not appear red or edematous, although significant bleeding and suppuration on probing are present. Smoking can mask the early signs of periodontal disease by suppressing the gingival inflammatory response.

Gingival pocketing tends to be proportionately greater in the anterior segments and maxillary lingual areas. There is often gingival recession, especially around the maxillary and mandibular anterior teeth. When recession occurs interdentally, it is often seen where gingival embrasures are constricted or narrow; the marginal gingiva tends to be thick and fibrotic with rolled margins (Fig 5-11). Frequently there is no relationship between the patient's periodontal status and plaque scores.

Smokers also respond differently when treated. In response to scaling, reduction of gingival pocket depth in smokers is minimal,[83] while repocketing within 1 year of surgical treatment is common.[84] Treated smokers tend to exhibit attachment loss over time while undergoing maintenance therapy. These findings are particularly interesting in view of recent analyses that showed that 86% to 90% of patients with refractory periodontitis were current smokers.[85,86] The efficacy of surgical treatment of current smokers needs to be evaluated because smoking, particularly heavy smoking, seems to be a contraindication for surgical treatment. These patients heal poorly and exhibit repocketing and continued attachment loss. Smoking-associated periodontitis should be considered a separate disease category, given the unique clinical appearance and behavior of the tissues of these patients.

References

1. Genco RJ. Current view of risk factors for periodontal diseases. J Periodontol 1996;67:1041–1049.

2. Daniel MA, Van Dyke TE. Alterations in phagoctye function and periodontal infection. J Periodontol 1996;67:1070–1076.

3. Grossi SG, Zambon JJ, Norderyd CM, et al. Microbiological risk indicators for periodontal disease. J Dent Res 1993;72:206.

4. Haber J, Wattes J, Crowley R. Assessment of diabetes as a risk factor for periodontitis [abstract]. J Dent Res 1991;70:414.

5. Mandell, RL, DiRienzo J, Kent R, Joshipura K, Haber J. Microbiology of healthy and diseased periodontal sites in poorly controlled insulin-dependent diabetics. J Periodontol 1992;63:274–279.

6. Mashimo PA, Yamamoto Y, Slots J, Park BH, Genco RJ. The periodontal microflora of juvenile diabetics. J Periodontol 1983; 54:420–430.

7. Zambon JJ, Reynolds H, Fisher JG, Shlossman M, Dunford R, Genco RJ. Microbiological and immunological studies of adult periodontitis in patients with noninsulin-dependent diabetes mellitus. J Periodontol 1988;59:20–31.

8. Manuouchehr-pour M, Spagnuolo PJ, Rodman HM, Biassada NF. Comparison of neutrophil chemotactic response in diabetic patients with mild and severe periodontal disease. J Periodontol 1981; 52:410–414.

9. Van Dyke TE, Horoszewicz HU, Cianciola LJ, Genco RJ. Neutrophil chemotaxis dysfunction in human periodontitis. Infect Immun 1980;27:124.

10. Grossi SG, et al. Response to periodontal therapy in diabetics and smokers. J Periodontol 1996;67:1094–1102.

11. Molvig J, Baek L, Christensen P, et al. Endotoxin-stimulated human monocyte secretion of interleukin 1, tumor necrosis factor alpha and prostaglandin E2 shows stable interindividual difference. Scand J Immunol 1988;27:706–716.

12. Todd JA. Genetic control of autoimmunity in type I diabetes. Immun Today 1990;11:122–129.

13. Katz J, Goultschin J, Benoliel R, Brautbar C. Human leukocyte antigen (HLA) DR 4 positive association with rapidly progressing periodontitis. J Periodontol 1987;58:607–610.

14. Hennessey PJ, Black CT, Andrassy RJ. EGF increases short-term type I collagen accumulation during wound healing in diabetic rats. J Pediatr Surg 1990;25:75–78.

15. Grotendorst GR, Martin GR, Pencer D, Sodek J, Harvey AK. Stimulation of granulation tissue formation by platelet-derived growth factor in normal and diabetic rats. J Clin Invest 1985;76:2323–2329.

16. Hennessey PJ, Black CT, Andrassy RJ. Epidermal growth factor and insulin act synergistically during diabetic healing. Arch Surg 1990;125:926–929.

17. Miller LS, Manwell MA, Newbold D, et al. The relationship between reduction in periodontal inflammation and diabetes control: a report of 9 cases. J Periodontol 1992;63:843–848.

18. Sastrowijoto SH, van der Velden U, van Steenbergen TJ, et al. Improved metabolic control, clinical periodontal status and subgingival microbiology in insulin-dependent diabetes mellitus. A prospective study. J Clin Periodontol 1990;17:233–242.

19. Worthington J, Saxe SR, McKean HE. Dental plaque in diabetic vs. non-diabetic patients [abstract]. J Dent Res 1991;70:1184.

20. Safkan SB, Anaimo J. Periodontal conditions in insulin dependent diabetes mellitus. J Clin Periodontol 1992;19:24–29.

21. Anaimo J, Lahtinen A, Vitto VJ. Rapid periodontal destruction in adult humans with poorly controlled diabetes. A report of 2 cases. J Clin Periodontol 1990;17:22–28.

22. Bay I, Anaimo J, Gad I. The response of young diabetics to periodontal treatment. J Periodontol 1974;45:806–816.

23. Kornman KS, Loesche WJ. Effects of estradiol and progesterone on *Bacteroides melaninogenicus* [abstract]. J Dent Res 1979;58A:107.

24. Gusberti FA, Mombelli A, Lang NP, Minder CE. Changes in subgingival microbiota during puberty. J Clin Periodontol 1990;17:685–692.

25. Holm-Pedersen P, Löe H. Flow of gingival exudate as related to menstruation and pregnancy. J Periodont Res 1967;2:13–20.

26. Cohen DW, Friedman L, Shapiro JA. A longitudinal investigation of the periodontal changes during pregnancy. J Periodontol 1969; 40:563–570.

27. Hasson E. Pregnancy gingivitis. Harefuah 1966;58:224–230.

28. Lundgren D, Magnussen B, Lindhe J. Connective tissue alterations in gingiva of rats treated with estrogens and progesterone. Odontol Rev 1973;24:49–58.

29. Löe H, Silness J. Periodontal disease in pregnancy. Acta Odontol Scand 1963;553.

30. Kornman KS, Loesche WJ. The subgingival microflora during pregnancy. J Periodont Res 1980;15:111–122.

31. Ojanotko-Harri AO, Harri MP, Hurttia HM, Sewon LA. Altered tissue metabolism of progesterone in pregnancy gingivitis and granuloma. J Clin Periodontol 1991;18:262–266.

32. Kornman KS, Loesche WJ. Effects of estradiol and progesterone on *Bacteroides melaninogenicus* and *Bacteroides gingivalis*. Infect Immun 1982;35:256–263.

33. Raber-Durlacher JE, Leene W, Palmer-bourva CCR, Raber J, Abraham-Inpijin L. Experimental gingivitis during pregnancy and post-partum: immunohistochemical aspects. J Periodontol 1993; 64:211–218.

34. O'Neill TCA. Maternal T-lymphocyte response and gingivitis in pregnancy. J Periodontol 1979;50:178–184.

35. Pindborg J. Atlas of Diseases of the Oral Mucosa. ed 4. Philadelphia: Saunders, 1985:228.

36. Alcox R. Biologic effect and radiation protection in the dental office. Dent Clin North Am 1978;22:517–532.

37. Rose LF. Sex hormonal imbalances, oral manifestations and dental treatment. In: Genco RJ, Goldman HM, Cohen DW (eds). Contemporary Periodontics. St. Louis: Mosby, 1990:221–227.

38. Lynn B. "The pill" as an etiologic agent in hypertrophic gingivitis. Oral Surg Oral Med Oral Pathol 1967;24:333–336.

39. el-Ashiry GM, el-Kafrawy AH, Nasr MD, Younis N. Effects of oral contraceptives on the gingiva. J Periodontol 1971;42:273–275.

40. Lindhe J, Bjorn AL. Influence of hormonal contraception on the gingiva of women. J Periodont Res 1967;2:1–6.

41. Kalkwarf KL. Effect of oral contraceptive therapy on gingival inflammation in humans. J Periodontol 1978;49:560–563.

42. Knight GM, Wade AB. The effects of hormonal contraception on the human periodontium. J Periodont Res 1974;14:18–22.

43. Moschil AI, Volozhin AI, Smetnik VP, Kangel'dieva AA. Status of tissue mineralization and the periodontium in women with impaired ovarian function. Akush Ginekol (Mosk) 1991;87:801.

44. Groen JJ, Menzel J, Shapiro S. Chronic destructive periodontal disease in patients with pre-senile osteoporosis. J Periodontol 1968;39:19–23.

45. Syrjanen J, Peltola J, Valtonen V, et al. Dental infections in association with cerebral infarction in young and middle-aged men. J Intern Med 1989;225:179–184.

46. Matila KJ, Nieminen MS, Valtonen VV, et al. Association between dental health and acute myocardial infarction. Br Med J 1989; 298:779–783.

47. Loesche WJ. Periodontal disease as a risk factor for heart disease. Compend Contin Educ Dent 1994;15:976–981.

48. Medically Compromised Patient—Cardiovascular Disorders. A Self Instructional Series in Rehabilitation Dentistry, Module IV, Unit A. Seattle: University of Washington, 1986.

49. ADA Oral Health Care Guidelines. Patients with cardiovascular disease. Chicago: American Dental Association, Oct 1993:1–15.

50. Thornton JB, Wright JT. Special and Medically Compromised Patients in Dentistry. Chicago: Yearbook, 1989:149–168.

51. Cash J, Raab RW, Coke JM. Understanding your patient with cardiac disease. J Colo Dent Assoc 1990;(Winter):16–19.

52. Dajani AS, Taubert KA, Wilson W, et al. Prevention of bacterial endocarditis: Recommendations by the American Heart Association. J Am Dent Assoc 1997;128:1142–1151.

53. Gerondontics. Fall Scientific Issue. Alpha Omegan 1986;79:34–41.

54. Rose LF. Cardiovascular disorders. In: Rose LF, Kaye D (eds). Internal Medicine for Dentistry. St. Louis: Mosby, 1990:505–514.

55. Kaplan NM. Clinical Hypertension. Baltimore, MD: Williams & Wilkins, 1978.

56. Montgomery MT. Dent Med Dig 1985;11:169–213.

57. Weindrin MC, Stason WB. Hypertension: A Policy Perspective. Cambridge, MA: Harvard University Press, 1976.

58. Redding S, Montgomery M. Dentistry in Systemic Disease: Diagnostic and Therapeutic Approach to Patient Management. Portland, OR: JBK Publishers, 1990.

59. Rose LF. Diseases of other organ or tissue systems with periodontal manifestations. In: Genco RJ, Goldman HM, Cohen DW (eds). Contemporary Periodontics. St. Louis: Mosby, 1990:251–267.

60. Burket LW. Histopathologic explanation for the oral lesion in the acute leukemias. Am J Orthod Oral Surg 1944;30:516.

61. Wentz FM, Anday G, Orban B. Histopathologic changes in the gingiva in leukemia. J Periodontol 1949;20:119.

62. Lindhe J. Textbook on Clinical Periodontology. Philadelphia: Saunders, 1983.

63. Carranza PA, et al. Histometric analysis of interradicular bone in protein deficient animals. J Periodont Res 1969;4:292.

64. Hemikson P, Wallenius K. The mandible and osteoporosis. J Oral Rehabil 1974;1:67.

65. Muzyka BC. Diagnosis and treatment of common oral manifestations associated with HIV disease. Penn Dent J 1993;60:30–31.

66. Murray PA. HIV disease as a risk factor for periodontal disease. Compend Contin Educ Dent 1994;15:1052.

67. Greenspan JS, Greenspan D, Winkler JR, Murray PA. Acquired immunodeficiency syndrome: Oral and periodontal changes. In: Genco RJ, Goldman HM, Cohen DW. Contemporary Periodontics. St. Louis: Mosby, 1990:319.

68. Hassell TM. Local and systemic actions of drugs and other chemical agents on periodontal tissues. In: Genco RJ, Goldman HM, Cohen DW. Contemporary Periodontics. St. Louis: Mosby, 1990:269.

69. Little JW, Falace DA. Dental Management of the Medically Compromised Patient. ed 4. St. Louis: Mosby, 1993:334.

70. Hassel TM. Local and systemic actions of drugs and other chemical agents on periodontal tissues. In: Genco RJ, Goldman HM, Cohen DW. Contemporary Periodontics. St. Louis: Mosby, 1990:273.

71. Petersen DE, Minah GE, Overholser CD, Suzuki JB, et al. Microbiology of acute periodontal infection in myelosuppressed cancer patients. J Clin Oncol 1987;5:1461–1468.

72. Stansbury DM, Peterson DE, Suzuki JB. Rapidly progressive acute periodontal infection in a patient with acute leukemia. J Periodontol 1988;59:544–547.

73. Wright WE. Periodontium destruction associated with oncology therapy. Five case reports. J Periodontol 1987;58:559–563.

74. Peterson DE. Pretreatment strategies for infection prevention in chemotherapy patients. Monogr Natl Cancer Inst 1990;9:61–71.

75. Council on Community Health, Hospital, Institutional and Medical Affairs. ADA Oral Health Care Guidelines. Patients receiving cancer chemotherapy. Chicago: American Dental Association, 1989.

76. Ratcliff PA. The relationship of the general adaptation syndrome to the periodontal tissues in the rat. J Periodontol 1956;27:40.

77. Shklar G. Periodontal disease in experimental animals subjected to chronic cold stress. J Periodontol 1966;37:377.

78. Stahl SS. Healing gingival injury in normal and systemically stressed young adult male rats. J Periodontol 1961;32:63.

79. Manhold JH, Doyel JL, Weisinger EH. Effects of social stress on oral and other bodily tissues. J Periodontol 1971;42:190.

80. Loesche WJ, et al. The bacteriology of ANUG. J Periodontol 1982;53:223.

81. Cogen RB, et al. Leukocyte function in the etiology of ANUG. J Periodontol 1983;54:402.

82. Zambon JJ, Grossi SG, Machtei EE, Ho AW, Dunford R, Genco RJ. Cigarette smoking increases the risk for subgingival infection with periodontal pathogens. J Periodontol 1996;67:1050–1054.

83. Preber H, Bergstrom J. The effect of non-surgical treatment on periodontal pockets in smokers and nonsmokers. J Clin Periodontol 1985;13:319–323.

84. Preber H, Bergstrom J. Effect of cigarette smoking on periodontal healing following surgical therapy. J Clin Periodontol 1990;17:324–328.

85. MacFarlane G, Herzberg M, Wolff L. Refractory periodontitis associated with abnormal polymorphonuclear leukocyte phagocytosis and cigarette smoking. J Periodontol 1992;63:908–913.

86. Bergstrom J, Blomlöf L. Tobacco smoking as a major risk factor associated with refractory periodontal disease [abstract 297]. J Dent Res 1972;71.

Treatment of Juvenile Periodontitis

Michael G. Newman, DDS
Perry R. Klokkevold, DDS, MS

CHAPTER 6

Despite improved understanding of the etiology, pathogenesis, and treatment of many forms of juvenile periodontitis, specific treatment protocols have not been firmly established nor universally practiced. The purpose of this chapter is to briefly review the rationale for treatment and to present specific recommendations for patient management.

Overview

Juvenile periodontitis is an inflammatory disease of the periodontium in young individuals. Clinically, juvenile periodontitis manifests as rapid alveolar bone loss around teeth; this bone loss may or may not be associated with minimal plaque, calculus, or inflammation. Bone loss can be localized to permanent first molars and mandibular incisors (classic presentation of localized juvenile periodontitis [LJP]), generalized to many permanent teeth, or nonspecific as to location of teeth affected. Bone loss may affect primary teeth, or it can occur in a combination of permanent and primary teeth.

Pathogenic bacteria, specifically *Actinobacillus actinomycetemcomitans* (*Aa*), have been implicated in the etiology and pathogenesis of LJP, as well as other forms of juvenile periodontitis. Genetic susceptibility, or a predilection for the disease, has also been implied in affected family members. Poor polymorphonuclear leukocyte chemotaxis and decreased phagocytosis are examples of phenotypic traits that could be inherited or induced. These white blood cell characteristics may be associated with an increased vulnerability to the disease, and, more importantly, they may be responsible for the severity of the clinical manifestations.

Historical Perspective

Alveolar bone loss of the type that has been associated with juvenile periodontitis was first described by Gottlieb,[1] in 1923, as a noninflammatory disease of the periodontium. Since its original description as a noninflammatory diffuse atrophy of the periodontium, the understanding of the etiology and pathogenesis of juvenile periodontitis has undergone many transformations, and the disease has undergone nearly as many name changes. Nomenclature for several of the manifestations of juvenile periodontitis has evolved to reflect current evidence.

Thoma and Goldman[2] later named the disease *paradontosis* to reflect their belief (in agreement with Gottlieb) that the disease was degenerative and not inflammatory. They described paradontosis to be a generalized involvement of the permanent dentition of young individuals (aged 14 to 25 years). Orban and Weinman[3] subsequently coined the English term, *periodontosis*, which remained for many years. They were the first to suggest a female predilection for the disease, a belief that has some evidence but has not been definitively determined.

In 1949, the Committee on Nomenclature of the American Academy of Periodontology defined periodontosis as a degenerative, noninflammatory destruction of the periodontium, originating in one or more of the periodontal structures, and characterized by migration and loosening of the teeth in the presence or absence of secondary epithelial proliferation and pocket formation or secondary gingival disease.[4] The 1966 World Workshop in Periodontics recognized that the 1949 definition lacked a statement regarding the health status of the affected individual and omitted discussion of the teeth involved. Additionally, they recognized that the migration and loosening of teeth were never early signs of periodontosis.[5]

Baer[6] reported the subsequent definition of periodontosis as a disease of the periodontium that is characterized by a rapid loss of alveolar bone about more than one tooth of the permanent dentition and occurs in an otherwise healthy adolescent. Two forms of periodontosis were thought to occur. One form was localized to the first molars and incisors while the other form was generalized to include several, if not most, other permanent teeth.

Several studies published in the mid-1970s provided evidence that bacterial plaque is associated with the localized form of periodontosis, which led to the current belief that the disease has a microbial etiology. Although the term *periodontosis* was still used by many to describe this advanced disease of adolescence, the understanding of an inflammatory component led to more common use of the term *juvenile periodontitis*. Waerhaug[7] described plaque-induced inflammation associated with localized juvenile periodontitis. He found a plaque front located 0.2 to 1.1 mm from the epithelial attachment along with a severe chronic inflammatory reaction and collagenolysis in the adjacent connective tissue. Newman et al[8–11] found and described five groups of bacteria associated with molar and incisor periodontal lesions. Their bacterial groups 2 and 3

contained *Actinobacillus actinomycetemcomitans* species. Since this original isolation of *Aa*, these bacterial species have received the most attention relative to their role in the etiology and pathogenesis of both LJP and other forms of periodontitis.

Diagnosis and Classification of Juvenile Periodontitis

Currently, the early-onset diseases of children and adolescents are classified into three distinct diseases, each of which has subclassifications. The diseases are primarily distinguished by age of onset and the number and type of teeth affected. Juvenile periodontitis patients are classified as having *prepubertal juvenile periodontitis*, *juvenile periodontitis*, or *postjuvenile periodontitis*. Each of these classifications is further subdivided into localized and generalized forms. Table 6-1 lists differential features of the three types of juvenile periodontitis.

Prepubertal Periodontitis

Prepubertal periodontitis affects the primary or mixed dentition of young individuals prior to the onset of puberty. It appears to be a rare form of the early-onset diseases, afflicting an unknown percentage of the population. By definition, children can be affected at any age, from after tooth eruption (1 to 3 years old) up to puberty (10 to 12 years old) or until they have completed the transition to permanent teeth. Most commonly, children are diagnosed with

Table 6-1   Differential features of various forms of juvenile periodontitis

Feature	Prepubertal	Juvenile	Postjuvenile
Age range	1–12 y	12–26 y	26–35 y
Sex ratio (F:M)	1:1	3:1	3:1
Location	Generalized or localized; primary or mixed dentition	LJP: Localized, first molars and incisors GJP: Generalized; permanent teeth	Variable
Inflammation	Variable	Minimal	Variable
Dental accretions	Minimal	Minimal	Variable
Caries index	Minimal	Minimal	Variable
Chemotaxis	Decreased	Decreased	?
Genetic factors	Yes	Yes	Yes

prepubertal periodontitis between the ages of 5 and 10 years. Cases of prepubertal periodontitis have been reported in the literature, and the clinical findings of the disease have been published as a distinct disease entity.[12]

Prepubertal periodontitis may be localized to a few teeth or generalized throughout the mouth.[13] The generalized form is associated with an acute, fiery-red proliferative gingival inflammation accompanied by rapid destruction of alveolar bone. The localized form is associated with little to no clinically observed gingival inflammation and slower periodontal bone destruction. Patterns of bone loss can be quite severe in advanced cases involving furcations. Dental accretions associated with the disease, such as bacterial plaque and calculus, are minimal. Caries incidence in individuals with prepubertal periodontitis is also low. Oral infections are often accompanied by otitis media, skin and upper respiratory tract infections, and some type of systemic disease. The ratio of males to females appears to be equal. Figures 6-1a to 6-1d show clinical and radiographic views of a child with the generalized form of prepubertal periodontitis.

Juvenile Periodontitis

The classic form of juvenile periodontitis, characterized by rapid bone loss localized to the permanent first molars and incisors, is diagnostic for this form of juvenile periodontitis. It is commonly referred to as *localized juvenile periodontitis.*

The disease is usually diagnosed when the patient is around the age of puberty, between the ages of 10 and 15 years. A definitive diagnosis of LJP is made when at least two sites (first molars and/or incisors) have lost 3 mm of attachment. As the disease progresses, severe bone loss around first molars and incisors is often seen bilaterally as mirror-image lesions.

A distinctive radiographic pattern is regarded as one of the classic diagnostic signs of LJP. Bone is often lost in an arc around first molars. Figures 6-2a to 6-2c show clinical photographs of a 17-year-old Hispanic boy with localized juvenile periodontitis. The radiographs exemplify the first molar and incisors bone loss pattern observed in localized juvenile periodontitis (Figs 6-2d to 6-2h).

In *generalized juvenile periodontitis* (GJP), the permanent first molars and incisors may be involved, but several other teeth are also affected. Patterns of bone loss are usually more horizontal. Individuals who are diagnosed later will have a slower progression of the disease than will those with active juvenile periodontitis.

Postjuvenile Periodontitis

Postjuvenile periodontitis patients are between 21 and 35 years old. These people most likely had undiagnosed and untreated juvenile periodontitis. For this reason, the clinical and radiographic appearance of postjuvenile periodontitis presents as a mix between the patterns of LJP and chronic

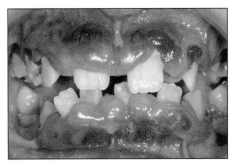

Fig 6-1a Patient suffering from generalized prepubertal juvenile periodontitis. (Courtesy of Dr P. Melnick.)

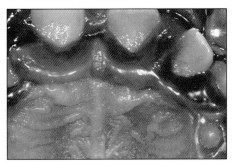

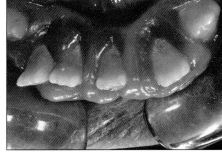

Figs 6-1b and 6-1c Maxillary and mandibular occlusal views of same patient. Note the degree of inflammation. (Courtesy of Dr P. Melnick.)

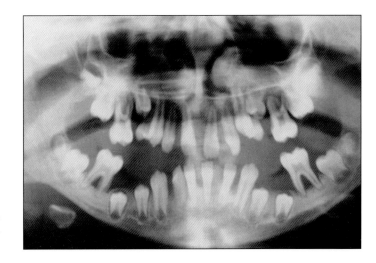

Fig 6-1d Panoramic radiograph of the same patient. Note the severe bone loss and premature loss of several primary teeth. (Courtesy of Dr P. Melnick.)

Figs 6-2a to 6-2c Patient with localized juvenile periodontitis.

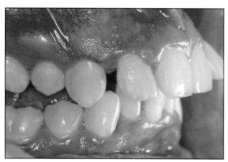

Fig 6-2a

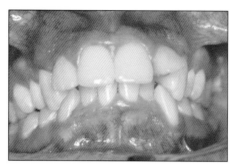

Fig 6-2b

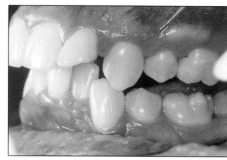

Fig 6-2c

Figs 6-2d to 6-2h Radiographic views of the same patient. Lesions are localized to maxillary first molars and incisors.

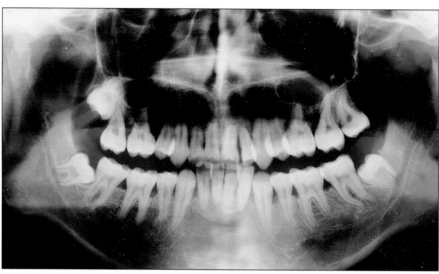

Fig 6-2d

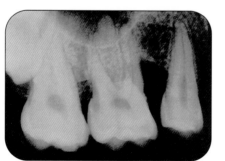

Fig 6-2e

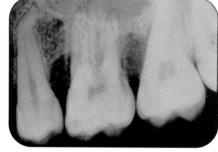

Fig 6-2f

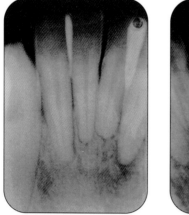

Fig 6-2g

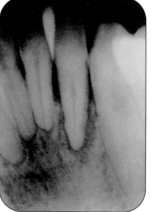

Fig 6-2h

adult periodontitis. Depending on the severity of the disease and previous treatment, patients may present with missing teeth and/or osseous defects with or without gingival recession. The bone loss often includes unilateral or bilateral arc-shaped defects around the first molars. Osseous defects can be localized to just the first molars and incisors or generalized throughout the permanent dentition.

The differences between juvenile periodontitis and postjuvenile periodontitis are primarily those of disease activity and the patient's age at the time of diagnosis. Because the disease activity in juvenile periodontitis often slows down by the time the individual reaches the early 20s, the patient's lesions are characterized by the term *burnout*. Burned out lesions may be considered to be arrested or may be converted into a chronic "garden variety" adult periodontitis. However, unlike patients with chronic adult periodontitis, individuals with postjuvenile periodontitis often have attachment loss and periodontal defects that are more advanced and difficult to manage and/or maintain. The caries rate is variable in the postjuvenile periodontitis patient. Plaque and calculus accretions are also variable but are always present in the patient with untreated postjuvenile disease.

Figures 6-3a to 6-3f depict a patient with postjuvenile periodontitis. She is a healthy African American woman with gingival recession and osseous defects around the first molars and incisors. Heavy calculus is evident around the mandibular incisors. Radiographs show chronic lesions localized around the first molars and incisors (Fig 6-3g).

Figs 6-3a to 6-3f Patient with postjuvenile periodontitis. Note the degree of gingival recession and the accumulation of heavy calculus. (Courtesy of Drs H. Takei and R. Grasu.)

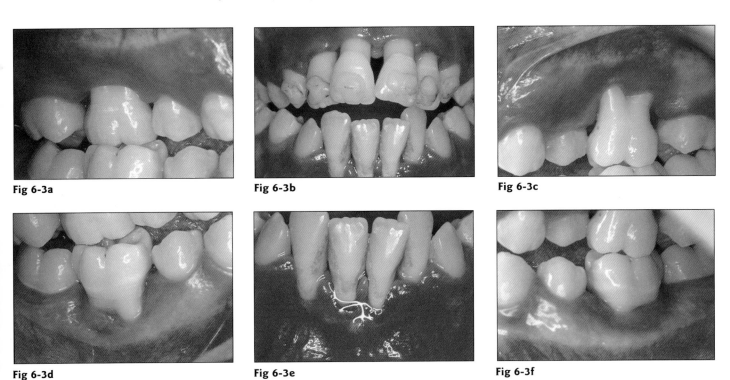

Fig 6-3a　　　　**Fig 6-3b**　　　　**Fig 6-3c**

Fig 6-3d　　　　**Fig 6-3e**　　　　**Fig 6-3f**

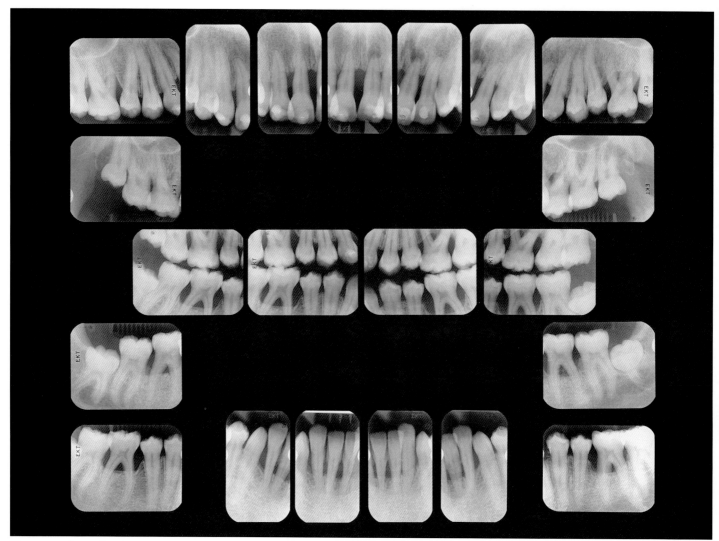

Fig 6-3g Full-mouth radiographs of the same patient. Bone loss is severe around the first molars and incisors. (Courtesy of Drs H. Takei and R. Grasu.)

Etiology and Pathogenesis of Juvenile Periodontitis

The etiology and pathogenesis of juvenile periodontitis are most likely multifaceted, which would help to explain the different presentations of the disease (localized versus generalized and prepubertal versus pubertal). Bacterial plaque, although usually minimal around affected teeth in LJP, has been implicated as the major etiologic factor in the alveolar bone destruction. The status of the immune system plays an important role in many, if not all, cases of early-onset juvenile periodontitis. Genetics has also been implicated as a factor in the susceptibility and severity of juvenile periodontitis.

Microbiology

Bacteria, specifically *Actinobacillis actinomycetemcomitans*, have been implicated in the etiology and pathogenesis of juvenile periodontitis.[15] Evidence for a specific bacterial etiology in localized juvenile periodontitis was first published by Newman et al.[8–11] In a series of studies, they found the microbial flora from localized juvenile periodontosis lesions to be composed of 78% gram-negative rods, predominated by *Aa*. Zambon et al[15,16] also found a high prevalence of *Aa* in subgingival plaque from LJP patients and implicated it as the major pathogen. Other investigators have implicated *Bacteroides gingivalis* (now called *Porphyromonas gingivalis*), *Bacteroides intermedius* (now called *Prevotella intermedia*), *Fusobacterium nucleatum*, *Eikenella corrodens*, *Capnocytophaga*, and spirochetes as part of the pathogenic flora in juvenile periodontitis.[17]

Actinobacillus actinomycetemcomitans is a pathogenic bacterium with destructive potential. It produces leukotoxin (neutrophil chemotaxis–inhibiting factor), lymphocyte-suppressing factor, lipopolysaccharide endotoxin, bone resorption–inducing toxin, acid/alkaline phosphotase, fibroblast-inhibiting factor, collagenase, and epitheliotoxin.[17] *Actinobacillus actinomycetemcomitans* may have tissue-invasive characteristics as well. Intragingival *Aa* has been observed in electron microscopic photomicrographs of gingival connective tissue of juvenile periodontitis lesions.[18-21]

Immunology

Systemic factors have long been implicated in the etiology and pathogenesis of juvenile periodontitis. Because the primary host defense against bacteria in periodontal infections is mediated by polymorphonuclear leukocytes (PMNs), it was a natural component of the immune system to investigate. Cianciola et al[22] measured two parameters of PMN function, chemotaxis and phagocytosis, and found that patients with localized juvenile periodontitis have significantly less function than do healthy controls. Monocyte chemotaxis is normal. They questioned whether the monocyte chemotaxis defect is preexisting or induced by the disease.[22] This question remains unanswered.

The results of that study initiated a series of investigations aimed at determining the basis of the abnormal PMN function. Genco[23] found that PMNs from most patients with LJP exhibit increased cellular adhesion. Subsequent studies revealed that PMNs from patients with LJP express a lower number of receptors for chemoattractants, altered signal transduction, and reduced intracellular killing of phagocytosed pathogens than do PMNs from healthy subjects.[24,25]

Genetics

It has long been recognized that underlying systemic diseases and their treatments predispose individuals to periodontal disease. Periodontitis has shown significant association with a number of disease conditions that have genetically inherited phenotypes, such as diabetes mellitus, Down syndrome, cyclic neutropenia, and Papillon-Lefèvre syndrome.

Several authors have suggested that juvenile periodontitis or a predilection for the disease has a familial inheritance. Familial occurrence of the disease is not absolute but significant enough to support the theory that familial inheritance plays some role in the etiology of juvenile periodontitis. The inheritable factor(s) may be autosomal recessive or X-linked dominant. It is also possible that multiple factors, in combination, ultimately lead to expression of the disease phenotype.

Examples of hereditary defects involving a variety of host tissues and responses associated with an increase in periodontitis include immune response variables (neutropenia, Chédiak-Higashi syndrome, trisomy 21, or diabetes), structural defects of the cementum (hypophosphotasia), structural defects of collagen (Ehlers-Danlos syndrome), and epithelial defects (Papillon-Lefèvre syndrome). The severe generalized prepubertal periodontitis with rapid alveolar bone loss associated with cyclic neutropenia underlines the importance of neutrophils as a major cellular defense against bacteria. Early-onset periodontitis associated with hypophosphotasia is believed to be related to cementum malformation. Papillon-Lefèvre syndrome is an autosomal-recessive condition characterized by aberrant epithelial development associated with severe early-onset periodontitis.

Treatment of Juvenile Periodontitis

Overall Treatment Strategy

The following treatment protocol is based on the evidence and reports available from the literature. It attempts to create a framework for decision making in the treatment of juvenile periodontitis. Clinicians are faced with a formidable challenge when attempting to correlate microbial tests with therapy and treatment results. *Patients with similar clinical presentations often have different microflora, and patients with similar pathogens may have very different clinical manifestations.* Clinical studies typically use classic periodontal parameters (probing depth and bleeding) to assess the success of treatment. Multiple factors are difficult to analyze and compare in clinical trials. For patients, however, all parameters must be considered in the assessment of disease and selection of therapy.

The diagnosis of juvenile periodontitis will lead the clinician through a series of treatments and evaluations. Because juvenile periodontitis sometimes undergoes spontaneous remission, or burnout, it is important to develop a disease activity rating that maps or documents the severity of clinical findings over time. If prior diagnostic information is available, it is important to obtain this information (radiographs, charting, etc) and use it to establish a baseline or reference disease activity level. When previous diagnostic information is not available or not conclusive, patients will often need to be treated and monitored before a definitive diagnosis or specific treatment pathway is chosen.

Diagnosis and Treatment Decision Pathway

The treatment algorithm begins with an identification of the patient's disease status (present or absent) (Fig 6-4). If no disease is found (A), the patient should be placed on regular maintenance therapy which includes prophylaxis, oral hygiene instructions, and monitoring every 4 to 6 months (B). If a subsequent reevaluation reveals signs of the presence of juvenile periodontitis, the patient will enter the treatment algorithm (C).

Following a preliminary diagnosis of juvenile periodontitis (C) and determination of the extent of disease (localized versus generalized), the patient will receive initial

Fig 6-4 Treatment flow chart.

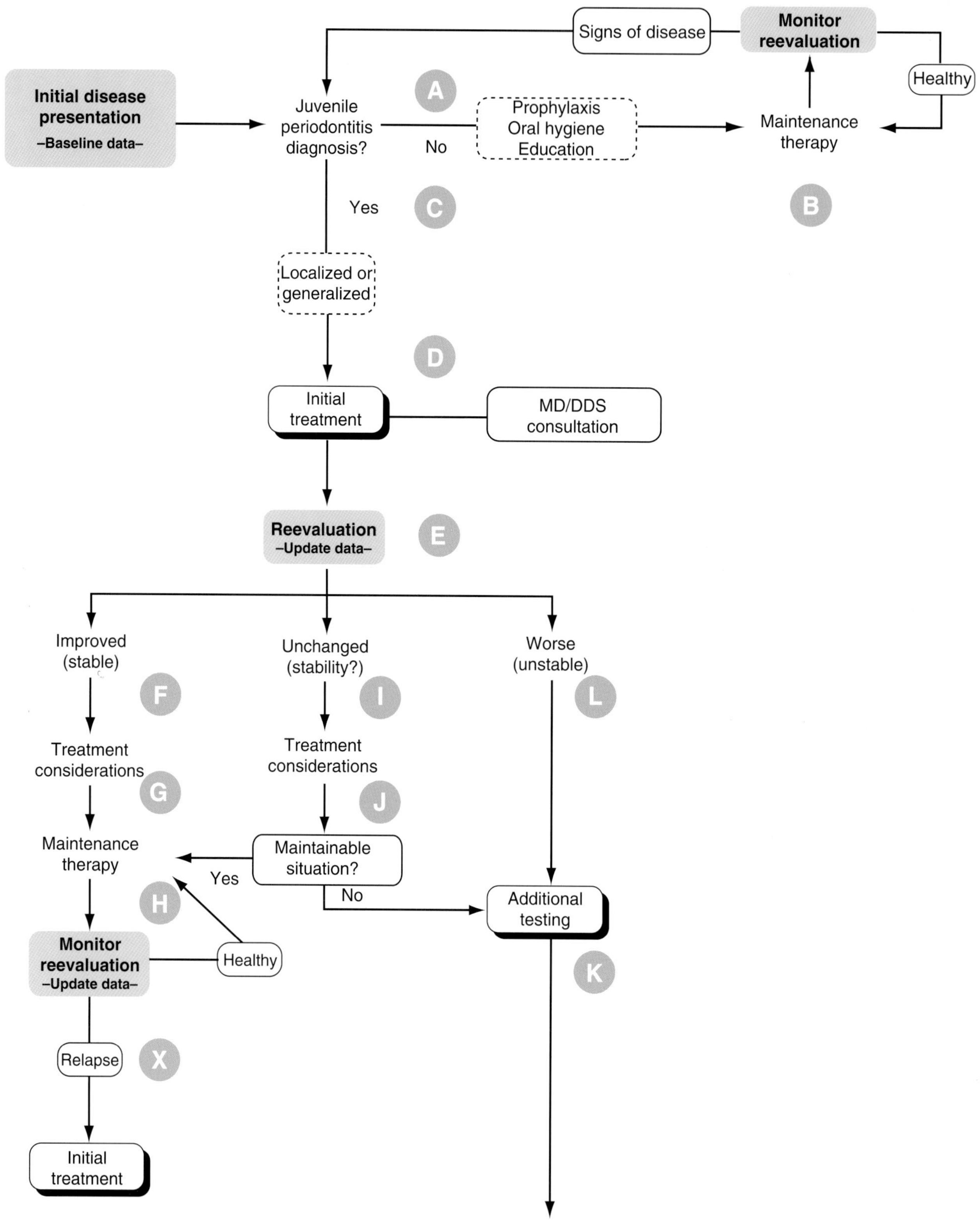

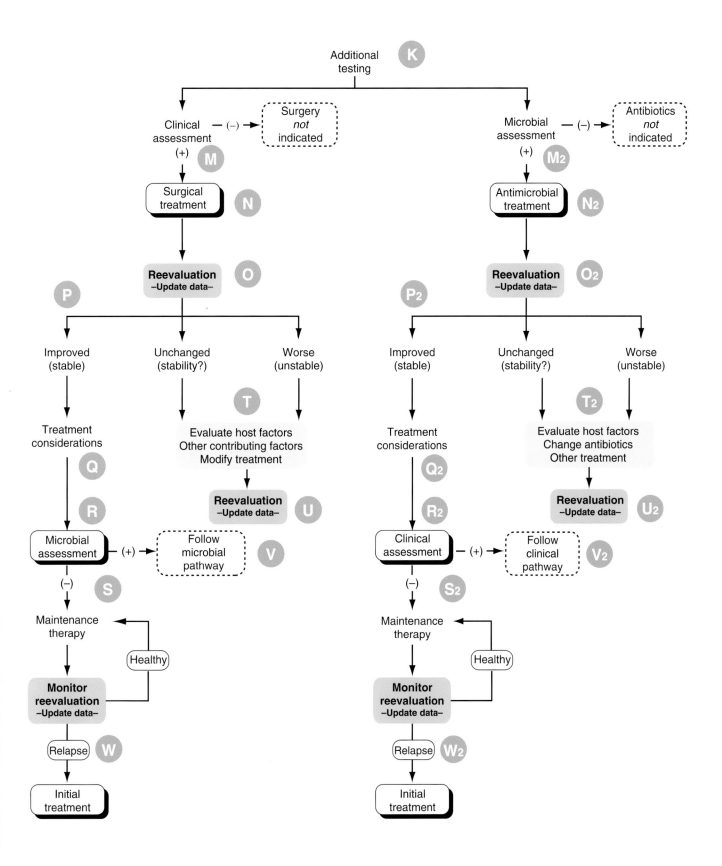

treatment (D), consisting of scaling and root planing, prophylaxis, oral hygiene instructions, disease education, and consultation with their physician and other dental specialists as needed. Family members should be informed about possible disease traits and encouraged to have an examination. Family trees should be developed and followed over the course of treatment. Early and consistent screenings of younger siblings at risk for juvenile periodontitis may lead to earlier diagnosis, intervention, and treatment. Following initial treatment, all patients should be reexamined to establish an activity level (E).

After initial treatment is completed, a reevaluation (E) is performed to determine whether the disease is improved/stable (F), unchanged (I), or worse (L). If the disease shows improvement or stability (F), additional treatment (G) will be based on correction of or improvement in the periodontal structures (ie, treatment to reduce pocket depth or regenerate lost tissues). If the clinical parameters appear to be unchanged or worse following initial therapy, additional testing (K) may be indicated. Clinical and microbiologic testing should be carried out simultaneously (M and M2).

Clinical assessment (M) is a judgment of whether a given condition is maintainable. When the clinical parameters (eg, probing attachment levels) worsen following initial therapy, surgical treatment (N) may be indicated to gain control of the disease. Areas of concern may be localized or generalized to many sites. Following surgical treatment, a reevaluation is completed (O), and clinical data are collected. These data become the new baseline data for future comparisons. If the disease continues to progress (T), host and local factors should be evaluated and treatment modification should be considered. Again, reevaluation and data collection are essential (U).

An improved or stable condition (P) will lead to consideration of adjunctive treatment (Q), intended to enhance maintenance therapy. Before maintenance therapy is begun, microbial tests must be evaluated (R). If microbial tests are positive for pathogens (V), then the treatment algorithm follows the microbial assessment pathway (M2).

Microbiologic assessment (M2) is indicated when the clinical parameters do not improve or become worse following initial therapy. Areas of concern may be localized or generalized to many sites. Antimicrobial treatment would be indicated as adjunctive therapy if microbial pathogens (especially Aa) were positive (N2). Negative test results would not indicate nor exclude antimicrobial therapy. Following antimicrobial therapy, a reevaluation (O2) is done to determine the effectiveness of the antibiotic. Data are again collected and compared to previous information. If pathogen levels are unchanged or worse (T2), a change in antibiotics and evaluation of host factors should be considered. Microbial data are reevaluated subsequent to the change in antibiotics, and the disease activity level is reassessed (U2).

An improved or stable microbiologic condition (P2) will lead to maintenance therapy. Before the patient enters maintenance therapy, clinical findings must be evaluated (R2). If additional treatment is deemed necessary (V2), then the treatment algorithm should return to clinical assessment and follow the surgical pathway (N). It is essential that both pathways are successfully passed before the patient enters maintenance therapy and monitoring (S or S2).

Successful treatment will lead to improved/stable disease activity levels and ultimately to the initiation of the maintenance and monitoring phase of the algorithm. *Every pathway has the potential to end in maintenance and monitoring (B, H, S, and S2). Constant reevaluation at maintenance visits allows for detection of increases in disease activity or relapses (W, W2, and X). Relapse to an increase in disease activity from any branch returns the patient to the beginning of the algorithm for initial treatment (D).*

Antimicrobial therapy may include topical chlorhexidine, local antibiotic delivery, systemic antibiotics, or a combination of these. Once again, the patient will be reevaluated following treatment. Clinical and microbiologic data are collected and compared to previous results.

Once the patient has improved, stabilized, and completed additional treatment, he or she will enter a cycle of maintenance and monitoring. However, if disease activity remains the same or worsens, additional tests should be considered and antimicrobials may need to be changed. Host factors should be evaluated. Table 6-2 lists factors that may modify specific treatment plans.

Each level in the treatment algorithm results in reevaluation or monitoring. Constant reevaluation and assessment of disease activity levels allows clinicians to "see" the progression or improvement in the disease and alter the course of treatment accordingly. At this point, current diagnostic information is collected and compared to previous data.

Further treatment or decision routes are determined not only by current clinical findings but also by a comparison of those findings to that individual's past disease indicators. Any given clinical sign (or microbial finding) may be indicative of improvement for one patient but mark destructive progression for another. Plotting data for each patient (and each area) on a simple graph showing clinical and microbiologic findings over time permits the clinician to "visualize" disease activity and treatment effectiveness. Figure 6-5 shows data collected over the course of treatment for one individual. In this manner, the unique disease activity profile for each patient will be accurately depicted and can be utilized in the treatment and decision-making process.

The reevaluation plot or graph should consist of relative values derived from clinical and microbiologic measurements. For example, a sum of probing attachment levels (minus baseline probing attachment levels) could be used as a clinical indicator. An increase in probing attachment loss would indicate disease activity, and a decrease might

Table 6-2 Factors that modify the treatment plan (see Fig 6-4)

Factor	Problem	Algorithm	Solution
Pathogen virulence	Antibiotic not effective	T2, U2	Change antibiotic
Poor host response	Treatment not as effective as expected	X, T, U, V, W, T2, U2	Use adjunctive therapy, such as antibiotics
Extensive bone loss	Excessive bone loss not amenable to treatment	D, G, J, N, Q, Q2	Consider extraction
Furcation involvement	Excessive bone loss not amenable to treatment	D, G, J, N, Q, Q2	Maintain with compromise or extract
Defect morphology	Excessive bone loss not amenable to treatment	D, G, J, N, Q, Q2	Attempt treatment with compromise or extract
Excessive tooth mobility	Impairs healing and worsens prognosis	D, G, J, N, Q, Q2	Rigidly splint (bond) to adjacent teeth or consider extraction
Unfavorable crown-root ratio	Poor prognosis	D, G, J, N, Q, Q2	Rigidly splint (bond) to adjacent teeth or consider extraction
Occlusal interferences	Impair healing and may contribute toward progression of disease	D, G, J, N, Q, Q2	Remove interferences or fabricate occlusal splint to protect contact teeth
Poor oral hygiene	Hinders control of disease factors	B, D, E, H, S, S2, X	Stress improvement in oral hygiene to patient
Poor general health	Impairs healing and worsens prognosis	D, I, L, T, T2, W, W2, X	Have medical consultation with physician and consider medical intervention treatment

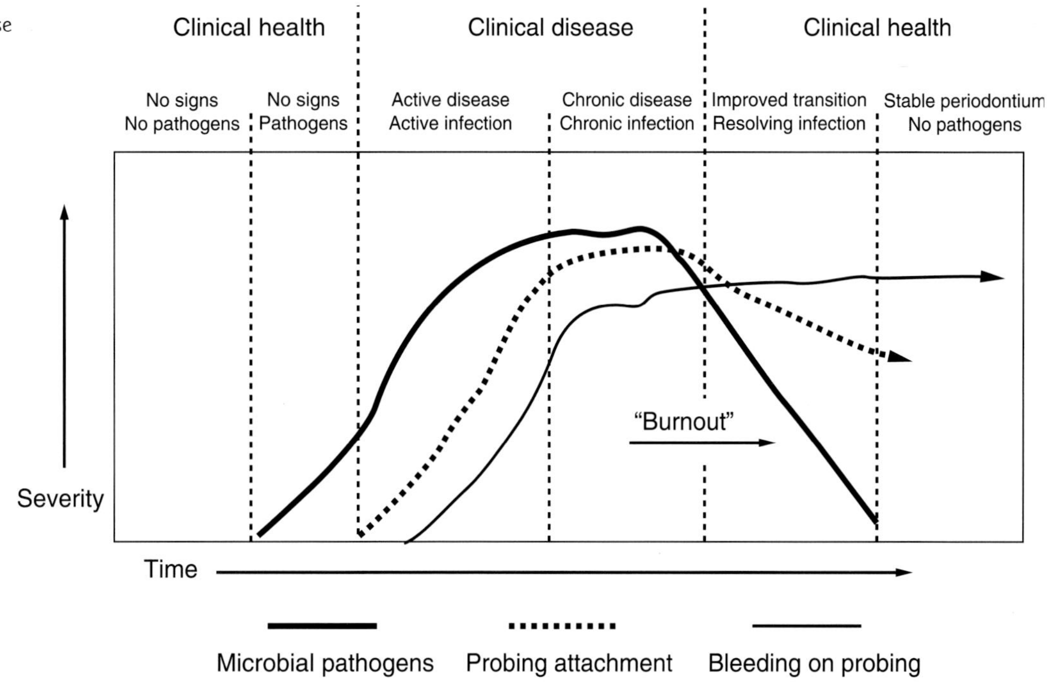

Fig 6-5 Example of a patient's disease activity over time.

111

indicate regeneration or reattachment and a decrease in disease activity. Bleeding on probing should also be charted by tooth area and charted as a factor of the number of bleeding sites. Although bleeding on probing is a less predictive measure, some specific patient decisions will be swayed by it.

Microbial assessment should consist of mapping the presence of one or more pathogens (especially *Aa*) multiplied by the number of positive sites. Constant or increasing levels of pathogens would indicate a potential for disease activity, and decreased levels would indicate a decreased potential. A site-specific evaluation of microbial and clinical measurements would give a risk assessment for each periodontal site. Ultimately, comparison of clinical and microbiologic measurements over time will provide a disease activity profile.

Nonsurgical Methods

The nonsurgical approach to the treatment of juvenile periodontitis consists of scaling and root planing of all areas that exhibit periodontal attachment loss. Oral hygiene instructions and plaque control are stressed. The access limitations for scaling and root planing, as well as oral hygiene, become increasingly more important and follow the same basic principles as with any other form of periodontitis. There are exceptions, however, that are an important part of the overall therapeutic strategy. Treatment of juvenile periodontitis should focus on meticulous plaque control and the eradication of periodontal pathogens, possibly with the aid of systemic and/or local antimicrobials.

Antimicrobial agents are important adjuncts to traditional mechanical, nonsurgical modes of treatment in these patients. Tetracycline has been considered the initial drug of choice when the treatment of juvenile periodontitis calls for systemic antibiotic therapy. Scaling and root planing used in conjunction with tetracycline therapy has been found to be more effective in eliminating *Aa* than scaling and root planing alone.[26] Given systemically, tetracycline concentrates in the gingival crevicular fluid at 2 to 10 times greater levels than in serum.[27,28] In addition, Slots et al[29–31] showed that most strains of *Actinobacillus actinomycetemcomitans* are sensitive to tetracycline. The anticollagenase activity produced by tetracycline[32] may also have a beneficial effect on wound healing.

Doxycycline, a semisynthetic tetracycline, has been used successfully in the treatment of juvenile periodontitis. The benefits of doxycycline include lower dosages (only once or twice a day) and compatibility with dairy products; patients experience fewer stomach problems and no photosensitivity. Patient compliance will likely be improved if there are fewer pills to take and fewer side effects. Another advantage for some patients is that its route of excretion is through the liver rather than the kidneys.

Novak et al[33,34] showed that tetracycline therapy is effective in the initial control of early juvenile periodontitis. Doxycycline has been shown to effectively eliminate *Aa* when used in conjunction with surgery.[35–37] Metronidazole has been found to be more effective than tetracycline in the suppression of *Aa*.[38] Metronidazole plus amoxicillin has been found to effectively eliminate *Actinobacillus actinomycetemcomitans* from infected subgingival pockets.[39] Other antibiotics, such as penicillin, have not been shown to be as effective.[40] Amoxicillin and clavulanic acid, used in combination, are not able to eliminate *Aa*.[41]

Local delivery of tetracycline has received a great deal of attention; impregnated fibers, gels, and resorbable antimicrobial chips have been used to deliver the drug to the infected pocket without the side effects associated with systemic administration of antimicrobial agents. Table 6-3 lists antimicrobials for the management of juvenile periodontitis.

Surgical Methods

The surgical approaches to management of juvenile periodontitis range from modified Widman flap, resective techniques, regenerative procedures, and extractions to autotransplantation. No single surgical therapy will be effective for every case of juvenile periodontitis. Each patient, and in fact each area, must be independently evaluated and assessed for treatment. Figure 6-6a shows a site with limited plaque and inflammation and no gingival recession. Yet, following flap reflection, severe localized destruction of bone is evident around the mandibular first molar (Fig 6-6b).

Lindhe and Liljenberg[42] used the modified Widman flap with 14 days of tetracycline to treat 16 patients with localized juvenile periodontitis. They found that successfully treated pockets were stable long term (5 years). Kornman and Robertson[26] compared surgical and nonsurgical therapies with and without tetracycline. The results indicate that surgical therapy, used along with tetracycline, reduces pockets, bleeding, and periodontal pathogens. When researchers compared surgery, local administration of tetracycline alone, and surgery plus doxycycline, they found that only surgery plus doxycycline is effective in reducing or eliminating *Aa*.[35,36]

Resective procedures are of limited value in the treatment of juvenile periodontitis because of the severity and defects of the disease. The therapeutic approach to the management of juvenile periodontitis, like most other periodontal diseases, has been forever changed by the success of regenerative periodontal therapy. Numerous reports of bone regeneration following treatment of lesions in juvenile periodontitis support a trend toward a conservative, regenerative therapy approach.

Regenerative procedures are directed toward preservation and reconstruction of the periodontium. Juvenile

Table 6-3 Antimicrobial agents for the management of juvenile periodontitis

Antibiotic type	Locally administered	Systemic route route	Adverse effects	Effective against *Aa*
	(Dose/mode)	(Dose/duration)		
Chlorhexidine gel	1% w/w / gingival irrigation	NA	Altered taste; stains teeth	Probably
Tetracycline	40% w/w / gingival application	250 mg, qid/ 14 days +	GI upset; photosensitivity	Yes
Doxycycline	?	100 mg, bid/ 14 days +	Minimal	Yes
Metronidazole	NA	200 mg, tid/ 10 days	GI upset; colitis	Variable
Penicillin	NA	250–500 mg, qid/ 10–14 days +	GI upset	No
Metronidazole + amoxicillin	NA	≤200 mg, tid, + 250–500 mg, qid/ 10–14 days	GI upset; colitis	Variable
Amoxicillin + clavulanic acid	NA	250–500 mg, qid/ 14 days +	GI upset	No

NA = not applicable.
GI = gastrointestinal.
? = Dosage and mode of local administration are being tested but remain unknown.

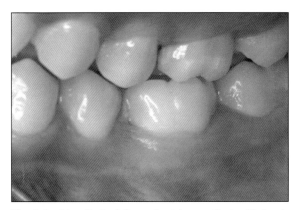

Fig 6-6a Mandibular left quadrant in a patient with localized juvenile periodontitis. Minimal plaque is present. The gingival margin appears pink and remains at a normal level without inflammation. (Courtesy of Dr P. Melnick.)

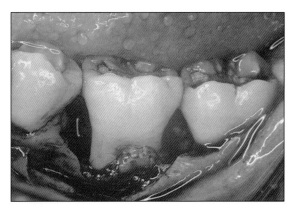

Fig 6-6b Defect around the first molar shown in Fig 6-6a. Flap reflection reveals that the signs of disease are not commensurate with the severity of the osseous defect. (Courtesy of Dr P. Melnick.)

periodontitis lesions conservatively treated with surgery have shown the potential to regenerate.[42,43] Figures 6-7a to 6-7d show an example of the regenerative potential around the diseased root surfaces in a young patient with localized juvenile periodontitis.[44] The principles of guided tissue regeneration can be applied to the regeneration of juvenile periodontitis lesions.[45] Bone grafting has been used successfully to regain bone and reduce probing depth.[46]

With any regenerative procedure, it is prudent to prevent microbial contamination by administering antibiotics. Treatment of the lesions of juvenile periodontitis is no exception. Although it is tempting to control the disease and regenerate lost tissue, it is probably important to control the disease and eliminate pathogens before regenerative procedures are employed.

As with many clinical entities, juvenile periodontitis is treated by various regimens of local and systemic therapy based on successful reports and current understanding. They are always modified on an individual basis. There are no special published treatment protocols for the treatment of juvenile periodontitis. This is probably due, at least in part, to the variations in response to different forms of therapy. Variations in pathogen virulence, timing and sequence of therapy, and host response certainly each play a role in the variable treatment outcome.

Maintenance Following Primary Therapy

The rationale for treatment is based on the current belief that bacterial plaque is the primary etiologic factor responsible for juvenile periodontitis. Thus, therapeutic efforts should be directed toward the control of pathogenic bacteria, especially *Actinobacillus actinomycetemcomitans*, with the potential for tissue invasion and destruction. Because genetic and/or local neutrophil and monocyte deficits may also exist and contribute toward disease susceptibility, use of chemotherapy is advised to assist host response.

The prognosis for each affected tooth and area must be assessed individually. As with any periodontally diseased tooth, the prognosis of the tooth with juvenile periodonti-

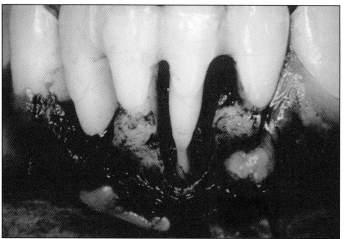
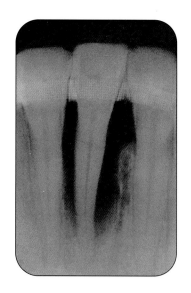

Figs 6-7a and 6-7b Severe osseous defect around the mandibular central incisor in a young, healthy patient with localized juvenile periodontitis. Bone loss extends to the apex of the tooth, and there are no supporting bony walls. (From Dodson.[44] Reprinted with permission.)

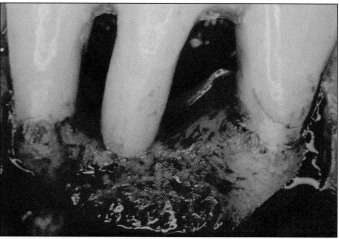
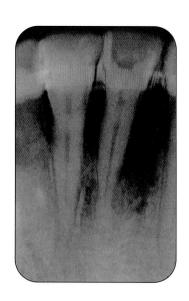

Figs 6-7c and 6-7d Same tooth, 1 year following treatment (splinting, antibiotics, scaling, root planing, and bone grafting with decalcified freeze-dried bone allograft.) (From Dodson.[44] Reprinted with permission.)

tis depends on multiple factors, such as the extent of bone loss, the presence of furcation involvement, the morphology of the bony defect, the degree of mobility, the crown-root ratio, the occlusion (interferences), and the oral hygiene and general health of the individual.

An essential element in the maintenance of patients with a history of juvenile periodontitis is monitoring or constant reevaluations. Clinical parameters should be evaluated and compared to previous data at every maintenance or monitoring visit. It is neither cost effective nor prudent to continue microbial testing for patients who have entered the maintenance phase of treatment. However, microbial testing should be done whenever a change in disease activity is evident from the clinical examination. One possible exception would be to continue microbial monitoring for patients whose disease is difficult to control and who continue to test positive for pathogens.

Future Prospects for Patients With Juvenile Periodontitis

Early Diagnosis and Prevention of Juvenile Periodontitis

Early screenings of individuals at risk for developing juvenile periodontitis may lead to earlier diagnosis, treatment, and intervention. Currently, younger siblings of diagnosed individuals can be tested for *Aa* and/or antibodies. Early detection of pathogens would support the initiation of antimicrobial and nonsurgical therapy that may prevent the disease from occurring in the first place. As the understanding of the etiology and pathogenesis of juvenile periodontitis improves, so will methods for early detection and intervention.

Implants

The recent success and acceptance of osseointegrated dental implants in the general population has provided many patients with a viable alternative for tooth replacement. The excitement of the potential for tooth replacement using implants in the patient with juvenile periodontitis is attenuated by undesirable osseous defects and a concern that implant sites will become infected with *Aa*.

Concern over the colonization of implant sites with *Aa* is valid considering its pathogenicity. An alternative that has been considered for patients with severe generalized juvenile periodontitis is removal of all affected teeth and administration of intense chemotherapy prior to the placement of dental implants. The theory is to eradicate *Aa* prior to implant placement to prevent colonization of implant sites.

Although it is tempting and feasible to include implants in the treatment planning of patients with juvenile periodontitis, it is still too early to make conclusions or recommendations about this therapy. Investigations and well-documented cases will undoubtedly shed light on this potential treatment option.

References

1. Gottlieb B. Die diffuse atrophie des alveolarknochens. Z Stomatol 1923;2:195–162.
2. Thoma KH, Goldman HM. Classification and histopathology of paradontal disease. J Am Dent Assoc 1937;24:1915–1928.
3. Orban B, Weinman JP. Diffuse atrophy of the alveolar bone (periodontosis). J Periodontol 1942;13:31–45.
4. Nomenclature and Classification Committee Report. J Periodontol 1950;21:40.
5. McCall JO. The World Workshop in Periodontics. J Periodontol 1967;38(6):555–557.
6. Baer PN. The case for periodontosis as a clinical entity. J Periodontol 1971;42:516.
7. Waerhaug J. Subgingival plaque and loss of attachment in periodontosis as observed in autopsy material. J Periodontol 1976;47:636.
8. Newman M, Williams R, Crawford A, Manganiello A, Socransky S. Predominant cultivable microbiota of periodontitis and periodontosis. III. Periodontosis [abstract 290]. J Dent Res 1973;52(special issue):131.
9. Newman M, Socransky S, Savitt ED, Propas DA, Crawford A. Studies of the microbiology of periodontosis. J Periodontol 1976;47:373.
10. Newman MG, Socransky SS. Predominant cultivable microbiota in periodontosis. J Periodont Res 1977;12:120.
11. Newman MG, Socransky SS, Savitt E, Krichevsky M, Listgarten MA, Lai W. Characterization of bacteria isolated from periodontosis. J Dent Res 1974;53(special issue):135.
12. Page R. Prepubertal periodontitis. I. Definition of a clinical disease entity. J Periodontol 1983;54:257–271.
13. Suzuki JB. Diagnosis and classification of the periodontal diseases. Dent Clin North Am 1988;32:195–216.
14. Socransky S. Relationship of bacteria to the etiology of periodontal disease. J Dent Res 1970;49:203–222.
15. Zambon JJ, Christersson LA, Slots J. *Actinobacillus actinomycetemcomitans* in human periodontal disease. Prevalence in patient groups and distribution of biotypes and serotypes within families. J Periodontol 1983;54:707–711.
16. Zambon JJ. *Actinobacillus actinomycetemcomitans* in human periodontal disease. J Clin Periodontol 1985;12:1–20.
17. Asikainen S. Occurrence of *Actinobacillus actinomycetemcomitans* and spirochetes in relation to age in localized juvenile periodontitis. J Periodontol 1986;57:537–541.
18. Gillett R, Johnson NW. Bacterial invasion of the periodontium in a case of juvenile periodontitis. J Clin Periodontol 1982;9:93.
19. Zhang JZ, Yang XX, Tong YH. Combined gu chi wan and spiramycin in the treatment of periodontal disease. Chung Kuo Chung Hsi I Chieh Ho Tsa Chih 1992;12:83–85, 68.
20. Saglie FR, Carranza FA Jr, Newman MG. The presence of bacteria within the oral epithelium in periodontal disease I. A scanning and transmission electron microscopic study. J Periodontol 1985;56:618–624.

21. Saglie FR, Smith CT, Newman MG, et al. The presence of bacteria in the oral epithelium in periodontal disease. II. Immunohistochemical identification of bacteria. J Periodontol 1986;57:492–500.

22. Cianciola LJ, Genco RJ, Patters MR, McKenna J, Van Oss CJ. Defective polymorphonuclear leukocyte function in human periodontal disease. Nature 1977;265:195–216.

23. Genco RJ. Neutrophil chemotaxis impairment in juvenile periodontitis. J Reticuloendothelial Soc 1981;28:81s–91s.

24. Van Dyke TE, Warbington M, Gardner M, Offenbacher S. Neutrophil surface protein markers as indicators of defective chemotaxis in LJP. J Periodontol 1990;61:180–184.

25. Agarwal S, Reynolds MA, Duckett LD, Suzuki JB. Altered free cytosolic calcium changes and neutrophil chemotaxis in patients with juvenile periodontitis. J Periodont Res 1989;24:149–154.

26. Kornman KS, Robertson PB. Clinical and microbiological evaluation of therapy for juvenile periodontitis. J Periodontol 1985;56:443–446.

27. Gordon JM, Walker CB, Murphy JC, et al. Tetracycline: levels achievable in gingival crevice fluid and in vitro effect on subgingival organisms. Part I. Concentrations in crevicular fluid after repeated doses. J Periodontol 1981;52:609.

28. Gordon JM, Walker CB, Murphy JC, et al. Concentration of tetracycline in human gingival fluid after single doses. J Clin Periodontol 1981;8:117.

29. Slots J, Evans RT, Lobbins PM, Genco RJ. In vitro antimicrobial susceptibility of Actinobacillus actinomycetemcomitans. Antimicrob Agents Chemother 1980;18:9.

30. Slots J, Reynolds HS, Genco RJ. Actinobacillus actinomycetemcomitans in human periodontal disease: A cross-sectional microbiological investigation. Infect Immun 1980;29:1013.

31. Slots J, Reynolds HS, Jobbins PA, Genco JF. Actinobacillus actinomycetemcomitans, selective culturing and oral ecology in patients with localized juvenile periodontitis [abstract 244]. J Dent Res 1980;59:328.

32. Golub LM, Wolff HM, Lee HM, et al. Further evidence that tetracyclines inhibit collagenase activity in human crevicular fluid and from other mammalian sources. J Periodont Res 1985;20:12–13.

33. Novak MJ, Polson AM, Adair SM. Tetracycline therapy in patients with early juvenile periodontitis. J Periodontol 1988;59:366–372.

34. Novak MJ, Stamatelakys C, Adair SM. Resolution of early lesions of juvenile periodontitis with tetracycline therapy alone: long-term observations of 4 cases. J Periodontol 1991;62:628–633 [erratum 1992;63:148].

35. Mandell RL, Tripodi LS, Savitt E, Goodson JM, Socransky SS. The effect of treatment on Actinobacillus actinomycetemcomitans in localized juvenile periodontitis. J Periodontol 1986;57:94–99.

36. Mandell RL, Socransky SS. Microbiological and clinical effects of surgery plus doxycycline on juvenile periodontitis. J Periodontol 1988;59:373–379.

37. Saxen L, Asikainen S, Kanervo A, Kari K, Jousimies-Somer H. The long-term efficacy of systemic doxycycline medication in the treatment of localized juvenile periodontitis. Arch Oral Biol 1990;35(suppl):227S–229S.

38. Saxen L, Asikainen S. Metronidazole in the treatment of localized juvenile periodontitis. J Clin Periodontol 1993;20:166–171.

39. van Winkelhoff AJ, Rodenburg JP, Goene RJ, Abbas F, Winkel EG, de Graaff J. Metronidazole plus amoxycillin in the treatment of Actinobacillus actinomycetemcomitans associated periodontitis. J Clin Periodontol 1989;16:128–131.

40. Kunihira DM, Caine FA, Palcanis KG, Best AM, Ranney RR. A clinical trial of phenoxymethyl penicillin for adjunctive treatment of juvenile periodontitis. J Periodontol 1985;56:352–358.

41. Vallcorba Plana N, Redondo Eleno M, Prieto Prieto J, et al. Microbiological changes in subgingival flora after treatment with amoxycillin-clavulanic acid. Av Odontoestomatol 1989;1:87–92.

42. Lindhe J, Liljenberg B. Treatment of localized juvenile periodontitis. Results after 5 years. J Clin Periodontol 1984;11:399–410.

43. Sewon L, Talonpoika J. Efficacy of bone-fill favoring treatment of juvenile periodontitis. Scand J Dent Res 1992;100:159–163.

44. Dodson SA, Takei HH, Carranza FA Jr. Clinical success in regeneration: Report of a case. Int J Periodont Rest Dent 1996;16:455–461.

45. Levine RA, Kutalek KM. Guided tissue regeneration in the treatment of localized juvenile periodontitis—a multidisciplinary approach in improving anterior esthetics: a case report. Compend Contin Educ Dent 1993;14:622–630.

46. Mabry TW, Yukna RA, Sepe WW. Freeze-dried bone allografts combined with tetracycline in the treatment of juvenile periodontitis. J Periodontol 1985;56:74–81.

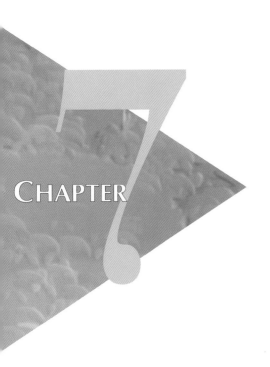

Nonsurgical Periodontal Therapy

Michael A. Brunsvold, DDS, MS

The role of nonsurgical methods in the management of periodontal disease is expanding rapidly. Use of adjuncts to scaling and root planing are greatly increasing the effectiveness of nonsurgical treatment. These adjuncts include systemic and local antibiotics, modified ultrasonic instruments, visual magnification, and fiberoptic illumination. When these methods are combined in the treatment of aggressive forms of periodontitis, the need for surgical treatment is often reduced. It is generally accepted that a tremendous amount of periodontal disease can be controlled by nonsurgical therapy and that almost all periodontal patients can benefit from it (Figs 7-1a and 7-1b).

The attention given to the Keyes technique in the 1980s and to soft tissue management in the current era serves to emphasize the value of nonsurgical treatment in the management of periodontal diseases. Claims that the Keyes technique replaces conventional periodontal therapy have been disproven,[1,2] but they stimulated a surge of interest in nonsurgical periodontal treatment, especially among general dentists and the public. The skills of scaling and root planing are not easy to acquire. Persistence and determination are necessary for the practitioner to become effective in this form of therapy.

Nonsurgical periodontal treatment includes not only scaling and root planing, but also emergency care, oral hygiene instructions, removal of plaque-retaining factors (such as overhangs), caries control, and occlusal adjustment. The main focus of this chapter is on scaling and root planing, the major part of nonsurgical treatment.

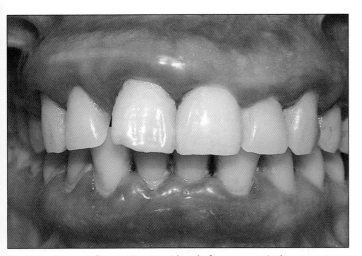

Fig 7-1a Severe inflammation is evident before nonsurgical treatment.

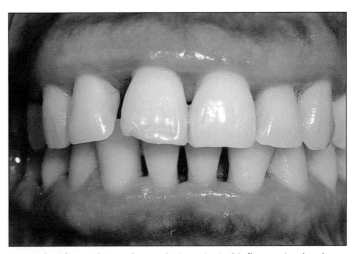

Fig 7-1b After scaling and root planing, gingival inflammation has been reduced.

Scaling is the removal of calculus, plaque, and stains from crowns and root surfaces. *Root planing* removes cementum or surface dentin that is contaminated by bacterial plaque, calculus, and bacterial products. The main difference in these procedures is that root planing aims at removing contaminated root surface tissues, while scaling removes only surface accumulations. Principles of instrumentation are the same for both scaling and root planing.

The purpose of nonsurgical periodontal treatment is the creation of a biologically acceptable root surface that is compatible with the health of adjacent periodontal tissues. A biologically acceptable root surface is defined as one that is smooth, hard, and completely divested of accrued substances and damaged tooth structure.

The objectives of nonsurgical therapy include *(1)* replacement of pathogenic microflora with the sparse flora found in health, *(2)* conversion of inflamed pathologic pockets to healthy gingival tissue, *(3)* shrinkage of the deepened pocket to a shallow, healthy sulcus, and *(4)* achievement of a root surface compatible with a healthy connective tissue and epithelial attachment.[3] Aspects of nonsurgical therapy discussed in this chapter include bacterial plaque and calculus detection, scaling and root planing instrumentation, effects of nonsurgical treatment, adjuncts, and limitations.

Detection and Removal of Bacterial Plaque

Supragingival plaque is best assessed with a disclosing solution or tablets. Disclosure of plaque with dyes should be performed at the *end* of the periodontal examination, so that the dye does not obscure color changes of the soft tissues. The severity of plaque can be greatly underestimated if disclosing agents are not used. Disclosed plaque shows the therapist how to individually modify the patient's plaque control methods for optimum results. Visualization of disclosed plaque by the patient in the dental office and at home can provide strong motivation for better oral hygiene efforts.

Because bacterial plaque is accepted as the primary etiologic agent of gingivitis and periodontitis, the control of its accumulation is paramount to the prevention and control of these diseases. Bacterial plaque almost always covers the surface of calculus. Plaque is usually removed by the therapist concomitantly with calculus; this is discussed later in this chapter. Removal of supragingival plaque by the patient is successfully performed with a variety of methods and instruments. These methods must include a mechanical device for interdental plaque control, such as dental floss or an interproximal brush.

The process of teaching and motivating patients to control supragingival plaque is one of the most important and challenging phases of periodontal therapy. Detailed instruc-

tions using the patient's own mouth as a visual aid, repeated reinforcement, and praise for positive progress are some of the keys in this process. Informing the patient of the relationship between bacterial plaque and bad breath is also a strong motivating factor to change the patient's behavior.

Chemical means, such as chlorhexidine mouthrinses, are sometimes used to control plaque in acute periodontal conditions and during postoperative healing but are not used routinely for indefinite periods. Chlorhexidine does not affect microorganisms within periodontal pockets; its effect is primarily supragingival. Supragingival plaque control can help to resolve gingival inflammation, but has little effect on subgingival microflora if pockets are 6 mm or deeper.[4]

Many local factors can contribute to plaque retention. These include calculus deposits, malposed teeth, palatogingival grooves, radicular grooves, open carious lesions, enamel extensions, overhanging restorations, subgingival restorations, defective proximal contacts, and gingival enlargement due to inflammation or drug therapy. Nonsurgical therapy includes the elimination of as many of these factors as possible. It also sometimes includes minor tooth movement and occlusal therapy.

Detection of Subgingival Calculus

Explorers

The ability to detect subgingival calculus is as important as the ability to remove it. Detection methods include the use of very fine, specially designed explorers, such as the Hu-Friedy No. 3-A explorer (Hu-Friedy, Chicago, IL) (Fig 7-2); compressed air to dry the teeth and displace the marginal gingiva; visual signs of gingival inflammation; and radiographs. None of these methods is very exact by itself.[5] The use of all four methods combined is recommended for best results. The fine explorer is the single-most useful method for detection of subgingival calculus.

Correct use of explorers to detect subgingival calculus requires training and practice. Tactile sensitivity to feel what cannot be seen is essential. This skill is best learned with supervised practice. The shape of the explorer is critical; not all explorers are suited for this task. The No. 23 shepherd's hook explorer, for example, is unsuitable for detection of subgingival calculus if pockets are deeper than 4 mm. Its design does not allow subgingival extension into deeper pockets, and it is often too thick for good tactile sensitivity.

The Hu-Friedy No. 3-A explorer is excellent for detection of calculus in deep pockets and furcations. Its fine tip allows for good tactile sensitivity, and its design permits good adaptation to all root surfaces. The No. 3-A explorer is the best single method for subgingival calculus detection.

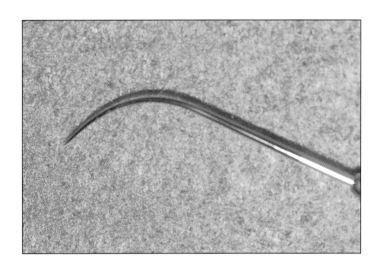

Fig 7-2 The No. 3-A explorer is a very fine explorer specially designed for detecting subgingival calculus.

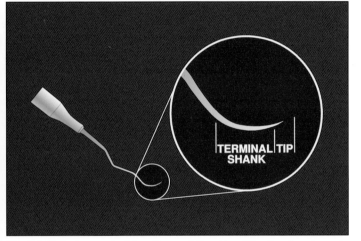

Fig 7-3 Only the terminal I to 2 mm of the side of the tip of explorers is used to detect subgingival calculus.

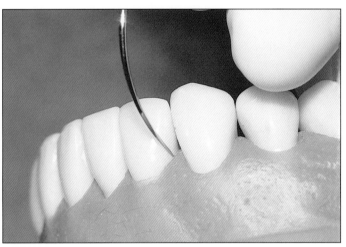

Fig 7-4 The terminal shank of the explorer should be positioned parallel to the root surface being examined so that the tip extends in an apical direction.

Other explorers suitable for this task include the No. 17, or Orban, explorer and pigtail-shaped explorers. Pigtail-shaped explorers are generally thin and have good tactile sensitivity. Their working ends are curved, permitting easy adaptation to most tooth surfaces. They must be long enough to extend into deep pockets. The No. 3 ML is an example of a good pigtail explorer.

Another excellent explorer is the O.D.U. No. 11-12 explorer. It is a highly sensitive instrument, adapted from the design of the Gracey 11-12 curette by faculty at Old Dominion University. It combines the pigtail design with a shank that is longer and straighter than that of most pigtail explorers.

The working end of an explorer is 1 to 2 mm long and is known as the *tip*. Only the terminal 1 to 2 mm of the side of the tip should be used to detect calculus (Fig 7-3). The terminal shank of the explorer should be positioned parallel to the root surface being examined so that the tip extends in an apical direction (Fig 7-4).

When explorers are being used to detect subgingival calculus, it is important to understand that subgingival calculus varies from thin, platelike deposits to thick, heavy ledges. Also, a thorough understanding of root anatomy and concavities[6] can greatly improve detection of subgingival calculus. A fine explorer should always be used toward the end of a root planing procedure to check the completeness of calculus removal. Curettes are inadequate for this step because they lack tactile sensitivity.

Compressed Air

Compressed air from an air-water syringe can be used to dry the tooth surface, making calculus more visible. Compressed air also displaces the marginal gingiva away from the tooth and thereby extends the clinician's vision deeper into periodontal pockets. Magnifying eye lenses and fiberoptic illumination can aid in detecting small deposits of subgingival calculus during this step of therapy. Compressed air is used most effectively toward the end of a root planing procedure but may have to be avoided in patients with thermal sensitivity.

Signs of Inflammation

Signs of inflammation, such as soft tissue swelling, redness, and bleeding, can also be very helpful in detecting subgingival calculus at the reevaluation stage of therapy. Differences in gingival contour and color caused by calculus and plaque-induced inflammation can aid the therapist in detecting deposits missed during previous debridement treatment (Figs 7-5a and 7-5b). A bluish gingival margin is a good indicator of subgingival calculus (Fig 7-6). Complete removal of calculus at reevaluation is especially important if surgical treatment is not planned for medical or other reasons.

Occasionally, gingival fenestrations are present (Fig 7-7). Their presence is almost always related to heavy subgingival calculus deposits and a thin periodontium.[7] Gingival fenestrations may disappear or persist after the removal of calculus, or the tissue coronal to the defect may be lost, converting the fenestration to a region of severe recession.[7]

Radiographs

Radiographs can help in calculus detection, but should not be the only method used. Detection of calculus by radiographs is influenced by the thickness of the deposits, the degree of mineralization, and the type of tooth. Calculus is usually not apparent radiographically on buccal and lingual tooth surfaces because of superimposed tooth structure. Buchanan et al[8] reported that radiographs do not detect existing calculus 56% of the time. Therefore, radiographs should be used only as an adjunct to other methods for the detection of subgingival calculus.

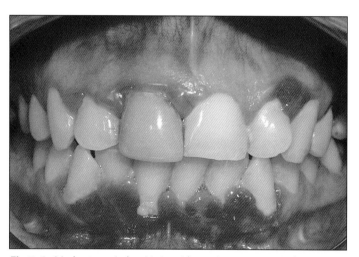

Fig 7-5a Moderate periodontitis is evident prior to nonsurgical treatment.

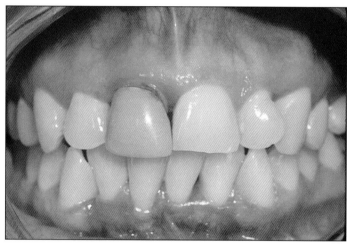

Fig 7-5b After nonsurgical therapy, the inflammation has been reduced, except in the mandibular incisor region, where residual calculus is present.

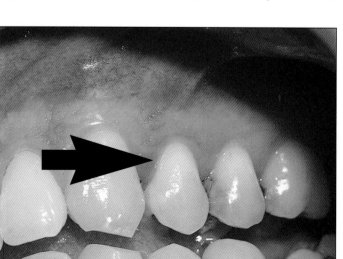

Fig 7-6 A bluish gingival margin is highly suggestive of the presence of subgingival calculus. The color of the gingiva between the maxillary canine and first premolar is related to subgingival calculus (arrow).

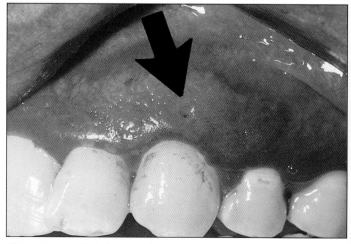

Fig 7-7 A gingival fenestration (arrow) is usually related to a heavy deposit of subgingival calculus.

Instrumentation

Careful selection, care, and application of instruments are extremely important aspects of effective nonsurgical treatment. Extensive texts have been written on these subjects,[9–11] and these are highly recommended for anyone seeking to increase his or her skills in nonsurgical therapy. In this chapter, only some of the most important concepts of instrumentation will be emphasized.

Instruments designed for scaling and root planing include curettes, sickle scalers, hoes, files, and ultrasonic devices. Curettes have long been considered the most effective instruments for root planing.

Curettes

Curettes are classified as either area specific or universal. Area-specific curettes are designed to be used on specific tooth surfaces. Gracey curettes are the most commonly used area-specific curettes. For example, the 11-12 Gracey is designed to be used specifically on the mesial surfaces of posterior teeth only. These curettes have only one cutting edge on each blade, so only one side of the blade requires sharpening (Fig 7-8). It is a good idea to memorize the specific areas for which each Gracey curette is designed so that these instruments are used efficiently (Table 7-1).

Universal curettes are designed so that each instrument can be adapted to all tooth surfaces. There are two cutting edges on each blade, and the curette blades are made at 90 degrees to the lower shank (Fig 7-8). The proper working angulation of universal curettes is determined by positioning the handle parallel to the surface being instrumented.

Subgingival instrumentation is a very difficult clinical skill because the blade cannot be seen as it is used. By learning to use the visual cues provided by the lower shank of a curette, the therapist can learn to apply the blade at the correct angulation without being able to see it. This principle is known as the *terminal shank rule* and is very important. It applies to both anterior and posterior teeth. The terminal, or lower shank should be parallel to the tooth surface for optimal angulation (Fig 7-9). If the terminal shank is leaning too far toward the tooth surface, the angulation will be too close to engage deposits during planing. However, leaning the terminal shank too far away from the tooth surface opens the angle of the blade to the tooth and also prevents effective deposit removal. Therefore, constant awareness of the position of the terminal shank is important.

Curette manufacturers have recently made modifications in design to improve subgingival effectiveness. These modifications include lengthening the terminal shank, shortening the blade, and thinning the blade. In addition, new curettes with accentuated angles are designed to permit better access to mesial, distal, and furcation surfaces of posterior teeth. Other innovations include the marking of the

Table 7-1 Specific teeth and surfaces for which Gracey curettes are designed

Gracey curette	Teeth (surfaces)
1-2	Anterior
3-4	Anterior
5-6	Anterior and premolar
7-8	Posterior (buccal and lingual)
9-10	Posterior (buccal and lingual)
11-12	Posterior (mesial)
13-14	Posterior (distal)

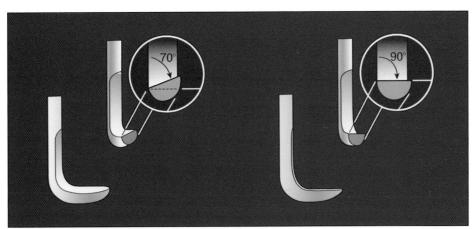

Fig 7-8 *(left)* The Gracey curette has only one cutting edge, and the face of the blade is aligned at 70 degrees to the terminal shank. *(right)* The universal curette has the face of its blade aligned at 90 degrees to the terminal shank and two cutting edges.

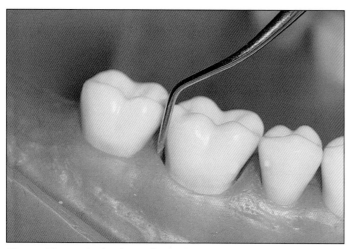

Fig 7-9 The terminal or lower shank of a curette should be parallel to the tooth surface being root planed.

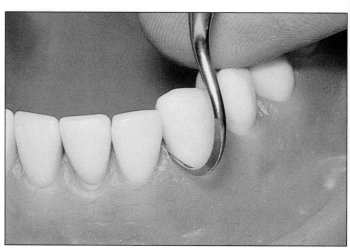

Fig 7-10 The sickle scaler is especially useful for removal of calculus where there is limited interproximal space between anterior teeth.

cutting edges of curettes for quick identification and the addition of millimeter markings on the terminal shank to allow visual assessment of probing depth during instrumentation. Also, the design features of Gracey curettes have now been combined with the efficiency of the universal curette blade. Clinical trials are needed to test the value of these new modifications.

Scalers

Scalers are designed primarily for supragingival calculus removal and can be used effectively only 1 to 3 mm subgingivally. The sickle scaler shown in Fig 7-10 is especially useful for removal of calculus in situations where there is limited interproximal space between anterior teeth. Scalers for posterior teeth are also available. Scalers are not useful for debridement of deep periodontal pockets.

Hoes

Hoes are rigid instruments used for removing heavy supragingival and subgingival calculus, mainly from the buccal and lingual surfaces of posterior teeth. They may also be used on proximal surfaces next to edentulous areas. There is a specific working end designed for each of the four tooth surfaces: mesial, distal, buccal, and lingual. The hoe is used only with a pulling stroke and is especially useful for removing heavy deposits on the distal surfaces of terminal molars.

Files

Files are also used to remove heavy and tenacious calculus. They are rigid, like hoes, and so lack tactile sensitivity. The file has multiple cutting edges that fracture and roughen the surface of calculus, making later removal with a curette easier. Like hoes, files are designed in sets of four, one for each tooth surface. Files are also especially useful for removing heavy, tenacious ledges of calculus on the distal surfaces of terminal molars. The design of the working end gives ideal access to these surfaces.

Ultrasonic Scalers

For many years, ultrasonic and sonic scalers were used as adjuncts to hand instruments in nonsurgical therapy. They were advocated for removal of gross calculus but, because of their bulky design, did not have good tactile sensitivity and were of limited use subgingivally. Recent modification of ultrasonic tips to make them narrower and straighter has made a big impact on nonsurgical therapy. Ultrasonic tips are now being used in an expanded role to remove plaque and calculus in deep periodontal pockets.[12]

Research has revealed that curettes have significant limitations in subgingival debridement, especially in deep pockets and furcations. Very often the size of the instrument does not allow access to a particular region. The majority of molar furcation entrances are smaller than the average width of a curette blade.[13] The concavities of root surfaces also limit curette access. In addition, debridement with a curette is a tedious, time-consuming, exacting procedure. Newly designed ultrasonic tips are easier to use than curettes and reach deeper into periodontal pockets.[12] They accomplish debridement faster than curettes and require no sharpening.[12]

Ultrasonic scalers convert electrical energy into mechanical energy, resulting in a high-frequency vibration of the instrument tip. The conversion of energy is performed by either a magnetostrictive or piezoelectric transducer. The rate of vibration is 25,000 to 42,000 cycles per second with a vibration amplitude of 7 to 28 μm. A significant amount of heat is produced in the conversion of energy. Water directed into the working area dissipates the heat and forms a fine spray from the energy release. The water spray helps to cleanse the work area and, with the vibration energy, may also have some bactericidal effects.[14] Removal of calculus from the root surface requires contact of the side of the tip against the calculus.

Ultrasonic devices are contraindicated for patients with older cardiac pacemakers because of the danger of interfering with the electrical mechanism of the pacemaker. Newer pacemaker designs with increased shielding may eliminate this concern. If the therapist is in doubt, he or she should consult with the patient's cardiologist. Patients with infectious diseases such as acquired immunodeficiency syndrome (AIDS), tuberculosis, and hepatitis should be treated with great caution with ultrasonic devices because of the aerosol produced in the treatment room. Airborne microorganisms increase 30-fold in the treatment room when ultrasonic instruments are used.

Guidelines for Use of Ultrasonic Devices

- Use enough water to avoid overheating the instrument and tooth surface.
- Apply the side of the instrument (not the tip) to the tooth surface.
- Move the tip continuously in a back-and-forth brush-like stroke, avoiding heavy pressure.
- Wear protective face mask and glasses during use.
- Check completeness of deposit removal with an appropriate explorer.
- Do not use ultrasonic devices on patients with cardiac pacemakers without consultation with their cardiologists; patients with infectious diseases such as AIDS, tuberculosis, and hepatitis should be treated with great caution.
- Flush water line for at least 2 minutes before use to decrease microbial contamination of the water lines and reservoir.
- Ultrasonic scalers produce bacteremias similar to those produced by hand scaling, so precautions are indicated for patients at risk for bacterial endocarditis.
- Ultrasonic devices should not be used near bonded veneer and cemented restorations.

Effective instrumentation for nonsurgical therapy involves the combined use of hand instruments and ultrasonic devices. Learning effective instrumentation takes patience and persistence.

Effects of Nonsurgical Treatment

Common questions related to nonsurgical periodontal therapy are: "What is the end point?" and "When is it completed?" The answers to these questions have been controversial. To provide a biologic answer, it is helpful to look at the specific effects of nonsurgical treatment on subgingival flora, soft tissues, root surfaces, bone, and tooth mobility.

Subgingival Flora

Alteration of the microflora in sites affected by periodontitis is a major goal of nonsurgical therapy. This therapy produces many of the other desirable effects of nonsurgical treatment. Complete eradication of microorganisms is not possible, however. The aim is to reduce the overall number of bacteria and replace a pathogenic flora with one that is sparse and compatible with health. The alteration in the microflora produced by scaling and root planing lasts from weeks to months, depending on the effectiveness of the oral hygiene of the patient. If patient plaque control is poor, the pathogenic plaque may return in as few as 4 weeks. In severe forms of periodontitis, bacteria invade the soft tissues, making complete eradication of bacteria more complicated.

Soft Tissues

Effects of scaling and root planing on soft tissues include the reduction of gingival inflammation and bleeding, gingival recession, and a reduction in probing depth. These effects occur mainly during the first month after nonsurgical therapy. Some continued improvement occurs over the next 9 to 12 months, but this improvement is small compared to that experienced during the first month.

The reduction in probing depth is in the range of 1 to 2 mm but may be more in very deep pockets. The reduction in probing depth is due to a combination of recession and an increase in clinical attachment. The gingival tissues are more resistant to penetration of the probe after nonsurgical treatment because of changes in the tissues that take place during wound healing. The inflammatory infiltrate is replaced by new collagen, which, when mature, will resist probe penetration.

Patients with moderate periodontitis and 5- to 6-mm pockets before treatment are sometimes treated definitively by scaling and root planing only. There is evidence that repeated instrumentation does not significantly improve the soft tissue response.[15] In moderate-to-severe periodontitis, bleeding on probing is greatly reduced by nonsurgical treatment but usually persists in localized pockets.[15] Gingival recession of 1 to 2 mm is common after debridement therapy and contributes to the pocket reduction.

Root Surfaces

Root surfaces are altered by nonsurgical treatment in several ways. These include the removal of plaque, calculus, and endotoxin. Calculus removal is rarely complete, but the reduction of the area covered by calculus is up to 10-fold.[5] Endotoxin, a product of plaque bacteria, has been found mainly on the root surface and is easily removed.[16] Root planing also removes cementum and dentin contaminated by plaque bacteria. Microorganisms are known to penetrate cementum in teeth affected by periodontitis.[17]

The major cemental changes associated with periodontal disease can be removed within 40 to 50 μm of the surface by 20 strokes of light scaling.[18] Following root planing, varying degrees of root surface roughness are found, depending on the type of instrument used. It has been shown that smooth surfaces promote significantly less subgingival colonization of bacteria than do rough surfaces.[19]

Bone

Changes in alveolar bone caused by nonsurgical treatment are not commonly documented, but significant long-term increases in bone density have been reported.[20] These changes are related to the remineralization of bone, which takes months to occur, and are therefore not practical as an indicator of disease activity. More research is indicated concerning this effect of nonsurgical treatment.

Tooth Mobility

Abnormal tooth mobility is commonly reduced by nonsurgical therapy in patients with severe forms of periodontitis. During wound healing following debridement therapy, the inflammatory infiltrate is slowly replaced by collagen fibers, which mature and eventually contribute to the stabilization of the teeth. A healthy gingival attachment to the teeth has been shown to contribute to tooth stability.

There is a consensus that the end point in scaling and root planing is a hard, smooth root surface. This goal seems to be sound, based on research findings.[21] However, because methods of detecting subgingival calculus are very inexact, careful assessment of the soft tissue inflammation, probing

depth, and attachment levels is also important. These factors should be considered together in deciding whether nonsurgical treatment is complete and if surgical therapy is indicated. Severe periodontitis, especially around posterior teeth, is treated most predictably by surgical procedures.

Adjuncts in Nonsurgical Therapy

Nonsurgical therapy is playing an increasing role in the overall management of periodontal disease, partly because of the use of adjuncts to enhance effectiveness. These adjuncts include the use of systemic and locally delivered antibiotics, visual magnification devices, fiberoptic illumination, and modified ultrasonic instruments. Correction of local factors, such as caries and defective restorations, was discussed earlier in the chapter.

Antibiotics

In aggressive forms of periodontitis, it appears that systemic antibiotics may enhance the effects of scaling and root planing.[22] Tetracycline and metronidazole are the antibiotics most commonly studied in clinical trials for this purpose. Both are concentrated in the gingival crevicular fluid to a much greater extent than in the bloodstream and are effective against a large number of periodontal pathogens.

Pathogens are known to invade the soft tissues in aggressive forms of periodontitis. In these cases, eradication of microorganisms is more complete with a combination of mechanical debridement and antibiotics. The ideal antibiotic regimen for this type of treatment has not been established, but use for 7 to 14 days is usually recommended. Aggressive forms of periodontitis include localized juvenile periodontitis and rapidly progressive periodontitis. Systemic antibiotics are not indicated to enhance the nonsurgical treatment of patients with slight-to-moderate adult periodontitis because clinical trials have shown no advantage for their use in these situations.

Local delivery of slow-release antibiotics as an adjunct to scaling and root planing is receiving a recent surge of interest. Tetracycline-impregnated fibers are a new, controlled, localized drug delivery method that can be used by therapists depending on the site, the patient, and the natural history of the disease process. Investigators who compared the efficacy of combined therapy (tetracycline fibers plus root planing) to that of root planing alone reported that combined therapy provides no additional clinical benefit with regard to reduction in probing depth or gain of clinical attachment in the treatment of adult periodontitis.[23] Similarly, Lowenguth et al[24] noted that combined therapy and root planing alone have suppressed pathogens at an equivalent amount of sites when patients are assessed 1 year after therapy. Others also have noted that scaling and fiber therapy result in a comparable suppression of pathogens and reduction of the number of infected sites.[25,26]

In contrast, Newman et al[27] found different results in a population of patients with recurrent periodontitis that did not respond to periodic root planing. Combined therapy often results in greater reduction in probing depth and gain in clinical attachment than does root planing.[27] Thus, it could be contended that it would have been more appropriate if tetracycline-impregnated fibers were labeled to be used in conjunction with scaling and root planing at sites that did not respond to conventional therapy.

Many articles have indicated that unnecessary use of antibiotics results in an increased prevalence of resistant bacterial strains. Accordingly, a basic tenet of periodontal therapy is to employ antibiotics only when necessary. Currently, there are limited data regarding the development of resistant strains after local drug delivery with tetracyclines.[28–30] The data indicate that increased resistance is often transient at treated sites. However, additional research is needed to determine the impact that single and multiple application of fibers will have on the development and selection of resistant strains. Of particular concern is the development of resistant bacteria at other intraoral sites that may be exposed to leakage of sublethal drug concentrations out of treated pockets.

With regard to selection of the appropriate antibiotic for patients not responding to conventional therapy, tetracycline is not the universal drug of choice for the treatment of periodontal diseases. Other drugs (eg, metronidazole, Augmentin) have been successfully used to treat patients with refractory periodontitis.[31] Therefore, in nonresponding patients, it is prudent to perform antibiotic sensitivity testing prior to the administration of drugs, to ensure the best results.

Another issue that warrants discussion concerns the advantages and limitations of local drug delivery and systemic administration of antibiotics. Local delivery can provide high concentrations of medications and decrease the incidence of adverse side effects. In contrast, systemic drug therapy is usually less expensive, easier to deliver, reduces chairside time, impacts on reservoirs of bacterial reinfection (eg, tonsils, saliva), and can affect tissue-invasive organisms (ie, *Actinobacillus actinomycetemcomitans*).[32] It is possible that a combination of both methods may be most efficacious, but there is no body of evidence to support this contention.

Many issues still need to be resolved regarding the potential use of tetracycline-impregnated fibers in the treatment of periodontal diseases. Undoubtedly, as additional research is completed, clearer indications for their utilization will become more apparent.

Magnification Devices

Eyestrain is a major cause of stress and fatigue in dentistry. Optimal vision is a prerequisite for effective nonsurgical treatment. Because of these two factors, many therapists are finding that magnification devices greatly increase the effectiveness and ease of treatment. These devices vary a great deal in design and cost. Headbands and clip-on lenses are the least expensive, ranging from $50 to $100. Other magnification aids may be custom designed with a specific magnification ratio, focal length, and depth of field (Fig 7-11). These vision aids cost from $500 to $1,500. Magnification of these lenses ranges from 2.5 to 5.0. They can greatly increase the completeness of nonsurgical treatment and are useful in many other areas of dentistry.

Fiberoptic Illumination

Fiberoptic illumination is another adjunct in tooth debridement procedures. The source may be provided with a freestanding light wand or attachments to a dental mirror, retractor, or suction device. Controlled studies indicate that fiberoptic devices significantly increase the thoroughness of root debridement.[33]

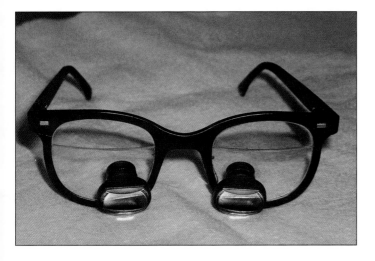

Fig 7-11 An example of a magnification aid that can be custom designed for the individual's requirements.

Modified Ultrasonic Instruments

Modified ultrasonic instruments are proving to be a very significant factor in increasing the effectiveness and importance of nonsurgical periodontal therapy. They are discussed in detail in the instrumentation section of this chapter.

These adjuncts are increasing the number of cases of periodontal disease that can be controlled by nonsurgical methods. They are reducing, but not eliminating, the need for periodontal surgical procedures.

Limitations

Scaling and root planing have significant limitations, especially in the treatment of posterior teeth affected by severe forms of periodontitis. These limitations include poor access to deep periodontal pockets, grooves, and concavities in roots, constricted access to furcations, and bacterial invasion of the gingiva and root surfaces. Pockets distal to terminal molars will usually not improve following scaling and root planing. The thick and often fibrous tissue in these areas does not readily shrink following debridement.

Clinical studies indicate that, as pockets get deeper, scaling and root planing are less effective.[34,35] Generally, pockets of 7 mm or greater are most predictably controlled by surgical treatment.[36] This is especially true in multirooted teeth. Grooves and concavities are found on the roots of all teeth, not just maxillary premolars, where they are most pronounced.[6] Once a plaque infection reaches these irregularities, it becomes much harder to control by patient and professional. The majority of hand instruments currently manufactured are too wide to fit into furcation areas for effective debridement. New designs in ultrasonic instruments and curettes appear to be improving this situation, however.

Bacterial invasion of the gingiva in severe forms of periodontitis makes it impossible to eliminate all microorganisms by scaling and root planing alone. Antibiotics and surgical procedures are necessary to control the progress of disease in these cases. Bacteria also penetrate into cementum and dentin. The effectiveness of removing bacteria from these tissues by scaling and root planing has not been thoroughly studied. Also, the significance of retention of microorganisms in these tissues needs further study.

Conclusion

Nonsurgical treatment, although effective in controlling a vast amount of periodontal disease, cannot be considered a panacea. Many adjunctive tools and refinements of scaling and root planing are being developed to overcome the limitations of this form of therapy. We should be constantly evaluating these in our clinical practice and by studying the dental literature. At present, surgical procedures are often necessary to overcome the limitations of nonsurgical therapy.

References

1. Cerra M, Killoy W. The effect of sodium bicarbonate and hydrogen peroxide on the microbial flora of periodontal pockets. A preliminary report. J Periodontol 1982;53:599–603.
2. West T, King W. Toothbrushing with hydrogen peroxide-sodium bicarbonate compared to tooth powder and water in reducing periodontal pocket suppuration and dark field bacterial counts. J Periodontol 1983;54:339–346.
3. Genco RJ, Goldman HM, Cohen DW. Contemporary Periodontics. St. Louis: Mosby, 1990:401.
4. Beltrami M, Bickel M, Baehni P. The effect of supragingival plaque control on the composition of the subgingival microflora in human periodontitis. J Clin Periodontol 1987;14:161–164.
5. Sherman PR, Hutchens LH, Jenson JG, Moriarty JM, Greco G, McFall WT. The effectiveness of subgingival scaling and root planing. I. Clinical detection of residual calculus. J Periodontol 1990;61:3–8.
6. Gher ME, Vernino AR. Root anatomy: A local factor in inflammatory periodontal disease. Int J Periodont Rest Dent 1981;1:53–63.
7. Lane J. Gingival fenestration. J Periodontol 1977;48:225–227.
8. Buchanan SA, Jendersech RS, Granet MA, Kircos LT, Chambers DW, Robertson PB. Radiographic detection of dental calculus. J Periodontol 1987;58:747–751.
9. Pattison AM, Pattison GL. Periodontal Instrumentation. 2nd ed. Norwalk, CT: Appleton and Lange, 1992.
10. Nield JS, Houseman GA. Fundamentals of Periodontal Instrumentation. 3rd ed. Baltimore: Williams & Wilkins, 1996.
11. Wasserman B. Root Scaling and Planing. Chicago: Quintessence, 1986.
12. Dragoo MR. A clinical evaluation of hand and ultrasonic instruments on subgingival debridement. Part I. With unmodified and modified ultrasonic inserts. Int J Periodont Rest Dent 1992;12:311–323.
13. Bower RC. Furcation morphology relative to periodontal treatment—furcation entrance architecture. J Periodontol 1979;50:23.
14. Baehni P, Thilo B, Chapis B, Pernet D. Effects of ultrasonic and sonic scalers on dental plaque microflora in vitro and in vivo. J Clin Periodontol 1992;19:455–459.
15. Baderstein A, Nilveus R, Egelberg J. Effect of nonsurgical periodontal therapy. III. Single versus repeated instrumentation. J Clin Periodontol 1983;11:114–124.
16. Hughes FJ, Smales FC. Immunohistochemical investigation of the presence and distribution of cementum associated lipopolysaccharides in periodontal disease. J Periodont Res 1986;21:660–667.
17. Daly CG, Seymour GJ, Kieser JB, Corbet EF. Histological assessment of periodontally involved cementum. J Clin Periodontol 1982;9:266–274.
18. Fukazawa E, Nishimura K. Superficial cemental curettage: Its efficacy in promoting improved cellular attachment on human root surfaces previously damaged by periodontitis. J Periodontol 1994;65:168–176.
19. Leknes KN, Lie T, Wikesjö UM, Bogle G, Selveg KA. Influence of tooth instrumentation roughness on subgingival microbial colonization. J Periodontol 1994;65:303–308.
20. Dubrez B, Graf JM, Vaagnat P, Amasoni G. Increase of interproximal bone density after subgingival instrumentation. A quantitative radiographical study. J Periodontol 1990;61:723–731.

21. Kaldahl WB, Kalkwarf KL, Patil KD. A review of longitudinal studies that compared periodontal therapies. J Periodontol 1993;64:243–253.

22. Loesche WJ, Schmidt E, Smith B, Morrison E, Caffesse R, Hujoel P. Effects of metronidazole on periodontal treatment needs. J Periodontol 1991;62:247–257.

23. Drisko C, Cobb C, Killoy R, Lowenguth R, et al. Clinical response to tetracycline fiber periodontal therapy [abstract 1637]. J Dent Res 1994;73:306.

24. Lowenguth R, Caton J, Chin I, Drisko C, et al. Evaluation of various treatments using controlled-release tetracycline fibers: microbiologic response [abstract 1639]. J Dent Res 1994;73:307.

25. Maiden MFJ, Tanner A, McArdle S, Najpauer K, Goodson JM. Tetracycline fiber therapy monitored by DNA probe and cultural methods. J Periodont Res 1991;26:452–459.

26. Goodson JM, Tanner A, McArdle S, Dix K, Watanabe SM. Multi-center evaluation of tetracycline fiber therapy. III. Microbiological response. J Periodont Res 1991;26:440–451.

27. Newman MG, Kornman KS, Doherty FM. A 6-month multi-center evaluation of adjunctive tetracycline fiber therapy used in conjunction with scaling and root planing in maintenance patients: Clinical results. J Periodontol 1994;65:685–691.

28. Goodson JM, Tanner A. Antibiotic resistance of the subgingival microbiota following local tetracycline therapy. Oral Microbiol Immunol 1992;7:113–117.

29. Preus HR, Lassen J, Aass AM, Ciancio SJ. Bacterial resistance following subgingival and systemic administration of minocycline. J Clin Periodontol 1995;22:380–384.

30. Larsen T. Occurrence of doxycycline resistant bacteria in the oral cavity after local administration of doxycycline in patients with periodontal disease. Scand J Infect Dis 1991;23:89–95.

31. Rams TE, Slots J. Antibiotics in periodontal therapy: an update. Compend Contin Educ Dent 1992;8:1130–1145.

32. Greenstein G. Treating periodontal diseases with tetracycline impregnated fibers: Data and controversies. Compend Contin Educ Dent 1995;16:448–455.

33. Reinhart RA, Johnson GK, Tussing GJ. Root planing with interdental papilla reflection and fiberoptic illumination. J Periodontol 1985;56:721–726.

34. Stambaugh R, Dragoo M, Smith D, Carasoli L. The limits of subgingival scaling. Int J Periodont Rest Dent 1981;1:30–41.

35. Rabbani G. Ash M, Caffesse R. The effectiveness of subgingival scaling and root planing in calculus removal. J Periodontol 1981;52:119.

36. Antczak-Bouckoms A, Joshipura K, Burdick E, Tullock J. Meta-analysis of surgical versus non-surgical methods of treatment for periodontal disease. J Clin Periodontol 1995;20:259–268.

CHAPTER 8

Treatment of the Periodontium Affected by Occlusal Traumatism

Paul A. Ricchetti, DDS, MScD

The effect of occlusion on the periodontium has been a topic of discussion among dentists, and periodontists in particular, since the beginning of this century. Debate has raged over the years regarding the influence or lack of influence of occlusal trauma on periodontal disease. Early studies without adequate controls implicated occlusal trauma in the formation of pockets and as the cause of gingival recession.[1-7]

Contemporary studies with adequate controls that limit variables have produced more objective data on occlusal trauma and its effect on the periodontium.[8-10] Within the scope of this chapter, the effect of occlusal force on the periodontium will be described to establish a biologic rationale for occlusal treatment in various clinical situations. The ability to link the clinical presentation and the biologic and histopathologic entity is the basis for clinical understanding and appropriate treatment planning.

The Effect of Force on the Periodontium

Any force applied to a tooth, whether a unilateral orthodontic-type force or a bilateral tooth-to-tooth "jiggling" force, has the potential to produce a pathologic effect on the attachment apparatus (cementum, periodontal ligament [PDL], and bone).[11,12] The pathologic lesion in the attachment apparatus that is established by trauma from force (occlusal trauma) causes a loss of alveolar and crestal lamina dura and a resultant widening of the periodontal ligament space (Figs 8-1a and 8-1b). Clinically, the occlusal traumatic lesion in the attachment apparatus presents as increasing tooth mobility over a period of time.[8,12]

Light Forces

If a force applied to a tooth is constant in intensity but within the adaptive range of the surrounding periodontium, the occlusal traumatic lesion in the attachment apparatus will resolve over time as the wound (occlusal traumatic lesion) heals.[8,13,14] As the pathologic inflammatory response in the attachment apparatus resolves, a permanent widening of the periodontal ligament space is established to compensate for the force.[8] The vascular reaction in the bone and PDL dissipates, along with the white cell response.[15] Healing occurs in the bone, but the PDL remains widened. The attachment apparatus returns to normal histologically, but with a widened PDL.[8,15] Clinically, the tooth will demonstrate increased mobility (Figs 8-2a and 8-2b) because the PDL has widened as a result of the morphologic change in the attachment apparatus in response to the force. As long as the intensity of the force does not increase, the PDL remains widened, but healed, and the mobility remains increased, but not increasing.[8,12]

If the force applied to a tooth is removed after an occlusal traumatic lesion has been established, the inflammatory lesion in the attachment apparatus will resolve, and the PDL will return to its original width prior to force application.[14] Bone apposition at the alveolar lamina dura occurs as the force is removed, allowing the PDL to return to its

Figs 8-1a and 8-1b Lesion of primary occlusal trauma. Clinical situation 1 presenting as primary occlusal trauma.

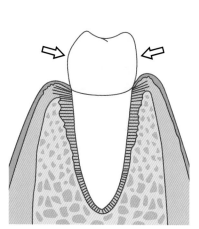

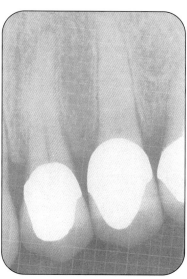

Fig 8-1a Widening PDL resulting from excessive force *(arrows)*.

Fig 8-1b Typical lesion of primary trauma with bone levels at or near the CEJ.

Figs 8-2a and 8-2b Adaptation of the attachment apparatus. Clinical situation 2 presenting as primary occlusal trauma.

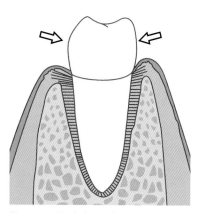

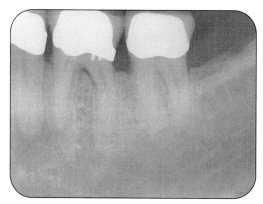

Fig 8-2a Healed attachment apparatus with widened PDL resulting from remaining force *(arrows)*.

Fig 8-2b Bone levels at or near the CEJ on teeth with widened PDL to accommodate increased, but not increasing, mobility.

pre–occlusal trauma width. Clinically, the tooth demonstrates increasing mobility as force is applied and then a return to preforce stability as the force is removed and the attachment apparatus repairs[16,17] (Figs 8-3a to 8-3c).

Clinical tooth-to-tooth contacts are more likely to generate lighter jiggling-type forces described in the literature.[10] Teeth subjected to these loads demonstrate milder, more subtle changes in mobility that can be difficult to discriminate clinically. Radiographic changes associated with teeth that are experiencing lighter occlusal traumatic loads also tend to be more subtle. There is a less obvious coronal and alveolar loss of lamina dura and a less obvious increase in PDL width.

Heavy Forces

The heavier the force applied to a tooth, the larger the resultant lesion in the attachment apparatus, the wider the PDL, and the larger the increase in mobility. If a heavy force exceeds the adaptive response of the attachment

Fig 8-3a Healing of the attachment apparatus as excessive force *(arrows)* creating primary occlusal trauma is reduced. The PDL returns to normal width as force is reduced.

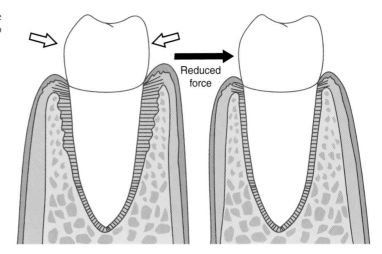

Reduced force

Figs 8-3b and 8-3c Healing of the attachment apparatus over a 2-year interval after elimination of primary trauma on the mandibular left second molar.

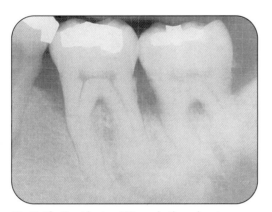

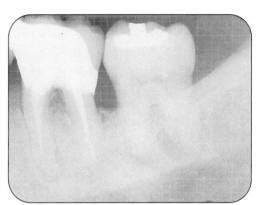

Fig 8-3b A widening PDL on both molars is exemplified by the nonprobing radiographic furcation involvement on the second molar.

Fig 8-3c The first molar class II buccal and lingual probing furcations have been treated surgically. Note the bone fill in the nonprobing furcation of the mandibular left second molar with healing of the attachment apparatus.

apparatus, the tooth can become increasingly mobile and never adapt.[9,18–20]

During orthodontic treatment, applied forces are heavy but are dissipated as energy in the wire is released to produce tooth movement.[11] Mobility of the tooth increases as the force from the wire is first applied but then decreases as the force in the wire dissipates and the tooth has moved to a new position (Figs 8-4a and 8-4b). If the wire is never changed and loses its ability to exert a force on the tooth, the "occlusal trauma–like" lesion in the attachment apparatus created by the force will resolve, and the tooth will stabilize in a new position dictated by the wire. Basically, the orthodontic effect on the periodontium can be interpreted as one of controlled occlusal trauma.[19,20] It allows tooth movement to occur through a series of controlled healing responses within the periodontium.[11]

With heavy forces similar to those in the orthodontic range, the lesion of occlusal trauma in the attachment apparatus can become extensive, severely widening the PDL and decreasing tissue resistance in the attachment apparatus.[9,20] Consequently, changes in mobility are more dramatic with heavier applied forces. This is less likely to occur when lighter forces overload an attachment apparatus. The amount of bone loss is less and the PDL less widened when resorption from a smaller occlusal traumatic lesion is induced by a lighter force.[10] The lighter the force, the less mobile the tooth will become to accommodate the applied force.

Pathologic Tooth Wear

When the effects of force on teeth are evaluated, it is important to consider pathologic dental wear in the overall diagnostic equation.[21] Each tooth likely has a threshold of force beyond which an occlusal traumatic lesion develops in the attachment apparatus.[22] This threshold force may be quite high yet may exceed a tooth's ability to resist wear. Occlusal and incisal wear may then occur, but mobility may or may not be present.[23,24] The extent of dental wear may not be directly related to the extent of the lesion of occlusal trauma in the attachment apparatus. If the focus of examination is restricted to mobility, tooth wear may be overlooked

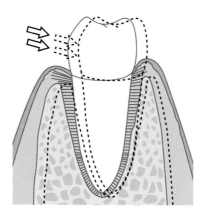

Fig 8-4a Alteration of the attachment apparatus caused by a heavy unilateral orthodontic force *(double arrows)*. *(dotted line)* New, stable position of the tooth and PDL.

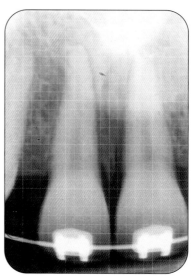

Fig 8-4b Teeth in primary trauma as a result of orthodontic forces. Note the general widening of the PDL and the subtle loss of coronal lamina dura, creating a radiographic picture of vertical bone loss without clinical loss of attachment or increased probing.

during the periodontal examination and during treatment planning for the affected periodontium.[25] Dental wear does affect the occlusal scheme and must be compensated for during occlusal treatment planning for the periodontally involved patient.[26]

Soft Tissues

Because the effects of occlusal force on the periodontium are limited to the attachment apparatus, occlusal force does not affect the supercrestal soft tissues of the periodontium.[8,12,27–31] The attached gingival soft tissues coronal to bone (the connective tissue attachment and the junctional epithelium) are not damaged by excessive force on a tooth.[8,12,14,32–36] Marginal soft tissue changes (recession and pocketing) are not initiated by the occlusal traumatic lesion.[8,12,14,32–36] Pocketing and recession are marginal disease entities (occlusal trauma is not a marginal disease) and as such are initiated by plaque-related pathosis beginning at the gingival margin.[37]

Theoretically, there are certain dental morphologic changes influenced by occlusal force that may affect the soft tissue attachment, although this has yet to be demonstrated scientifically. It is possible that heavy occlusal forces that cause dental wear, and more specifically cervical abfractions, may, by damaging tooth structure cervically at the interface of the soft tissue attachment, create attachment loss that presents clinically as gingival recession.[38–43] If this phenomenon is possible, it is likely to be noted in those patients who clinically demonstrate cervical erosion (abfractions) and in whom the extent of gingival recession present may not correlate with the degree of plaque-related disease alone.

In fact, it may be possible that as cervical abfraction of a tooth occurs due to force, increased plaque retention may develop as a result of poor access in the abfracted area. Plaque-related recession can then occur secondary to the morphologic tooth alteration from force.

Biologic Rationale for Occlusal Intervention

Two types of occlusal trauma are encountered clinically.[44] *Primary occlusal trauma* occurs when increasing mobility is caused by an excessive force on a tooth (see Figs 8-1a and 8-1b). *Secondary occlusal trauma* occurs when increasing mobility is caused by inadequate bone support (Figs 8-5a to 8-5c) rather than excessive force. Mobility in secondary occlusal trauma is secondary to the bone loss. Occlusal forces encountered in secondary occlusal trauma are acceptable to the attachment apparatus. It is the lack of adequate bone support in secondary trauma that allows the tooth to become increasingly more mobile or to migrate.

Figs 8-5a to 8-5c Lesion of secondary occlusal trauma. Clinical situation I presenting as secondary occlusal trauma.

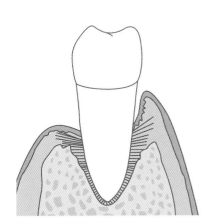

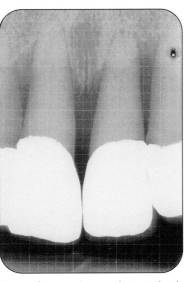

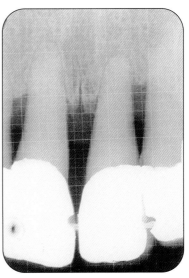

Fig 8-5a Widening PDL caused by inadequate bone support. Plaque-related disease, represented by pocketing on the right half of the tooth, is separated from the more apical lesion of occlusal trauma by the intact connective tissue attachment.

Fig 8-5b Typical secondary occlusal traumatic situation demonstrating vertical bone loss caused by widening of the PDL. Pocketing does not extend into the area of radiographic bone loss.

Fig 8-5c Radiograph taken 16 months later. The healing of the attachment apparatus after wire splinting is indicated by loss of the vertical lesions (widening PDLs) shown in Fig 8-5b.

If no primary or secondary occlusal trauma is present, the occlusion is labeled *physiologic*. A patient with physiologic occlusion may have mobile teeth, but the mobility is not increasing. There is no occlusal traumatic lesion in the attachment apparatus in a physiologic occlusion. The PDL width is stable; it may be increased, but it is not increasing.[8,15]

Primary Occlusal Trauma

Diagnosis and Treatment

Because primary occlusal trauma is caused by excessive force, its treatment is predicated on reduction of force to a level acceptable to the attachment apparatus. Excessive force can be reduced by altering the occlusion. After occlusal alteration, the lesion in the attachment apparatus can resolve, PDL width can return to preforce levels, and mobility will be reduced.

Clinically, a tooth in primary trauma will demonstrate increasing mobility, migration, and/or fremitus. Radiographically, a tooth in primary trauma may demonstrate vertical bone loss due to widening of the PDL. This radiographic bone loss representing the occlusal traumatic lesion in the attachment apparatus should not be confused with radiographic bone changes related to loss of attachment from marginal plaque–related disease. With heavy force or longstanding primary trauma, thickening of the

alveolar lamina dura or root resorption may be noted radiographically.[11,45]

Primary occlusal trauma can be encountered in conjunction with plaque-related bone loss that is not advanced enough to create secondary trauma. If a tooth has reduced bone support that is not advanced enough to permit mobility, the increasing mobility may be caused by excessive force. Under these circumstances, the tooth will demonstrate clinically increasing mobility, and/or migration, and/or fremitus just like a tooth in primary trauma without loss of attachment. Radiographically, however, teeth with loss of attachment not advanced enough to create secondary trauma but that are under heavy enough force to cause primary trauma will demonstrate various forms of vertical and horizontal bone loss, depending on the extent of attachment loss from plaque-related disease and the extent of PDL widening created by force.

Occlusal treatment of this clinical situation is the same as treatment for primary trauma without attachment loss. If excessive force is reduced by altering the occlusion, mobility will return to the preforce levels after resolution of the occlusal traumatic lesion in the attachment apparatus and return of the widening PDL to its preforce width. Any plaque-related bone loss in primary trauma is not affecting mobility.

A diagnostic dilemma can develop when evidence of primary trauma and advancing plaque-related bone loss is encountered on the same tooth because these situations can be confused with secondary trauma. It is also possible that mobility of teeth with bone loss from plaque-related disease can represent an adaptive response of the attachment apparatus to force rather than primary or secondary trauma. Mobility can also simply represent a clinical response to plaque-related inflammation without the presence of excessive force or bone loss.[46–48]

To assist in establishing the correct diagnosis and the appropriate occlusal treatment, it is imperative that a strict treatment sequence be followed initially in periodontal treatment. Control of the plaque-related inflammatory lesion must be the first course of treatment when significant mobility and bone loss caused by plaque-related disease are both evident.[16,17,46–49] After control of the marginal plaque–related lesion through nonsurgical or surgical periodontal treatments, the effect of plaque-related inflammation on the mobility patterns may be ruled out. If mobility is under control after elimination of marginal inflammation, then plaque-related inflammation can be designated as the cause of tooth mobility. If, however, mobility patterns have not stabilized (dissipated or reduced) after control of the marginal plaque–related inflammatory lesion, and occlusal contacts are extraordinary, the clinician may consider alteration of the occlusion to reduce excessive occlusal force, permitting the lesion to resolve in the attachment apparatus and the PDL to return to normal width.[46,50]

The timing of occlusal alteration in the treatment sequence can be dictated by the degree of mobility and the nature of the occlusal contacts. Obvious, heavy occlusal interferences on teeth with severe mobility can be adjusted during initial nonsurgical periodontal preparation.[51–53] Under other circumstances, occlusal adjustment in any form should be delayed until plaque-related inflammation is under control, unless the occlusion must be altered for a restorative or other course as part of the comprehensive treatment plan.

Because the attachment apparatus can adapt to force, as evidenced by increased but not increasing mobility, it may be difficult after control of the plaque-related inflammatory lesion to determine if the mobility still present is actually increasing or increased, and if occlusal alteration is indicated or adaptation has occurred. Reevaluation of mobility can be delayed for 6 to 12 months after control of the plaque-related inflammatory lesion to better determine if mobility is still only increased or is yet increasing and occlusal trauma is present. This 6- to 12-month delay in diagnosis permits the attachment apparatus to heal.[54–56] If mobility does not increase over 6 to 12 months, an active lesion of occlusal trauma in the attachment apparatus can be ruled out. As plaque-related inflammation is controlled and its effect on mobility is ruled out, healing in the attachment apparatus can proceed.[13,57] If the PDL adapts to occlusal forces present in a widened dimension or heals with a return to normal width, mobility will be unchanged or reduced, respectively, after 6 to 12 months, and correc-

tion of occlusal contacts is not indicated. If mobility is increasing after 6 to 12 months, then occlusal correction should be performed.

For dentitions requiring restorative dentistry in which the occlusal or guiding surfaces are being altered, it may be prudent to institute occlusal correction earlier in treatment, regardless of the mobility patterns, to provide an occlusal scheme compatible with the restorative plan. For dentitions in which mobility is determined to be increased but not increasing, it may be prudent to pursue occlusal correction if occlusal contacts are obviously influencing mobility patterns and alteration of such contacts would reduce or eliminate mobility.

Differential Diagnosis

There are four clinical situations that present features of primary occlusal trauma (Table 8-1); the clinician must distinguish among them. In the *first clinical situation*, the patient presents with increasing mobility caused by excessive force and bone levels at or near the cementoenamel junction (CEJ). This combination is indicative of the classic case of primary occlusal trauma (see Figs 8-1a and 8-1b). In this situation, the treatment indicated is occlusal alteration to eliminate excessive force. The reduction in force results in decreased mobility because of resolution of the occlusal traumatic lesion in the attachment apparatus and a resultant decrease in PDL width to normal.

A *second clinical situation* (see Figs 8-2a and 8-2b) that may seem to be primary occlusal trauma occurs when mobility is increased (not increasing) because of excessive force with bone levels at or near the CEJ. This is the classic entity compatible with adaptation to force in the attachment apparatus. This situation is not primary occlusal trauma. Mobility has increased but is not increasing. The PDL has widened but is not widening. There is no longer pathosis in the attachment apparatus indicative of the occlusal traumatic lesion. The attachment apparatus has changed morphologically by increasing the PDL width to accommodate the increased force on the tooth. No treatment is necessary, because there is no pathosis. The PDL is healthy in a widened state.

Mobility is a sign of disease, not a disease entity that requires treatment. Mobility is a sign of morphologic change—the change in width of the PDL. Mobility may be reduced in the second clinical situation that presents as primary occlusal trauma by altering the occlusion if a restorative or other course dictates, but occlusal correction is not biologically necessary for periodontal management if the clinical situation (force and mobility) remains unchanged.

When teeth adapt to force, the mobility present is historical evidence of an excessive force that caused the PDL to widen. Because the force is in the adaptive range of the periodontium, the lesion of occlusal trauma in the attachment apparatus has healed and the mobility represents the

Table 8-1 Clinical entities presenting features of primary occlusal trauma

	Clinical situation 1 (Fig 8-1)	Clinical situation 2 (Fig 8-2)	Clinical situation 3 (Fig 8-6)	Clinical situation 4 (Fig 8-7)
Force	Increased	Increased	Increased	Increased
Bone support	Normal	Normal	Reduced	Reduced
Mobility	Increasing	Increased	Increasing	Increased
Periodontal ligament	Widening	Widened	Widening	Widened
Diagnosis	Primary occlusal trauma	Physiologic occlusion	Primary occlusal trauma	Physiologic occlusion
Treatment	Occlusal correction	Monitor	Occlusal correction	Monitor
Outcome	Reduced force, mobility, and periodontal ligament	Adaptation of attachment apparatus	Reduced force, mobility, and periodontal ligament	Adaptation of attachment apparatus

adaptation to the ongoing force. The clinical outcome with respect to mobility and force remains unchanged if the occlusion is not altered. If the occlusion is altered after the teeth have adapted to an occlusal force, and bone levels are at or near the CEJ, reduced mobility can be expected.

The *third clinical situation* that may present as primary trauma occurs when reduced bone support is not influencing increasing tooth mobility that is caused by excessive force (Figs 8-6a to 8-6c). This situation *is* one of primary occlusal trauma, and treatment of this entity is similar to that of the first clinical situation of primary trauma. With occlusal alteration, the lesion of occlusal trauma resolves and the PDL width decreases, resulting in a clinical outcome of reduced mobility and force. Any plaque-related lesion is treated separately. The plaque-related lesion does not involve the attachment apparatus, so it exists as a separate entity not affecting the mobility.[32] Two distinct pathologic lesions, the lesion of occlusal trauma in the attachment apparatus and the plaque-related lesion coronal to this, are acting on the tooth independent of each other.

The *fourth clinical situation* that may seem to present as primary occlusal trauma occurs when reduced bone support is not influencing increased (but not increasing) mobility caused by an excessive force (Figs 8-7a to 8-7c). In this situation, the attachment apparatus has adapted to the force. Primary occlusal trauma is not present.[58] The lesion of occlusal trauma in the attachment apparatus has healed, but the PDL remains widened to accommodate the remaining force on the tooth. As in the second clinical situation presenting as primary occlusal trauma, no occlusal treatment has to be pursued because there is no pathosis in

the attachment apparatus. If the occlusion is altered for a restorative or other course to control the clinical parameters of the occlusal scheme, reduced mobility and force can be expected.

Secondary Occlusal Trauma

Diagnosis and Treatment

Secondary occlusal trauma is caused by the loss of adequate bone support rather than excessive occlusal force. Treatment is predicated on splinting. If splinting is not required to control increasing mobility, a diagnosis of secondary occlusal trauma should not be made. Splinting in secondary occlusal trauma compensates for inadequate bone support and permits the lesion of occlusal trauma in the attachment apparatus to resolve, the PDL to narrow, and mobility to be reduced.[16,58,59] The purpose of the splint is to inhibit the increasing lesion of occlusal trauma in the attachment apparatus and permit a healing response that allows the PDL to narrow by bone apposition along the crestal and alveolar lamina dura.

All teeth to be splinted must be fixed permanently to prevent any tooth movement that would allow the PDL to continue widening.[16] If a tooth is not fixed in all planes in space, then splinting to control increasing mobility will not be accomplished. Removable prostheses and nonfixed precision or semiprecision attachments, therefore, do not splint. They do not permit healing in the attachment apparatus because they do not hold a tooth in a totally fixed

Figs 8-6a to 8-6c Primary occlusal traumatic lesion in a reduced periodontium. Clinical situation 3 presenting as primary occlusal trauma.

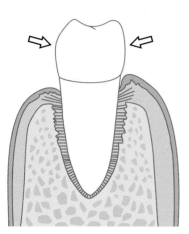

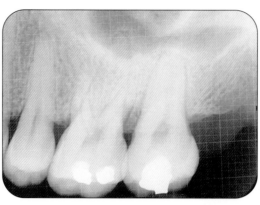

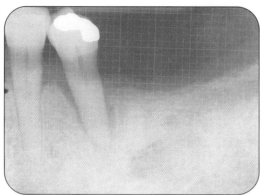

Figs 8-6b and 8-6c Lesions of primary occlusal trauma in a reduced periodontium. The subtly widening PDLs are indicative of the occlusal traumatic lesion in the attachment apparatus resulting from excessive force generated by occlusal interferences. The probe does not extend beyond the marginal crest of bone. Note the radiographic evidence of cervical abfraction in Fig 8-6c.

Fig 8-6a Widening of the PDL with loss of lamina dura is similar to that seen in other lesions of occlusal trauma. Pocketing on the right half of the tooth is separated from the lesion of occlusal trauma by the intact connective tissue attachment. (arrows) Excessive force.

Figs 8-7a to 8-7c Adaptation of the attachment apparatus in a periodontium not reduced enough to create secondary trauma. Clinical situation 4 presenting as primary occlusal trauma.

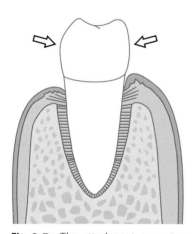

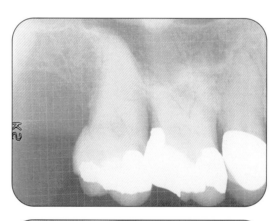

Fig 8-7b Teeth with reduced bone support where the attachment apparatus has adapted to force. Mobility of teeth is increased.

Fig 8-7a The attachment apparatus has healed with a widened PDL, but excessive force remains (arrows).

Fig 8-7c Radiograph taken 4 years later. The attachment apparatus remains unchanged without occlusal treatment over the 4-year period. Mobility remains increased but is not increasing.

position that can allow the PDL to become narrower and mobility to be reduced. Splinting is an occlusal treatment that controls mobility that has been created by force in the normal range of function on teeth that have less than adequate bone support.

Teeth in secondary trauma that are permanently splinted with cast restorations or temporarily splinted with bonded wire or mesh[60] will demonstrate reduced mobility or no mobility after splinting.[61] As long as occlusal forces remain in the normal range and attachment levels are maintained, mobility patterns of the splint will remain predictably stable.[62,63]

Individual teeth that are provisionally splinted with acrylic resin crowns for at least 6 to 12 months may demonstrate reduced or no mobility when the provisional splint is removed.[61] If a provisional acrylic resin complete-crown splint is removed before the final restoration is placed, but after PDL healing has occurred, it may erroneously be assumed that individual tooth stability encountered is permanent and that further splinting is not required. Attempts to discontinue splinting in this circumstance will result in increasing mobility as secondary trauma is reinstituted. Because occlusal trauma is secondary to bone loss when splinting is required and bone levels remain inadequate to support the teeth without splinting, mobility will return to the increasing presplint levels if splinting is interrupted.

If splinting is interrupted and individual mobility does not return to presplint levels over a period of time, secondary occlusal trauma was a misdiagnosis. The mobility was related instead to inflammation, to primary trauma that was corrected by alteration of occlusal surfaces on the splint, or to the presence of an attachment apparatus adapted to force generated on a reduced periodontium that was not sufficiently reduced to create secondary trauma.

A tooth in secondary occlusal trauma presents with increasing mobility but with occlusal forces in the normal range of function. Radiographically, a tooth in secondary trauma will demonstrate reduced bone levels that are inadequate to support the tooth without increasing mobility, migration, or fremitus under a normal load. The desired clinical outcome of splinting is tooth stability without increasing mobility, and the desired radiographic outcome is PDL narrowing through repair of crestal and alveolar lamina dura from bone apposition. Any radiographic evidence of vertical bone loss related to the widening PDL is eliminated.

Differential Diagnosis

There are three clinical situations that present features of secondary occlusal trauma (Table 8-2). In the *first clinical situation*, increasing mobility is present and there is radiographic evidence of reduced bone support that is not ade-

Table 8-2 Clinical entities presenting features of secondary occlusal trauma

	Clinical situation 1 (Fig 8-5)	Clinical situation 2 (Fig 8-8)	Clinical situation 3 (Fig 8-9)
Force	Normal	Normal	Increased
Bone support	Reduced	Reduced	Reduced
Mobility	Increasing	Increased	Increasing
Periodontal ligament	Widening	Widened	Widening
Diagnosis	Secondary occlusal trauma	Physiologic occlusion	Primary trauma if mobility reduced by occlusal correction; secondary trauma if splinting required after occlusal correction
Treatment	Splinting	Monitor	Occlusal correction; splinting if mobility not reduced after occlusal correction
Outcome	Reduced mobility and periodontal ligament	Adaptation of attachment apparatus	Reduced force, mobility, and periodontal ligament

Figs 8-8a to 8-8c Adaptation of the attachment apparatus in a periodontium reduced enough to expect secondary trauma. Clinical situation 2 presenting as secondary occlusal trauma.

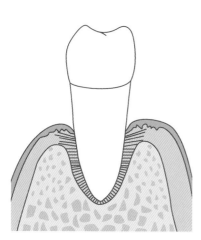

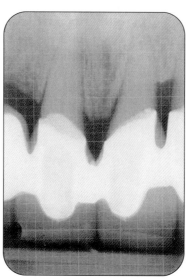

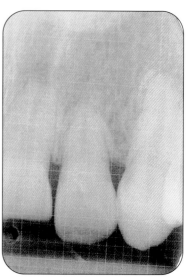

Fig 8-8a The PDL is widened because of a lack of adequate support, but is not widening.

Fig 8-8b Splinted teeth with widened PDLs representing adaptation of the attachment apparatus after elimination of secondary trauma through splinting. Clinical mobility has remained increased over many years because of the reduced periodontium but is not increasing.

Fig 8-8c Attachment apparatus adapted to loss of support from root resorption. Mobility is increased over 5 years but is not increasing.

quate to maintain tooth stability (see Figs 8-5a to 8-5c). The occlusal scheme and contacts are within the normal range and cannot be altered to reduce occlusal force on the teeth. This is the classic case of secondary occlusal trauma, for which the indicated treatment is fixed stabilization of the teeth through splinting. Clinically, reduced mobility should be expected after splinting. The occlusal traumatic lesion in the attachment apparatus resolves as occlusal force is dissipated throughout the splint,[64,65] allowing the periodontal ligament space to be reduced.

In a *second clinical situation*, which may simulate secondary occlusal trauma, there is radiographic evidence of reduced bone support that appears inadequate to maintain tooth stability and tooth mobility is increased but not increasing. The occlusal scheme, contacts, and force are within the normal range (Figs 8-8a to 8-8c). No treatment is necessary because mobility patterns are a result of a widened PDL in the adapted attachment apparatus of a reduced periodontium. A diagnosis of secondary trauma is not indicated, and alteration of the occlusion to reduce force is not possible. Splinting in this situation may be performed based on restorative needs, but is not necessary to treat the occlusion because no lesion of occlusal trauma exists in the attachment apparatus. Reduced mobility will be obtained if the clinician elects to pursue splinting for restorative or other purposes.

In the *third clinical situation*, mobility is increasing because excessive force is superimposed on radiographically

evident reduced bone support that appears inadequate to maintain tooth stability. The occlusal scheme may require correction, and excessive occlusal contacts require adjustment to reduce force on the teeth (Figs 8-9a to 8-9c). In this situation, it may be difficult to discriminate between the diagnoses of primary and secondary trauma. Because there are occlusal interferences generating excessive force, occlusal correction can be initiated to determine if excessive occlusal force is the cause of mobility. After occlusal adjustment, reevaluation of mobility should be delayed for 6 to 12 months[54–56,66] to permit adequate healing time in the attachment apparatus and possible narrowing of the PDL.

If mobility patterns are reduced after 6 to 12 months and are now in the increased rather than increasing mode, further occlusal treatment through splinting is not necessary, and a final diagnosis of primary trauma can be made. If, however, mobility patterns are still increasing 6 to 12 months after occlusal adjustment, splinting should be pursued because additional alteration of the occlusion to further reduce force is not possible. Increasing mobility in this case is clearly due to loss of bone support, and a diagnosis of secondary occlusal trauma can be made. The occlusal adjustment assists in establishing an ultimate diagnosis by either ruling out or verifying excessive occlusal force as the cause of mobility.

If it is determined that splinting is necessary in this third clinical situation, but the extent of splinting necessary to stabilize multiple loose teeth cannot be determined easily, a

Figs 8-9a to 8-9c Periodontium reduced enough to create secondary occlusal trauma in conjunction with excessive force *(arrows)* capable of creating primary occlusal trauma. Clinical situation 3 presenting as secondary occlusal trauma.

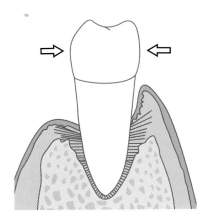

Fig 8-9a Widening PDL in a significantly reduced periodontium.

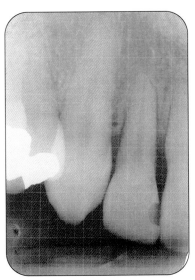

Fig 8-9b Reduction of the periodontium is extensive enough to warrant splinting, but clinical evidence indicates that occlusal force is excessive enough to also warrant a diagnosis of primary trauma.

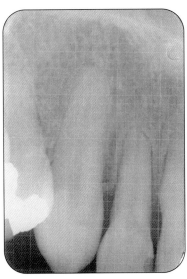

Fig 8-9c Situation 2 years after occlusal adjustment by selective grinding. Clinical mobility 2 years later is less than it was, yet still increased, but not increasing, ruling out the need for splinting.

provisional splint can be fabricated utilizing minimal abutments. The stability of this provisional splint can be evaluated after 6 to 12 months to determine if additional abutments will be needed.[61] The stability of the splint would be indicated by a reduction in mobility, an absence of mobility, or the presence of increased (but not increasing) mobility after 6 to 12 months.[61–63] If the mobility of the splint utilizing minimal abutments is increasing after 6 to 12 months, additional abutments can be incorporated in the splint to gain the degree of stability desired or possible.

In most situations such as these, it is best for the long-term prognosis to splint to such an extent that no mobility of the splint is evident immediately at splint fabrication or after 6 to 12 months. If the splint can be made immobile, then there is less chance that a misdiagnosis has occurred and that an increasing mobility of the splint will be encountered later when it may be difficult to correct. Because clinical evaluations of mobility are inexact, discriminating between increased and increasing mobility patterns can be difficult and can easily lead to misdiagnosis.

In the third clinical situation described, reduced mobility can be expected whether the ultimate treatment is occlusal adjustment or splinting.

The Concept of Co-destruction

In the past, some clinicians and researchers believed that a co-destructive process, whereby attachment loss is enhanced, occurs when occlusal trauma affects a tooth involved with plaque-related loss of attachment.[27,67–72] Under these circumstances, occlusal adjustment would be indicated whenever clinical loss of attachment and excessive force are encountered on the same tooth. Other clinicians and researchers took the opposite view, that co-destruction does not occur and that the lesion of occlusal trauma does not affect marginal plaque-related disease.[31,34,73,74]

In recent years, animal studies have been completed that help to explain the concept of co-destruction and how or when it may occur. When a heavy occlusal force with an intrusive component acts on a tooth, the occlusal traumatic lesion in the attachment apparatus can become extensive.[8,9,18] The PDL correspondingly can become extensively widened and present radiographically as an extensive periradicular radiolucency. Animal studies have demonstrated that, when this extensive occlusal traumatic lesion is active on a tooth with marginal plaque–related loss of attachment,

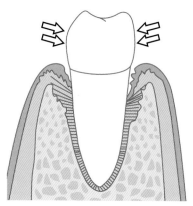

Fig 8-10a Possible mechanism of co-destruction. The plaque-related marginal lesion may combine with the occlusal traumatic lesion in the attachment apparatus after breakdown of the connective tissue attachment by an acute plaque-related episode on an attachment apparatus severely compromised by occlusal trauma.

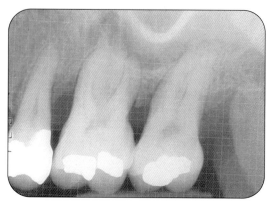

Fig 8-10b First molar possibly involved with a co-destructive lesion. Pulp tests indicate that the tooth is vital. Pocket depth is severe but not into the apical extent of the periradicular radiolucency. Mobility is severe, and occlusal force on the first molar is heavy.

the plaque-related disease is exacerbated and the marginal loss of attachment is increased several fold.[9,18,20] The larger extension of the plaque-related lesion may result from the decreased tissue resistance created throughout the attachment apparatus by the advanced lesion of occlusal trauma.[20,75] Because the forces required to generate this type of lesion must be of the orthodontic level or heavier,[19,76] it is rare for co-destruction to occur in cases where occlusal trauma is generated by tooth contacts.

Researchers observing the effects of lighter occlusal forces have been able to demonstrate a lack of co-destructive effect in most cases.[10,31,35,73,74] These occlusal loads are likely to be more in line with those encountered most frequently in daily clinical practice, ie, those generated by tooth-to-tooth contacts. Research in animals indicated that when occlusal trauma is induced by lighter loads on teeth with marginal plaque–related loss of attachment, co-destruction is unlikely to occur except when host resistance is decreased.[73]

When occlusal trauma is induced by lighter forces more compatible with routine tooth-to-tooth contact, the lesion in the attachment apparatus remains independent of the marginal plaque–related lesion. These two independent lesions, indefinitely separated by the connective tissue attachment, can act on the same tooth.[33,34,37] When teeth are acted on by heavier, intrusive, orthodontic-level forces and marginal plaque–induced disease is present, the marginal lesion and the lesion in the attachment apparatus may coalesce to some degree by a more rapid breakdown of the con-

nective tissue attachment that has been separating the two lesions. This coalescence of the marginal lesion and the more apical occlusally induced lesion of the attachment apparatus creates the co-destructive effect[18–20] (Figs 8-10a and 8-10b).

By extrapolating from the animal research, it would seem reasonable to assume that if co-destruction were to occur in humans, it would be more likely to occur in the patient who is undergoing active orthodontic treatment and who has untreated marginal plaque–induced loss of attachment during the course of tooth movement.[19,76] Some clinicians have been reluctant to pursue orthodontics in a periodontally involved dentition for fear of creating a co-destructive response. If plaque-related marginal disease is completely treated through the surgical phase of treatment prior to orthodontics, this possibility is greatly reduced. Animal studies have demonstrated that occlusal trauma induced on a healthy but reduced periodontium (a successfully treated periodontal case) has no different effect on the periodontium than occlusal trauma induced on a healthy periodontium with normal bone levels.[32,58,77] Patients with bone loss but no significant marginal inflammation or probing depth after definitive periodontal therapy respond to orthodontics in a manner similar to that of patients without bone loss or marginal inflammation.

Host resistance may also modify a patient's ability to develop a lesion of co-destruction.[73,78] Although co-destruction may be encountered clinically in humans, certain parameters (heavy force, decreased host resistance, and/or decreased local tissue resistance) are likely necessary for it to occur. In a patient whose resistance to disease may have been compromised either locally or systemically,[9,18,31,32,34,48,73,77,78] forces generally greater than those encountered by routine tooth-to-tooth contacts may still be required in conjunction with plaque-induced marginal loss of attachment to produce a co-destructive lesion.

Evaluation of the Occlusion

Occlusal examination is the clinical process of collecting occlusal data for evaluation in conjunction with data from the clinical and radiographic dental and periodontal examinations. These data are then used to arrive at a diagnosis based on the existing pathosis demonstrated by the examinations. The diagnosis is used to develop a treatment plan capable of delivering a planned biologic response.

Data to be collected by the occlusal examination should pertain to both dynamic and static tooth relationships (Fig 8-11). Static relationships include Angle's classification, skeletal relationships, incisal relationships, presence of ante-

rior coupling, tooth migration, tooth position, occlusal plane characteristics, vertical alterations of the occlusion, dental wear, and missing teeth. Dynamic relationships should include centric relation–centric occlusion discrepancies, excursive relationships, and fremitus. These data must be integrated with tooth mobility patterns from the periodontal examination (Fig 8-12) to evaluate the effect of tooth contacts and the force they may generate on the periodontium.

Thorough occlusal evaluation includes a diagnostic mounting on at least a semiadjustable articulator with an accurate facebow and centric relation record (Figs 8-13a and 8-13b).[79] With an accurate diagnostic mounting, a diagnostic or trial equilibration can be completed in conjunction with a diagnostic waxup and orthodontic tooth setup to determine the extent of treatment by selective grinding, orthodontics, restoration, or extraction required to provide an occlusal scheme compatible with health and stability over the long term.[80,81]

Patients with a history of occlusal habits or muscle dysfunction may require a biteplane appliance to facilitate occlusal deprogramming and muscle relaxation[82–91] prior to fabrication of centric records. A centric relation maxillary or

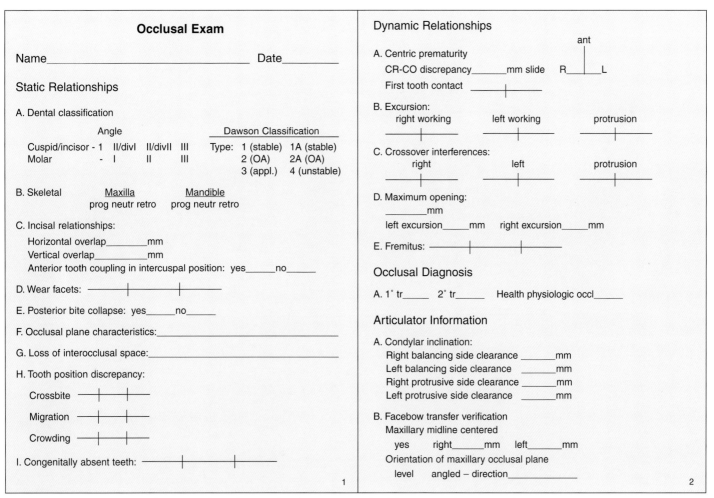

Fig 8-11 Occlusal examination form, providing adequate data for accurate occlusal diagnosis and treatment planning.

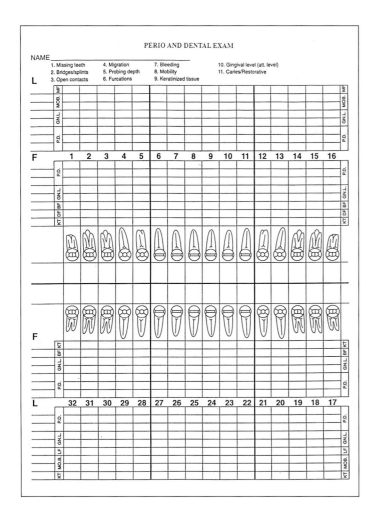

Fig 8-12 Periodontal chart, providing documentation of tooth mobility patterns.

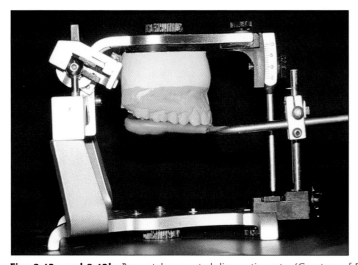 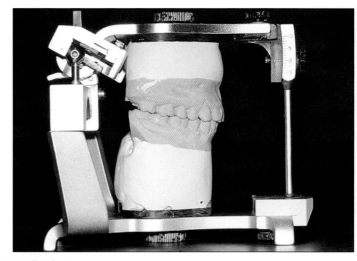

Figs 8-13a and 8-13b Accurately mounted diagnostic casts. (Courtesy of Dr Darell Fisher.)

mandibular biteplane fabricated with a flat posterior component, point centric posterior contacts, and a compatible anterior guidance can be worn by the patient for a varying amount of time to facilitate loss of proprioceptive response, muscle release, and ease of mandibular manipulation in centric record fabrication.[80,83–91] More accurate examination of tooth contacts intraorally and more accurate collection of clinical data can then be accomplished to pursue the correct diagnosis and to establish an appropriate treatment plan. After a diagnosis of primary occlusal trauma, an occlusal scheme should be developed to provide a centric relation occlusion and an acceptable anterior guidance incapable of generating forces beyond the adaptive levels of the attachment apparatus of the involved teeth.[25,49,79,81,92–98]

In patients with Angle Class I occlusion, a canine-guided occlusion generally will provide the most stable tooth relationships.[79–81,97,99–100] Angle Class II and Class III occlusions may not permit a canine-guided scheme to be developed because mesio-occlusal and disto-occlusal landmarks have been shifted anteriorly or posteriorly, respectively. A group function can be acceptable in the lateral excursions of these patients,[99,100] as long as tooth contacts that are developed are not influencing mobility patterns, fremitus, or a migratory component.[79]

Tooth contacts generating primary occlusal trauma must be reduced to the adaptive levels of the attachment apparatus in centric and excursive movements to provide occlusal stability and a good prognosis.[52,101,102] If a diagnosis of secondary occlusal trauma has been made, occlusal contacts introduced by the restorative splinting procedure must be compatible with the adaptive levels of the attachment apparatus in centric and excursive movements.[79] Ideally, the anterior and lateral guidance in patients with secondary occlusal trauma should be as flat as possible to diminish the lateral force on the splinted dentition.[25,79,102–105]

The anterior guidance in all occlusally involved dentitions must be thoroughly evaluated and managed for long-term success. The importance of the anterior guidance in controlling the occlusal scheme and occlusal force cannot be overemphasized. The anterior guidance is the "transmission" of a good occlusion. It protects the contacting parts from abuse by overload or overuse, and it provides a means of smooth transition for the teeth in various movements of the mandible.

For all patients with occlusal trauma, but especially those in whom tooth position or skeletal relationships do not permit development of an ideal occlusal scheme, the goal of occlusal treatment should be to axially load teeth in centric relation occlusion and to minimize lateral tooth contacts while developing an acceptable disocclusive scheme of the posterior dentition. This approach to therapy will minimize vertical and horizontal forces on the teeth and more predictably keep occlusal forces within the adaptive range of the periodontium.[25,79,80,97,99–101,104,105]

Because altering the occlusal scheme may not be necessary in periodontally involved dentitions where occlusal trauma is not part of the diagnosis, the existing occlusal scheme can be accepted as physiologic.[81,97] If the occlusion is altered for restorative purposes in patients with a physiologic occlusion, the occlusal scheme and occlusal contact subsequently developed by the restoration must remain in the adaptive range of the attachment apparatus or occlusal trauma may be iatrogenically introduced.[25]

A full and thorough occlusal examination is always a necessity.[80,81] In patients with a physiologic occlusion, it may wrongly be assumed, either because of the lack of mobility or because of the lack of increasing mobility, that complete evaluation of the occlusal scheme and individual occlusal contacts is unnecessary. A physiologic occlusion often can be restored at the current occlusal scheme without alteration.[81] However, if it is restored beyond the tenets of the existing occlusion, and individual forces on certain teeth are unknowingly increased by the alteration of tooth contact or the occlusal scheme is altered by a restoration, then the adaptive capacity of the attachment apparatus may be exceeded and an occlusal traumatic lesion may be produced in the attachment apparatus.

Even for a healthy physiologic occlusion, it is always important to be cognizant of the limits of the occlusal scheme for each particular patient and to be mindful not to violate the adaptive range of any tooth. It is for this reason that return to a repeatable centric relation occlusion is usually recommended in the construction of any prosthesis that will affect an eccentric excursion or where multiple centric stops must be recaptured.[79–81,94–96,98,101,105] Fabrication of a prosthesis in centric relation occlusion with a compatible anterior guidance, as dictated by properly mounted working casts on a semiadjustable articulator, permits restoration of the occlusion within the parameters of the existing occlusal scheme, the gnathostomatic system, and the adaptive range of the attachment apparatus.[79,106]

Altering the Occlusion

Altering the occlusion through occlusal adjustment to reduce force on teeth under occlusal traumatic load can be accomplished by addition procedures (occlusal restoration), subtraction procedures (selective grinding or extraction), and/or combinations of the two (orthodontics and/or orthognathic surgery).

Many patients require combinations of these procedures to obtain an occlusal scheme incorporating correct occlusal landmarks, proper tooth position for axial loading, and an anterior–posterior skeletal relationship that permits anterior tooth coupling and disocclusion. All too often, occlusal adjustment is limited to a selective grinding procedure that cannot compensate for the compromises in an occlusal scheme that may be produced by poor tooth position, skeletal malrelationships, bite collapse, occlusal and incisal wear, or missing teeth.[25,26,81,107,108]

Because selective grinding entails reshaping of cusps, cuspal inclines, incisal edges, and the guiding inclines of anterior teeth, it is not an effective course of therapy when recapturing of occlusal contact is necessary to restrict occlusal force by axial loading or alteration of the lateral guidance. Cast restorations are indicated for occlusal correction when selective grinding may be excessive or recapturing contact is necessary. However, restorative addition procedures can limit the occlusal result when key teeth are missing or malposed to a degree that the restoration results in overcontouring, inadequate retention, or violation of the periodontal status interproximally or subgingivally. Orthodontics can enhance the occlusal result obtained by selective grinding and restorative dentistry in those cases where changes in tooth position are necessary to recapture or alter occlusal contacts to the most ideal occlusal scheme.[44,109]

If a complete occlusal examination including thorough clinical documentation and properly mounted casts is always pursued, a better understanding of the intricacies and needs of each occlusion will be developed. In this way, the necessary occlusal treatment, providing predictable, long-term, stable results, will be recommended and pursued.

The Effect of Trauma on the Postoperative Course

The effect of occlusal trauma on the healing response after periodontal surgery has often been debated. Whether this effect is positive or negative has not yet been determined. It has been speculated that occlusal trauma may delay the healing response[57,77,110–113] or that it may not have an effect on the healing response at all.[32,33,56,114] More than likely, the interaction is more complicated than previously thought (Table 8-3). Whether occlusal traumatism influences the healing response may still be debated for some time.

Surgical trauma itself may have an effect on the status of the attachment apparatus and the postoperative course. When osseous recontouring procedures are incorporated into a periodontal surgical procedure, the involved teeth tend to demonstrate postoperative increases in mobility.[54,55] Mobility patterns may increase two- or three-fold.[56] With the completion of healing 3 to 12 months postoperatively, these increases in mobility tend to dissipate, and the mobility of the surgically treated teeth returns to preoperative levels.[54–57,66] The clinician must be aware of this effect of surgery on the periodontium and the resultant clinical changes in mobility that may accompany it. With proper evaluation, misconceptions or misdiagnoses regarding postoperative increases in mobility from surgical trauma can be avoided, along with any resulting compromised or inappropriate treatment.

Conclusion

A good understanding of occlusal trauma and its effect on the periodontium can provide a sound rationale for accurate diagnosis and predictable treatment planning for the periodontally compromised patient. In today's health care environment, patients seek and demand stable, long-term results. Failure to understand the biologic consequences of occlusal force can cause the practitioner to pursue an inadequate or unjustified treatment course. Treatment that is not based on biologic principles that provide predictable outcomes is likely to be neither cost effective nor successful.

Table 8-3 Effect of occlusal trauma and treatment on the periodontium

Treatment	Mobility	Bone	Attachment level	Probing depth
Healthy				
Decrease OT	Decreased	Increased vol and ht	No change	No change
Gingivitis				
Decrease OT	Decreased	Increased ht but not vol	No change	No change
Decrease inflammation	Decreased or no change	Increased vol but not ht	No change	No change
Decrease OT and decrease inflammation	Decreased	Increased vol and ht	No change	No change
Periodontitis				
Decrease OT	Decreased	Increased ht but not vol	No change	No change
Decrease inflammation	Decreased or no change	Increased vol but not ht	Increased or no change	Decreased
Decrease OT and decrease inflammation	Decreased	Increased vol and ht	Increased or no change	Decreased
Reduced healthy				
Decrease OT	Decreased	Increased vol and ht	No change	No change

OT = occlusal trauma, vol = volume; ht = height.

References

1. Box H. Experimental traumatogenic occlusion in sheep. Oral Health 1935;25:9.

2. Stones H. An experimental investigation into the association of traumatic occlusion with periodontal disease. Proc R Soc Med 1938;31:479.

3. Stillman PR. What is traumatic occlusion and how can it be diagnosed and corrected? J Am Dent Assoc 1926;12:1330.

4. McCall JO. Traumatic occlusion. J Am Dent Assoc 1939;26:519.

5. Vaughan OB. Functional analysis of occlusion as it relates to periodontal conditions. Northwest Univ Bull 1951;52:18.

6. McCollum BB, Stuart CE. Gnathology. A Research Report. South Pasadena, CA: Scientific Press, 1955.

7. Nepola SR. Treatment of periodontal pockets caused by traumatic occlusion. Dent Radiogr Photogr 1961;34:31.

8. Svanberg G, Lindhe J. Experimental tooth hypermobility in the dog. Odontol Rev 1973;24:269.

9. Lindhe J, Svenberg G. Influence of trauma from occlusion on progression of experimental periodontitis in the beagle dog. J Clin Periodontol 1974;1:3.

10. Meitner S. Co-destructive factors of marginal periodontal disease and repetitive mechanical injury. J Dent Res 1975;54:c78.

11. Reitan K. The initial tissue reaction incident to orthodontic tooth movement. Acta Odontol Scand 1951;9(suppl):6.

12. Wentz F, Jarabak J, Orban B. Experimental occlusal trauma imitating cuspid interferences. J Periodontol 1958;29:117.

13. Kantor M, Polson A, Zander H. Alveolar bone regeneration after removal of inflammation and traumatic factors in chronic periodontal disease. J Periodontol 1976;47:687.

14. Polson A, Meitner S, Zander H. Trauma and progression of periodontal disease in squirrel monkeys. IV. Reversibility of bone loss due to trauma superimposed upon periodontitis. J Periodont Res 1976;11:290.

15. Svanberg G, Lindhe J. Vascular reactions in the periodontal ligament incident to trauma from occlusion. J Clin Periodontol 1974;1:58.

16. Lindhe J, Nyman S. Role of occlusion in periodontal disease and biologic rationale for splinting in treatment of periodontitis. Oral Sci Rev 1977;10:11.

17. Polson A. The relative importance of plaque and occlusion in periodontal disease. J Clin Periodontol 1986;13:423.

18. Nyman S, Lindhe J, Ericsson I. Effect of progressive tooth mobility on destructive periodontitis in the dog. J Clin Periodontol 1978;5:213.

19. Ericcson I. The combined effects of plaque and physical stress on periodontal tissues. J Clin Periodontol 1986;13:918.

20. Ericcson I, Lindhe J Effect of longstanding jiggling on experimental marginal periodontitis in the beagle dog. J Clin Periodontol 1982;9:497.

21. Fradeani M, Bottacchiari RS, Tracey T, et al. The restoration of functional occlusion and esthetics. Int J Periodont Rest Dent 1992;12:63.

22. Williams WN, Low SB, Cooyser WR, Cornell CF. The effect of periodontal bone loss on bite force discrimination. J Periodontol 1987;58:236.

23. Baer PN, Kakehashi S, Littleton NW, et al. Alveolar bone loss and occlusal wear. Periodontics 1963;1:91.

24. Hanamura H, Houston F, Rylander H, et al. Periodontal status and bruxism—A comparative study of patients with periodontal disease and occlusal parafunctions. J Periodontol 1987;58:173.

25. Lytle J. The clinician's index of occlusal disease: definition, recognition and management. Int J Periodont Rest Dent 1990;10:103.

26. Rosenberg E, Simons J, Gualini F. Clinical aspects and treatment of posterior bite collapse due to accelerated wear. Int J Periodont Rest Dent 1987;7(1):67.

27. Macapanpan L, Weinman J. Influence of injury to the periodontal ligament on spread of gingival inflammation. J Dent Res 1954;33:263.

28. Goldman H. Gingival vascular supply in induced occlusal trauma. J Periodontol 1956;9:939.

29. Cohen DW, Keller G, Feder M, et al. Effects of excessive occlusal forces on the gingival blood supply. J Dent Res 1960;39:677.

30. Waerhaug J. Pathogenesis of pocket formation in traumatic occlusion. J Periodontol 1955;26:107.

31. Comar MD, Kollar JA, Gargiulo AW. Local irritation and occlusal trauma as co-factors in the periodontal disease process. J Periodontol 1969;40:193.

32. Ericcson I, Lindhe J. Lack of effect of trauma from occlusion on the recurrence of experimental periodontitis. J Clin Periodontol 1977;4:115.

33. Lindhe J, Ericsson I. The effect of elimination of jiggling forces on periodontally exposed teeth in the dog. J Periodontol 1982;53:562.

34. Waerhaug J. The infrabony pocket and its relationship to trauma from occlusion and subgingival plaque. J Periodontol 1979;50:355.

35. Polson A, Zander H. Effect of periodontal trauma upon infrabony pockets. J Periodontol 1983;54:586.

36. Budtz-Jorgenson E. Bruxism and trauma from occlusion. An experimental model in Macaca monkeys. J Clin Periodontol 1980;7:149.

37. Waerhaug J. The angular bony defect and its relationship to occlusal trauma and downgrowth of subgingival plaque. J Clin Periodontol 1979;6:61.

38. McCoy G. Dental compression syndrome. A new look at an old disease. Presented at Congress XV of the International Academy of Gnathology. Coronado, CA, 18–22 Sept 1991.

39. Lee WC, Eakle WS. Possible role of tensile stress in the etiology of cervical erosive lesions of teeth. J Prosthet Dent 1984;52:3.

40. Grippo J. Abfractions: A new classification of hard tissue lesions of teeth. J Anesthet Dent 1991;3:1.

41. Hand JS, Hunt A, Reinhardt JW. The prevalence and treatment implications of cervical abrasion in the elderly. Gerodontics 1986;2:167–170.

42. McCoy G, et al. The etiology of gingival erosion. J Oral Implantol 1982;X:3.

43. Selna LG, Shillingburg HT, Kerr PA. Finite element analysis of dental structures—Axisymmetric and plane stress idealizations. J Biomed Mater Res 1975;2:237–252.

44. Hoag PM. Occlusal treatment. In: Nevins M, Becker W, Kornman K (eds). Proceedings of the World Workshop in Clinical Periodontics. Chicago: American Academy of Periodontology, 1989:III-1.

45. Itoiz ME, Carranza FA, Cabrini RL. Histologic and histometric study of experimental occlusal trauma in rats. J Periodontol 1963;34:305.

46. Polson A, Kantor M, Zander H. Periodontal repair after reduction of inflammation. J Periodont Res 1979;14:520.

47. Khoo KK, Watts TL. Upper anterior tooth mobility. Selected association in untreated periodontitis. J Periodontol 1988;59:231.

48. Polson A. Interrelationship of inflammation and mobility in pathogenesis of periodontal disease. J Clin Periodontol 1980;7:351.

49. Levinson E. Periodontal postulates for the prosthodontist. Int J Periodont Rest Dent 1989;8(1):45.

50. Jin LJ, Cao CF. Clinical diagnosis of trauma from occlusion and its relation with severity of periodontics. J Clin Periodontol 1992;19:92.

51. Youdelis R, Mann WU. Prevalence and possible role of nonworking contacts in periodontal disease. Periodontics 1965;3:219.

52. Ramfjord S, Ash M. Significance of occlusion in the etiology and treatment of early, moderate, and advanced periodontal disease. J Periodontol 1981;52:511.

53. Moozah MB, Suit SR, Bissada NF. Tooth mobility measurements following two methods of eliminating non-working side occlusal interferences. J Clin Periodontol 1981;8:424.

54. Galler C, Selipsky H, Phillips C, Ammons W. The effect of splinting on tooth mobility. II. After osseous surgery. J Clin Periodontol 1979;6:317.

55. Selipsky H. A longstanding study of osseous surgery and plaque control in perio treatment and their effects on mobility. Dent Clin North Am 1976;20:79.

56. Persson R. Assessment of tooth mobility using small loads. IV. Effect of gingivoplasty and flap procedures. J Clin Periodontol 1981;8:88.

57. Polson AM, Adams RA, Zander HA. Osseous repair in the presence of active tooth hypermobility. J Clin Periodontol 1983;10:370.

58. Perrier M, Polson A. The effect of progressive and increasing tooth hypermobility on reduced but healthy supporting tissues. J Periodontol 1982;53:152.

59. Smukler H, Lemmer J. A rationale for the stabilization of mobile teeth in advanced periodontal disease. J Dent Assoc South Afr 1975; 30:543–546.

60. Kleyer A. Compromised periodontal treatment for teeth with advanced bone loss. Int J Periodont Rest Dent 1988;8(2):35.

61. Nyman S, Lindhe J. Considerations on the design of occlusion in prosthetic rehabilitation of patients with advanced periodontal disease. J Clin Periodontol 1977;4:1.

62. Nyman S, Lindhe J, Lundgren D. Role of occlusion for stability of fixed bridges in patients with reduced periodontal support. J Clin Periodontol 1975;2:53.

63. Nyman S, Ericsson I. The capacity of reduced periodontal tissues to support fixed bridgework. J Clin Periodontol 1982;9:409.

64. Glickman I, Stein RS, Smulow JB. Effect of increased functional forces on splinted and non-splinted teeth. J Periodontol 1961;32:290.

65. Glickman I, Roeber FW, Brion M, et al. Photoelastic analysis of internal stresses in the periodontium created by occlusal forces. J Periodontol 1971;41:30.

66. Nyman S, Lindhe J. Persistent tooth hypermobility following complications of periodontal treatment. J Clin Periodontol 1976;3:81.

67. Glickman I, Smulow J. Alterations in the pathway of gingival inflammation by excess occlusal forces. J Periodontol 1962;33:7.

68. Glickman I. Inflammation and trauma from occlusion, co-destructive factors in periodontal disease. J Periodontol 1963;34:5.

69. Glickman I, Smulow J. Further observations on effects of trauma from occlusion in humans. J Periodontol 1967;38:280.

70. Glickman I, Smulow J. Adaptive alterations in the periodontium of rhesus monkeys in chronic trauma from occlusion. J Periodontol 1968;39:101.

71. Glickman I, Smulow J. Effect of excess occlusal forces upon pathway of inflammation in humans. J Periodontol 1965;36:141.

72. Glickman I, Smulow J. The combined effects of inflammation and trauma from occlusion in periodontics. Int Dent J 1969;19:393.

73. Waerhaug J, Hansen E. Periodontal changes incident to prolonged occlusal overload in monkeys. Acta Odontol Scand 1966;24:91.

74. Stahl S. The responses of the periodontium to combined gingival inflammation and occlusion—functional stresses in four human specimens. Periodontics 1968;6:14.

75. Neidrud AM, Ericsson I, Lindhe J. Probing pocket depth at mobile/non-mobile teeth. J Clin Periodontol 1992;19:754.

76. Ericsson I, Thilander B, Lindhe J. The effect of orthodontics on periodontal tissues of infected and non-infected dentition in dogs. J Clin Periodontol 1977;4:278.

77. Lindhe J, Ericsson I. The influence of occlusal trauma on reduced but healthy periodontal tissues in dogs. J Clin Periodontol 1976;3:110.

78. Socransky S, Haffajee A, Goodson J, Lindhe J. New concepts of destructive periodontal disease. J Clin Periodontol 1984;11:21.

79. Keough B. Occlusal considerations in periodontal prosthesis. Int J Periodont Rest Dent 1992;12:359.

80. Dawson PE. Evaluation, Diagnosis and Treatment of Occlusal Problems. ed 2. St. Louis: Mosby, 1989.

81. Lytle J, Skurow H. An interdisciplinary classification of restorative dentistry. Int J Periodont Rest Dent 1987;7(3):9.

82. Clark GT. A critical evaluation of orthopedic interocclusal appliance therapy: Design, theory, and overall effectiveness. J Am Dent Assoc 1984;108:359.

83. Greene CS, Laskin DM. Splint therapy for myofascial pain dysfunction (MPD) syndrome: A comparative study. J Am Dent Assoc 1972;40:563.

84. Carraro J, Caffesse R. Effect of occlusal splints on TMJ symptomatology. J Prosthet Dent 1978;40:563.

85. Shore NA. A mandibular autorepositioning appliance. J Am Dent Assoc 1967;75a:908.

86. Clark GT, Beemsterboer PL, Rugh JD. Nocturnal masseter muscle activity and the symptoms of masticatory dysfunction. J Oral Rehabil 1981;8:279.

87. Clark GT, Beemsterboer PL, Solberg WK, Rugh JD. Nocturnal electromyographic evaluation of myofascial pain dysfunction in patients undergoing occlusal splint therapy. J Am Dent Assoc 1979;99:607.

88. Solberg WK, Clark GT, Rugh JD. Nocturnal electromyographic evaluation of bruxism patients undergoing short term splint treatment. J Oral Rehabil 1975;2:215.

89. Agerberg G, Carlsson GE. Late results of treatment of functional disorders of the masticatory system. J Oral Rehabil 1974;1:309.

90. Clark GT. Occlusal therapy: Occlusal appliances. In: American Dental Association. The President's Conference on the Examination, Diagnosis, and Management of Temporomandibular Disorders. Chicago: American Dental Association, 1983:144.

91. Moller E, Sheik-Ol-Eslam A, Lous I. Deliberate relaxation of the temporal and masseter muscles in patients with functional disorders of the chewing apparatus. Scand J Dent Res 1971;79:478.

92. Ramfjord S, Ash M. Occlusion. ed 3. Philadelphia: Saunders, 1983:390-391.

93. Lundgren D. Prosthetic reconstruction of dentitions seriously compromised by periodontal disease. J Clin Periodontol 1991;18:390.

94. Schuyler CH. Fundamental principles in correction of occlusal disharmony, natural and artificial. J Am Dent Assoc 1935;22:1193.

95. Dawson PE. Optimum TMJ condyle position in clinical practice. Int J Periodont Rest Dent 1985;5(3):11.

96. Celenza FV. The theory and clinical management of centric positions. II. Centric relation and centric relation occlusion. Int J Periodont Rest Dent 1984;4(6):63.

97. Skurow H, Nevins M. The rationale of the preperiodontal provisional biologic trial restoration. Int J Periodont Rest Dent 1988;8(1):9.

98. Cohen LA. Integrating treatment procedures in occlusion—rehabilitation. J Prosthet Dent 1957;7:511.

99. Lundeen HC. Occlusal morphologic considerations for fixed restorations. Dent Clin North Am 1971;15:649–661.

100. Okeson JP. Fundamentals of Occlusion and Temporomandibular Disorders. St. Louis: Mosby, 1985:113.

101. Amsterdam M. Periodontal prosthesis: Twenty-five years in retrospect. Alpha Omegan 1974,67:9.

102. Svanberg G. Influence of trauma from occlusion of the periodontium of dogs with normal and inflamed gingiva. Odontol Rev 1974;25:165.

103. Katona TR. The effects of cusp and jaw morphology on the forces on teeth and the temporomandibular joint. J Oral Rehabil 1989; 16:219–221.

104. Kay H. Postsurgical prosthetic management. In: Rosenberg MM, Kay HB, Keough B, Holt R (eds). Periodontal and Prosthetic Management of Advanced Cases. Chicago: Quintessence, 1988:390–391.

105. Schuyler CH. An evaluation of incisal guidance and its influence in restorative dentistry. J Prosthet Dent 1959;9:374.

106. Pavone BW. Bruxism and its effect on the natural teeth. J Prosthet Dent 1985;54:110.

107. Schaffer H, Richter M. Functional preprosthetic orthodontics and prosthetics reconstruction with resin bonded fixed partial dentures. Int J Periodont Rest Dent 1991;11:127.

108. Wise R, Nevins M. Anterior tooth site analysis (Bolton Index): How to determine anterior diastema closure. Int J Periodont Rest Dent 1988;8(6):9.

109. Melsen B, Agerback N. Orthodontics as an adjunct to rehabilitation. Periodontology 2000 1994;4:148.

110. Flezar TJ, Knowles JW, Morrison EC, et al. Tooth mobility and perio therapy. J Clin Periodontol 1980;7:495.

111. Kerry GJ, Morrison EC, Ramfjord SP, et al. The effect of periodontal treatment on tooth mobility. J Periodontol 1982;53:635.

112. Burgett F, Ramfjord S, Nissle R, et al. A randomized trial of occlusal adjustment in the treatment of periodontitis patients. J Clin Periodontol 1992;19:381.

113. Ericsson I, Lindhe J. Lack of significance of increased tooth mobility in experimental periodontitis. J Periodontol 1984;55:447.

114. Ericsson I, Giargia I, Lindhe J, Neidrud AM. Progression of periodontal tissue destruction at splinted/non-splinted teeth. An experimental study in the dog. J Clin Periodontol 1993;20:693.

Interaction of Periodontal and Orthodontic Treatment

CHAPTER 9

John R. Bednar, DMD
Roger J. Wise, DDS

Practitioners of orthodontics and periodontics have often been at odds as a consequence of their lack of comprehensive knowledge of the other discipline. Combined education has produced a wealth of knowledge regarding the benefits of treating periodontal disease through a combination of surgical intervention and tooth movement.

The diseased periodontium can often be enhanced through orthodontic therapy, which includes uprighting, extrusion, intrusion, rotation, and a host of other tooth movements. It is critical for the dentist who becomes involved in combined therapy to have a comprehensive knowledge of the treatment of periodontal disease and orthodontic mechanotherapy. The presence of periodontal disease may make it necessary to consider compromising ideal orthodontic end points of therapy in favor of more practical treatment objectives. Achieving a functional occlusion in a periodontally compromised patient may be a more practical and secure approach than the pursuit of a perfect occlusion at the expense of long-term periodontal stability. This realization must be coupled with a profound understanding that the adult patient is distinctly different from the adolescent or child patient.

One of the most important factors in the orthodontic treatment of the periodontal patient is the immediate elimination of active inflammation prior to the initiation of tooth movement. Once this has been accomplished, it is extremely important to determine the sequence of definitive treatment that will produce the most predictable result for the patient. Some patients will benefit from the initiation of orthodontic therapy before periodontal treatment, and others may realize the most benefits through a reversal of these procedures.

Proper sequencing may often not only improve the periodontal stability of the affected area, but also be critical to the esthetic considerations in the patient's treatment. Periodontal intervention prior to orthodontic therapy may help avoid significant pitfalls that often present themselves in patients with limited soft tissue protection and osseous defects.[1] Preorthodontic gingival grafting or other forms of soft tissue enhancement, sometimes in conjunction with osseous regeneration, may prevent a number of problems that can result from hard and soft tissue loss during orthodontic tooth movements.[2] These procedures may also help improve resistance to inflammation that may occur during the orthodontic therapy.[3]

The dentist who has a proper understanding of periodontal problems may elect to decrease active orthodontic treatment time, thereby reducing the strain that extensive orthodontic therapy may exert on a compromised periodontium. The trauma of vertical loading of teeth, as they are moved occlusally and/or distally, may be reduced through selective occlusal equilibration. This simple procedure may help to significantly reduce problems that may result from traumatic occlusion in a periodontally diseased patient.

The periodontally informed dentist, recognizing the osseous constraints posed by the fragile interseptal bone between the maxillary first and second molars and the limited bone distal to the second molars, may select an extraction treatment plan rather than attempt maxillary molar distalization in an adult patient. Extraction therapy may also significantly reduce overall treatment time and, consequently, help to reduce the adult patient's exposure to periodontal risks.

Orthodontic treatment time might also be reduced in the adult patient by selecting interproximal stripping in the mandibular anterior region to achieve the space necessary for alignment.[4] Occasionally, the extraction of one mandibular incisor for the resolution of extensive mandibular anterior crowding may be the best approach, even though incisal guidance may be sacrificed in the resulting occlusion.[5] A proper evaluation of the length of incisor contact points and the extent of interproximal bone between the incisors may affect the decision to perform interproximal stripping rather than the extraction of one mandibular anterior tooth. This decision is also determined by other factors, which may include the Bolton Index, the overjet, the vertical dimension of occlusion, the extent of the crowding, and the presence of severe periodontal complications involving one or more teeth.

Special orthodontic considerations should always include the patient's desires. Many adult patients do not seek orthodontic therapy for the attainment of an ideal occlusion. Their goal may be to realize some of the mutual benefits that can be achieved through combined orthodontic and periodontal intervention. Quite often, orthodontic therapy may also be a prerequisite to prosthetic restoration of a functional occlusion.

The dentist who becomes involved in orthodontic and periodontal treatment of a patient must first collect the necessary diagnostic data prior to formulating a treatment plan and initiating therapy. The data should include both a comprehensive evaluation of the patient's present periodontal status and an overall evaluation of the existing adult malocclusion. A determination of the level of activity of the periodontal disease must be made prior to initiation of tooth movement. Probing data, soft tissue quality, the quantity and character of osseous defects, and root status (size, length, and form) are just some of the details that are critical components in the formation of a treatment plan.

This information, tempered by an understanding of why the patient is seeking orthodontic therapy, should lead to a functional treatment plan that may or may not vary from the orthodontic ideal. The primary objective is to maintain a functionally sound occlusion supported by a healthy periodontium. A compromised periodontium is a determinant to be considered when a treatment plan is formulated, and only after examining this aspect should the dentist initiate the orthodontic therapy. Theoretical and clinical consideration of these factors will be addressed in the treatment modalities discussed in this chapter. The central theme will be to consider information that will provide the practitioner with practical insight into the combined periodontal-orthodontic treatment of adult patients.

Pathologic Migration

The first notable clinical sign of advancing periodontal disease may be pathologic migration. Pathologic migration may include extrusion, labial flaring (tipping), or rotation of anterior teeth.

Pathologic migration may or may not be accompanied by an existing malocclusion. A patient may present with pathologic migration of the maxillary incisors but also have an intact, stable posterior dentition (Figs 9-1a to 9-1c). The mandibular incisors may undergo extrusion, creating a stepped occlusion accompanied by a severely accentuated curve of Spee. Frequently, clinicians associate flared incisors with a "collapsed bite," which is identified by missing posterior teeth and the resultant mesial tipping of molars and distal tipping of premolars (Fig 9-1b). It is also possible to have pathologic migration of anterior teeth with a superimposed "collapsed bite" in the posterior region.

When maxillary or mandibular anterior spacing is corrected, it is important to determine whether orthodontic or periodontal treatment should be rendered first. Developing the treatment sequence challenges the clinician to understand the interrelationships of orthodontics and periodontics in terms of periodontal disease activity.[6] Prior to the initiation of therapy, it is essential to establish goals for definitive periodontal care, final esthetics, and functional occlusion.

When pathologic spacing is present, esthetic limitations may complicate pocket elimination in the maxillary anterior segment. It may behoove the periodontist to provide orthodontic correction of the maxillary anterior spacing and permanent stabilization prior to periodontal surgery (Figs 9-2a to 9-2c). This stabilization may also be accomplished by constructing a provisional acrylic resin fixed prosthesis to provide the foundation for permanent stabilization and esthetics.

The goals of periodontal therapy and the type of interventions may have to be altered or compromised to satisfy esthetic and phonetic goals. Some possible alternatives to definitive surgery may include closed root planing and/or placement of antibiotic fibers in the gingival sulcus.[7] The surgery may have to be modified with a palatal approach, thus leaving a high labial curtain of tissue with some significant probing depth.

It is important that the orthodontic therapy result in stability and esthetics with minimum detriment to the periodontium. The health of the interproximal periodontium must be assessed (especially at the buccal line angles of the maxillary incisors) to determine if any cosmetic disfigurement may result from the orthodontic and periodontal therapy.

It is essential to collate the radiographic and clinical data to establish a working treatment plan. If one incisor

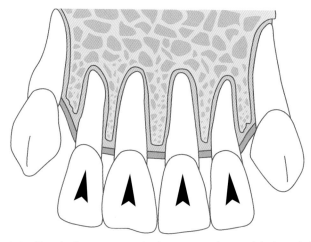

Fig 9-4a Angular bony topography between canines and incisors before intrusion *(arrows)*.

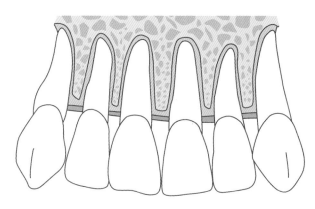

Fig 9-4b Leveling of bone after intrusion.

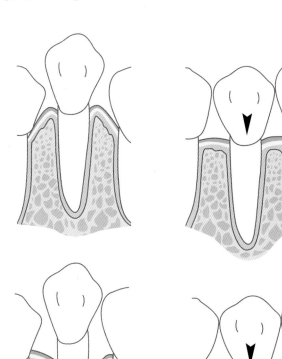

Fig 9-5a Intrusion *(arrow)* of erupted tooth with normal periodontium.

Fig 9-5b Exacerbation of periodontal lesion during intrusion *(arrow)* of diseased root structure.

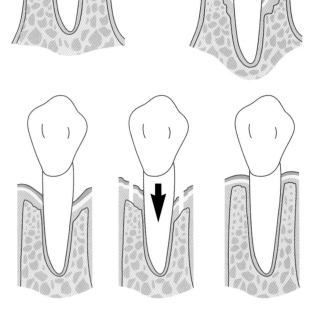

Fig 9-5c Surgical cutting of fibers and root debridement prior to intrusion *(arrow)* to gain reattachment.

intrusion. If the dentoperiosteal fibers are present in patients with periodontal disease, intrusion does not result in coronal regeneration of the bone, cementum, and periodontal ligament (Fig 9-5b). Theoretically, this would only be possible if the crestal fibers were removed to alleviate crestal resorption. Intrusion would then increase the level of connective tissue attachment, even in the presence of an altered cementum on a diseased root (Fig 9-5c). Shortening of the clinical crown and deepening of the gingival sulcus may accompany intrusion. There is the additional possibility of undetectable apical root resorption.[13]

Clinicians should remain cognizant of the possible esthetic complications that can result from initiating periodontal surgery prior to intrusion in patients having diseased root structures in the maxillary incisor segment. It may be difficult to predict the posttreatment results because of the limitation of two-dimensional radiographs and clinical probings. The orthodontist should work closely with the periodontist to intercept periodontal changes that develop during the treatment. The patient must also understand that orthodontic space closure and stabilization bear a certain degree of periodontal liability.

Tipping

A certain periodontal risk accompanies the tipping that occurs when pathologically diseased incisors are retracted. Infrabony pocketing on the lingual or palatal aspect of the incisors may worsen during orthodontic retraction. Definite consideration should be given to preorthodontic periodontal surgical intervention, ranging from root planing to regenerative procedures in patients presenting with vertical osseous lesions.

Rotation

The pathologic labial migration of teeth may be further complicated by rotation of the affected teeth. Orthodontic realignment, including the derotating of the incisors in conjunction with retraction, is followed by permanent stabi-

lization to prevent relapse. It has been suggested that a circumferential fiberotomy may be useful in stabilizing the corrected portions of previously rotated teeth.[14] It is difficult and risky to perform a circumferential fiberotomy in patients who have periodontal disease because of the problem of gaining access to the crestal gingival fibers while, for esthetic reasons, simultaneously attempting to maintain the tissue level with an increased probing depth in the maxillary incisor region. Consequently, consideration must be given to the potential for both periodontal and orthodontic relapse when rotations resulting from pathologic migration are corrected.

Each case of pathologic migration must be diagnosed individually, and treatment must be customized. The formula for determining success will vary because of the myriad treatment factors that must be considered. Overall, the treatment objective is not only stabilization with preservation of esthetics but also simultaneous control of periodontal disease activity. Some patients require a compromise in the periodontal treatment plan to satisfy their esthetic and phonetic needs.

Tooth Size Discrepancy (Bolton Index)

Another factor to consider before space closure of the maxillary incisors is tooth size. This is a critical factor in determining whether space closure is possible without restorative intervention to augment the width of the incisors. A normal value of a 77% ratio represents the ideal balance of total mandibular incisor and canine mesiodistal widths relative to the maxillary incisor and canine widths in a Class I occlusion with minimal overjet and overbite (Fig 9-6a).[15,16] A ratio greater than 77% indicates that the mandibular incisors are too wide and/or the maxillary incisors are relatively too narrow. A ratio of less than 77% reflects narrow mandibular incisors and/or wide maxillary incisors.

Failure to understand this Bolton relationship could lead a clinician to recommend orthodontic space closure when the spacing is not related to pathologic migration but rather

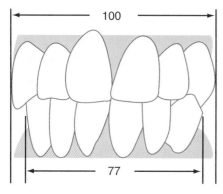

Fig 9-6a Normal Bolton Index.

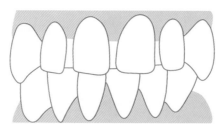

Fig 9-6b Abnormal Bolton Index.

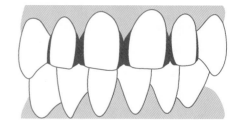

Fig 9-6c Maxillary anterior teeth requiring restorative increase of mesiodistal widths to achieve space closure.

is the result of an abnormality in the size of the maxillary and mandibular incisors (Fig 9-6b). In patients with pathologic migration and a superimposed Bolton irregularity, orthodontic retraction or intrusion may have to be combined with the application of restorative materials to increase the mesiodistal widths of the incisors and canines (Fig 9-6c). It is important to determine whether the spacing has always existed or is a recent development.

Bite Collapse

Adult patients often present with a compromised occlusion as a result of missing posterior teeth. The loss of posterior teeth may result in the loss of critical supporting structures that are essential to the integrity of the well-functioning dental unit. Within the same arch, the loss of one or more teeth allows others to drift; consequently, spacing between the remaining teeth becomes evident. As interproximal contact is lost, neighboring teeth tip into the existing spaces and the dental arch inevitably begins to collapse. The acute inclination of these teeth makes it difficult for the patient to cleanse the areas; as a consequence, vertical osseous defects often develop, presenting a significant periodontal risk. If the process is left unattended, the combination of the adverse inclination of the teeth, the active inflammation, the progressing vertical osseous defects, and traumatic occlusion can frequently lead to loss of additional teeth.

The loss of occlusal support for the opposing arch may soon follow. Tipped teeth lose contact with opposing teeth, resulting in extrusion (see Fig 9-1b) that can become severe enough to lead to traumatic occlusal forces on the opposing teeth. This collapse may result in the eventual loss of vertical dimension, leading to a deepening of the anterior overbite. This can then result in spacing between maxillary

anterior teeth if the mandibular incisors drive into the cingula of the maxillary anterior teeth (see Fig 9-1c). Frequently, it is when the esthetic problems become evident that the patient seeks treatment. It is to be hoped that the destruction in the supporting structures of the posterior periodontium is not so severe as to prevent the possibility of reconstruction of a functional occlusion.

Establishing a Functional Occlusion

Restoration of a functional occlusion is not a simple process. Treatment planning data must include the severity of the existing malocclusion, the number of missing dental elements, and the level of active periodontal disease. Initial preparation is critical, so that inflammation can be eliminated before the patient is subjected to the controlled trauma that is inevitable with orthodontic intervention.

An existing malocclusion may be a result of missing teeth and their liabilities within an arch, or it may be a superimposition of this problem on a malocclusion that was present prior to the loss of teeth. The practitioner is faced with a choice of selecting as a goal the ideal correction of the compete malocclusion or the simple restoration of function and esthetics. As posterior teeth begin to drift, opposing teeth often display extrusion beyond the practical orthodontic level of reintrusion. Intrusion of excessively extruded teeth may place excessive strain on periodontally damaged anchorage units. A practical approach may involve reduction of the crown and possible endodontic therapy, followed by restorative treatment to achieve the proper plane of occlusion (Figs 9-7a and 9-7b). If necessary, ostectomy can be performed to level the bone.

Closure of spaces in the maxillary anterior segment can present an equally challenging dilemma to the practitioner. Adequate clearance must be available for retraction of the

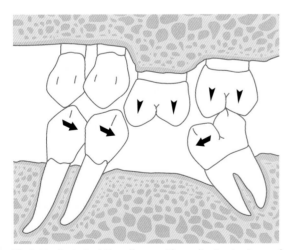

Fig 9-7a Posterior bite collapse with resultant extrusion and tipping of teeth (arrows) caused by loss of arch integrity.

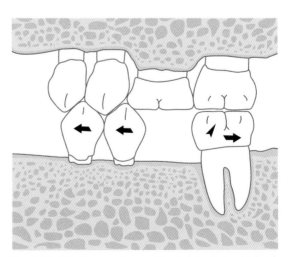

Fig 9-7b Maxillary molar equilibrated back to occlusal plane (arrows). Ostectomy and endodontic therapy may be required.

incisors as spaces are closed. This clearance is often unavailable in malocclusions that display incisor spacing caused by posterior bite collapse, bite deepening, and the resulting mandibular incisor impingement on the palatal surfaces of the maxillary anterior teeth. Retraction of the maxillary teeth and space closure is impeded by the increased overbite. Proper treatment sequence mandates restoration of the posterior vertical dimension, correction of the bite collapse, and, eventually, incisor gathering and space closure as bite opening is achieved.

Space Closure Versus Uprighting

Space Closure

The practitioner is often faced with the difficult decision about how to treat the spacing that has resulted from one or more missing teeth. Spaces are often distributed between posterior teeth that may be severely inclined. The mandibular dental midlines are frequently shifted toward the available spaces, the overjet and overbite are obviously increased, and normal occlusal relationships are lost. The comprehensive treatment plan must collate the orthodontic data and the assessment of the damage to the periodontium.

Is it possible to consider closure of the posterior spaces? Considerable vertical osseous defects may be present adja-

cent to tipped teeth and these would prevent, or, at best, make it risky to consider, movement of adjacent teeth. Movement into osseous defects could lead to additional bone loss, increased vertical osseous defects, or even furcation involvement.[17] Longstanding extraction spaces may have undergone considerable bone atrophy. Tooth movement into a ridge with atrophied buccolingual dimension may lead to significant buccal or lingual dehiscence (Fig 9-8). It has been radiographically demonstrated that patients with a healthy periodontium exhibit 2 to 3 mm loss of crestal alveolar bone when extensive protraction (10+ mm) is attempted.[18]

Even if adequate bone is present, consideration must be given to the fact that tooth movement may be very slow and complete space closure may not be possible. Inadequate space closure may lead to areas that are difficult for the patient to maintain and thereby predispose the patient to future periodontal breakdown. Retaining closure of these spaces may be impossible without fixed retention or splinting.

Protraction of tipped molars may exacerbate an existing malocclusion as mandibular incisor anchorage is tested, dental midlines shift, and, inevitably, overjet and overbite increase. Achieving and maintaining proper axial inclination of these posterior teeth as they are uprighted and moved mesially may be difficult, if not impossible.

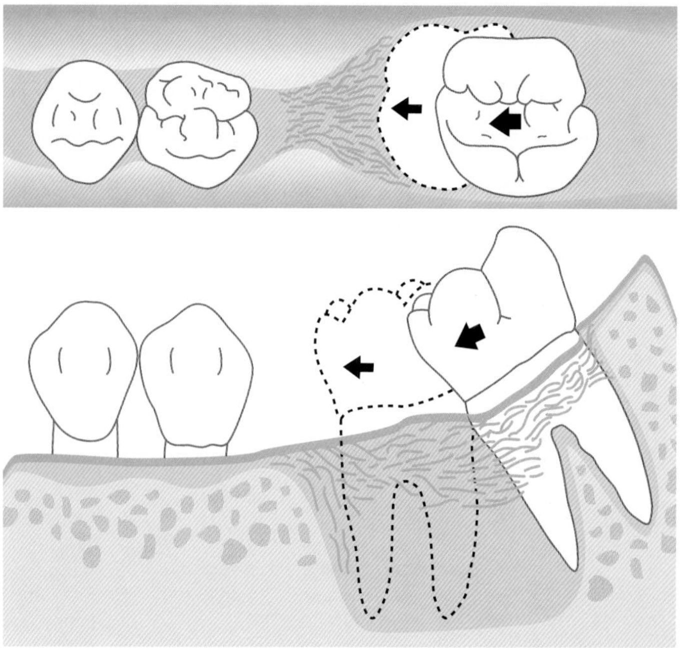

Uprighting

A more predictable and pragmatic approach to handling spaces resulting from missing posterior teeth may be simple uprighting of the adjacent teeth followed by restoration with fixed partial dentures or implants. The utilization of orthodontic treatment to upright mesially tipped second molars came into vogue in the 1970s.[19] The overall objective was to achieve an environment that was easily maintained by the patient and periodontally sound as the teeth were restored to their proper axial inclination (at a right angle to the interproximal bone).

From the standpoint of mechanotherapy, uprighting of abutments presents a set of favorable conditions. Classic orthodontic uprighting mechanotherapy between the teeth abutting the space results in a desirable action-reaction equation. As the tipped teeth are uprighted, reciprocal forces precipitate closure of any generalized spacing that may have occurred in the anterior segments. The reaction force will also frequently help to restore a shifted dental midline and reduce overjet as the anterior portion of the arch is returned to its original position. Moreover, the infrabony defect on the mesial aspect of an orthodontically uprighted molar becomes less pronounced as the mesial

Fig 9-8 Tooth movement *(arrows)* into atrophied ridge, leading to loss of crestal bone and possible buccal and/or lingual dehiscence and fenestration.

surface of the tooth is extruded during the procedure[20] (Fig 9-9a). After the uprighting has been completed, any remaining mesial periodontal defect can be surgically corrected. Molar uprighting provides the clinician with an improved surgical access to the osseous defect.

A comparative estimate of the treatment time for uprighting versus space closure (protraction) would be within the range of a 4:1 ratio. Normally, uprighting tipped abutment teeth can be accomplished in approximately 6 months, whereas space closure could necessitate full fixed orthodontic therapy for 2 years. This considerable discrepancy in treatment time may be a deciding factor in the patient's choice of treatment plans.

Unfortunately, molar uprighting also has its own set of consequences and liabilities. As mesially inclined posterior teeth are uprighted, they undergo extrusion, and this leads to premature contact with the opposing arch. This problem is compounded as the teeth upright distally and are wedged into the narrowing angle formed between the maxilla and mandible. This combination of factors may lead to excessive vertical loading on the uprighted teeth (Figs 9-10a and 9-10b). Traumatic occlusion becomes inevitable, and careful occlusal equilibration of these teeth is critical to pre-

vent additional destruction of the supporting apparatus (see Fig 9-9b). As previously noted, severely extruded teeth may even require endodontic treatment prior to their reduction back to the level of the occlusal plane.

Molar uprighting requires careful monitoring to prevent the extreme consequences of the orthodontic uprighting system. As the mandibular anterior teeth return to their proper anteroposterior positions, obvious labial forces are exerted on the cortical plate of bone in the incisor and canine areas. Prior to activation of the orthodontic system, these areas must be evaluated for any pretreatment soft tissue grafting requirements.[21]

Consideration must also be given to the nature and quality of soft tissue surrounding the second and third molars, if they are present. As tipped molars are uprighted, they are driven distally into the existing hard and soft tissues surrounding these teeth. Frequently, bunching of soft tissues occurs as the molar crowns are pushed posteriorly, and these areas can readily become inflamed. Left unchecked, this inflammation may result in significant bone destruction, followed by the unavoidable loss of additional teeth.

Careful evaluation of these distal areas, prior and during uprighting procedures, can help to avoid these sequelae. As

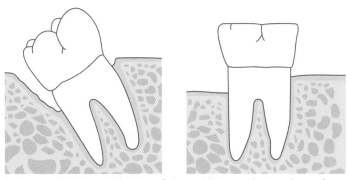

Fig 9-9a Selective equilibration of the uprighting molar to enhance favorable osseous changes during the uprighting process.

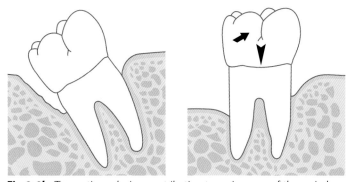

Fig 9-9b Traumatic occlusion contributing to an increase of the periodontal defect on an uprighting *(arrow)* molar.

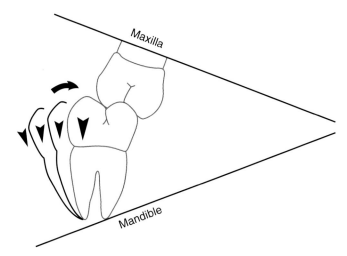

Fig 9-10a Molar uprighting *(arrows)* resulting in vertical loading.

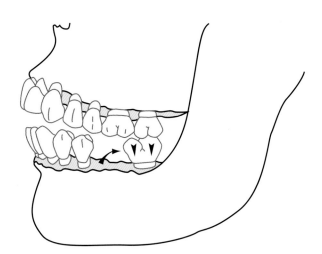

Fig 9-10b Molar uprighting *(arrows)* resulting in bite opening.

mesially inclined molars are uprighted to their proper axial inclination, the third molar is frequently displaced severely in a lingual or buccal direction. If, during uprighting, it is determined that there is inadequate space for the third molar, it should be extracted. Excessive soft tissue should be reduced or eliminated prior to the undesirable occurrence of acute periodontal disease.

When uprighting and space consolidation have been achieved, a proper restorative plan can then be finalized for the areas of missing teeth. Quite often, the restorative procedure of choice will include fixed prostheses that will simultaneously replace the missing teeth and stabilize the uprighted abutments. Under ideal conditions, a dental implant might serve as the necessary prosthetic replacement. Implant placement is dependent on the extent of abutment restoration required coupled with existing osseous conditions.

Bodily Movement

Wennström et al[17] explored the possibilities of orthodontic bodily movement of teeth into periodontal defects in beagle dogs. They were unable to show an increase in attachment following mesial movement into a periodontal defect. Previously a similar monkey study was performed by Polson et al,[22] who created infrabony defects on the mandibular incisors and were unable to gain connective tissue attachment on the root by orthodontic movement into the defect. However, Geraci et al[23] were able to demonstrate connective tissue attachment by moving maxillary teeth into proximal defects in the monkey.

Based on this research, extreme caution should be exerted by any clinician who anticipates eradicating a periodontal defect by orthodontically moving a tooth mesially or distally. Despite the unfavorable results in animals, many clinicians attempt to orthodontically move teeth displaying diseased root structures. In the event of horizontal bone loss, the consequences may be minimal. However, such movements may worsen vertical defects. (Figs 9-11a and 9-11b)

Consequently, the question arises as to whether a periodontist should attempt a regenerative procedure in a periodontal defect either prior to or following orthodontic tooth movement. In some cases, initiating treatment with orthodontic therapy may enhance the possibility of regeneration by lessening the size of the lesion, increasing the proximity of the progenitor cells in regeneration, and improving access to the lesion. In other cases, periodontal intervention prior to orthodontic space closure may be the treatment of choice (Figs 9-12a to 9-12e).[24]

To date, there is no recognized controlled research demonstrating whether or not there is true regeneration (bone, cementum, and periodontal ligament), as opposed to formation of a long junctional epithelium, with bone repair in such a combined periodontal-orthodontic treatment.[24] However, because regeneration by itself is a proven entity, the practitioner, bearing in mind the aforementioned risks and limitations, should be aware of the possibility of combined treatment of an infrabony defect.

There is a paucity of data regarding osseous grafting to achieve ridge augmentation prior to movement of healthy teeth through an area once devoid of bone. It is possible to regenerate bone in edentulous ridges previously decimated by periodontal disease before initiating orthodontic treatment (Figs 9-13a to 9-13f). An alternative approach might involve orthodontic alignment of the teeth in the defect area followed by permanent stabilization and periodontal refinement (Figs 9-14a to 9-14e).

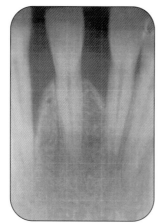 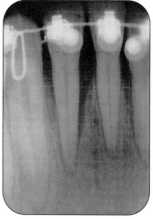

Fig 9-11a and 9-11b Orthodontic tooth movement into a vertical defect, resulting in additional bone loss.

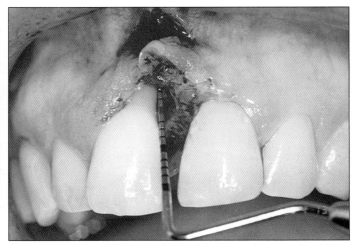

Fig 9-12a Infrabony defect on the mesial aspect of a rotated maxillary right central incisor.

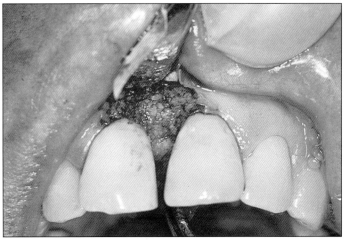

Fig 9-12b Regeneration procedure using a decalcified freeze-dried bone allograft, performed in conjunction with guided tissue regeneration.

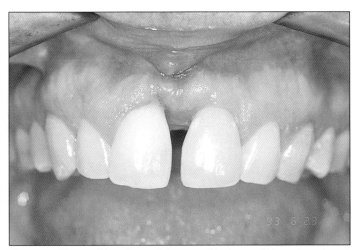

Fig 9-12c The mesial surfaces of the central incisors will be reshaped, and orthodontic treatment will be performed to close a diastema.

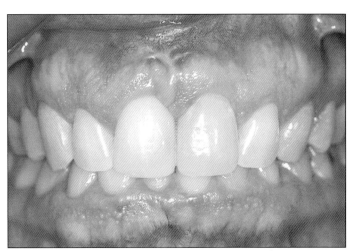

Fig 9-12d The posttreatment open gingival embrasure has been closed by dental bonding. Retention is via palatal intracoronal wire and resin composite.

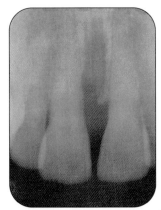
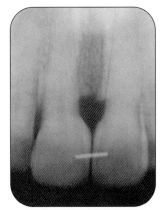

Fig 9-12e There appears to be bone regeneration occurring in the defect, which probed 7 mm pretreatment.

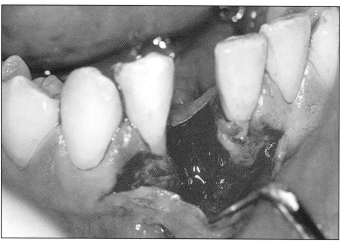

Fig 9-13a Extraction of a mandibular right incisor with severe loss of buccal and lingual plate because of endodontic-periodontal infection.

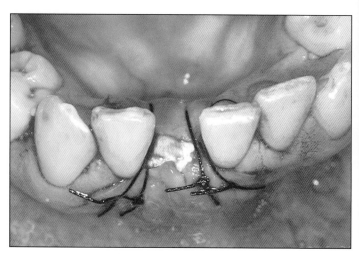

Fig 9-13b Guided tissue regeneration procedure to restore the ridge anatomy prior to initiation of orthodontic therapy.

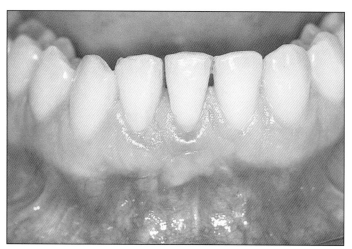

Fig 9-13c Completion of orthodontic therapy, initiated following 2 months of healing.

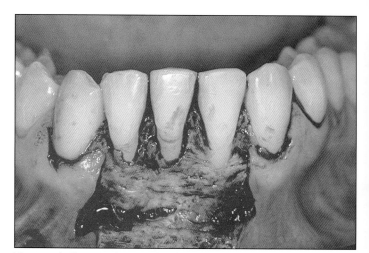

Fig 9-13d Flap raised 6 months after orthodontic therapy was completed, revealing that bone is 1 mm below the level of the cementoenamel junction.

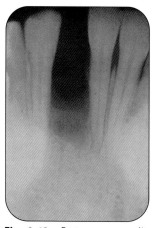

Fig 9-13e Pretreatment radiograph.

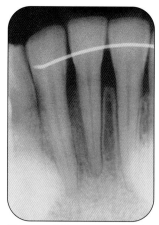

Fig 9-13f Posttreatment radiographs of the defect, showing ridge and interproximal septum regeneration following orthodontic therapy.

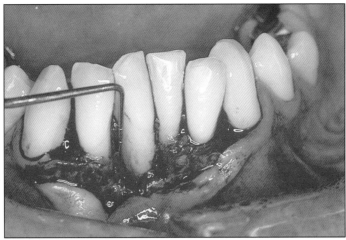

Fig 9-14a Strategic extraction of a mandibular right central incisor with a severe periodontal defect. The septa were very narrow interproximally between the remaining teeth.

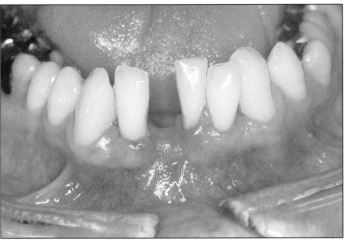

Fig 9-14b Ridge after 1 month of healing. Orthodontic therapy was initiated at this time.

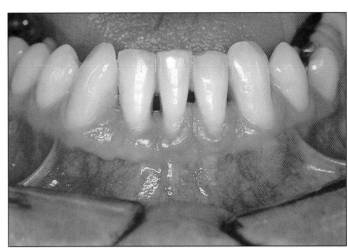

Fig 9-14c Orthodontic realignment of the remaining mandibular incisors with permanent stabilization.

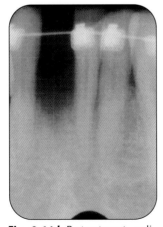

Fig 9-14d Pretreatment radiograph.

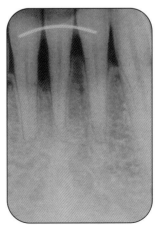

Fig 9-14e Posttreatment radiograph demonstrating that the original 50% bone level in the extraction site was maintained during treatment. The narrow pretreatment embrasures and interproximal bone septa now are widened after orthodontics.

161

Stripping

Although interproximal stripping may result in tight embrasures and narrow interproximal septa, it is frequently utilized to resolve limited tooth size–arch size discrepancies. It can be a very useful clinical tool for resolving crowding when there is accompanying loss of supporting bone (Fig 9-15a). Stripping can provide space for the elimination of crowding without necessitating complex bodily movement. The loss of interproximal bone, coupled with the conical root morphology, presents a favorable compromise in embrasure form as the stripping is performed. This desirable phenomenon can serve to provide a well-maintainable interproximal architecture as the teeth are aligned (Fig 9-15b).

Forced Eruption (Extrusion)

Forced eruption can be used to aid in the leveling of an infrabony defect[25,26] because it avoids potential problems of regeneration or repair normally associated with a diseased root structure. With forced eruption, dentoperiosteal fibers at the base of an infrabony defect are stretched, stimulating deposition of bone along their length. The level of bone that occurs with extrusion in the area of the defect may be significant enough to obviate the need for periodontal surgery. However, surgeons often utilize forced eruption, wait until approximately 6 months after maturation of the bone, and then perform finite soft or hard tissue revisions.

Canine studies have demonstrated that forced eruption allows the bone to follow the dentoperiosteal fibers even in

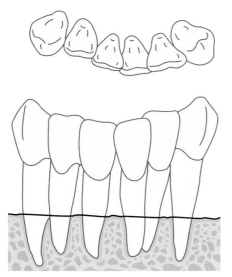
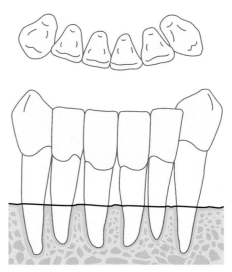

Fig 9-15a Crowding accompanied by bone loss.

Fig 9-15b Interproximal stripping to provide space for alignment. Bone loss and root anatomy may create a favorable interproximal architecture as teeth are aligned.

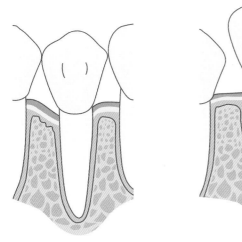

Fig 9-16a Osseous changes during extrusion *(arrow)* of teeth with a normal bone level and a periodontal defect.

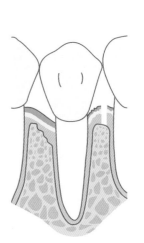
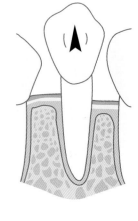

Fig 9-16b Cutting fibers on the normal side prevents an angular defect. Uncut fibers on the lesion side produce leveling of the bone defect during extrusion *(arrow)*.

the presence of inflammation.[27,28] This information is clinically useful when forced eruption is contemplated as a vehicle to eliminate periodontal defects. During the eruption, simple root planing to maintain inflammatory control will continue to produce a positive response at the level of the crestal bone. The calculus present will become more visible and easily removed as the tooth is orthodontically extruded. This phenomenon is not a possibility during intrusion and bodily movement.

When trying to eliminate a defect via forced eruption, the clinician must consider the possibility that reverse osseous topography will be created on another surface of the tooth (Fig 9-16a). This problem may be eliminated via a selective crestal fiberotomy[29] (Fig 9-16b), thereby inhibiting any undesirable osseous increase on the normal side. Each patient will demonstrate individual variation and must be treated accordingly.

Forced eruption is useful in the modification of irregular gingival architecture and should be considered to control esthetics in the maxillary incisor region.[20] Esthetic deformities may result when a tooth that is fractured at or below the level of bone is surgically uncovered, resulting in an unsightly long tooth. Utilizing forced eruption first and then performing ostectomy may be a good treatment alternative. Forced eruption will allow the bone and gingiva to extrude with the fractured root structure, thereby creating a more favorable topography. Following a 2- to 3-month retention period, the root that has been extruded can undergo ostectomy and/or gingival positioning to allow proper exposure without the esthetic liabilities that would result from surgical crown exposure alone.

One risk of this treatment is that extrusion followed by ostectomy reduces the clinical root supported in bone and may result in a mobile tooth. As the bone is reduced in an apical direction, there is the tendency to open up embrasure space, which may require closure via restorative material or a subepithelial connective tissue graft to restore the papilla.

Conclusion

Clinicians confronted with malocclusions with superimposed periodontal disease are faced with the difficult task of making complex clinical decisions involving the integration of periodontal and orthodontic therapies. The sequence of treatment, design of surgical procedures, choice of tooth movement, and orthodontic mechanotherapy, are just some of the options which must be considered and integrated. The therapies discussed in this chapter are not the only therapeutic possibilities for resolution of these clinical complexities. However, the combined therapies are founded in repeated clinical successes that have provided patients with pleasing esthetics, healthy function, and increased longevity of their natural dentitions. Patients will continue to benefit from the combination of research and shared clinical information that the specialties of orthodontics and periodontics will provide.

References

1. Geiger AM. Mucogingival problems and the movement of mandibular incisors: A clinical review. Am J Orthod 1980;78:511–527.
2. Wehrbein H, Bauer W, Diedrich P. Mandibular incisors, alveolar bone, and symphysis after orthodontic treatment. A retrospective study. Am J Orthod Dentofac Orthop 1996;110:239–246.
3. Lang M, Löe H. The relationship between the width of keratinized gingiva and gingival health. J Periodontol 1972;43:623.
4. Tuverson DL. Anterior interocclusal relations. Part I. Am J Orthod 1980;78:361–370.
5. Tuverson DL. Anterior interocclusal relations. Part II. Am J Orthod 1980;78:371–393.
6. Greenstein G, Caton J. Periodontal disease activity: A critical assessment. J Periodontol 1990;61:543–552.
7. Newman MG, Kornman KS, Doherty FM. A 6 month multi-center evaluation of adjunctive tetracycline fiber therapy used in conjunction with scaling and root planing in maintenance patients: Clinical results. J Periodontol 1994;65:685–691.
8. Artun J, Urbye KS. The effect of orthodontic treatment on periodontal bone support in patients with advanced loss of marginal periodontium. Am J Orthod Dentofac Orthop 1988;93:143–148.
9. Lynch SE. Methods for evaluation of regenerative procedures. J Periodontol 1992;63:1085–1092.
10. Melsen B, Agerbaek N, Eriksen J, Terp S. New attachment through periodontal treatment and orthodontic intrusion. Am J Orthod Dentofac Orthop 1988;94:104–116.
11. Melsen B, Agerbaek N, Mardenstam G. Intrusion of incisors in adult patients with marginal bone loss. Am J Orthod Dentofac Orthop 1989;96:232–241.
12. Murakami T, Yokota S, Takahama Y. Periodontal changes after experimentally induced intrusion of the upper incisors in Macaca Fuscata monkeys. Am J Orthod Dentofac Orthop 1989;95:115–126.
13. Wehrbein H, Fuhrmann RAW, Deidrich PR. Periodontal conditions after facial root tipping and palatal root torque of incisors. Am J Orthod Dentofac Orthop 1994;106:455–462.
14. Edwards JG. A long-term prospective evaluation of the circumferential supracrestal fiberotomy in alleviating orthodontic relapse. Am J Orthod Dentofac Orthop 1988;93:380–387.
15. Bolton WA. Disharmony in tooth size and its relation to the analysis and treatment of malocclusion. Am J Orthod 1958;28:113–130.
16. Wise RJ, Nevins M. Anterior tooth size analysis (Bolton Index): How to determine anterior diastema closure. Int J Periodont Rest Dent 1988;8:9–23.
17. Wennström JL, Stokland BL, Nyman S, Thilander B. Periodontal tissue response to orthodontic movement of teeth with infrabony pockets. Am J Orthod Dentofac Orthop 1993;103:313–319.
18. Hom BM, Turley PK. The effects of space closure of the mandibular first molar area in adults. Am J Orthod Dentofac Orthop 1984;85:457–469.
19. Brown IS. The effect of orthodontic therapy on certain types of periodontal defects. I. Clinical findings. J Periodontol 1973;44:742–750.
20. Wise RJ, Kramer GM. Predetermination of osseous changes associated with uprighting tipped molars by probing. Int J Periodont Rest Dent 1983;3:69–81.

21. Artun J, Krogstad O. Periodontal status of mandibular incisors following excessive proclination. Am J Orthod Dentofac Orthop 1987; 91:225–232.

22. Polson A, Caton J, Polson AP, Nyman S, Novak J, Reed B. Periodontal response after tooth movement into intrabony defects. J Periodontol 1984;55:197–202.

23. Geraci TF, Nevins M, Crossetti HW, Drizen K, Ruben MP. Reattachment of the periodontium after tooth movement into an osseous defect in a monkey. Part I. Int J Periodont Rest Dent 1990; 10:185–197.

24. Nevins M, Wise RJ. The use of orthodontic therapy to alter infrabony pockets. Part II. Int J Periodont Rest Dent 1990;10:199–207.

25. Ingber JS. Forced eruption. Part I. A method of treating isolated one and two infrabony osseous defects—rationale and case report. J Periodontol 1974;45:199–206.

26. Ingber JS. Forced eruption. Part II. A method of treating nonrestorable teeth—periodontal and restorative considerations. J Periodontol 1976; 47:203–216.

27. Van Venrooy JR, Yukna RA. Orthodontic extrusion of single-rooted teeth affected with advanced periodontal disease. Am J Orthod Dentofac Orthop 1985;87:67–74.

28. Vanarsdall RL, Van Venrooy JR. Tooth eruption: Correlation of histologic and radiographic findings in the animal model with clinical and radiographic findings in humans. Int J Adult Orthodont Orthognath Surg 1987;2:235–247.

29. Pontoriero R, Celenza F Jr, Ricci G, Carnevale G. Rapid extrusion with fiber resection: A combined orthodontic-periodontic treatment modality. Int J Periodont Rest Dent 1987;7:31–43.

CHAPTER 10

Intracoronal and Extracoronal Stabilization

James J. Hanratty, DDS

The periodontally compromised dentition offers many opportunities to debate the efficacy of splinting. It frequently addresses the therapeutic goals of treatment, including patient comfort with mastication and retention of teeth after orthodontic intervention. This chapter does not address minimal mobility as an issue but limits this clinical exercise to teeth in secondary occlusal trauma or those with an increasing mobility pattern. A continued increase in mobility can be devastating in the presence of a reduced periodontium. In such situations, normal or physiologic forces can no longer be tolerated and a change in the attachment apparatus occurs.[1–4]

In clinical practice, the treatment of mobile anterior teeth seems to be one of the most common and most challenging situations practitioners face. Splinting stabilizes the teeth as a unit by including healthy teeth, and redirects the forces from individual teeth to the new unit as a whole. Including the healthier teeth results in a new increase in crown-root ratio and a net decrease in force to the individual tooth, especially in a horizontal direction. Horizontal forces are believed to be more traumatic than axial forces.[5,6]

The most important aspect of splint design is to secure the teeth in all planes.[7] Many times this principle necessitates crossarch stabilization. This ensures tooth stability without increasing mobility and allows the periodontal ligament of each tooth to increase in surface area,[8] thus providing long-term retention.[9]

The selection of the form of splinting will be affected by the problem at hand. It has been suggested that splints be categorized by the length of time they will be used.[10]

Classification of Splints

A *temporary splint* is used on a short-term basis to stabilize teeth during periodontal therapy or after a traumatic episode.

A *provisional splint* is used for several months to several years for diagnostic information. Provisional splints allow the clinician time to observe the healing response to treatment and to make changes based on patient response; this enables the clinician to properly design a more permanent and biologically acceptable form of stabilization.

A *permanent splint* is used indefinitely. Permanent splints are usually used in a more reduced periodontium.

In the periodontal patient, application of splints frequently crosses the planned perimeters of use and may create several gray zones. The etiology of mobility, the degree of mobility, esthetics, tooth contours, tooth position, the coronal condition of the teeth, and embrasure morphology are some of the factors to be considered in choosing the type of splint.

Splints of all three categories can be further subdivided into extracoronal and intracoronal forms.

Intracoronal Splints

Intracoronal splints are the most commonly used type of splint. As the name implies, the technique entails making a cavity preparation into the lingual, palatal, or occlusal surface. This preparation is used to increase strength and retention of the restorative material. The preparation can be continuous (Fig 10-1) or discontinuous (Fig 10-2). The continuous splint is generally used in the mandibular segment because of the relatively short mesiodistal dimension of mandibular incisors. The discontinuous splint is more commonly used in the maxillary segment.

The teeth must first be evaluated as stable abutments. If the canines are periodontally sound, it is not necessary to include additional teeth in the splint. If the canines are not periodontally sound, additional teeth should be added, or use of a complete-coverage provisional splint should be considered.

Indications

1. Teeth with a more reduced periodontium (Figs 10-3a and 10-3b)
2. Dentition with a deep overbite
3. Teeth with very short roots or resorbed roots (Fig 10-4)
4. To evaluate potential abutment teeth
5. Teeth with root amputations and mobility
6. To avoid dislodgment during regenerative procedures
7. Postorthodontics, especially in cases involving intrusions, extrusions, rotations, pathologic migrations, or molar uprighting
8. When teeth with advanced mobility cannot be treated any other way (eg, the patient has medical or financial problems)

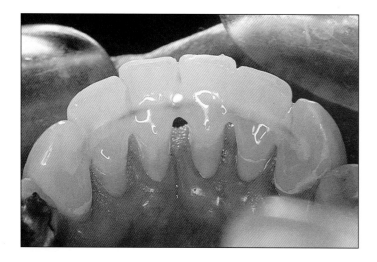

Fig 10-1 Continuous splint.

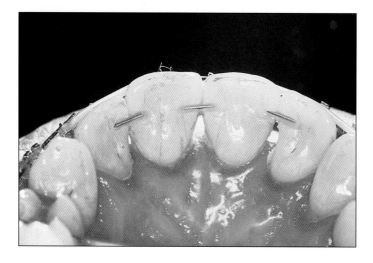

Fig 10-2 Discontinuous splint.

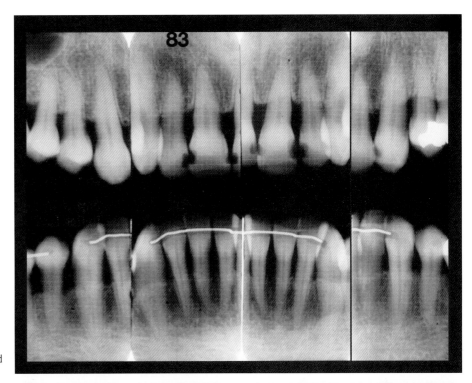

Fig 10-3a Intracoronal splint in teeth with advanced periodontal disease.

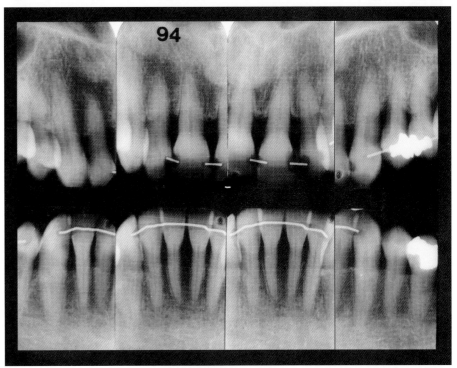

Fig 10-3b Same patient, 11 years later, with additional splint in maxilla.

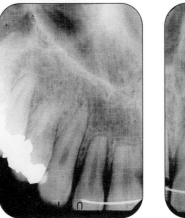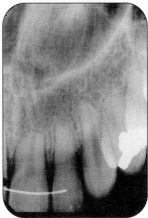

Fig 10-4 Splint in place in teeth with short roots and widened periodontal ligament.

167

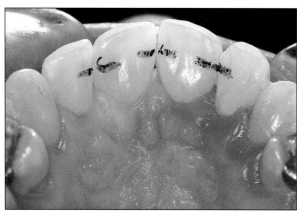

Fig 10-5a Lines drawn on teeth to demonstrate where preparations will be made. Lines also identify the thickest part of the contact area.

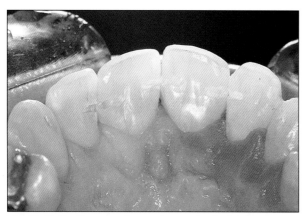

Fig 10-5b Tooth preparation made to a depth of 2.0 mm.

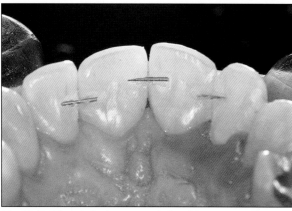

Fig 10-5c Threaded wires cut and placed into preparations.

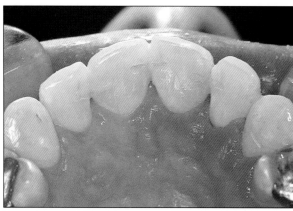

Fig 10-5d Splint finished and polished.

Technique

Step 1. Evaluate occlusal contacts. This is especially important in maxillary anterior teeth. Try to avoid centric occlusion and centric relation contacts to minimize damage or breakage of material.

Step 2. Evaluate proximal contacts (Fig 10-5a). If possible try to design preparation in the thickest part of the contact area. This will aid in strength, retention, and comfort.

Step 3. Make cavity preparations with a No. 699 bur. Refine later with a No. 33⅓ bur. The depth of the preparation is 1.5 to 2.0 mm (Fig 10-5b). For the continuous splint, it is best to prepare one tooth at a time, beginning at one proximal surface and ending at the other. At the distal end, it is best to stop one half to two thirds the width of the tooth, so as not to leave unsupported tooth structure.

Step 4. Cut wire or mesh to match the cavity preparation and try in place (Fig 10-5c). The wire thickness can vary from 0.018 to 0.030 in diameter, depending on the strength needed and the proximal contact width. Threaded wire is recommended for increased surface area.

Step 5. Apply etchant, dentin bonding agents, and adhesives according to their manufacturers' specifications. Layer material and secure wire or mesh. Layering is especially important, to ensure complete curing, if a light-cured material is used. The use of a rubber dam or wooden wedges is recommended to keep a dry field and prevent excess material from blocking interproximal spaces or injuring tissue.

Step 6. All occlusal contacts are checked for prematurities. It is especially important to check protrusive and lateral protrusive contacts. If left unchecked, these forces will cause early failure of the splint. In teeth that have supererupted, it may be necessary to perform odontoplasty so that the incisal edges provide evenly distributed surfaces for posterior disocclusion in protrusive movements.

Step 7. Refine form and polish. All excess material should be removed, and embrasures should be opened enough to allow routine hygienic procedures (Fig 10-5d).

As with all splints, the integrity of the splint and the patient's ability to perform adequate oral hygiene should be evaluated within a 4- to 6-week period.

The major advantage of intracoronal splinting is the ease with which it can be done, without disruption of occlusal harmony or function. It is also more comfortable, more esthetically pleasing, and less irritating to the gingival tissues. The disadvantages of intracoronal splinting are the risk of pulpal injury during cavity preparation and the risk of caries if material breaks or loosens.

Extracoronal Splints

Extracoronal splints are usually temporary in nature, although, with today's materials, they can be considered provisional or permanent splints. In contrast to the intracoronal splint, this type of splint does not involve any tooth preparation. Similar to the intracoronal splints, extracoronal splints can be reinforced with wire or mesh if additional strength is needed. Use of extracoronal splints is usually confined to anterior teeth.

Indications

1. Anterior teeth with moderate mobility
2. Postorthodontic retention without mobility, especially where retainer compliance is a concern (Figs 10-6a to 10-6c)
3. To provide stability in cases of acute trauma and allow for healing of the periodontal ligament, remodeling of alveolar bone, maintenance of tooth position, and comfort during function
4. Regenerative procedures, where mobility may temporarily increase
5. Endodontic-periodontic lesions

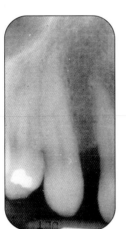 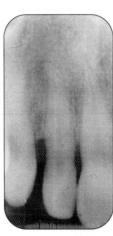 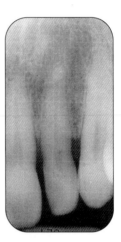 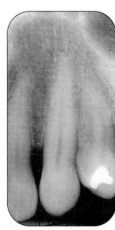

Fig 10-6a Radiographs taken before orthodontic treatment.

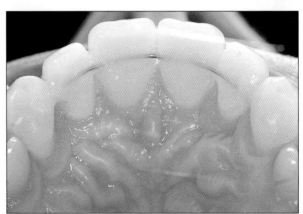

Fig 10-6b Splint in place.

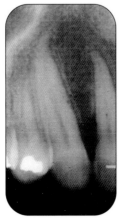 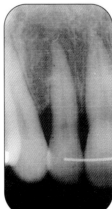 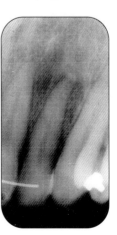 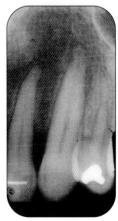

Fig 10-6c Radiographs taken 5 years postorthodontic treatment.

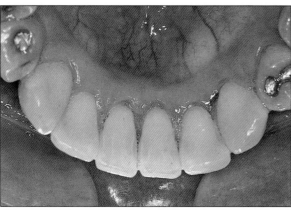

Fig 10-7a Preoperative view to evaluate proximal contacts.

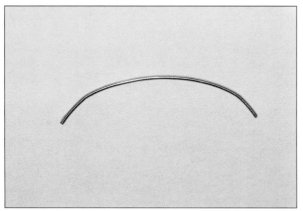

Fig 10-7b Threaded wire, demonstrating compensatory bend for canine.

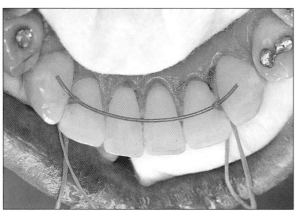

Fig 10-7c Threaded wire held in place with floss.

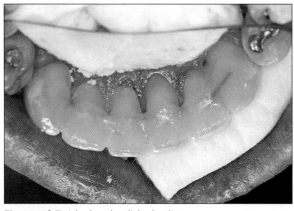

Fig 10-7d Finished and polished splint.

Technique

Step 1. Evaluate occlusal contacts. This technique is contraindicated in patients with deep overbites or minimal posterior occlusion.

Step 2. Evaluate proximal contacts. This will indicate the amount of material that can be flowed onto lingual surface without creating unsupported material or an unsightly situation (Fig 10-7a).

Step 3. Try in wire or mesh. Tight adaptation of material is very important for strength and thickness of material. Floss may be used to hold the material in place while the wire or mesh is secured (Fig 10-7b). If canines are included in a continuous splint, it is usually necessary to place a slight offset bend between the lateral incisor and canine to compensate for the larger lingual dimension of the canine (Fig 10-7c).

Step 4. Apply etchant, dentin bonding agent, and adhesives according to their manufacturers' specifications. Layer material; if possible, flow a small amount of material into the interproximal areas to provide additional resistance to dislodgment.

Step 5. Check occlusal contacts.

Step 6. Refine and polish (Fig 10-7d).

Extracoronal splints offer advantages over intracoronal splints: They require less time because no tooth preparation is necessary, and are more reversible. The disadvantage of extracoronal splints is initial compromise of phonetics and comfort. They may also limit the patient's ability to perform oral hygiene.

Materials

The materials used in splint construction come in a variety of forms. The most commonly used materials are resin composite, acrylic resin, and amalgam.

Resin composite is the most popular material used today in both extracoronal and intracoronal stabilization for several reasons: ease of application, strength, esthetics, and relatively simple repair. The biggest disadvantage to resin composite is the bond strength. The newer materials are much stronger but must still be monitored for breakage, which can allow teeth to migrate or caries to form.

Acrylic resin is used primarily in the provisional type of stabilization. The main advantages of acrylic resin are: esthetics and strength (especially with crossarch design). The disadvantages of acrylic resin are that it is difficult to repair and stains easily.

Amalgam is rarely used today because it fractures more easily and is very difficult to repair.

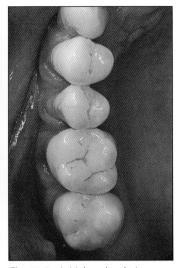

Fig 10-8a Initial occlusal view.

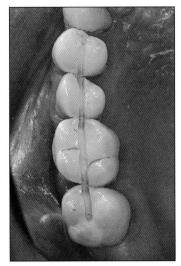

Fig 10-8b Tooth preparation.

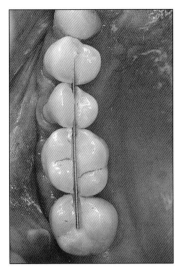

Fig 10-8c Threaded wire fitted to place.

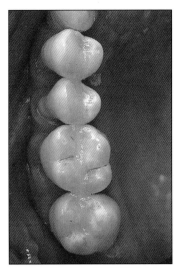

Fig 10-8d Finished splint.

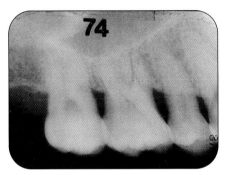

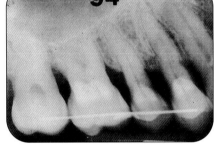

Fig 10-8e Radiographs taken 20 years apart.

Conclusion

The value of splinting has been debated for decades. Most of the data about splinting come from clinical observations rather than from scientific studies, but that does not mean that these findings should be discounted altogether. Certainly Fleszar et al[11] have demonstrated that nonmobile teeth heal much better than mobile teeth, and most clinicians treating advanced disease would agree (Figs 10-8a to 10-8e).

Splinting in any form, temporary, provisional, or permanent, provides the clinician with invaluable information during the course of treatment. At the same time, splinting increases the patient's comfort and function. Splinting should be considered, therefore, as part of an overall treatment plan in patients with moderate-to-severe tooth mobility.

References

1. Nyman S, Lindhe J. Considerations of patients with advanced periodontal disease. J Clin Periodontol 1977;4:1.

2. Nyman S, Lindhe J, Lundgren D. Role of occlusion for stability of fixed bridges in patients with reduced periodontal support. J Clin Periodontol 1975;2:53.

3. Nyman S, Ericsson I. The capacity of reduced periodontal tissues to support fixed bridgework. J Clin Periodontol 1982;9:409.

4. Nyman S, Lindhe J. Persistent tooth hypermobility following complications of periodontal treatment. J Clin Periodontol 1976;3:81.

5. Gibbs GH, Lundeen MC. Jaw movements and forces during chewing and swallowing and their clinical significance. In: Advances In Occlusion. PSG, 1982:

6. Smyd ES. The role of torque, torsion, and bending in prosthodontic failures. J Prosthet Dent 1961;11:95.

7. Lindhe J, Nyman S. Role of occlusion in periodontal disease and biologic rationale for splinting in treatment of periodontitis. Oral Sci Rev 1977;10:11.

8. Polson AM, Kantor ME, Zander HA. Periodontal repair after reduction of inflammation. J Periodont Res 1979;14:520.

9. Jin LJ, Cao CF. Clinical diagnosis of trauma from occlusion and its relation with severity of periodontitis. J Clin Periodontol 1992;19:92.

10. Lemmerman K. Rationale for stabilization. J Periodontol 1976; 47:405.

11. Fleszar TJ, Knowles JW, Morrison EC, Nissle RR, Ramfjord SP. Tooth mobility and periodontal therapy. J Clin Periodontol 1980;7:495.

Osseous Surgery: The Resective Approach

Michael P. Mills, DMD, MS
Howard T. McDonnell, DDS, MS

The use of the term *osseous surgery* usually brings forth visions of bone removal around periodontally diseased teeth to eliminate the osseous defect and the periodontal pocket. In reality, osseous surgery includes resective (subtractive) procedures, regenerative (additive) procedures, and a combination of both procedures, any of which may be employed to modify the bony support of the teeth. This chapter, however, will be limited to a discussion of the resective approach. The objectives will be to provide the therapist with *(1)* a review of significant anatomic relationships that exist between the hard and soft tissues of the oral cavity, *(2)* a conceptual understanding of the extent to which these tissues can be effectively altered, *(3)* the essential elements of wound healing as it relates to osseous surgery, and *(4)* the technical aspects of treating various types of osseous defects. As this chapter develops, the reader will soon begin to understand why true practitioners of this time-honored modality of treatment often refer to it as a distinctive blend of both the science and the art of periodontics.

The Evolution of Osseous Resective Therapy

For nearly a century, the need for surgical therapy to gain access to diseased root surfaces and the underlying alveolar bone has been recognized. The introduction of the mucoperiosteal flap in the early 1900s allowed for the removal of diseased bone thought to be infected and necrotic. Although this concept was not universally accepted, it prevailed until

1935, when Rudolf Kronfeld[1] demonstrated that bone affected by periodontal disease was neither necrotic nor infected. This led to a waning of interest in osseous resective techniques and a rekindling of one of the oldest surgical procedures in periodontics, the gingivectomy.

The gingivectomy was an extremely popular treatment modality during the early and mid-1900s, but it was not without its critics. In a classic 1949 article, Saul Schluger[2] expressed concerns about the frequent recurrence of periodontal pockets during the healing period following a gingivectomy procedure. He maintained that the gingivectomy failed to account for aberrations in the underlying osseous topography and, for this reason, could not totally achieve stable pocket eradication. Based on astute clinical observations, Schluger presented what are considered to be the first sound principles of osseous resective surgery, which provided the guidance for several clinicians who later modified and expanded the techniques to those that are followed today.

In 1955, Nathan Friedman[3] introduced the concept of using osteoplasty and ostectomy to achieve the desired physiologic osseous contours, as well as pocket elimination. Later, the rationale and technical aspects of the surgical approach to successful osseous resection were presented in an excellent series of articles,[4-7] authored by well-respected masters in osseous resective therapy: Clifford Ochsenbein, Harry Bohannan, Leonard Tibbets, and Dan Loughlin. Their presentations of the palatal and lingual approaches to osseous resective therapy provide the basis from which the concepts promoted in this chapter have evolved. Although today's approach to resective therapy is somewhat more conservative, with a greater emphasis on compromise, very little has changed in the techniques described several years ago by these insightful clinicians.

Rationale for Osseous Surgery

For decades, a great controversy has brewed over the use of osseous resective surgery to treat the ravages of periodontal disease. Opponents of this treatment modality have long held that removal of supporting bone provides no significant advantage over other surgical flap procedures, such as the modified Widman flap. Indeed, longitudinal studies cited by this group tend to demonstrate that gains in clinical attachment levels are greater with the modified Widman procedure.[8–10] Proponents, on the other hand, have shown that osseous resection, combined with an apically positioned flap, provides a more predictable reduction in probing depth over the long term.[11,12] These reduced probing depths are generally thought to be important in establishing an environment in which access for plaque control and supportive periodontal therapy (maintenance) is greatly facilitated.

Regardless of which treatment technique is selected, the common denominators most closely associated with the long-term maintenance of a functional, healthy dentition are excellent oral hygiene demonstrated by a compliant patient and professional supportive periodontal therapy provided at regular intervals. What is vastly more important to the clinician who practices periodontics is that he or she become proficient in several modalities of therapy to provide patients with the best quality of care that satisfies the patient's expectations and the therapist's treatment goals.

The Essentials of Wound Healing

The thickness or thinness of the bone that surrounds a tooth prior to surgical modification could be the single-most important determinant for a successful outcome to a case treated with osseous resective procedures. Thick bone may be characterized as trabecular bone containing marrow interposed between the outer cortical plate of the alveolar process and the alveolar bone proper of the tooth. Thick bone has a greater capacity for regeneration because the marrow is an excellent source of regenerative cells and vascular support. In contrast, thin bone contains minimal or no trabecular bone between the cortices of the alveolar process and alveolar bone proper. Such bone has very little capacity for regeneration.

These concepts of bone healing are supported by Wilderman et al,[13] who performed a histologic investigation of 23 human block sections that were removed following staggered healing periods of 0 to 18 months. Osteoplasty and ostectomy were performed according to a specific surgical design on the buccal surfaces of primarily single-rooted teeth demonstrating either thin, medium, or thick bone. If the preoperative radicular bone was thin, the authors noted that postoperative resorption occurred on the periodontal surface of the bone, ie, alveolar bone proper. If the radicular bone was thick, then resorption occurred on the bone surfaces facing the marrow spaces and haversian systems. Depending on the bone thickness, the amount of resorption ranged from 0.14 to 4.47 mm (average of 1.2 mm); resorption was followed by alveolar repair, ranging from 0.14 to 1.15 mm (average of 0.4 mm).

Another critical factor to consider is the amount of bone that is left exposed following flap placement and suturing and its subsequent effect on repair or regeneration. Less than 2 mm of crestal bone exposure may not result in a significant loss of attachment, provided that the bone is initially protected with a clot.[14] This finding is supported by the fact that the periodontal ligament is a primary source of granulation tissue during healing, with a regenerative capacity extending up to 2 mm beyond the alveolar crest. However, if larger areas of bone exposure occur, human and animal studies have shown that significant resorption will predictably occur.[15] In this scenario, only one half of the bone resorbed in the radicular area may be expected to regenerate, whereas nearly complete restoration will usually occur in the interdental and interradicular areas because of the presence of an abundant and broad base of marrow bone.

Thus, the degree to which the bony support of the teeth may be modified without jeopardizing additional attachment is dependent on the quality and quantity of the bone. It is wise for the clinician who is performing osseous resection to evaluate the thickness of the bone on all tooth surfaces prior to any removal.

The Nature of Osseous Defects

The general patterns of bone loss associated with destructive periodontal disease may be considered horizontal, vertical, or, more commonly, a combination of the two. These patterns of bone loss may affect multiple teeth in all sextants or be localized to a few teeth or even a single tooth. Practitioners of osseous resection have further developed a set of terms that descriptively identify specific types of osseous defects based on their morphologic appearance, anatomic location, or resemblance to commonly known structures, as in a fenestration (window) or moat. Discussion in this section will emphasize the factors that influence the type(s) of osseous defects that might be encountered surgically, along with special reference to those defects best corrected with a resective technique.

It is well established that putative periodontal pathogens within the subgingival plaque are responsible for the destructive nature of periodontal disease. As tissue attachment is lost along the root, pathogenic species will eventually colonize these newly exposed surfaces. This so-called migrating plaque front appears to have a zone or "sphere of influence" within which bone resorption may occur.

Histologic observation of periodontally involved teeth has suggested that the sphere of influence of the plaque has a range of between 0.5 and 2.7 mm.[16,17] Clinical observations strongly support these histologic findings.

It thus becomes evident that the topography of various types of osseous defects would be significantly influenced by the location and surface area of the plaque and any factor that might contribute to its lateral or apical extension, such as calculus deposits, restoration overhangs, and marginal placement, or anatomic aberrations, such as enamel pearls or cervical enamel projections. But perhaps the most important factor that determines the predilection for a particular defect shape is the quantity of bone within the destructive range of the plaque. Simply stated, the thickness or thinness of bone on any given surface of a tooth or between the teeth is the key factor. Bone quantity appears to be directly influenced by the structural anatomy of the mandible and maxilla; the form, size, and position of the roots and the inclination of the teeth; tooth-to-tooth relationships in the arch; and the presence of osseous ledges and exostoses.

Areas where thick bone predominates are predisposed to various forms of vertical defects, such as the intrabony defects, one-wall or hemiseptal defects, circumferential or moat defects, and vertical components of advanced furcation invasions. Areas of thin bone are typically associated with varying degrees of horizontal bone loss (Table 11-1). There is a direct correlation between the width of the interdental septum and the frequency of intrabony defects. Complete horizontal destruction of interproximal bone is more likely with narrow interdental septa, ie, less than 1.6 mm, and intrabony defects are more likely to occur if the interdental distance is wider, ie, greater than 2.6 mm.[18]

Although the idea is controversial, many clinicians believe that traumatogenic occlusion has the potential to be a significant modifier in the destructive patterns associated with periodontitis. These defects are typically circumferential and have a proclivity for the lingual surface of teeth. This is particularly true for the premolar teeth, which have been demonstrated to have the highest incidence of interferences from a centric relation to a centric occlusion position.

One descriptive categorization of osseous defects is based on the number of remaining bony walls surrounding the area of destruction.[19] The one-wall defect presents with either one proximal wall (hemiseptal) or one linguopalatal or buccolabial wall (Fig 11-1). These defects are generally not amenable to regenerative therapeutic approaches. Resective therapy, with the goal of creating a physiologic osseous architecture, will provide a more predictable and stable long-term result.

Two-wall defects are bordered by either two proximal walls, a buccal/labial and proximal wall or a buccal/labial and lingual wall. A two-wall defect consisting of a buccal/labial and lingual/palatal wall is commonly referred to as an *interdental* or *osseous crater* (Fig 11-2). According to a study by Manson and Nickolson,[20] the interdental crater constitutes approximately one third of all intrabony defects and as many as two thirds of all mandibular defects. The management of these defects is often dictated by the vertical depth of the crater, thickness of the crater walls, location

Table 11-1 Anatomic factors influencing bone quantity

Determining factor	Thick bone	Thin bone
Structural anatomy of the maxilla	Malar process Palatine process Buccal exostoses/ledges	Labial/buccal/palatal fossae
Structural anatomy of the mandible	External oblique ridge Exostoses/ledges	Labial/buccal/lingual fossae
Maxillary tooth position	Buccal surface of second molars	Mesiobuccal root of first molars Buccal surface of premolars Labial surface of incisors
Mandibular tooth position	Buccal surface of second molars Lingual surface of premolars	Mesial root of first molars Buccal surface of premolars Labial surface of incisors
Maxillary tooth inclination	Buccal surface of second molars	Labial surface of incisors
Mandibular tooth inclination	Lingual surface of premolars/molars	Labial surface of incisors
Root proximity	Distant	Close
Root form	Tapering and/or divergent	Thickened and/or convergent

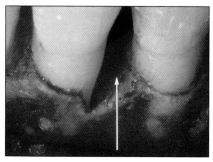

Fig II-I One-wall interproximal osseous defect. One proximal wall *(arrow)* remains adjacent to the distal mandibular premolar.

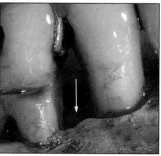

Fig II-2 Two-wall interproximal osseous defect (interdental crater). Only buccal and lingual osseous walls remain between the mandibular first molar and second premolar. Base of the crater *(arrow)*.

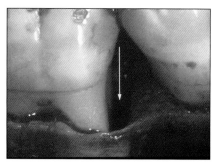

Fig II-3 Three-wall interproximal osseous defect. Buccal, lingual, and proximal walls enclose the interproximal defect. Base of the defect *(arrow)*.

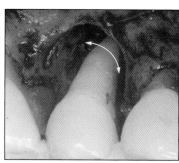

Fig II-4 Circumferential defect *(arrow)* around the palatal root of a maxillary premolar. The osseous defect involves the mesial, distal, and palatal surfaces of the root.

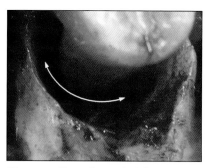

Fig II-5 Circumferential defect *(arrow)* involving the buccal, distal, and lingual root surfaces of a mandibular second molar.

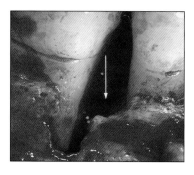

Fig II-6 Combination interproximal osseous defect. Three osseous walls encompass the apical extent of the defect. Coronally, either one or two osseous walls remain, depending on what area of the defect is being considered.

in the dental arch, tooth type, and, if multirooted teeth are involved, root trunk length. Osseous resective therapy is best applied to shallow (1- to 2-mm-deep) and moderate (3- to 4-mm-deep) interdental craters. Craters greater than 5 mm in depth may be more suited for regenerative procedures.

Three-wall intrabony defects are characterized as having three osseous walls; the tooth surface constitutes the fourth wall (Fig 11-3). These defects may be localized to one proximal or midradicular surface or may be circumferential (Figs 11-4 and 11-5), involving two or more root surfaces. Osseous therapy to treat these types of alveolar defects is aimed at reconstruction of the periodontium either through open flap curettage, osseous or alloplastic grafting techniques, and/or guided tissue regeneration procedures.

A total resective approach is generally contraindicated in three-wall defects.

Surgical therapy frequently exposes osseous defects that are composed not purely of one, two, or three walls but rather a combination of these (Fig 11-6). The apical aspect of a combination defect often consists of three walls, while more coronally the defect is bordered by one wall, two walls, or a combination of both. The therapeutic approach for these types of defects is based on defect depth and the proportion of the defect comprised by either the one-, two-, or three-wall component.

The resultant configuration of the osseous defect plays a significant role in the ability to eliminate it or reduce its extent through a resective approach or, perhaps, the need to select another treatment modality.

Osseous Resective Procedures

The primary objective of osseous resective procedures is to create a bony base that will be compatible with the overlying gingival tissue. It may not be possible to completely eliminate all osseous defects and their bizarre configurations without adversely affecting the prognosis for furcated teeth, creating reverse bony architecture, or surgically removing significant amounts of attachment. A greater understanding of normal anatomic relationships and their influence on the resective approach will successfully guide the clinician through most procedures.

Anatomic Concepts and Considerations

Several anatomic features and relationships among the teeth, bone, and investing soft tissues must be reviewed and understood by the clinician before he or she can properly perform osseous resective surgery. If the clinician will consider these anatomic manifestations as being unique for each patient, he or she will be able to attain an architectural pattern that is compatible for all tissues in any given situation. The preconceived notion that "one pattern fits all" must be forgotten.

Positive Architecture

In health, the gingival margin and the crest of the alveolar bone parallel the cementoenamel junction (CEJ) of the teeth (Fig 11-7). This means that the gingiva and the bone occupy a more apical position over the radicular surfaces of the teeth and a more coronal position interdentally. Considering the various anatomic shapes of the teeth, it

follows that the difference between marginal and interdental tissue levels will be greatest for the incisors and least for the molars. This architectural pattern has been commonly described as being *scalloped*. If the mesiodistal dimension of the crown is also included in this relationship, the scalloping associated with the incisors could be described as being accentuated, while the scalloping around most molars would almost be flat. On the proximal surfaces of the teeth, the bone assumes a different but important architectural pattern that again parallels the CEJ and is influenced by the buccal/labial-to-lingual/palatal dimensions of the teeth. The proximal bone generally assumes a pyramidal shape for incisor teeth and a convex or parabolic shape for premolar and molar teeth. A final relationship among the tooth, gingiva, and bone is created by the contacts of the anterior and posterior teeth within an arch. Viewed from either the labial/buccal or lingual/palatal, the interproximal septa of the incisor and premolar teeth will usually be pyramidal to convex, whereas the interproximal septa between molars will be predominantly flat. Together, relationships reflect what many clinicians refer to as *positive architecture.*

As a general rule, many therapists attempt to recreate a positive architectural form during the correction of various types of osseous defects because it is accepted as the norm. It might be more appropriate to consider positive architecture as merely a guide to treatment and not necessarily an end point that must be reached. Assuming normal alignment and position of the teeth within the arch, tooth form and tooth-to-tooth relationships will be key factors in determining the degree of scalloping that might exist in any given patient (Table 11-2). For example, the tissue scalloping associated with square anterior teeth would be characterized as being flat or less accentuated than the contours of tissue scalloping around oval anterior teeth. Although a flat

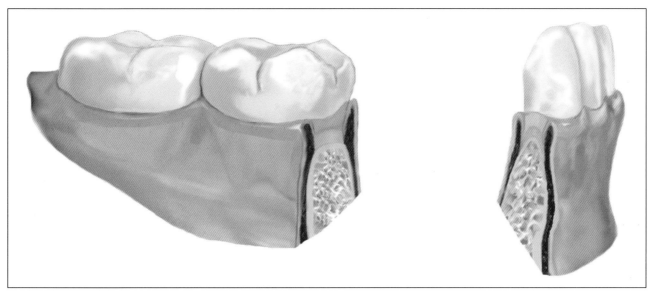

Fig 11-7 Normal anatomic relationships among the CEJ, gingiva, and bone.

Table 11-2 Factors affecting the degree of osseous scalloping

Determining factor	Pronounced osseous scallop	Flat osseous scallop
Gingival scalloping	Pronounced	Flat
Tooth form	Square	Ovoid
Interdental space	Narrow	Wide
Interdental bone	Narrow	Wide
Prominent roots	Yes	No
Root proximity	Convergent	Divergent

scalloped contour for the anterior teeth may not fit the mold of a positive architectural form, it would be a normal finding for patients presenting with this particular tooth shape. Because anatomic variation can usually be expected between patients and in some cases even within different areas in the same patient, it is more important that the clinician consider what is normal for the patient and not attempt to impose an ideal standard.

Anatomic Determinants for Postresective Architecture

Bone. Many clinicians harbor the misconception that the architectural pattern of the bone determines the contours of the gingival tissue. In health, it may be very difficult to argue against this concept because the contours of the bone and gingiva do parallel each other, as has previously been described. However, in moderate-to-advanced periodontal disease, the resultant patterns of bone destruction may be quite bizarre, yet the overlying gingiva still assumes its original architectural pattern. This occurs because, as bone is lost to periodontitis, it is replaced by a reparative tissue, composed almost entirely of connective tissue and epithelium, which supports the gingiva in its original position relative to the teeth. In a more simplistic way, the teeth should be thought of as creating an anatomically comfortable environment for the gingiva. The gingiva will accept change in this environment, as long as it is within normal anatomic variation and is dictated by the teeth and not the bone.

As a further explanation, let us consider a case scenario involving shallow two-wall intrabony defects (craters) between posterior teeth. The teeth are anatomically normal and in good alignment. The overlying gingival tissue demonstrates an average scalloped architecture with interdental tissue margins located more coronally than radicular margins. Surgical incisions are made which follow the outline of the marginal gingiva. Surgical flaps are reflected and osseous resective techniques are chosen to eliminate the crater walls of the bony defects. However, no resection is performed on the radicular bone margins, leaving them at their original position on the root. A flat bony architecture has now been created with radicular bone at the same level as interdental bone. Surgical flap margins are positioned at the bony crest and stabilized with sutures. During the next several months of healing, interdental papillae are observed to be reforming coronally. They begin to fill most of the embrasure space that had been opened as a result of surgery. Probing depths are found to increase interdentally approaching pretreatment recordings. The therapeutic end point in this case scenario is a result of a scalloped gingival form being adapted to a flat bony architecture. The scalloped positive architectural pattern which characterized the gingiva presurgically had been ignored.

It may be stated that the architectural pattern established in the bone should generally follow and be consistent with those contours common to the gingiva. This is another basic tenet that the clinician may use as a guide when designing flap incisions, modifying the bony architecture, and determining final flap placement. Where this rule applies with few exceptions is in the elimination of shallow osseous defects, reduction of exostoses and ledges, and in prerestorative crown lengthening procedures.

The correction of moderate osseous defects will often result in bone levels that are located more apically on the root surfaces of the teeth. The true measures of success for these procedures are the elimination of the defect with minimal or no removal of alveolar bone proper and the adaptation of the gingival tissue to this new environment without the re-formation of deep probing depths. Factors other than gingival form alone must now be used by the clinician to determine the extent to which the bone may be modified or sculptured in expectation of what the gingiva will accept as a compatible base. Important additional factors include the tooth-related determinants of root morphology, position of the roots in the arch, and root proximity.

Roots. As the roots of adjacent teeth taper apically, the interdental septum naturally becomes wider. If the level of the interdental crest is surgically placed in a more apical location relative to the adjacent roots, then the interdental space will be wider and the gingival papilla that occupies it will be flat or blunted in contour. Thus, greater distances between teeth dictate a flatter architectural form for the gingiva. An analogous example previously described is the difference in the shape of the interdental gingiva of anterior and posterior teeth, ie, pyramid-shaped papillae in narrow spaces and flat or blunted papillae in wide spaces. Other examples in the normal periodontium can be seen with diastemas, open contacts, or orthodontically created spaces. What this means clinically is that minimal or no alveolar bone (proper) need be resected to create a scalloped bony architecture to accommodate the original gingival scallop. A flat bony contour will be quite acceptable to the gingiva and not result in deep residual probing depths.

Another factor to consider is the prominence of the roots in the arch. Where roots are positioned well within the alveolar process, the bone is normally thicker and the gingival scalloping is flatter; when the roots are prominent and the bone is thin to absent, the gingival scalloping is usually more pronounced. When roots are prominent, the removal of additional radicular bone to maintain a positive architecture relative to the interdental bone is usually not indicated because the prominence itself provides an "imposed" natural scalloping as a result of the thinness of the overlying bone and gingiva. Vertical grooving techniques have been advocated as a means of creating prominent roots and thus reducing the amount or need for radicular ostectomy.[21]

Root proximity presents quite another dilemma for the clinician, especially in multirooted teeth. Wide separation of molar roots on the buccal surfaces may require the clinician to treat the roots as if they were those of two adjacent premolar teeth. The flat gingival architecture usually associated with the molars at the CEJ will now require a slightly scalloped form. The palatal roots of maxillary molars may also be treated as those of single-rooted teeth and will require more scalloping as the radicular bone crest becomes located farther apically. The opposite holds true for the lingual surfaces of mandibular molars, which will tolerate a flatter gingival architecture because of the broader crest or ledge of bone encountered in this region.

When the roots of multirooted teeth or adjacent teeth begin to closely approximate each other, a very narrow septum of bone is encountered; this is very difficult to manage because it will not readily support a normal papillary form. Heins and Wieder[22] have reported that septal widths of less than 0.5 mm consist of cortical bone with no cancellous bone widths of less than 0.3 mm consist of adjacent periodontal ligaments and no bone. Clinical situations such as these can be managed effectively by creating a broad, arch-shaped scallop with the narrow septum located in the middle; thus, if narrow interradicular bone exists on a multirooted tooth or narrow interdental bone between adjacent teeth, then the arched scallop would extend from the mesial surface of one root to the distal surface of the adjacent root.

In dealing with more advanced forms of bone loss, the clinician is now faced with the further dilemma of correcting the osseous defects without sacrificing significant periodontal attachment, while still trying to create a harmonious relationship between the gingiva and bone so that reduced probing depths can be established and maintained. Is this a realistic goal? The answer is, not usually. In these situations, the clinician must be willing to compromise, utilizing additional treatment modalities, such as regenerative techniques, tooth resection, flap curettage, or combinations of techniques.

These are but a few of the many variations which exist in the anatomic relationships among the teeth, gingiva, and bone. If the clinician has a profound understanding of these and other basic principles, he or she will be able to apply them to almost any scenario and reach an acceptable end point, albeit a compromise under some circumstances.

Approaches to Osseous Resection

Two approaches to osseous resection have been described in much detail and with great clarity by Ochsenbein and Bohannan[4,5] and Tibbets et al.[6] These authors advocate a palatal approach and a lingual approach, respectively, to eliminate shallow interproximal two-wall (crater) defects, the most common posterior defect. The most important rationale for both of these approaches is to avoid exposing the buccal furcations of molar teeth, especially when anatomic factors dictate a more effective and natural approach. The reluctance of many surgeons to treat defects from the palatal or lingual side primarily reflects an aversion for dealing with areas that they find difficult to visualize and access. A detailed understanding of anatomic features and their influence on the prospective treatment of the osseous defect, along with improved techniques of surgical flap management, will do much to quell their concerns.

Palatal Approach

The advantages of the palatal approach are related to the anatomic structure of the posterior maxilla, the quantity and quality of bone, the abundance of keratinized mucosa, tooth morphology, operator convenience, and access for oral hygiene.

Advantages of the Palatal Approach[5,6]

- Avoids surgical exposure of buccal furcations and possible root fenestrations or dehiscences
- Avoids dealing with a shallow vestibule
- More cancellous bone
- All keratinized tissue
- Wider interdental space
- Greater access for grooving or contouring the tooth
- Natural cleansing action of the tongue

A shallow vestibular depth may be associated with the posterior maxilla in the region of the first and second molars, depending on the prominence of the malar process. Wherever a shallow vestibule is found, there is normally a narrower band of attached gingiva on the radicular surfaces of the teeth bordering it which does not permit any resection of the gingival margin. A shallow vestibule also precludes the apical positioning of the surgical flap at the alveolar crest because the muscles tend to move the flap coronally, thus negating any gain in probing depth reduction postoperatively. However, this problem is not encountered on the palatal side where the abundant keratinized tissue can be scalloped and thinned in order that the flap margin be more apically located. As a result, presurgical probing depths may be reduced provided that proper osseous resection has also been performed.

The bone over the buccal roots of the posterior teeth is typically thin, which means that little or no cancellous bone is present. On the other hand, the bone on the palate has anatomically been determined to be thicker, and cancellous bone is abundant. As healing studies have proven,[13,15] more permanent resorption can be expected where thin bone exists, and virtually complete regeneration can be expected where thick bone is found. Therefore, a greater degree of osseous contouring may be accomplished from the palate with little postoperative detriment to the remaining attachment.

As discussed in previous sections of this chapter, tooth morphology not only plays a key role in determining the type and location of the osseous defect, but also influences the clinician's decision on "how much" and "where" the bone can be effectively modified to eliminate defects and reduce probing depths. Because the gingiva and bone parallel the CEJ, the normal bone pattern in the posterior region displays a gradual coronal-to-apical incline toward the palate. With just a single molar root to the palate, the interdental spaces become wider, affording better operator access for osseous and tooth contouring. Such an anatomic arrangement may also improve patient access for oral hygiene procedures and the natural cleansing action of the tongue.

Another key feature of tooth morphology is the location of the furcations. The mesiobuccal and distobuccal root separation have been found to be more apical than the

buccal furcation entrance.[7] Therefore, the risk of furcation exposure resulting from resective procedures would be greatest on the buccal surface. However, this does not imply that osseous resection is not performed on buccal surface. The root trunk and crater depth will play a significant role in determining the extent and location of resective procedures.

Lingual Approach

The advantages of the lingual approach are directly related to the structural anatomy of the mandible, the quantity and quality of the bone, the morphology and axial inclination of the posterior teeth, and access for oral hygiene.

Advantages of the Lingual Approach[6]

- Avoids surgical exposure of buccal furcations
- Avoids dealing with a shallow vestibule
- Base of defects is usually located lingually
- Thicker bone
- Slightly wider embrasures
- Natural cleansing action of the tongue

Like the malar process in the maxilla, the external oblique ridge of the mandible usually presents the clinician with a difficult therapeutic challenge. This ridge courses from the anterior border of the ramus toward the tubercle of the mental foramen, forming a thick shelf of bone buccal to the alveolar process. The more closely the height of the external oblique ridge approximates the height of the alveolar process, the flatter will be this shelf of bone and the shallower the vestibular depth. This situation occurs primarily in association with the second and third molars and less often with the first molar. To the clinician, this means that any osseous resection performed on the buccal surface may prove to be ineffective in reducing probing depths postoperatively, if the surgical flap cannot be positioned apically as a result of either a shallow vestibule or an inability to scallop because the band of marginal gingiva is narrow. The bone becomes much thinner over the mesial root of the first molar and both premolars. Additional thinning of this bone could result in significant resorption during the healing phase, creating reversed architecture or exposing furcations.

On the lingual surface, a thick shelf of bone may be encountered because of the location and prominence of the mylohyoid ridge and the axial inclination of the mandibular teeth. Proceeding from the second premolar to the molar teeth, the average axial inclination is 9 to 20 or more degrees[6] to the lingual. Because of this axial inclination, osseous defects, which often develop directly beneath the contacts of the teeth, tend to be located closer to the lingual surface; furcations will be positioned farther apically on the lingual aspect; and an apical ramping of the interproximal bone will be found from the buccal to the lingual as the bone parallels the CEJ. These anatomic relationships can be translated into the following clinically relevant information, which supports the lingual approach to osseous resection: *(1)* thick lingual bone allows greater osseous reduction with less permanent postoperative resorption; *(2)* defects located closer to the lingual surface should logically be treated from the lingual aspect; *(3)* a lingual furcation that is located more apically than the buccal furcation reduces the probability of significant furcation exposure; *(4)* a thicker postresective marginal bone permits a flatter gingival architecture pattern postsurgically than does thinner buccal bone.

The mesiodistal dimensions of the crown and root trunk on the buccal surfaces compared to the lingual surfaces of posterior teeth generally results in a slightly wider lingual embrasure, affording somewhat better access. Whether this greatly improves operator access, patient access for oral hygiene aides, or both could be considered a controversial issue. However, there are various instrument designs that greatly facilitate the performance of lingual osseous resective procedures. The effectiveness of plaque control measures is most dependent on patient compliance with oral hygiene instructions and supportive periodontal care.

The Influence of the Root Trunk and Crater Depth on Resective Techniques

As discussed in the previous sections, nearly all shallow two-wall bony defects (craters) may be completely eliminated or significantly reduced from a palatal or lingual approach. This is made possible by the more apical location of the mesial and distal furcations of maxillary molars and the lingual furcations of mandibular molars as compared to buccal furcations. However, as crater depths increase, anatomic and therapeutic limitations may preclude the total elimination or reduction of the crater walls from only one side of the arch. In these situations it would be advantageous to reduce some of the defect depth by removing buccal bone as well. The extent to which osteoplasty and ostectomy may be performed from the buccal side depends on the location of the furcation entrance relative to the base of the bony crater. This relationship between crater base and furcation is directly influenced by the length of the root trunk.[7]

Table 11-3 summarizes the average root trunk dimensions for the maxillary and mandibular molars measured from the CEJ to the buccal furcation. Table 11-4 demonstrates the relationship between crater depth, root trunk

Table 11-3 Molar root trunk length measured from the CEJ*

Classification	Maxillary	Mandibular
Short	3 mm	2 mm
Medium	4 mm	3 mm
Long	≥ 5 mm	≥ 4 mm

*From Ochsenbein.[7] Reprinted with permission.

Table 11-4 Influence of root trunk length on crater reduction from the palatal, lingual, and buccal approaches*

| Root trunk length | Crater depth | | |
	Shallow (1–2 mm)	Medium (3–4 mm)	Deep (> 5 mm)
Short	Palatal/lingual approach only	Palatal/lingual approach only	Minimal palatal/lingual, no buccal, and/or alternative modality
Medium	Palatal/lingual and minimal buccal	Palatal/lingual and minimal buccal	Minimal palatal/lingual and buccal and/or alternative modality
Long	Palatal/lingual and buccal	Palatal/lingual and buccal	Palatal/lingual and buccal and/or alternative modality

*From Ochsenbein.[7] Reprinted with permission.

length, and crater wall reduction. This information may be interpreted to mean that in the presence of a short root trunk, the base of a shallow crater may typically be level with the entrance of the buccal furcation so that practically all of the osseous reduction would need to be performed on the palatal or lingual crater wall to avoid exposing the furcation. But as the root trunk length increases, reduction of the buccal crater wall could now be done provided that some marginal bone remains coronal to the buccal furcation following the establishment of a positive architecture. What should be remembered is that regardless of root trunk length, if the base of the crater is located at the same level as the furcation entrance or apical to it, then no bone can be removed from the buccal wall without risking a reverse

architecture or exposing the furcation. The clinician must utilize diagnostic radiographs to estimate the length of the root trunk, ie, CEJ to furcation, and surgically determine the depth of the crater relative to the buccal furcation entrance.

Resective Procedures

The surgical steps and instrumentation involved in osseous resective therapy are outlined in Tables 11-5 and 11-6. The rationale for the palatal and lingual approaches and the importance of root trunk length in guiding the extent of resection for the crater (two-wall) defect have been

Table 11-5 Instruments for osseous resective procedures

Instrument	Indications for use
Ochsenbein chisel Nos. 1 and 2	Ostectomy: Radicular bone/widow's peaks
Ochsenbein chisel No. 3	Ostectomy: Interproximal bone
Ochsenbein chisel No. 4	Ostectomy: Radicular bone
Schluger bone file 9/10 (curved)	Osteoplasty: Interproximal bone
Sugarman bone file 3s/4s (straight)	Osteoplasty: Interproximal bone
Wedelstadt chisel	Ostectomy: Radicular/interproximal bone
Tracy scaler by Koblitz	Ostectomy: Interproximal bone at line angles
Rhodes chisel 35/36	Ostectomy: Interproximal bone at line angles
Burs: Surgical-length round Nos. 4, 6, 8	Osteoplasty
Burs: Surgical length end cutting	Ostectomy: Radicular/interproximal bone at line angles
Burs: Surgical-length finishing (round, flame-shaped)	Osteoplasty/odontoplasty
Burs: Diamonds (various shapes)	Osteoplasty/odontoplasty

Table 11-6 Surgical steps for osseous resective procedures

Step	Goal	Instrumentation
1	Bulk reduction of osseous ledges, exostoses, and thick bone: Osteoplasty	Surgical round burs
2	Subtle interdental fluting: Osteoplasty	Surgical round burs and finishing burs
3	Elimination or reduction of crater walls: Osteoplasty	Surgical round burs, Ochsenbein chisel No. 3, Wedelstadt chisel, Schluger bone file 3s/4s, Sugarman bone file 9/10 (straight)
4	Thinning of marginal radicular bone: Osteoplasty	Surgical round burs
5	Removal of widow's peaks: Ostectomy	Ochsenbein chisels Nos. 1 and 2, Tracy scaler, Rhodes chisel 35/36, surgical end cutting burs
6	Removal of radicular bone to achieve physiologic architecture: Ostectomy	Ochsenbein chisels Nos. 1 and 2, Ochsenbein chisel No. 4, Wedelstadt chisel, surgical end cutting burs
7	Final shaping and smoothing of alveolar bone: Osteoplasty	Various chisels and finishing burs

previously discussed. Although it is crucial to remember those points when envisioning the final osseous contours, the basic steps involved in osseous resection usually remain the same: bulk reduction of thick osseous ledges, exostoses, and osseous margins; mild interdental fluting; elimination or reduction of the wall(s) of the osseous defect; resection of marginal bone to achieve the desired physiologic anatomy; and final reshaping to obtain smooth alveolar contours, allowing proper flap adaptation. For instructional purposes, the procedures are presented as distinct steps. In reality, clinical application of these techniques often results in the individual steps being blended together and some even being accomplished simultaneously.

The initial osteoplasty or bulk reduction of alveolar bone is best accomplished with high-speed instrumentation using surgical-length round burs (Fig 11-8). Copious irrigation is essential to prevent overheating of bone and to allow the bur to cut more efficiently. The extent of osteoplasty is determined by the thickness of the periodontium. Thin radicular bone and/or prominent roots usually reduce or totally eliminate the need for initial osteoplasty. Excessive thinning of the alveolar bone should definitely be avoided. If indicated, interdental vertical grooving or fluting should be kept subtle (Figs 11-9 and 11-10). The goal is to create contours that allow the appropriate adaptation of the flap to the marginal bone and root surface. Extensive grooving is unnecessary and should be avoided.

Elimination of the wall(s) of the osseous defect is also completed through osteoplasty (Figs 11-10 and 11-11). Again, the ability to completely eliminate a defect is determined primarily by the relationship between the base of the defect and the furcation entrance. In a shallow-to-moderate crater defect at a tooth with a medium or long root trunk, the bony walls can usually be reduced to the defect base.

Fig 11-8 Bulk reduction of mandibular lingual tori with a surgical-length round bur. Depth grooves have been placed to guide the extent of the initial osteoplasty.

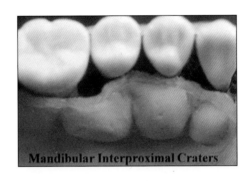
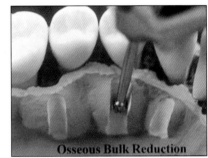

Fig 11-9 Interdental fluting or grooving with a surgical-length round bur in facial and lingual interproximal areas.

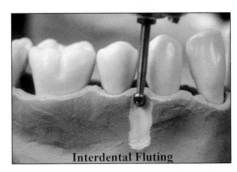
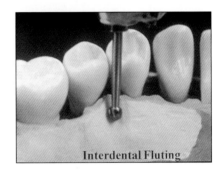

Fig 11-10 *(left)* Completed interdental fluting. *(right)* Remaining osseous defect. The premolar has been removed to enhance the view of the base (in red) of the interdental craters. The marginal aspect of the crater walls is highlighted in yellow.

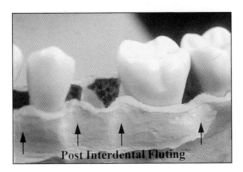
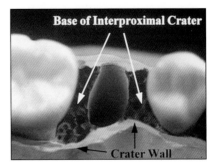

183

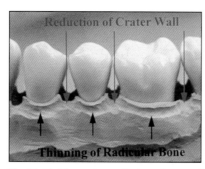
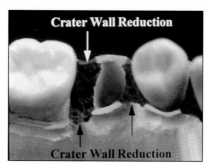

Fig 11-11 The crater walls have been reduced to a level approximating the base of the interdental crater. Marginal radicular bone has also been thinned. Care must be taken not to lower the base of the defect.

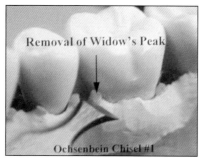
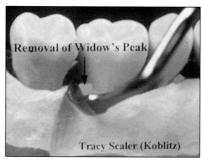

Fig 11-12 Thinned radicular bone and widow's peaks are removed with hand instruments. *(left)* Use of the Ochsenbein chisel to remove a buccal widow's peak. *(right)* Application of a Tracy scaler.

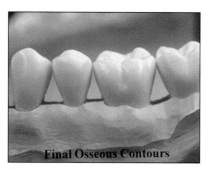
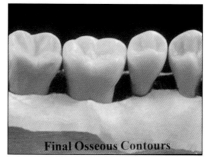

Fig 11-13 Final osseous contours have been achieved. Positive bony architecture is shown; interdental bone is at a more coronal level than is radicular bone. Radicular bone has been scalloped to parallel the cementoenamel junction.

Care must be taken not to lower the base of the defect itself. Generally, the interdental septum is sloped lingually or palatally no more than 10 degrees to avoid the need for accentuated scalloping of the marginal bone.[7]

Following the removal of the lateral or crater walls of the defect, a reverse architecture is often created in the marginal bone. To surgically establish a more physiologic form, marginal radicular bone, as well as spikes of bone left at the proximal line angles (ie, "widow's peaks"), must be removed (Fig 11-12). Use of a round bur to thin the radicular bone prior to ostectomy procedures will facilitate the use of hand instruments in obtaining the final osseous contour. Table 11-6 outlines some common hand instruments utilized to perform resective techniques. Care must be

taken not to create gouges in the root with inappropriate use of chisels. If the working edge of the chisel is used perpendicular to the root surface, a gentle back-and-forth twisting motion will aid in the atraumatic removal of supporting bone. If the chisel is used parallel to the tooth surface, the working edge is placed between the bone and root so that the beveled edge is facing out. A similar twisting motion is applied to outfracture the thin radicular supporting bone.

The last step involves minor osteoplasty to smooth the bone and achieve the final contours before the mucoperiosteal flaps are placed at a level approximating the new position of the alveolar crest (Fig 11-13). As in any flap surgery, copious amounts of sterile saline are used to irrigate under the flap prior to closure. Suturing can be accomplished with a variety of different techniques, as long as they allow the apical positioning of the tissues.

With experience and a clear vision of the desired outcome, the surgeon can perform resective therapy quickly. Each movement should be purposeful and definitive. Adequate access, obtained through proper flap management, is of paramount importance. Visibility of the surgical field can be enhanced with the use of fiberoptic headlamps and surgical optics. In addition, sharp instruments, appropriate irrigation with sterile saline, and evacuation of irrigants, saliva, and blood are extremely important to the final surgical outcome.

Conclusion

Osseous resection is but one of many modalities of therapy available to the clinician in the treatment of the various types of periodontal disease. Its success is directly related to the appropriate application of the normal anatomic relationships that exist among the teeth, bone, and gingiva to re-create an architectural pattern harmonious with all of these structures. The result will be significantly reduced probing depths, which are usually more easily maintained by both the patient and therapist. If the techniques are properly performed, it becomes a very predictable therapy.

Note: The views expressed in this chapter are those of the authors and do not reflect the official policy or position of the United States Air Force or the Department of Defense.

References

1. Kronfeld R. The condition of the alveolar bone underlying periodontal pockets. J Periodontol 1935;6:22–29.

2. Schluger S. Osseous resection—A basic principle in periodontal surgery. Oral Surg 1949;2:316–325.

3. Friedman N. Periodontal osseous surgery: Osteoplasty and ostectomy. J Periodontol 1955;26:257–269.

4. Ochsenbein C, Bohannan HM. Palatal approach to osseous surgery. I. Rationale. J Periodontol 1963;34:60–68.

5. Ochsenbein C, Bohannan HM. Palatal approach to osseous surgery. II. Clinical application. J Periodontol 1964;35:54–68.

6. Tibbetts L, Ochsenbein C, Loughlin D. Rationale for the lingual approach to mandibular osseous surgery. Dent Clin North Am 1976;20:61–78.

7. Ochsenbein C. A primer for osseous surgery. Int J Periodont Rest Dent 1986;6(1):8–47.

8. Rosling B, Nyman S, Lindhe J, Jern B. The healing potential of the periodontal tissues following different techniques of periodontal surgery in plaque-free dentitions. J Clin Periodontol 1976;3:233–250.

9. Knowles JW, Burgett FG, Nissle FR, Schick RA, Morrison EC, Ramfjord SP. Results of periodontal treatment related to pocket depth and attachment level. Eight years. J Periodontol 1979;50:225–233.

10. Hill RW, Ramfjord SP, Morrison EC, Appleberry EA, Caffesse RG, Kerry GJ, Nissle RR. Four types of periodontal treatment compared over two years. J Periodontol 1981;52:655–662.

11. Lindhe J, Nyman S. Long-term maintenance of patients treated for advanced periodontal disease. J Clin Periodontol 1984;11:504–514.

12. Olsen C, Ammons W, van Belle G. A longitudinal study comparing apically repositioned flaps with and without osseous surgery. Int J Periodont Rest Dent 1985;5(4):11–33.

13. Wilderman MN, Pennel BM, King K, Barron JM. Histogenesis of repair following osseous surgery. J Periodontol 1967;41:551–565.

14. Pfeifer J. The growth of tissue over denuded bone. J Periodontol 1963;34:10–16.

15. Wilderman MN. Exposure of bone in periodontal surgery. Dent Clin North Am 1964;8:23–35.

16. Waerhaug J. The angular bone defect and its relationship to trauma from occlusion and downgrowth of subgingival plaque. J Clin Periodontol 1979;6:61–82.

17. Waerhaug J. The infrabony pocket and its relationship to trauma from occlusion and subgingival plaque. J Periodontol 1979;50:355–365.

18. Tal H. Relationship between the interproximal distance of roots and the prevalence of intrabony pockets. J Periodontol 1984;55:604–607.

19. Goldman HM, Cohen DW. The infrabony pocket: Classification and treatment. J Periodontol 1958;29:272–291.

20. Manson JD, Nickolson K. The distribution of bone defects in chronic periodontitis. J Periodontol 1974;45:88–92.

21. Selipsky H. Osseous surgery—How much need we compromise. Dent Clin North Am 1976;20:79–106.

22. Heins PJ, Wieder SM. A histologic study of the width and nature of interradicular spaces in human adult premolars and molars. J Dent Res 1986;65:948–951.

CHAPTER 12

Flap Design and Suturing in Periodontal Surgery

Nicholas M. Dello Russo, DMD, MScD

Every periodontal surgical procedure begins with an incision, and the manner in which that incision is designed, executed, and sutured will have an enormous impact on its success. Periodontists have at their disposal a wide variety of surgical procedures to augment, regenerate, and reconstruct the soft and hard tissues of the human periodontium. Each of these surgical procedures has specific requirements regarding the type of flap access that is indicated and the manner in which it must be sutured. This chapter will discuss the various types of periodontal flaps, their indications and contraindications, and the ways these flaps may be sutured to achieve the desired therapeutic result.

Periodontal Flaps

Definitions

A *periodontal flap*[1] may be defined as that part of the gingiva and oral mucosa that is separated from the teeth and alveolar bone by horizontal and/or vertical incisions, yet remains attached to the rest of the alveolar mucosa in at least one area. This means that a free gingival graft[2,3] would not be considered a flap because it is completely separated from its surrounding mucosa, but that a pedicle graft is a type of flap because it remains attached to the rest of the oral mucosa at its base. Flaps may be either full thickness or partial (split) thickness, depending on whether the periosteum is incorporated into the flap or left on the bone.[4] If vertical incisions are used, the flap is termed *relaxed*; if no vertical incisions are used, it is termed an *envelope flap*. Each of these flaps, and their modifications, will be discussed in the following sections.

Envelope Flaps

Envelope flaps have no vertical incisions and begin and end within the gingival sulcus of contiguous teeth (Fig 12-1). Vertical incisions may interfere with the lateral blood supply to a flap. Because envelope flaps have no vertical incisions, they are quicker to heal and are associated with less postoperative pain and bleeding. Envelope flaps are used primarily in situations where esthetics is a major consideration or where the buccal and lingual flaps are meant to be sutured tightly to each other to achieve primary closure or healing. The maxillary anterior region is one of the most challenging areas of the mouth on which to operate because of the esthetic demands of the area. Envelope flaps are often used here to achieve a pleasing gingival architecture and to preserve the interdental papillae.

Two disadvantages of envelope flaps are that they limit access to the bony tissues and they cannot be easily moved or repositioned to other locations.

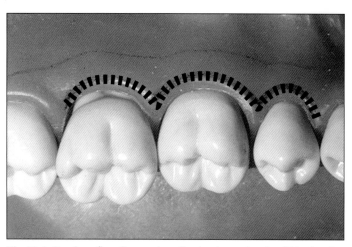

Fig 12-1 Envelope flap. An envelope flap begins and ends within the gingival sulci of contiguous teeth. Because it has no vertical incisions, it cannot be moved to a different position. It is used when the flap will be replaced in its starting position.

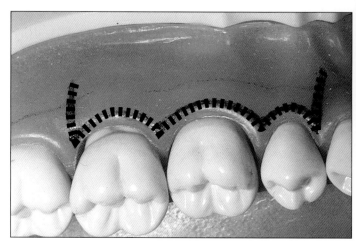

Fig 12-2 Relaxed flap. A relaxed flap has one or more vertical incisions, which allow easier access to the underlying periodontal tissues and make it possible to move or position the flap to a different location. Note, in this illustration, that the vertical incisions are placed at the line angles of the teeth. Vertical incisions usually extend beyond the mucogingival junction to offer not only the best access but also flap mobility. If the flap is to be moved laterally, the vertical incisions are angled in the direction toward which the flap will be positioned.

Relaxed Flaps

Relaxed flaps have vertical incisions and offer the periodontist tremendous flexibility in terms of access and tissue control (Fig 12-2). Vertical incisions have potential disadvantages including delayed healing and the potential for greater postoperative pain and bleeding. Nevertheless, vertical incisions are often essential and the skilled periodontist should not be shy about using them.

The two great advantages offered by vertical incisions are greatly improved access to the osseous tissues and the ability to move or position the flap to a new location. Vertical incisions must be used if the osseous defect is very deep or if it is isolated to one or two teeth. To gain an equal degree of access with an envelope flap, the incision would have to be extended to include several additional teeth on either side of the osseous defect. This would mean that perfectly healthy teeth would have to be included in the surgical field. Vertical incisions help the periodontist limit the surgical field to only those teeth that are pathologically involved.

Vertical incisions also allow the periodontist to move the flap to another position without causing excessive tension. A flap may be positioned coronally to achieve primary coverage over a surgical site, it may be positioned apically to eliminate a pocket, or it may be moved laterally to cover an exposed root or increase the zone of attached gingiva. Vertical incisions allow each of these maneuvers to be made in a neat, elegant manner.

Incision Design

The two basic types of periodontal incisions are horizontal incisions, which generally follow the occlusal plane of the teeth, and vertical incisions, which are perpendicular to the long axis of the tooth. All other incisions are modifications of these.

Horizontal Incisions

Horizontal incisions are made parallel to the occlusal plane of the teeth, somewhere between the free margin of the gingiva and the mucogingival junction. Using the gingival margin and the mucogingival junction as landmarks, the surgeon can make the incision in the gingival sulculus (sulcular incision) or at some point between the gingival margin and the mucogingival junction (subsulcular incision). The determining factor is the width of the attached gingiva relative to the pocket depth. In areas with shallow-to-moderate pockets and wide bands of attached gingiva, the incision may be made several millimeters apical to the gingival margin, sacrificing a small amount of attached gingiva to eliminate the pockets. Areas with moderate-to-deep pockets and narrow bands of attached gingiva require incisions closer to the gingival margin to preserve the zone of attached gingiva. In these situations, the flap must be sutured apically to eliminate the pocket.

An incision that aims for and touches the highest point of the alveolar bone is termed a *crestal incision*, and these are

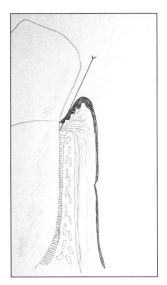

Fig 12-3 Sulcular incision. When a sulcular incision is made, the scalpel is placed within the sulcus surrounding the teeth and extends down to the periodontal ligament. The incision is carried interproximally as far as possible, severing the circular and transseptal fibers. The epithelium lining the sulcus remains on the inside of the flap and will be replaced against the tooth when the flap is sutured. Therefore, this type of incision is made only when the sulcular epithelium is healthy, such as when a pedicle graft is performed or an implant is placed. This incision is usually followed by a full-thickness flap.

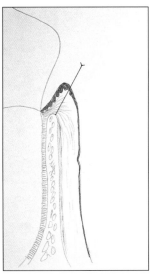

Fig 12-4 Extrasulcular incision. This incision is made at some point between the gingival crevice and mucogingival junction, the determining factors being the probing depth and the amount of attached gingiva. If, for example, the pockets are deep and there is a large dimension of attached gingiva, the incision may be made or scalloped several millimeters apical to the free gingival margin. If the pockets are shallow or the amount of attached gingiva is minimal, the incision is made as illustrated, just lateral to the gingival sulcus. This preserves as much of the attached gingiva as possible.

usually made when a full-thickness flap is being performed. In full-thickness flaps, the periosteum is reflected away from the alveolar bone and becomes part of the flap. This is accomplished by blunt dissection with a periosteal elevator. In partial-thickness flaps, the periosteum is left on the bone; this is achieved by using a scalpel blade to sharply dissect through the attached gingiva and alveolar mucosa. The lamina propria of the gingiva and alveolar mucosa is thereby split; some connective tissue remains with the flap and the rest is left on the bone to serve as periosteum.

Sulcular incision. The sulcular incision is the easiest to perform and is accomplished by placing the scalpel blade into the gingival sulcus and severing both the epithelial and connective tissue attachments from the tooth (Fig 12-3). It is usually followed by a full-thickness flap, which is relatively easy to reflect and suture. The sulcular incision might be used when the surgeon is extracting a tooth or a root fragment, placing a dental implant, or performing an apicoectomy.

The major disadvantage is that the epithelial lining of the gingival sulcus is incorporated into the flap and is then sutured back onto the root when the flap is closed. This might be acceptable as long as the gingival attachment is healthy, but if a periodontal pocket is present and the sulcular epithelium is diseased, a sulcular incision is contraindicated.

Extrasulcular incision. The extrasulcular, or subsulcular, incision is made at some point between the gingival margin and the mucogingival junction (Fig 12-4). The factor that determines where the incision is made is the depth of the pocket relative to the amount of attached gingiva. For example, if pocket elimination is the surgical objective, and a large dimension of attached gingiva is present, the initial incision can be made just apical to the base of the pocket without compromising the zone of attached gingiva. This situation is common on the lingual or palatal surfaces of teeth.

The subsulcular incision is also called the *crestal-anticipation incision* because it aims for, or anticipates, the crest of the alveolar bone. The amount of attached gingiva is often quite narrow on the labial and facial aspects of teeth, and the subsulcular incision must be made just lateral to the periodontal pocket to preserve as much of the keratinized mucosa as possible.

Vertical Incisions

Vertical incisions are made perpendicular to the occlusal plane and parallel to the long axis of the tooth. They extend from the horizontal incision to a point beyond the mucogingival junction and are used to allow greater access and mobility of the flap. They should always be placed at the line angles of teeth and never (except in rare instances, such as a double papilla flap) over the height of contour of

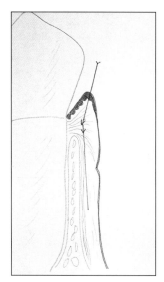

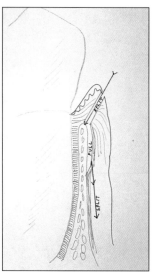

Fig 12-5 Partial-thickness flap. This is also called a *split-thickness flap* and begins with an extrasulcular incision. Once the initial incision is made, the flap reflection is accomplished by a sharp dissection with a scalpel blade. In this way, the connective tissue's lamina propria is split: Part of the tissue remains on the bone, to serve as periosteum, and the rest becomes the wall of the flap. This differs from a full-thickness flap, which is performed by blunt dissection with a periosteal elevator, which is used to separate all the connective tissue from the bone.

Fig 12-6 Combination flap. This is also termed a *split-full-split flap*. The first incision is of the subsulcular type, splitting (bisecting) the connective tissue lateral to the periodontal pocket. This is followed by a blunt dissection for several millimeters, which is the full-thickness portion of the flap. Apical to this, the remainder of the flap is again split with a sharp dissection. This type of flap offers the periodontist the ease of a full-thickness flap to treat the bone and the flexibility of a split-thickness flap for periosteal suturing and tissue positioning.

the root. Placing vertical incisions at the proximal line angles accomplishes two things: It protects the interdental papilla adjacent to the surgical site, and it allows the vertical incision to be sutured without having to stretch the flap over the cervical convexity of the tooth.

Vertical incisions may also be used to move a flap laterally, such as when a pedicle flap is used to cover the surface of an adjacent root. In this situation, the vertical incision is made at an acute angle to the horizontal incision, in the direction toward which the flap will move, placing the base of the pedicle at the recipient site. This is termed a *cutback incision.*

Vertical incisions are always sutured to prevent postoperative bleeding and to align the flap in a proper mesiodistal direction. It is a good idea to suture the vertical incisions before the horizontal portion of the flap, to align the interdental papillae with the interproximal spaces.

Flap Reflection

Once the initial incisions have been made, the body of the flap is reflected in one of three ways: a full-thickness flap, a partial-thickness flap, or a combination flap.

Full-Thickness Flap

A full-thickness flap is performed by a blunt dissection of the oral mucosa away from the teeth and alveolar bone. This is done with a periosteal elevator, or another blunt

instrument, and is termed *full thickness* because the connective tissue covering the bone (periosteum) is stripped away from the bone to become the base of the flap.

Full-thickness flaps have several advantages:

1. They are easier to perform than split-thickness flaps.
2. They offer improved visibility of the alveolar bone.
3. They are generally associated with less bleeding and postoperative pain.

Full-thickness flaps are used in procedures that require access to and visibility of the alveolar bone and when primary wound closure is essential, for example, implant surgery and guided tissue regeneration procedures. Other procedures that are usually performed with full-thickness flaps are distal wedges, open flap curettage (Widman flaps), and the so-called excisional new attachment procedure, which is a curettage done with a scalpel blade. Full-thickness flaps may be performed on either the buccal or lingual aspect of the teeth.

Partial- (Split-) Thickness Flap

Partial- or split-thickness flaps are accomplished by using a scalpel to sharply dissect through the lamina propria of the gingiva and alveolar mucosa (Fig 12-5). In this way, part of the mucosal lamina propria remains with the flap and the rest remains on the alveolar bone. Partial-thickness flaps are technically demanding but offer an unparalleled degree of surgical flexibility. Several periodontal surgical procedures require that periosteum remain on the bone, either to serve as a blood supply for a graft, as with free gingival grafts or pedicle grafts, or to aid in suturing with periosteal sutures. In areas of prominent roots where dehiscences or fenestrations are anticipated, partial-thickness flaps should be used to prevent permanent root exposure.

Split-thickness flaps are generally limited to the buccal surfaces. Palatal and lingual surfaces, with their wide zones of attached gingiva and thick alveolar bone, do not require split-thickness flaps. Instead, a scalloped, subsulcular incision is made to the crest of the alveolar bone.

Combination Flap

A useful variation of these two flaps is the combination, or "split-full-split," flap (Fig 12-6). This is done when the periodontist wants the surgical access of a full-thickness flap, to perform osseous surgery, but would like to use periosteal sutures to close the wound. First, a subsulcular incision is made lateral to the periodontal pocket and down to the crest of alveolar bone (split). Next, a periosteal elevator is used to bluntly dissect the flap down to the approximate level of the mucogingival junction (full). Last, the scalpel is again used to split the alveolar mucosa apically beyond the mucogingival junction (split). This type of flap design exposes several millimeters of alveolar bone, which can then be recontoured or augmented, while it maintains periosteum in the apical part of the surgical site to aid in suturing and flap reattachment.

All of the types of flaps discussed may and should be modified, depending on the specific surgical situation. For example, a surgical procedure may require a single horizontal incision and anywhere from no to several vertical incisions. The key points to remember are that no single technique is suited to every surgical situation and that the skilled periodontist must be thoughtful and creative in designing every incision.

Suturing Periodontal Flaps

Almost all periodontal surgical wounds are closed with sutures, and a wide variety of suturing techniques have been developed to aid the surgeon in achieving the surgical objectives.[5] Successful suturing is an exercise in tissue control, and different surgical procedures will require different types of suture materials and suturing methods.[6]

Many periodontal surgical procedures, such as bone grafting, placement of dental implants, and guided tissue regeneration, require primary closure over the surgical site, which means that the flaps must be drawn up tightly so that the wound edges approximate each other. Primary wound closure allows the flap edges to knit quickly to each other, sealing the wound and reducing the likelihood of bacterial contamination of the wound site. Other types of surgical procedures, such as pedicle grafts or apically positioned flaps, require that the flaps be positioned at a site distant from which they originated, and specific suturing procedures are required to position these flaps in a precise manner.

Sutures

There are two general methods of suturing periodontal flaps: interrupted suturing and continuous suturing.[7] With interrupted sutures, each interdental papilla is sutured separately from the others; with continuous sutures, several papillae are sutured together with one knot. There are several variations within these two categories.

Simple Interrupted Suture

The simple interrupted suture is the easiest suture to perform. It is used to rejoin a buccal interdental papilla and a lingual interdental papilla that have been separated by a flap (Fig 12-7a). Beginning on the buccal aspect, the suture needle is passed through the interdental papilla, leaving approximately 2 cm of free suture material on the buccal aspect. This is called the *tag* end of the suture. The needle is then passed, back end first so as not to dull the point, through the same interdental space to the lingual aspect, where the lingual flap is engaged in a similar manner (Fig 12-7b). Finally, the needle is once again passed through that interdental space, and a knot is tied on the buccal aspect. As a general rule, sutures are always tied with the knot on the facial or buccal surfaces of the teeth. This makes them easier to remove and protects the tongue from soreness or ulceration (Fig 12-7c).

Simple interrupted sutures are used to reposition the flap to its initial starting position or to position flaps coronally, the difference depending on the extent of the flap dissection. If the flap reflection is limited to the area coronal to the mucogingival junction, the flap cannot be positioned coronally (or apically) and may only be returned to its original position. A flap that is dissected beyond the mucogingival junction and into the much more malleable and elastic alveolar mucosa may be repositioned to a new site. This is true with either full- or partial-thickness flaps.

Continuous Suture

As the name implies, continuous sutures are used to join two or more interdental papillae of the same flap. They are usually used when the buccal flap is sutured separately from the lingual flap or when no lingual flap is performed. In a continuous suture, the suture needle is first passed through an interdental papilla on the buccal aspect of a flap (Fig 12-8a). The needle is then passed through the interdental space to the lingual aspect, where it does not engage the lingual tissue. Instead, the needle is passed around the tooth, either mesially or distally, and through the adjacent interdental space back to the buccal aspect. Here the buccal flap is

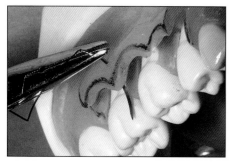

Fig 12-7a Simple interrupted suture, buccal view. The needle enters the buccal flap through the interdental papilla and exits under the flap. The needle is then passed through the interdental space to engage the lingual flap.

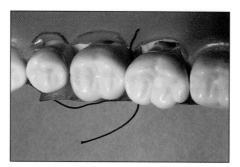

Fig 12-7b Simple interrupted suture, lingual view. The suture needle enters and exits the lingual flap in the same manner as on the facial surface. The needle enters the flap at the midpoint between the adjacent teeth. This ensures that the flap will be centered perfectly in a mesiodistal dimension once it is tied.

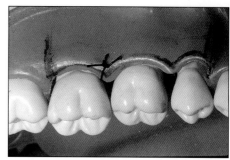

Fig 12-7c Simple interrupted suture, tied. After the lingual flap is engaged, the needle is passed back through to the buccal aspect and tied. Sutures are almost always tied on the buccal aspect, which makes them easier to remove and prevents the knots from irritating the patient's tongue. The simple interrupted suture is used when the flap is repositioned coronally to achieve primary wound closure. It is not indicated to position a flap apically or laterally.

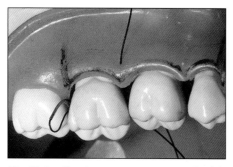

Fig 12-8a Continuous suture, step 1. In this illustration, the suture is started at the mesial aspect of the second molar. The buccal flap is engaged, and the needle is passed through the interdental space between the first and second molars. The needle is then passed around the lingual aspect of the tooth to the distal aspect and passed through the interdental space between the second and third molars back to the buccal aspect, where the buccal flap is again engaged.

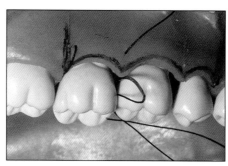

Fig 12-8b Continuous suture, step 2. The needle is passed back around the lingual aspect of the tooth, where it emerges in the interdental space between the first and second molars. At this point, the buccal flap has been engaged twice, but the needle has not penetrated the lingual tissues.

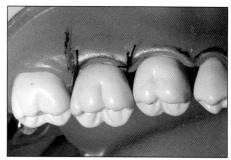

Fig 12-8c Continuous suture, tied. The suture is tied on the buccal aspect. The tightness of the knot will determine the position of the flap in an apico-occlusal dimension. If the knot is tied tightly, the flap will be pulled coronally; if the knot is tied loosely, the flap will be draped apically.

again engaged (Fig 12-8b). The needle is once again passed through the interdental space and back around the tooth, to emerge at the position from which the suture began. The suture is tied at this point (Fig 12-8c).

Continuous sutures are very useful in a variety of different clinical situations. For example, they may be used to suture a barrier membrane over the buccal surface of a tooth. The overlying flap may then be sutured coronally with a separate continuous (or interrupted) suture.

In addition, continuous sutures may be used to position flaps either coronally or apically, depending on the tightness of the knot.[8] Assuming the flap extends beyond the mucogingival junction, a tight knot will pull the flap coronally, while a loose knot will allow the flap to be draped apically.

Continuous sutures may be used to suture flaps that extend from two to several interdental spaces. If the flap encompasses many teeth, it is tied in a different way. First,

a knot is tied at the most distal extent of the flap. Then, instead of threading the suture needle back through all the interdental spaces to tie it to the tag end from which it started, the surgeon may tie the suture at the mesial end by leaving some slack in the last loop and using this loop of suture material as the tag end with which to tie a knot.

Mattress Suture

Periodontal flaps that are contained within the zone of attached gingiva, and do not extend beyond the mucogingival junction, are sutured through the interdental papillae with papillary sutures. In this type of suture, the needle enters the flap through the papilla and exits under the free margin of the flap. These flaps cannot be sutured coronally, apically, or laterally because they are bound down at the mucogingival junction, limiting their movement.

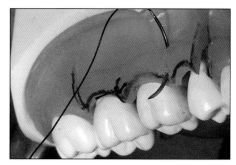

Fig 12-9a Mattress suture, buccal view. The mattress suture enters the buccal flap at or near the mucogingival junction and exits the flap through the interdental papilla. The needle is then passed through to the lingual aspect, where it engages the lingual flap in a similar manner.

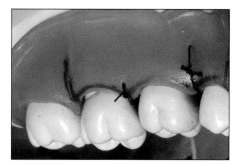

Fig 12-9b Mattress suture, tied. The mattress suture is so named because much of the suture material lies on top of rather than under the flap. This presses the flap onto the underlying bone or periosteum, facilitating flap reattachment. Mattress sutures are also used with periosteal sutures. Compare the two sutures in the illustration, the one on the right is a simple papillary suture, while the one on the left is a mattress suture.

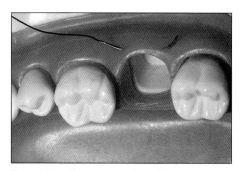

Fig 12-10a Criss-cross suture. The suture needle enters the buccal flap at the mesiobuccal line angle and travels horizontally under the flap to exit at the distobuccal line angle. The same maneuver is done on the lingual; the needle enters the flap at the mesiolingual line angle and exits at the distolingual line angle.

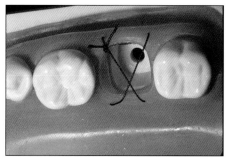

Fig 12-10b Criss-cross suture, tied. When this suture is tied, it crosses over the surgical field. This suture may be used over edentulous spaces or at the buccal or lingual surfaces of teeth.

Flaps that involve dissection beyond the mucogingival junction (either split- or full-thickness flaps) require the use of a mattress suture (Fig 12-9a). This suture enters the flap at or near the mucogingival junction and exits the flap through the interdental papilla. In this way, much more of the suture lies on top of the flap, and it is able to hold the full extent of the flap in close contact with the underlying bone or periosteum (Fig 12-9b). This aids in healing and flap reattachment and reduces the chance of postoperative bleeding. If the surgeon merely relies on the periodontal dressing or a primary blood clot to hold the flap in contact with the bone or periosteum, postoperative complications, such as bleeding under the flap, flap detachment, or flap necrosis, may occur.

Mattress sutures are also used in periosteal suturing[9] when a split-thickness flap is extended beyond the mucogingival junction. In this situation, the needle enters the flap at or near the mucogingival junction, passes through the underlying periosteum, and exits the flap through the interdental papilla. In this way the flap is bound down to the periosteum, resulting in precise positioning and an abundant blood supply. In areas of prominent roots where dehiscences or fenestrations are anticipated, split-thickness flaps and periosteal sutures are almost mandatory to protect the connective tissue attachment.

Mattress sutures may be either interrupted or continuous.[10,11]

Cross (Criss-Cross) Suture

This is a useful variation of a continuous mattress suture. Here, the mattress sutures are placed horizontally, not vertically. For example, at an edentulous space with buccal and lingual flaps, the suture needle enters the buccal flap at the distobuccal line angle and exits the buccal flap at the mesiobuccal line angle (Fig 12-10a). The same maneuver is duplicated on the lingual or palatal aspect; the needle enters the flap at the distobuccal line angle and exits through the mesiobuccal line angle. The knot is then tied and will form a cross on top of the flap (Fig 12-10b).

This type of suture is an elegant way to close a wound over an edentulous saddle area and is particularly helpful in mucogingival surgery, where root coverage is desired.

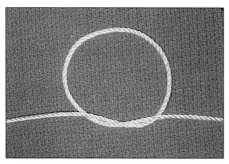

Fig 12-11 Overhand knot. This knot is a simple loop made by crossing the free end of the suture over the standing part one time. It is the basis for all other surgical knots.

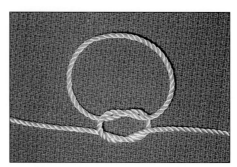

Fig 12-12 Square knot. This suture knot is made by tying two overhand knots, each done in opposite directions. For example, the first knot could be made by making a loop over the jaws of the needle holder and the second knot by making a loop under the jaws of the holder. This knot is easy to tie, but may tend to loosen when synthetic or monofilament sutures are used.

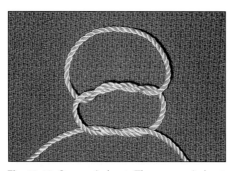

Fig 12-13 Surgeon's knot. The surgeon's knot is a modified square knot in which the first overhand knot is doubled. Two loops are made over the jaws of the needle holder and tightened, and then one loop is made under the jaws of the needle holder in a direction opposite from the first loops. This is the standard knot for suturing of periodontal flaps. When synthetic or resorbable sutures are used, one or more additional overhand knots can be added to the surgeon's knot to keep it from unraveling.

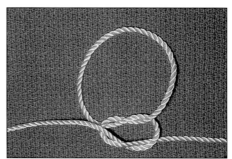

Fig 12-14 Granny or slip knot. The granny knot is similar to a square knot, in that it is made with two overhand knots, but both knots are made in the same direction. With a needle holder, one overhand knot is made so that the loop goes over the jaws of the needle holder and then tightened; a second overhand knot is then made so that the loop goes in the same direction over the needle holder and tightened. The great advantage of this knot is that, once the second overhand knot is tied, the knot can be tightened even further. The knot can then be locked into place with one or two additional overhand knots going in opposite directions.

Knots

The purpose of knots is to join the two ends of the suture in a secure but gentle way. Knots are held by the friction of the suture material, and different types of suture material will require different types of knots. Knots must be placed tightly enough to prevent slippage and loosening of the flap but not so tightly as to blanch the tissues, which may compromise the blood supply and cause flap necrosis. Knots are generally placed on the buccal aspects of flaps, where they are less apt to irritate the patient's tongue.[12]

There are three types of knots that are useful to the periodontal surgeon: the square knot, the surgeon's knot, and the slip or "granny" knot.

Square Knot

This is a simple knot to tie and consists of two overhand knots,[13] each done in opposite directions (Fig 12-11). The first overhand knot is made by making a loop over the jaws of the needle holder, grabbing the tag end of the suture material, and pulling the knot snugly to the flap. A second overhand knot is then made by making a loop under the jaws of the needle holder again, grabbing the tag end of the suture, and pulling the two ends of the suture (the one held by the needle holder and the one held in the surgeon's hand) tight (Fig 12-12).

The advantages of the square knot are that it is quick and simple. It is useful when the surgeon is using silk suture, which has good frictional resistance to loosening, and in situations when there is no tension on the flaps. If the flaps are not lying passively against the bone, but are pulling away from each other, the square knot cannot be used because the tension on the flaps will pull them apart between the time the first and second overhand knots are made.

Surgeon's Knot

The surgeon's knot is a modified square knot with two overhand knots, each done in opposite directions (Fig 12-13). The first knot, however, is a double overhand knot, and the second one is a single. This doubling of the first overhand knot prevents slippage and loosening, especially if the flaps are under tension. This is probably the most commonly used knot in periodontal surgery. It is quick and simple to tie and can hold flaps securely, even if they are under slight or moderate tension.

When silk suture material is used, only two overhand knots are needed, because of the superior frictional resistance of silk. However, some of the newer, synthetic suture materials are very slippery and have poor frictional resistance to loosening. These will require several additional overhand knots to be added to the basic surgeon's knot to prevent loosening.

Slip Knot

This extremely useful knot is sometimes called the *granny knot* (Fig 12-14). It too is a variation of the square knot made with two single overhand knots; with the slip knot, however, both overhand knots are made in the same direction. The first overhand knot is made by making a loop over the needle holder, grabbing the free end of the suture, and pulling the ends tight. The second overhand knot is made the same way, so that the loop again goes over the needle holder.

The great advantage of the slip knot is that, once it is tied, it can be tightened further. Once it is tightened to the desired extent, it can be locked into place by another overhand knot, made in the opposite direction of the first two. This ability to be tightened makes the slip knot enormously useful in many surgical situations. For example, it can be used to stretch flaps to achieve primary healing over a surgical site. It is also very helpful to control bleeding where hemostasis is a problem. The slip knot should be part of the repertoire of every periodontal surgeon.

Suture Materials

Suture materials are generally divided into two types, resorbable and nonresorbable.[14,15] Each type has a place in periodontal surgery, and most offices have an assortment of sutures to be used in different surgical situations.

Resorbable Sutures

Catgut sutures. Catgut, or surgical gut, is the classic resorbable suture[16] and has been used as a suture material for more than 100 years. It is still useful for periodontal surgery today, as long as its limitations are recognized and it is used in appropriate situations. Despite its name, catgut sutures are not made from cats, but from the purified connective tissue collagen found in the intestinal mucosa of large animals, such as sheep or cattle. In the mouth, plain gut sutures will remain in place for 7 to 10 days, and gut that has been treated with chromic salts (chromic gut) will last for up to 14 days.

Gut sutures are moderately difficult to handle; they hold a knot poorly and require a surgeon's knot with several additional overhand knots to prevent loosening. Gut sutures are resorbed by enzymatic breakdown and phagocytosis, and because they are composed of foreign proteins, they may induce a robust inflammatory response. Despite these limitations, gut sutures are useful in situations when suture removal would be difficult or impossible. These would include frenectomies, some free gingival or connective tissue grafts, and areas of soft tissue biopsies. Gut sutures should not be used when an excessive degree of inflammation would compromise the surgical result, such as with bone grafts, guided tissue regeneration, implants, or where esthetics is a major consideration.

Synthetic resorbable sutures. To overcome the deficiencies of surgical gut, synthetic resorbable sutures have been developed. Two that are useful in periodontal surgery are Dexon (Ethicon, Johnson & Johnson) and Vicryl (Davis & Geck). Dexon is made of polyglycolic acid and Vicryl of polyglactin. Both are easier to handle and hold a knot better than surgical gut, although they also require additional overhand knots to be added to the surgeon's knot. Both are resorbed by hydrolysis, which is generally complete in 14 to 30 days; Vicryl is resorbed more quickly than Dexon.

Because these synthetic resorbable sutures cause much less tissue inflammation than surgical gut, they can be used in a wider variety of surgical situations. However, they should be removed if they do not resorb with 10 days because plaque will build up on the suture material itself, which is braided, and on the knot. This buildup of plaque could delay the healing of the surgical wound.

Nonresorbable Sutures

Silk sutures. The classic nonresorbable suture material, and the one to which all other sutures are compared, is surgical silk. Silk sutures are made from the silk protein secreted by silkworms in making their cocoons. The individual threads of silk are braided to make a suture. Silk has been used as a suture material since ancient times and offers the surgeon a material with superb handling properties. Silk sutures are easy to tie and, because they are soft and pliable, are very comfortable for the patient. Knots tied with silk sutures are exceptionally strong,[17] and silk is particularly well suited to tying slip knots.

In spite of its excellent handling properties, silk sutures cause a great deal of inflammation in the mucosal tissues, which may compromise the surgical result. Being a foreign protein, silk elicits a local inflammatory response that is directly related to the amount of suture material under the flap in direct contact with the submucosal tissues. The periodontal surgeon should use the fewest number of sutures possible consistent with proper wound closure, hemostasis, and flap stability. Mattress sutures are useful when silk is used because more of the suture material lies on top of the flap rather than under it. Because silk suture is made up of several individual strands that are braided, it acts as a wick, drawing oral fluids and plaque down under the flap, causing further inflammation.

Because of the amount of inflammation silk sutures induce in the surrounding mucosal tissues, the following guidelines should be followed:

1. Silk sutures should be removed as soon as healing allows, generally within 5 to 7 days and never later than 10 days.
2. The least amount of suture material possible should be under the flap. Mattress sutures are useful in achieving this goal, and it is important to use only as many sutures as the surgical situation requires.
3. Silk sutures should not be used when inflammation would compromise the surgical result, such as with bone grafts, guided tissue regeneration, or osseointegrated implants.

In spite of these limitations, silk remains a valuable, cost-effective suture material that is useful in many surgical situations.

Braided polyester sutures. To overcome the negative aspects of silk while retaining its superior handling characteristics, braided polyester sutures have been developed. These sutures are extremely strong and are similar to silk in their handling properties. Because they are braided, they lie comfortably against the tissues and are easy to remove. They also cause less tissue inflammation than silk.

The better polyester sutures are coated with polybutilate, silicone, or polytetrafluoroethylene. Two examples of these are Ethibond (Ethicon) and Ti-Cron (Davis & Geck), both of which are coated with silicone. The silicone coatings make these sutures much smoother and easier to handle and markedly reduce the amount of soft tissue inflammation. These coated polyester sutures are very useful to the dental surgeon. Knots made in coated sutures tend to slip, however, and require two or more overhand knots in addition to the standard surgeon's or slip knot.

Monofilament sutures. One other suture that is used in periodontal surgery is the Gore-Tex suture (WL Gore). This is a monofilament suture made of polytetrafluoroethylene. It has excellent handling characteristics and causes very little tissue reaction. In fact, Gore-Tex is so well accepted by the body that if it is left in too long it tends to become embedded in the mucosal tissues, making removal difficult. Gore-Tex sutures are used most commonly in guided tissue regeneration procedures. Several other monofilament sutures are available, such as Surgilene (Davis & Geck), which is made of propylene, and Ethilon (Ethicon), which is a nylon suture.

These sutures exhibit excellent strength and cause very little tissue reactivity. Because they are monofilaments, however, their cut ends do not lie flat against the mucosal tissues but tend to stick straight up and will abrade the patient's lips and cheeks if they are not covered with periodontal dressing.

Suture Needles

All suture needles that are used in periodontal surgery are made of stainless steel that has been hardened and sharpened to a precision point. These needles vary in size and shape, and their sizes are matched to the suture material to which they are attached. Suture sizes 3-0 and 4-0 are the ones most commonly used in periodontal surgery; the 3-0 is slightly wider in diameter than the 4-0. Sutures smaller than 5-0 are difficult to handle with conventional surgical instruments and require microsurgical instruments and techniques.

Suture needles also vary in shape from straight to ¾ circle, but the two shapes that are most useful in periodontal surgery are the ¼ and ⅜ circle. The ¼ circle is used for the more delicate procedures, such as pedicle grafts and free gingival grafts, while the ⅜ circle needle is most often used in flap surgery, wound closure after placement of osseointegrated implants, and guided tissue regeneration procedures.

The keratinized oral tissues are surprisingly dense, and piercing attached gingiva with a round needle would be very difficult. To facilitate suturing, most oral surgical needles are sharpened on three of their edges to give them three cutting surfaces (Fig 12-15). If one of the cutting surfaces is on the inside curve of the needle it is termed a *cutting needle*. The sharpened edges allow it to pass through attached, keratinized gingiva without pulling or tugging. However, because one of the cutting surfaces is on the inside curve of the needle, upward pressure on the needle during suturing will slice through the flap, making an undesired vertical incision.

Reverse cutting needles were developed to eliminate this problem. These needles also have three cutting edges, one on each side and the third on the bottom of the needle. Viewed in cross section, reverse cutting needles resemble

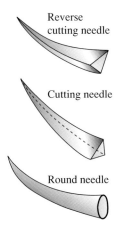

Reverse
cutting needle

Cutting needle

Round needle

Fig 12-15 Suture needles. A reverse cutting needle has three cutting edges, to ease its passage through dense collagenous tissues, but none of the cutting edges is on the inside curve of the needle. The cutting needle also has three cutting edges, but one of the edges is on the inside curve of the needle. By using a cutting needle, the periodontal surgeon risks cutting through the flap, in essence making an unintended vertical incision. A round needle is not generally used in periodontal surgery because it is difficult to pass through keratinized mucosa.

a triangle with its apex on the bottom. Reverse cutting needles are the only ones that should be used in periodontal surgery.

Conclusion

Several types of surgical procedures have been discussed, along with different incision designs and the various ways sutures are used to close these incisions. An amateur learns one technique and tries to apply it to all situations, whereas a skilled surgeon is knowledgeable in many techniques, keeping them in his or her repertoire, ready to use at the appropriate time. The techniques discussed in this chapter should be the starting point for any dentist interested in developing his or her surgical skills, which are then honed over a lifetime of study, analytic observation, and practice.[18]

References

1. Bahat O, Handelsman M. Periodontal reconstructive flaps—classification and surgical considerations. Int J Periodont Rest Dent 1991; 11:481.

2. Miller PD. Root coverage using the free soft tissue autograft following citric acid application. III. Int J Periodont Rest Dent 1985;5(2):15.

3. Holbrook T, Ochsenbein C. Complete root coverage of denuded root surfaces with a one-stage gingival graft. Int J Periodont Rest Dent 1983;3(3):8.

4. Kramer GM, Kohn JD. A classification of periodontal surgery: An approach based on tissue coverage. Periodontics 1966;4:80.

5. Dahlberg WH. Incisions and suturing. Some basic considerations about each in periodontal flap surgery. Dent Clin North Am 1969;13:149.

6. Halsted WS. Ligature and suture material. JAMA 1913;60:1119.

7. Morris M. Suturing techniques in periodontal surgery. Periodontics 1965;3:84.

8. Johnson RH. Basic flap management. Dent Clin North Am 1976;20:3.

9. Kramer GM, Nevins M, Kohn JD. The utilization of periosteal suturing in periodontal surgical procedures. J Periodontol 1970;41:457.

10. Corn H. Mucogingival surgery and associated problems. In: Goldman HM, Cohen DW (eds). Periodontal Therapy, ed 5. St Louis: Mosby, 1973:638–751.

11. Rosner D. A continuous simultaneous interdental suture technique. J Periodontol 1977;48:792.

12. Levin MP. Periodontal suture materials and surgical dressings. Dent Clin North Am 1980;24:767.

13. Lenin MP, Bhaskar SN, Frisch J. Use of sutures and periodontal dressings following surgical procedures. In: Ward HL (ed). A Periodontal Point of View. Springfield, IL: Thomas, 1973:281–310.

14. Meyer RD, Antonini CJ. A review of suture materials. Part I. Compend Contin Educ Dent 1989;10:260.

15. Meyer RD, Antonini CJ. A review of suture materials. Part II. Compend Cont Educ Dent 1989;10:360.

16. Prichard JF. Advanced Periodontal Disease. Philadelphia: Saunders, 1972.

17. Heijl L, Wennström J, Lindhe J. Periodontal surgery: Techniques for periodontal pockets. In: Lindhe J (ed). Textbook of Clinical Periodontology. Copenhagen: Munksgaard, 1983:370–392.

18. Nevins N, Becker W, Kornman K (eds). Proceedings of the World Workshop in Clinical Periodontics. Chicago: American Academy of Periodontology, 1989.

CHAPTER 13

Treatment of Mandibular Furcations

Myron Nevins, DDS
Emil G. Cappetta, DMD

The treatment of multirooted teeth offers a challenge to all practitioners because the posterior position of these teeth in the dental arch limits access for diagnostics, therapy, and cleansing by the patient. The loss of periodontium in the interradicular areas, referred to as a *furcation invasion*, occurs with remarkable frequency. A study of 83 cadavers revealed the loss of bone in more than 70% of furcations in specimens over the age of 35 years.[1] Once exposed to the oral cavity, these areas are difficult to clean and frequently demonstrate continued deterioration. The etiology of the furcation invasion may involve plaque-related inflammatory disease, endodontics, occlusion, root fractures, root perforations, and combined lesions.[2] Available treatment modalities include pocket reduction; root resection; extraction; nonsurgical therapy; tunnel preparation; surgical regeneration procedures, including grafting, membranes, and root conditioning; anti-infective therapies; and various combinations of these therapies.[3]

The significant difference between mandibular and maxillary molars is that the mandibular furcation opens to the buccal and lingual directions. Therefore, no matter how advanced the loss of bone, it does not damage the interdental bone for the adjacent teeth (Figs 13-1a and 13-1b). The maxillary molars have mesial and distal furcations, and inflammatory lesions can result in the loss of interdental bone on adjacent teeth.

Anatomy of Mandibular Molar Roots

The mandibular molars usually present with distinct mesial and distal roots. Their buccolingual width, together with their relative inaccessibility interradicularly, present problems to both the patient and the dental team.[4–24] Indeed, even their replacement with implants is precarious because of the proximity to the inferior alveolar nerve.

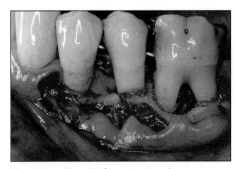

Fig 13-1a Class III furcation involvement on a mandibular molar. The furcation opens to the buccal and lingual surfaces, and therefore the advanced bone loss in the furcation area does not damage the interdental bone of the adjacent teeth.

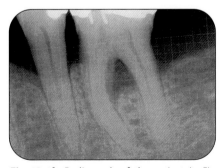

Fig 13-1b Radiograph of the patient in Fig 13-1a. The adjacent interdental bone is not affected by the furcation invasion.

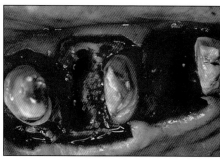

Fig 13-2 The residual extraction socket reveals the shape of the mesial root of the mandibular molar to be similar to that of a biconcave disk. Note the significant concavity on the distal aspect of the mesial root. The distal root is more oblong and presents flat mesial and distal surfaces. It is more parallel to the premolars.

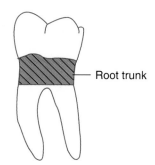

Root trunk

Fig 13-3 The root trunk is defined as that area that extends from the cementoenamel junction to the furcation.

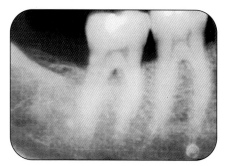

Fig 13-4a There is a class III complete furcation involvement of both mandibular molars. The radiograph indicates there is a short root trunk with long roots.

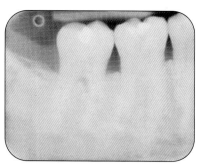

Fig 13-4b Disease progression in the furcation region after 6 years.

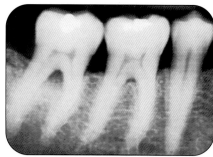

Fig 13-4c The same molars, 12 years later. A molar with long roots and a short trunk may be more vulnerable to furcation invasion, but can be more safely committed to observation over a period of time. It is now time to intervene before additional bone is lost.

The mesial root is thin and shaped like a biconcave disk; the distal concavity is usually more prominent (Fig 13-2). The two root canals are located buccally and lingually, and connected in the pulp chamber. The apical portion of the root demonstrates a distal curvature that is an obstacle to extraction, especially when the tooth is sectioned (see Fig 13-1b) and only the mesial root is to be removed.

The distal root is more oblong and presents flat mesial and distal surfaces. It has one root canal and is easier to manage prosthetically because it is more parallel to the premolars (see Figs 13-1b and 13-2). This root is a realistic candidate for a post and core buildup because of its perimeter morphology and its root canal system.

The root trunk is described as that part of the tooth that extends from the cementoenamel junction to the furcation, or the separation of the two roots (Fig 13-3). A molar with a short trunk and long roots is more vulnerable to a furcation invasion but can be more safely committed to observation (Figs 13-4a to 13-4c). A small loss of bone will not worsen the prognosis of root sectioning dramatically. In contrast, a molar with a long trunk and short roots may prove to be untreatable by root sectioning (Fig 13-5).

A significant percentage of molar teeth display enamel projections that alter the level of attachment apparatus to the tooth as the enamel enters the interradicular area (Figs 13-6a to 13-6c). The enamel projection can never have a connective tissue attachment because it is an ectodermal derivative and is covered only by epithelium; therefore, enamel projections can make a molar more vulnerable to inflammatory disease. The presence of enamel projections is significant in molar teeth, and the incidence of furcal invasion in those teeth demonstrating vertical enamel projections is high (82% to 90%). The extent of the enamel projection is directly proportional to the amount of furcation involvement.[25–30]

As the alveolar process widens to accommodate the larger root form of these teeth, the larger interdental septa are prone to interdental craters and deeper forms of vertical intrabony pockets. The most compelling periodontal problem relating to mandibular molars is the partial or complete loss of the periodontium between the two roots. The healthy interradicular root surface is covered by cementum to which Sharpey's fibers are connected. These connective tissue fibers join the tooth to the alveolar process and are oriented at oblique angles or perpendicular to the tooth surface. The periodontal ligament is of the same dimension as on the periphery of the root (Fig 13-7).[31]

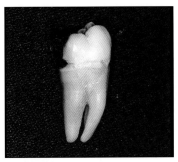

Fig 13-5 Extracted molar with a long trunk and short roots. This anatomic variation may prove to be untreatable by root sectioning. The root is too short from the furcation to the apex to be a good candidate for root resection therapy.

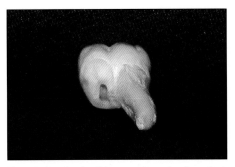

Fig 13-6a Grade IV enamel projection that extends almost from buccal to lingual. The enamel projection never has a connective tissue attachment and is more vulnerable to inflammatory disease.

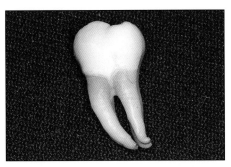

Fig 13-6b The facial view of the molar demonstrates the enamel projection entering the furcation area.

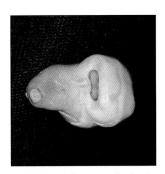

Fig 13-6c Bifurcational ridge in the interradicular area.

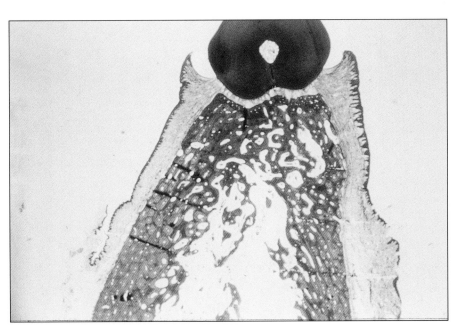

Fig 13-7 Histologic section demonstrating the periodontium of a normal interradicular area.

Classification of Furcation Involvement

The interradicular horizontal loss of periodontium is considered a furcation invasion (Fig 13-8), the extent of which is expressed by a gradation system:

1. Class I. Incipient or early loss of attachment.
2. Class II. A deeper invasion and loss of attachment that does not extend to a complete invasion. This category has many shades of gray and myriad treatment options.
3. Class III. Complete loss of periodontium, extending from the buccal surface to the lingual surface (Fig 13-9). It is usually diagnosed by radiographic analysis and clinical probing with an explorer.

Ricchetti[32] proposed a linear classification that provides horizontal and vertical measurements and establishes a meaningful clinical tool to determine a treatment approach for the incipient and class II models (Fig 13-10). His class I and class Ia furcations are incipient and will respond to pocket elimination treatment on both the buccal and lingual surfaces. Tooth preparation in the form of odontoplasty will eliminate the dentinal hood of tooth structure over the furcation and provide a smooth surface from the seam of root surface and bone to the occlusal surface of the tooth when the tooth has been prepared for a crown (Figs 13-11a to 13-11c). As the deeper horizontal (class II) furcation invasion is encountered, odontoplasty continues to be useful for teeth with divergent roots, but the end result is problematic for most teeth. It is necessary to observe the tooth preparation and consider the possibility of constructing a crown that will fit and that the patient and hygienist can keep clean (Fig 13-12).

The Ricchetti class III furcation denotes furcal invasion half the distance from the buccal surface to the lingual surface. It is too deep to resolve by odontoplasty and must be considered a candidate for periodontal regeneration, maintained as is, or hemisected (see Fig 13-11b).

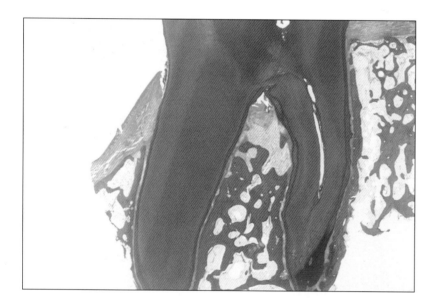

Fig 13-8 Histologic section of an extracted mandibular molar. Note the loss of interradicular bone and the disruption of the connective tissue attachment to the underside of the furcation.

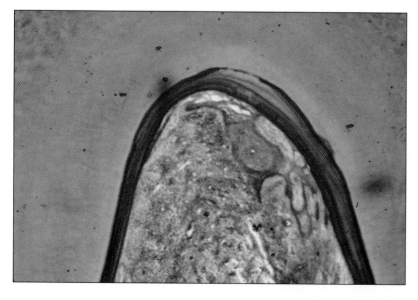

Fig 13-9 Histologic section demonstrating the replacement of the connective tissue attachment with epithelium. It is a class III, or complete, furcation invasion.

Fig 13-10 Mandibular molar demonstrating the pocket configuration and bone loss generally found with furcation invasion:

Class I: 1 mm of horizontal measurement—the root furrow.

Class Ia: 1 to 2 mm of horizontal invasion—earliest damage.

Class II: 2 to 4 mm of horizontal invasion—observe or perform odontoplasty.

Class IIa: 4 to 6 mm of horizontal invasion—observe, section, or attempt regeneration.

Class III: more than 6 mm of horizontal invasion—must section.

(left) Occlusal view of mandibular molar. *(right)* Mesial view of distal half of mandibular molar section through the interradicular septum after section of mesial root.

This furcation classification is most useful when the clinician is considering the treatment of early and intermediate furcation invasions. (From Ricchetti.[32] Reprinted with permission.)

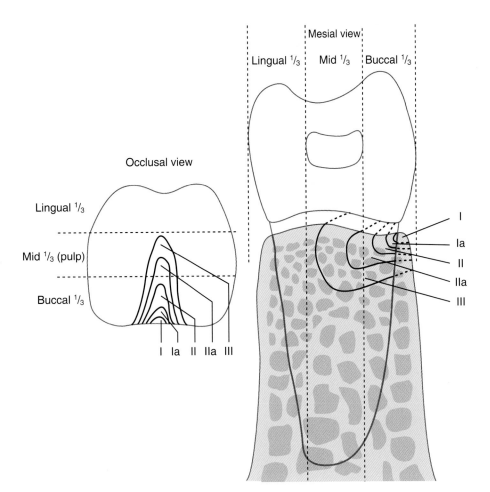

Fig 13-11a

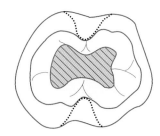

Fig 13-11b

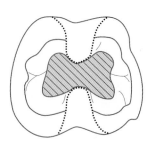

Fig 13-11c

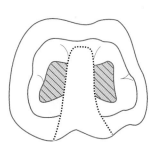

Fig 13-12

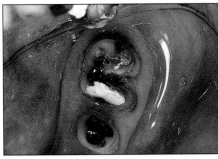

Fig 13-11a The treatment of a tooth that has been prepared for a complete-coverage crown includes odontoplasty to remove the hood of tooth structure that covers the interradicular furcation invasion. This procedure eliminates a difficult cul de sac and allows complete debridement.

Fig 13-11b Odontoplasty is ineffective when the furcal invasion has proceeded so far that only a small isthmus of periodontium remains. The prosthetic procedures coupled with the patient's inability to cleanse will likely result in a complete furcation involvement from the buccal surface to the lingual surface.

Fig 13-11c This configuration cannot be treated successfully by odontoplasty. (Courtesy of Dr Howard M. Skurow.)

Fig 13-12 The furcation invasion is too significant for odontoplasty to be effective. It is impossible to construct a well-fitting restoration that can be maintained by the patient and the hygienist.

Treatment of Furcation Invasion

Regeneration

It is always preferable to regenerate the lost periodontium; however, the predictability for regeneration in the case of a through-and-through furcation is low (Figs 13-13a and 13-13b).[33] It is extremely time consuming and expensive, and continued failure is likely to erode the patient's confidence in periodontal treatment. The defects with the most promising prospects for regeneration have a vertical wall of bone buccal to the furcation and divergent roots to allow proper root debridement (Figs 13-14a to 13-14e, and 13-

15a to 13-15d).[34,35] This is rare, because the distance between the roots is smaller than the size of a periodontal curette 58% of the time.[13,14] Ultrasonic instruments can be used but also have limitations.

Treatment Considerations

The furcation that extends more than two thirds the buccolingual dimension of the tooth, or completely, can only be treated by maintenance or root resection. Because a mandibular molar rarely presents a proximal furcation, adjoining teeth will suffer no damage as a result of the furcation problem that is diagnosed but not treated (Fig 13-16). In fact, even if all the bone is lost between the roots, a

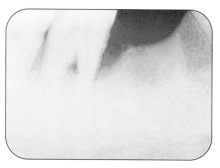

Fig 13-13a Osseous defect on the mesial surface and complete furcation invasion on the mandibular molar (1966).

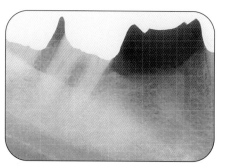

Fig 13-13b The osseous defect and the furcation responded to periodontal regeneration and, most importantly, continue to be successful after 29 years (1995).

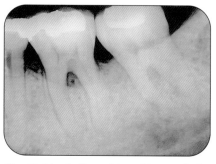

Fig 13-14a Radiographic evidence of the furcation invasion on the mandibular first and second molars. The presence of the external and internal oblique ridges hides the extensive furcation involvement of the second molar. (Courtesy of Dr Marcelo de Costa Camelo.)

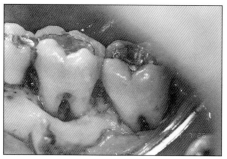

Fig 13-14b The lingual furcations have both horizontal and vertical components. There are osseous craters in the interproximal region.

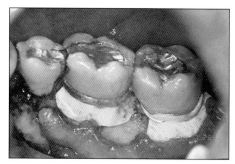

Fig 13-14c Demineralized freeze-dried bone has been used in the furcation regions, and Gore-Tex e-PTFE barrier membranes (WL Gore, Flagstaff, AZ) have been placed into position to cover the furcation involvements.

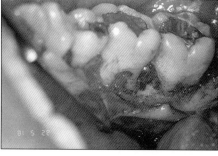

Fig 13-14d A 6-month reentry into the site reveals complete fill in the furcation of both molars.

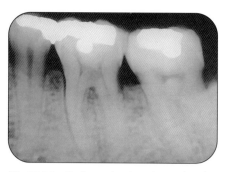

Fig 13-14e Radiograph taken 6 months after surgery.

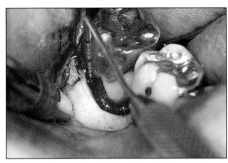

Fig 13-15a The furcation involvement has both horizontal and vertical components. Note the 5-mm vertical probing depth of the defect. The defect has been decorticated to establish communication with the cancellous bone.

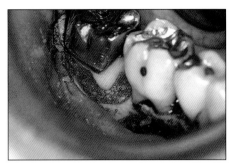

Fig 13-15b A freeze-dried bone allograft fills the defect.

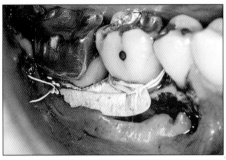

Fig 13-15c A Gore-Tex barrier membrane is fitted to cover the interproximal and facial furcation defects. It is difficult to manage at the distobuccal line angle of the second molar because of the lack of a vestibule.

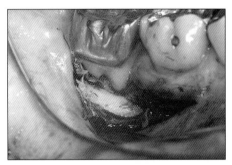

Fig 13-15d Reentry reveals the complete fill in the furcation of the mandibular second molar.

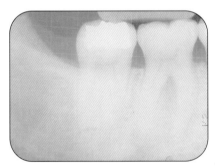
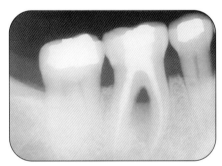

Fig 13-16 *(left)* An early furcation invasion of this vital mandibular first molar was misdiagnosed and treated endodontically. *(right)* The interradicular bone has continued to be lost until the tooth is no longer a candidate for resection, but there is no damage to the interproximal bone of adjacent teeth.

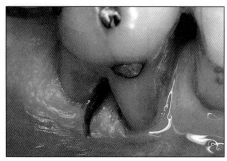

Fig 13-17a An instrument has been placed into the lingual furcation and emerges through the buccal furca. The patient tries to be compliant but caries is present on the inferior surface of the trunk.

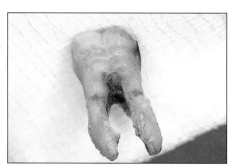

Fig 13-17b Extraction of the molar in Fig 13-17a reveals caries in the furcation. Few patients maintain on open furcation satisfactorily.

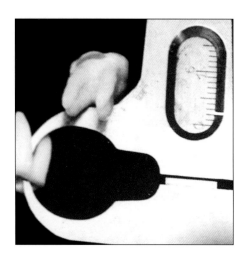

Fig 13-17c Root caries in the furcation is almost untreatable because there is very little tooth structure on the pulpal floor.

fixed partial denture can be constructed to replace the failed tooth. A molar with a through-and-through furcation should not be selected as an abutment for a fixed partial denture but can continue to service a dentition for a long time (see Figs 13-4a to 13-4c).

It is preferable to treat complete furcation invasions non-surgically or by hemisection. Pocket reduction surgery is not appropriate for a complete mandibular furcation invasion, because exposure of the interradicular area requires skill and diligence on the part of the patient and frequently leads to disappointment. Root caries is rarely manageable because of the small amount of tooth structure that exists between the pulp chamber and the furcation (Figs 13-17a to 13-17c). Few patients are able to maintain an open furcation, and continued inflammation results in additional loss of attachment apparatus.

The long-term survival rate of furcated teeth could potentially lead to a position of false security. The decline of a compromised furcation is subject to many factors, and a humble approach is most appropriate.[15-21] Minor problems have the potential to worsen unexpectedly and result in untreatable situations. It is necessary to consider the following:

1. Is this tooth strategic to the future of the dentition in question?
2. What is the ratio of root trunk to root length?
3. Is the patient a realistic candidate for compliance with periodontal maintenance with a periodicity that will result in an opportunity to recognize a worsening of the defect?
4. How old is the patient? How long will this tooth service the dentition?

Periodontal Abscess

The presence of a periodontal abscess adjacent to a furcation is indicative of a serious problem. Incision and drainage alleviate symptoms but can hardly address bone loss. If the tooth is nonvital, endodontic therapy should be carried out immediately. This may result in remarkable radiographic resolution of the problem without periodontal treatment (Figs 13-18a to 13-18d). but a vital tooth requires careful periodontal analysis. Because the furcation is normally within 3 to 4 mm of the cementoenamel junction,[31] aggressive treatment is indicated to prevent worsening of the problem.

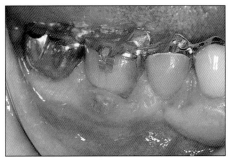

Fig 13-18a The patient presents with a fistula on the facial aspect of the mandibular first molar. It is necessary to determine the etiology of the lesion before treatment. If the tooth is nonvital, endodontics should be performed immediately.

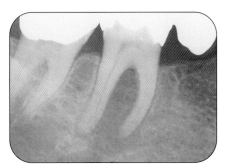

Fig 13-18b Extensive radiolucency in the furcation region extending periapically.

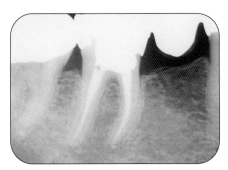

Fig 13-18c Endodontic treatment has been completed. The 1-year radiograph provides evidence of the resolution of the defect.

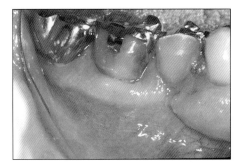

Fig 13-18d One year postoperatively. There has been complete resolution of the lesion. The fistula has healed and the area appears to be healthy.

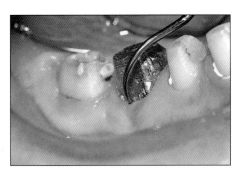

Fig 13-19a Clinical examination reveals furcation involvement of the mandibular first molar. Do not be deluded by pink tissue and an absence of bleeding.

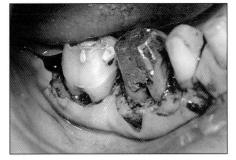

Fig 13-19b Clinical-surgical examination reveals that both molars have furcation invasion. It is incorrect to lengthen the crown by building the coronal portion of a tooth as is demonstrated by the poor gingival margin of the alloy. Calculus is found subgingivally in the furcation area of the second molar. Instrumentation is difficult between the roots of multirooted teeth.

Clinical and radiographic examination is essential after the resolution of the symptoms of a periodontal abscess adjacent to a furcation. When there is a probing depth of 5 mm after abscess resolution, it should be interpreted as the loss of some bone between the roots of the tooth. A flap should be elevated to provide access for root planing and osteoplasty, if indicated, because chronic adult periodontitis is a microbial-based disease process, and it is crucial to develop an environment that is cleansable. This is especially true because there is no accurate method of predicting patient susceptibility or patient compliance at the outset of treatment. Therefore, the treatment of the early furcation offers an opportunity to avoid treatment of an advanced defect. Clinicians should not be deluded by pink tissue and an absence of bleeding[36] (Figs 13-19a and 13-19b).

Root-Sectioning Procedures

Root-sectioning procedures have endured as a predictable means of creating an environment that is cleansable and have proven to be efficacious[37-44] (Fig 13-20a). A thorough

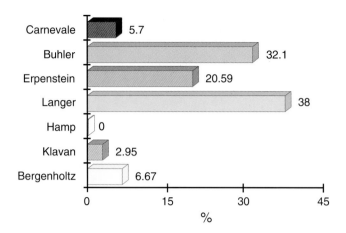

Fig 13-20a Comparison of failure after root amputation procedures.[37] (Figs 13-20a and 13-20b from Carnevale.[37] Reprinted with permission.)

Author		Root/Tooth fracture	Periodontal	Endodontic	Caries cement washout	Total failures	Total cases
Carnevale	1990	12	3	4	9	28	488
Buhler	1988	1	2	5	1	9	28
Erpenstein	1983		1	6		7	34
Langer	1981	18	10	7	3	38	100
Hamp	1975					—	87
Klavan	1975		1			1	34
Bergenholtz	1972		2			3	45

Fig 13-20b Retrospective analysis of failures after root amputation. In these six studies, failures are categorized as caries, root fracture, endodontic complication, and periodontal disease. Collectively, most failures are caused by problems other than periodontal disease. This underscores the need to evaluate the ability to complete a root canal successfully, to ascertain the effect of occlusion on the resected molar, and to evaluate whether a tooth is a candidate for root resection therapy by analysis of the root anatomy and the dentist's ability to restore the sectioned root.

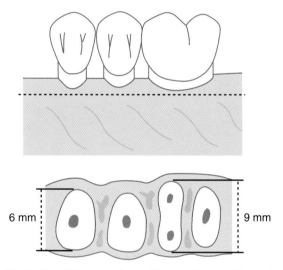

Fig 13-21a A hemisected mandibular molar is not identical to two premolars. The embrasure is wider buccolingually and complicated by root concavities.

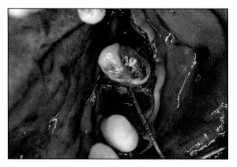

Fig 13-21b The mesial root has been extracted and offers an opportunity to measure the narrow interradicular embrasure. This is insufficient space to fit restorations or to allow debridement by the patient or the health professional.

review of the available evidence to date would suggest root resection to be a technique-sensitive procedure, requiring a careful diagnostic process for selection of those teeth that would likely be successful candidates, followed by meticulous interdisciplinary treatment. Reported failures are categorized as caries, root fracture, endodontics, and periodontal disease, but the etiology of most failures is nonperiodontal (Fig 13-20b).[37–44] This underscores the need to evaluate the patency of the root canal system for successful root canal therapy; the occlusal forces relating to the opposing arch; the length of the edentulous span; and the length, width, and shape of the root.

The retrospective longitudinal studies available to date have observed the fate of sectioned teeth for time frames ranging from 3 to 12 years and have reported success rates ranging from 100% to 62%. None found a periodontal failure rate of greater than 10%. Carnevale et al[37] evaluated 488 root-resected teeth for periods ranging from 1 to 11 years; they reported a failure rate of only 5.7%. Only three sectioned teeth, 0.61% of the total, were extracted because of periodontal disease among the 28 failures. The study by Langer et al[38] included 100 teeth, of which 10 failed periodontally. The study by Blomlöf[43] evaluated 159 resected molars in 80 patients. In this study the success rate after 10 years of observation ranged from 56% to 89%.

Surgical decisions bear some of the responsibility for failures. A hemisected molar is not identical to two premolars because the size and anatomy of the roots are so different. Mandibular premolars have more rounded roots with less extensive buccolingual embrasures and are more accessible for debridement (Figs 13-21a and 13-21b). The embrasure between the two roots of a mandibular molar is very small

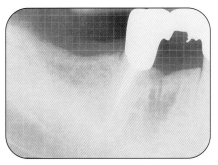

Fig 13-22a The radiographic image of this sectioned mandibular molar shows that too much tooth structure has been removed during routine endodontics. This leaves too little dentin, and the root is susceptible to occlusal forces.

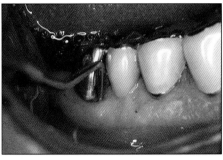

Fig 13-22b A probing depth of 10 mm is discovered at a periodontal maintenance visit. This occurred 6 years after the completion of treatment.

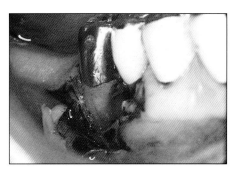

Fig 13-22c A vertical fracture appears on the facial aspect of the distal root. This tooth failed because of the root fracture.

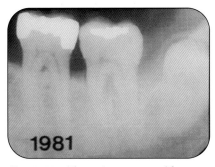

Fig 13-23a The patient presented for treatment in 1981. There is a complete furcation invasion of the first and second molars. The first molar is stable; the second molar has a mobility of 2+.

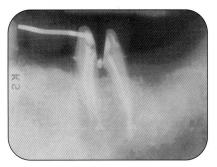

Fig 13-23b The first molar has been hemisected and the second molar has been extracted.

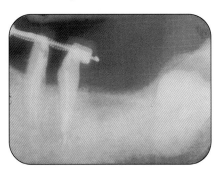

Fig 13-23c The two roots of the first molar are orthodontically separated.

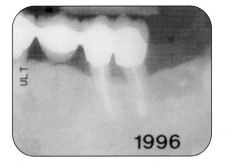

Fig 13-23d Fifteen years later, the two roots provide the only posterior support for the mandibular fixed partial denture.

mesiodistally and very wide buccolingually. In addition, the distal root concavity on the mesial root is difficult to manage prosthetically and difficult for the patient to deplaque (see Figs 13-1b and 13-2). It is rare to be able to crown both roots and provide a workable embrasure.

It is very important to be judicious when performing endodontics for a sectioned root. The removal of too much dentin results in a weak structure that may fracture prematurely under the occlusal load (Figs 13-22a to 13-22c).

Minor tooth movement is effective to separate the two roots and open the embrasure but requires proximal space and is of most value when the adjacent tooth is absent (Figs 13-23 and 13-24). Because such treatment integrates the disciplines of periodontics, endodontics, orthodontics, and restorative dentistry, it is both complicated and expensive and requires specific organization of the treatment plan. This approach must now be evaluated as it compares to the prognosis of osseointegration, but deserves strong consideration when the volume of bone to place implants is deficient or the anatomic obstacle of the nerve is foreboding. A single sectioned root of a mandibular molar will offer a better prognosis when a short edentulous span is being restored (Figs 13-25a to 13-25d, and 13-26a and 13-26b). The longer span is more problematic and should be reevaluated for osseointegrated implants (Figs 13-27a and 13-27b, and 13-28a to 13-28d) unless the remaining root is large.

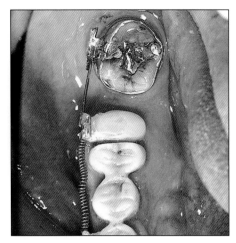

Fig 13-24a The mandibular first molar has been hemisected and orthodontically treated to move the distal root distally. This will result in an embrasure that can be easily restored and cleansed by the patient.

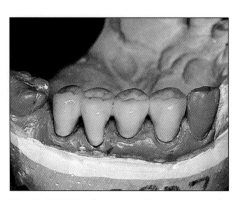

Fig 13-24b The final restoration on the working cast reveals the embrasure between the sectioned first molar roots, which can be adequately cleaned by the patient.

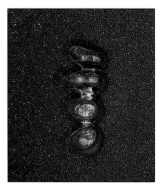

Fig 13-24c Underside of the casting. Note the size of the embrasure between the hemisected roots and the internal anatomy of the casting, which reflects the tooth preparation of the hemisected molar.

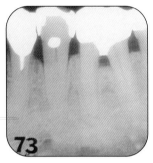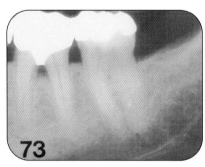

Fig 13-25a and 13-25b Series of radiographs that spans 23 years. In 1973, the patient presented with a complete (class III) furcation invasion of the mandibular first molar and class II furcation invasion of the second molar. The presence of the external oblique ridge, as well as the thickness of the cortex, precludes a definitive diagnosis of furcation involvement on the second molar. Clinical diagnosis is of critical importance.

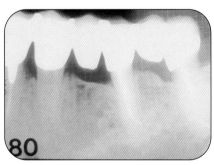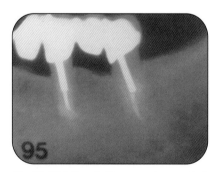

Fig 13-25c Seven-year observation after the mesial roots were sectioned and the prosthesis was constructed using the distal roots (1980).

Fig 13-25d Result 22 years after surgical and prosthetic care.

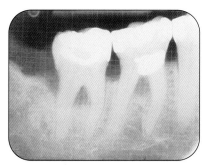

Fig 13-26a Class III (complete) furcation invasion on both mandibular molars (1972).

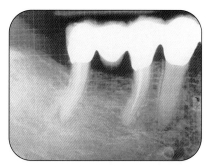

Fig 13-26b Hemisection procedures resected the distal roots to resolve the molar furcations. This radiograph was taken 23 years postoperatively (1995).

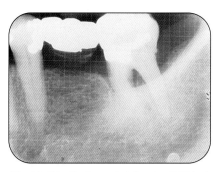

Fig 13-27a Radiograph taken in 1972 just prior to definite therapy involving hemisection and construction of a fixed partial denture. The distal root is small and mobile and there is less support.

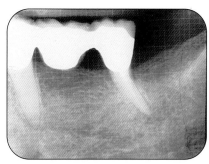

Fig 13-27b Radiograph taken 23 years later. This is a long span for the average size of the clinical root but was the decision of choice before osseointegration.

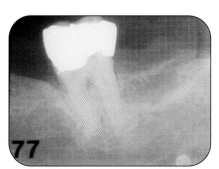

Fig 13-28a The patient presented in 1977 with furcation involvement of this mandibular molar.

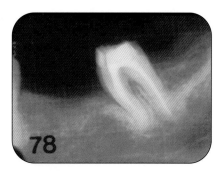

Fig 13-28b Endodontic therapy has been completed before sectioning of the tooth.

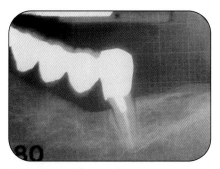

Fig 13-28c The single root supports a long edentulous span in the prosthetic rehabilitation of the mandibular dentition.

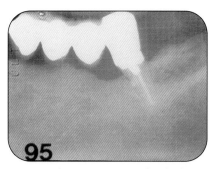

Fig 13-28d Seventeen years after the hemisection procedure was completed (1995). Although this molar has been in service for 18 years, present-day treatment planning would consider a fixture-assisted prosthesis using osseointegrated implants.

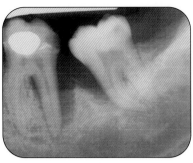

Fig 13-29a There is extensive loss of attachment on the distal root of the mandibular first molar as well as class III furcation involvement; the mandibular third molar has tipped mesially and is untreatable (1975). The patient is financially compromised and there is no restorative treatment plan.

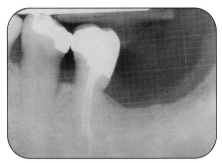

Fig 13-29b Twenty years after the hemisection of the first molar (1995). The mesial root has been retained as a single-rooted tooth, endodontic treatment has been completed, and the tooth has been restored with an alloy.

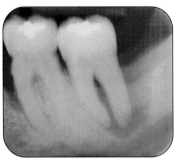

Fig 13-30a There is extensive loss of attachment on the mesial root of the mandibular first molar, and the second molar has been condemned because of extensive attachment loss and mobility (1981).

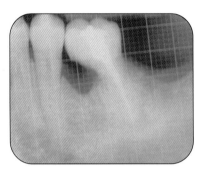

Fig 13-30b Thirteen years after the mesial root was amputated (1994). The tooth was restored with an alloy restoration. The root is stable and in no need of splinting.

It is more common to extract one root of one or both of the first and second mandibular molars when sectioning than to try to keep both roots (see Figs 13-25 to 13-28). The following factors should be considered when deciding which root to keep:

1. Mobility
2. State of repair of the tooth structure
3. Morphology of periodontal defects
4. Endodontics
5. Edentulous span
6. Root anatomy

It is important to acknowledge that sectioned teeth are included in the treatment plan for financially compromised patients (Figs 13-29a, 13-29b, 13-30a, and 13-30b). Not every sectioned tooth requires a crown and, if stable, it does not have to be splinted (see Figs 13-29 and 13-30).

The restorative margin must be placed on sound tooth structure, including the area apical to the pulp chamber (Fig 13-31). Thus, deep caries or a root fracture may negate the use of a root that is periodontally sound. The thin tooth structure of the mesial root together with the two small root canals make the construction of a post and core a questionable procedure that may result in a fractured root. The single-canal distal root is a better candidate for post and core (Figs 13-32 and 13-33).

It is easier to include a distal root in a prosthesis because it is more parallel to the premolars (see Figs 13-25a to 13-25d, 13-32a, and 13-32b). However, it is more difficult to extract mesial roots because of the root morphology of the mesial root. The distal root is straight and easy to remove, but the apical curve on the mesial root requires that it be elevated distally, and it will then collide with the distal root. Therefore, it is delivered buccally with a forceps after

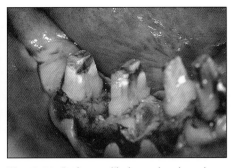

Fig 13-31 Both mandibular molars have been sectioned, and the distal roots have been retained. Note the sound tooth structure available on the mesial surfaces to place a restorative margin apical to the pulp chamber.

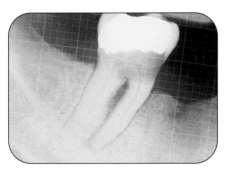

Fig 13-32a Extensive carious involvement of the mandibular molar and an osseous defect in the zone of the furcation (1971). The mesial root was sectioned, and a bone graft was performed to regenerate lost periodontium.

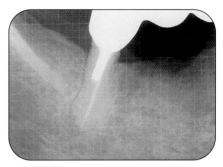

Fig 13-32b The tooth has been treated endodontically and restored as part of a five-unit restoration (1993). A longer span is more problematic but agreeable when there is a large root. This slide represents a 22-year observation. The patient died in 1993.

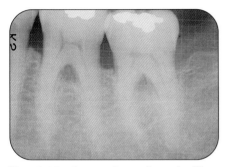

Fig 13-33a Preoperative radiograph. Note the long, thin roots and the distal angulation of the apical portion of the mesial root on the second molar.

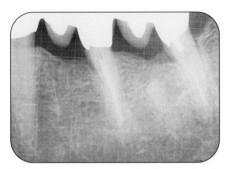

Fig 13-33b The dentition has been restored prosthetically, and hemisection procedures were utilized to retain the distal roots of each molar. The mesial root of the mandibular second molar has broken. The provisional prosthesis was allowed to remain 4 to 6 months to allow the complete healing of the extraction socket before the restoration was delivered in 1989. At times it may be best to advise the patient of the remaining root tip and leave it rather than to compromise the bone support to the adjacent teeth by attempting to remove the broken root.

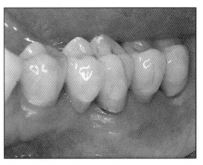

Fig 13-33c The sectioning of both molars and the removal of the mesial roots result in a series of premolar-sized teeth with pontics interposed.

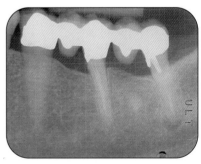

Fig 13-33d Radiograph taken 8 years after the hemisection procedure was completed.

it is mobilized with an elevator. When the premolars are present, the embrasure problem is resolved by retaining the distal roots and removing the mesial roots (see Figs 13-25 and 13-33).

If the tip of a mesial root breaks it may be best to advise the patient and leave it, rather than compromise the bone support for adjacent teeth (Figs 13-33a to 13-33d). If so, the provisional prosthesis should be allowed to remain for 4 to 6 months to ensure the complete healing of the extraction socket.

It is important to consider the mobility of both roots after sectioning when tooth restorability is not a factor, and it is logical to use the more stable root. It is unreasonable to section a mobile tooth and expect one root to be stable.

The presence of extensive periodontal defects will affect the selection of a root, as will the limitations of endodontics. The most fragile portion of the tooth for endodontic treatment is the distal surface of the mesial root just apical to the trunk. Access is difficult, and repeated instrumentation may result in perforations or the removal of too much

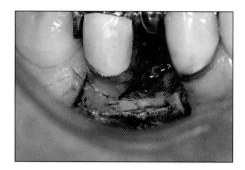

Fig 13-34 This molar has been hemisected to correct a complete (class III) furcation invasion; however, overhanging tooth structure remained at the time of sectioning, which was performed nonsurgically. It is important to remove the furcation to create an environment that can be cleansed.

dentin, and weakens the tooth. This must be considered as an issue in the failure of sectioned mandibular molars.[38]

Vital sections are seldom indicated for mandibular molars unless a combination of events precludes an accurate diagnosis. The customary regimen of treatment would suggest total pulpal extirpation before sectioning. The root that remains is finished endodontically after the periodontal surgery.

When the periodontal problems are more extensive than determined presurgically, and the removal of a root becomes the treatment of choice, it is unnecessary and unacceptable to close the procedure, wait for endodontic therapy, and then repeat the surgery. The pulpal tissues can be left in place at the time of sectioning or removed. An endodontic appointment should be arranged for 2 weeks later. It has been determined that pulpal tissues remain vital and without resorptive changes.[45,46] If there is a provisional prosthesis, it is recemented; if not, the periodontal pack appears to offer sufficient insulation.

There are reasonable interdisciplinary guidelines that must be observed when mandibular molars are sectioned. Sectioned multirooted teeth should respond to the recipe of treatment offered for single-rooted teeth, but all the aforementioned complications must be considered. It is necessary to select the most predictable treatment for the problem at hand and then perform it in an exacting fashion. It may be that a premolar occlusion resolves the problem and

the mandibular molars can stay in place untreated until they are impossible to maintain. It may be that the mandibular molars would be best replaced by dental implants or a removable partial denture.

Guidelines for Sectioning Mandibular Molars

- Do *not* section excessively mobile teeth.
- Try *not* to section heavily restored teeth.
- Remove *all* overhanging tooth structure at the time of sectioning (Fig 13-34).
- Do *not* be aggressive with endodontic instrumentation.
- Do *not* use post and core restorations for mesial roots of mandibular molars.
- Do *not* use internalized tooth preparations. There is no need to make room for ceramics in the tooth preparation. It can be done in the casting, and the restoration can have a gold collar.
- Do *not* construct large occlusal tables.
- Recognize the moment when it is too late to section the tooth successfully.

It is mandatory to consider all treatments and select a plan that will provide predictable, long-lasting results without the need for continual active treatment encounters to nurse the area.

References

1. Purisi T. [thesis]. Boston University, 1980 (unpublished).

2. Carnevale G, Pontoriero R, Hurgeler M. Management of furcation involvement. Periodontology 2000 1995;9:69.

3. Kalkwarf K, Kadahl WB, Patel KD. Evaluation of furcation region response to periodontal therapy. J Periodontol 1988;59:794.

4. Stambaugh R, Dragoo M, Smith DM, Cerasali L. The limitations of subgingival scaling. Int J Periodont Rest Dent 1981;1(5):30.

5. Nordland P, Garrett S, Kiger R, Vanooteghem R, Hutchens LH, Egelberg J. The effect of plaque control and root debridement in molar teeth. J Clin Periodontol 1987;14:231.

6. Leon LE, Vogel RI. A comparison of the effectiveness of hand scaling and ultrasonic debridement in furcation as evaluated by darkfield microscopy. J Periodontol 1987;58:86.

7. Gher ME, Vernino AR. Root morphology—Clinical significance in pathogenesis and treatment of periodontal disease. J Am Dent Assoc 1980;101:627.

8. Gher ME, Vernino AR. Root anatomy—A local factor in inflammatory periodontal disease. Int J Periodont Rest Dent 1981;1(5):52.

9. Fleischer HC, Mellonig JT, Brayer WK, Gray JL, Barnett JD. Scaling and root planing efficacy in multirooted teeth. J Periodontol 1989;60:402.

10. Matia JI, Bissada NF, Maybury JE, Ricchetti P. Efficiency of scaling of the molar furcation area with and without surgical access. Int J Periodont Rest Dent 1986;6(6):24.

11. Paraskis AO, Anagnour-Varetzides A, Demetriou N. Calculus removal from multirooted teeth with and without surgical access. II. Comparison between external and furcation surfaces and effect of furcation entrance width. J Clin Periodontol 1993;20:71.

12. Svärdström G, Wennström JL. Furcation topography of maxillary and mandibular first molars. J Clin Periodontol 1988;15:271.

13. Bower RC. Furcation morphology relative to periodontal treatment—Furcation entrance architecture. J Periodontol 1979;50:23.

14. Bower RC. Furcation morphology relative to periodontal treatment—Furcation root surface anatomy. J Periodontol 1979;50:366.

15. Hamp SE, Nyman S, Lindhe J. Periodontal treatment of multirooted teeth—Results after five years. J Clin Periodontol 1975;2:126–135.

16. Hirschfeld L, Wasserman B. A long term survey of tooth loss in 600 treated periodontal patients. J Periodontol 1978;49:225–237.

17. Bjorn AL, Hjort P. Bone loss of furcated mandibular molars—A longitudinal study. J Clin Periodontol 1982;9:402–408.

18. McFall WT. Tooth loss in 100 treated patients with periodontal disease—A long term study. J Periodontol 1982;53:539–549.

19. Goldman MJ, Ross IF, Goteiner D. Effect of periodontal therapy on patients maintained for 15 years or longer—A retrospective study. J Periodontol 1986;57:347–353.

20. Becker W, Berg L, Becker BE. The long term evaluation of periodontal treatment and maintenance in 95 patients. Int J Periodont Rest Dent 1984;4(2):54–71.

21. Ross IF, Thompson RH. A long term study of root retention in the treatment of maxillary molars with furcation involvement. J Periodontol 1978;49:238–244.

22. Martin M, Gantes B, Garrett S, Egelberg J. Treatment of periodontal furcation defects. I. Review of the literature and description of a regenerative surgical technique. J Clin Periodontol 1988;15:227–331.

23. Wang HL, Burgett FG, Shyr Y, Ramfjord S. The influence of molar furcation involvement and mobility of future clinical periodontal attachment loss. J Periodontol 1994;65:25–29.

24. Becker W, Berg L, Becker BE. Untreated periodontal disease—A longitudinal study. J Periodontol 1979;50:234.

25. Bissada NF, Abdelmalek RG. Incidence of cervical enamel projections and its relationship to furcation involvement in Egyptian skulls. J Periodontol 1973;44:583–585.

26. Larato DC. Some anatomical factors related to furcation involvements. J Periodontol 1975;46:608–609.

27. Leib AM, Berdon JK, Sabes WR. Furcation involvements correlated with enamel projections from the cemento-enamel junction. J Periodontol 1967;38:330–334.

28. Grewe JM, Meskin LH, Miller T. Cervical enamel projections—Prevalence, location and extent; with associated periodontal implications. J Periodontol 1965;36:460–465.

29. Masters DH, Hoskins SW. Projection of cervical enamel into molar furcations. J Periodontol 1964;35:49–53.

30. Swan RH, Hurt WC. Cervical enamel projections as an etiologic factor in furcation involvement. J Am Dent Assoc 1976;93:342–345.

31. Wheeler RC. A Textbook of Dental Anatomy and Physiology. Philadelphia: Saunders, 1968: chap 12.

32. Ricchetti P. A furcation classification based upon pulp chamber–furcation relationships and vertical radiographic bone loss. Int J Periodont Rest Dent 1982;2(5):51.

33. Pontoriero R, Lindhe J. Guided tissue regeneration in the treatment of Degree II furcations in maxillary molars. J Clin Periodontol 1995;22:756–763.

34. Schallhorn R, McClain P. Combined osseous composite grafting, root conditioning and guided tissue regeneration. Int J Periodont Rest Dent 1988;8:9–31.

35. McClain P, Schallhorn R. Long term assessment of combined osseous composite grafting, root conditioning and guided tissue regeneration. Int J Periodont Rest Dent 1993;13(1):9.

36. Dragoo M, Grant D, Gutberg S, Stambaugh R. Experimental periodontal treatment in humans. I. Subgingival root planing with and without chlorhexadine gluconate rinses. Int J Periodont Rest Dent 1984;4(3):9–29.

37. Carnevale G, DiFebo G, Tonelli MP, Marin C, Fuzzi MA. Retrospective analysis of the periodontal-prosthetic treatment of molars with interradicular lesions. Int J Periodont Rest Dent 1991; 11:189–205.

38. Langer G, Stein SD, Wagenberg B. An evaluation of root resection—A 10 year study. J Periodontol 1981;52:719–722.

39. Klavan B. Clinical observation following root amputation in maxillary molar teeth. J Periodontol 1975;46:105.

40. Bergenholtz A. Radectomy of multirooted teeth. J Am Dent Assoc 1972;85:870.

41. Erpenstein HJ: A three year study of hemisected molars. J Clin Periodontol 1983;10:1–10.

42. Buhler H. Evaluation of root resected teeth—Results after 10 years. J Periodontol 1988;59:805–810.

43. Blomlöf L, Jansson L, Applegren R, Ehnevid H, Lindskog S. Prognosis and mortality of root-resected molars. Int J Periodont Rest Dent 1997;17:191–201.

44. Basten CH-J, Ammons WF Jr, Persson R. Long term evaluation of root resective molars: A retrospective study. Int J Periodont Rest Dent 1997;16:207–219.

45. Haskell T, Stanley H. A review of vital root resection. Int J Periodont Rest Dent 1982;2(6):29.

46. Smukler H, Tagger M. Vital root amputation—A clinical and histologic study. J Periodontol 1976;47:324–330.

CHAPTER 14

Treatment of the Maxillary Furcation

Myron Nevins, DDS
Emil G. Cappetta, DMD

The maxillary molars present unique diagnostic, therapeutic, and maintenance problems to the astute clinician because the proximal furcations endanger the supporting bone of adjoining teeth. The etiologic factors for furcation involvement must be identified early so an accurate treatment approach can be used to resolve the problem. The etiology of furcation invasion includes the possibilities of endodontics, occlusion, plaque-related inflammatory disease, combined lesions, root fractures, and root perforations.[1] There is great benefit to recognizing the incipient inflammatory lesion and making a definitive treatment approach to correct it. Treatment modalities include nonsurgical therapy, tunnel preparation, regenerative techniques, anti-infective therapies, root conditioning, coronal positioning of surgical flaps, various combinations of these therapies, root resection, and extraction.[1,2]

Anatomy of Maxillary Molar Roots

The treatment of these three-rooted teeth requires a thorough knowledge of their root anatomy. The length of the root trunk is the distance from the cementoenamel junction (CEJ) to the opening between the roots and is variable from one surface to another.[3] Any pocketing deeper than the length of the root trunk should be immediately evaluated for correction before the loss of periodontium opens the space between the roots (Fig 14-1). A tooth with a long trunk or fused roots may allow more time to consider the treatment decision.

The mesial root is oblong, resembles the mesial root of the mandibular molar, and has a distal concavity (Figs 14-2 and 14-3). The shape of the root places the mesial furcation

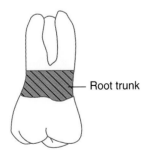

Fig 14-1 The distance from the CEJ to the furcation varies from one surface to another. A probing depth deeper than the length of the root trunk should be immediately evaluated. This is no longer early disease, and intervention is necessary before the loss of periodontium opens the spaces between the roots, compromising plaque control procedures.

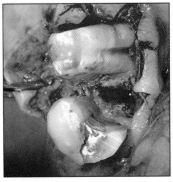

Fig 14-2 The mesial root is oblong, and the mesial furcation is about two thirds the buccopalatal surface of the tooth toward the palate. The mesial root should be removed if there is inadequate embrasure space between the maxillary molars.

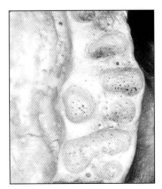

Fig 14-3 This skull demonstrates the shape of the roots of the maxillary posterior teeth. The mesial root is oblong and the distal root is round. Note the distal concavity present on the mesial root of the maxillary first molar.

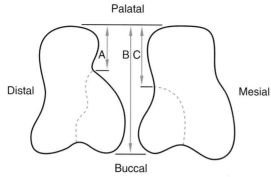

Palatal

Distal

Mesial

Buccal

Fig 14-4 Relationship of the maxillary first and second molars. *(A)* The distance from the palatal surface of the maxillary molar to the mesial furcation; *(B)* The total buccopalatal width of the interdental space between two maxillary molars; *(C)* The distance from the palatal surface of the maxillary molar to the distal furcation. Removal of the distal root of the first molar will result in a distal concavity on the mesial root and another concavity between the mesial and palatal roots, which will make plaque removal difficult. If the goal is to open an embrasure between these two teeth, the mesial root of the second molar should probably be removed because this is wider buccolingually. This area will be easier to clean in a straight-action fashion, rather than the back-action method that would be necessary to remove plaque from the concavity behind the prominent mesial root.

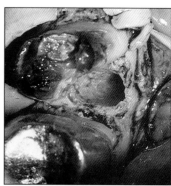

Fig 14-5 Distobuccal root amputation. The distal root is round, and the distal furcation is found midway between the buccal and palatal surfaces. The remaining infrabony defect will be eliminated with ostectomy.

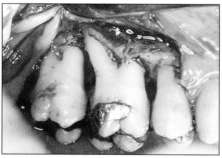

Fig 14-6 The distobuccal root of the maxillary first molar frequently diverges toward the mesiobuccal root of the second molar. The embrasure lessens as bone is lost.

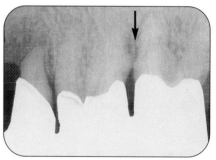

Fig 14-7 Root proximity between the maxillary molars. Note the interproximal radiolucency between the roots *(arrow)*.

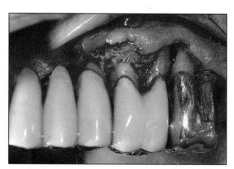

Fig 14-8 It is not unusual for the distobuccal root of the first molar to diverge toward the second molar, resulting in a smaller embrasure apically along the root surface. This root proximity increases the level of difficulty of plaque control (see Fig 14-7).

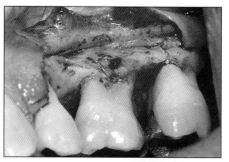

Fig 14-9 Although the distobuccal root of the maxillary first molar diverges toward the mesial root of the second molar, there is a wide embrasure. Therefore, plaque control is easier for the hygienist, as well as the patient.

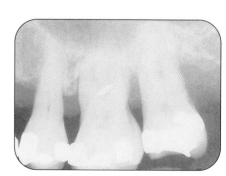

Fig 14-10 The selection of an old curette to fit in a small space can result in the dilemma of a broken instrument that is difficult to remove.

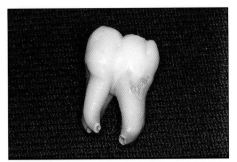

Fig 14-11 A cervical enamel projection is present in the furcation of this molar.

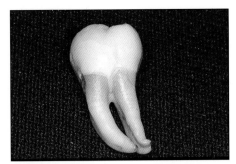

Fig 14-12 A cervical enamel projection and a bifurcation ridge are present in this mandibular molar.

about two thirds the buccopalatal surface of the tooth to the palate (Fig 14-4). The distal root is round, and the distal furcation is found midway from the buccal to the palatal surfaces (Figs 14-4 and 14-5). It is not unusual for the distobuccal root of the first molar to diverge toward the second molar, resulting in a embrasure that is smaller as it proceeds apically (Figs 14-6 to 14-8). This increases the level of difficulty of plaque control for both the hygienist and the patient, and it may preempt fixed restorative dentistry.

As a general rule, molars with a large embrasure enable easier diagnostics, access for treatment, and cause fewer periodontal debridement problems (Fig 14-9). The irregular surface of the interfurcal area is difficult to cleanse with available instrumentation.[4-11] In fact, the standard curette is larger than the entrance of the interradicular area 58% of the time[12-14] (Fig 14-10).

Furcation Invasion

The loss of bone between the roots of a multirooted tooth is referred to as a *furcation invasion*. Enamel projections into the furcation preclude connective tissue attachment from the moment of eruption and destine the areas to be problematic. Cervical enamel projections are common in molar teeth, and the incidence of furcation invasion in those teeth demonstrating cervical enamel projections is high (82% to 90%). The grade of enamel projection is directly related to the amount of furcation involvement[15-20] (Figs 14-11 and 14-12). The compromised furcation is best treated when bone loss is early, a class I furcation, and unresponsive when it connects all three areas, a trifurcation. The recent past has demonstrated some regeneration success with buccal class II furcations, which are described as being somewhere between an incipient lesion and a complete invasion extending from one interradicular area to another.[21-23]

There is little information about the frequency of furcation problems in the adult population with chronic periodontitis, but one cadaver survey of 83 skulls found an involvement of 26% of the furcations in the 29- to 35-year-old group and an involvement of approximately 70% of the furcations in the group older than this age. The clinician must be on guard and examine the maxillary molar area carefully.[24]

The ultimate goal of corrective periodontal treatment is to create an environment that is accessible to periodontal maintenance care by both the patient and the dental hygienist. The control of the inflammatory lesion should coincide with arrest of the disease. A review of the findings of previous retrospective studies indicates that this is more difficult to achieve with multi-rooted teeth. Attachment loss and tooth extraction are considerably higher for furcated molars than for single-rooted teeth with treatment modalities ranging from root planing to flap surgery with and without ostectomy; some studies reporting as much as 30% to 57% of teeth demonstrating furcation invasion.[25-34]

The most frequently used diagnostic tools are the periapical radiograph and the periodontal probe. Computerized tomography provides a valuable adjunct to other diagnostic methods when available, but it presents financial and irradiation considerations (Figs 14-13 to 14-15). Computerized tomograms better prepare the clinician for the problem at hand. Periapical films should be made carefully with accurate horizontal and vertical angulations. It is possible to determine the loss of bone by a triangle of radiolucency between two roots and to observe root structure that has lost periodontium and the vertical bone position relative to the length of the root trunk (Figs 14-16a and 14-16b). Determination of periodontal attachment loss and probing depths, used in conjunction with radiographic information, enhances diagnostic skills and allows for a thoughtful diagnosis, but the surgical procedure itself will continue to be both investigative and therapeutic (Figs 14-17a and 14-17b).

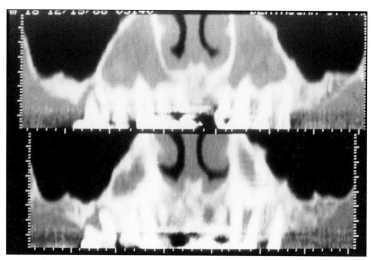

Fig 14-13 The panoramic view of a computerized tomography scan. Note the furcation invasion of the maxillary right molar. This diagnostic method is not routinely suggested because of financial and irradiation considerations.

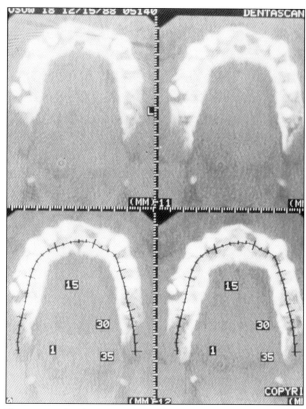

Fig 14-14 The furcation is noted on the maxillary right first molar in the axial view of the computerized tomography scan.

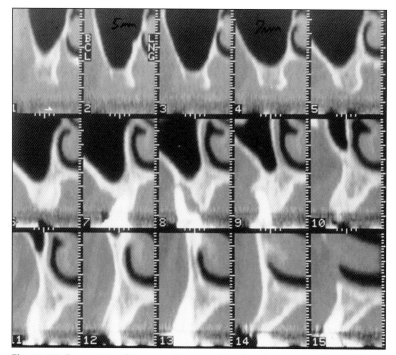

Fig 14-15 Computerized tomography scan depicting the cross-sectional oblique images. The image in the center shows a furcation involvement of a maxillary molar. The sagittal views confirm the compromised periodontium of the maxillary molar.

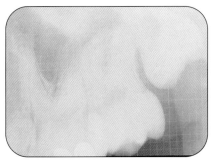

Fig 14-16a A radiograph that is not diagnostic. It is not possible to determine the extent of bone loss and furcation involvement.

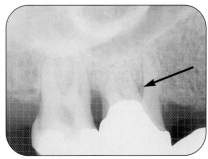

Fig 14-16b A radiograph with proper vertical and horizontal angulation. It is possible to determine the loss of bone, which presents as a triangle of radiolucency *(arrow)* between the two roots, and to observe the vertical bone loss on the individual roots.

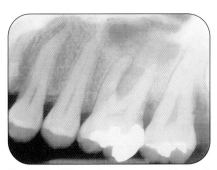

Fig 14-17a The patient presents with distal and buccal furcation invasion of the vital first molar. The distal root was amputated as a vital section to provide an opportunity to investigate the periodontal health between the two remaining roots. Endodontic therapy was performed 2 weeks later.

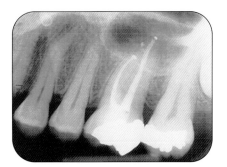

Fig 14-17b The tooth continues to be a useful member of this dentition 12 years later. It is not splinted because it is stable.

Root-Sectioning Procedures

Success Rates

A thorough review of the available evidence to date suggests that root resectioning is a technique-sensitive procedure requiring a careful diagnostic process to select those teeth that are likely to be successful candidates.[35–42] Reported failures are categorized as being caused by caries, fractures, endodontic complications, and periodontal disease, but the etiology of most failures is nonperiodontal. This underscores the need to evaluate the ability to negotiate the root canal system for successful endodontic therapy; the occlusal forces relating to the opposing arch; the length of the edentulous span; the length, width, and shape of the root; and dental caries.

Retrospective longitudinal studies have observed the fate of sectioned teeth for time frames ranging from 3 to 12 years and have found success rates ranging from 62% to 100%. None has found a periodontal failure rate greater than 10%.[35–42] Carnevale et al[35] evaluated 488 root-resected teeth from 1 to 11 years and found only a 0.6% periodontal failure rate and a total failure rate of 5.7%. Among the total of 28 failures, only three sectioned teeth were extracted because of periodontal disease. Langer's 10-year study[36] included 100 teeth, of which 10 failed periodontally. The results of these studies are compared in Figures 13-20a and 13-20b (see p. 208).

Treatment Considerations

Any thought of root sectioning must be considered in light of mobility. A three-legged stool that is wobbly will not be stabilized by the removal of one or two legs. Because proximal furcations between approximating maxillary molars share a narrow septum of bone, it is necessary to resolve a mesial or distal furcation problem before it extends to the next tooth and before bone is lost between the other two roots of the tooth (see Figs 14-3, 14-5, 14-6, and 14-7). A mesial furcation on the first molar can compromise the bone between the molar and the second premolar, but it may be far enough toward the palate to be self-limiting (Figs 14-18a to 14-18h).

It is very important to make the decision to section a root to solve a deep furcation invasion before all of the bone is lost between the two remaining roots (Figs 14-19a to 14-19e). It is easy to commit to a sectioning procedure

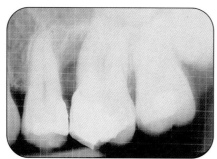

Fig 14-18a There is significant radiographic bone loss on the mesial root of the maxillary molar. The furcation must be involved, as determined by the vertical loss of bone apical to the furcation entrance. This procedure is performed as a vital section to assay the furcation between the palatal and distobuccal roots. Note the apex of the mesial root curves distally.

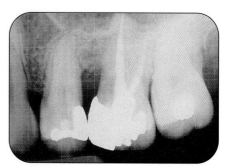

Fig 14-18b Radiograph made 10 weeks after surgery. A mesiobuccal root amputation has been performed, and endodontic treatment was completed 2 weeks later.

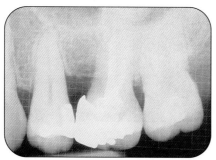

Fig 14-18c The radiograph made 8 months after surgery demonstrates a significant resolution of the interdental osseous problem and suggests that a crown can be constructed.

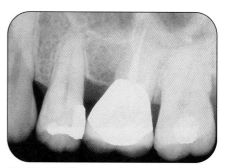

Fig 14-18d Crown in place 17 years later.

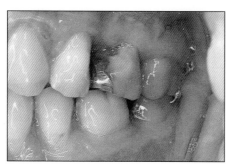

Fig 14-18e Clinical view of the tooth 8 months after resection of the mesial root. The crown morphology after odontoplasty suggests the form of a crown to the restorative dentist.

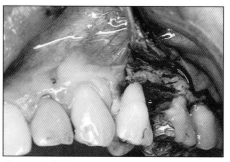

Fig 14-18f The reopening 8 months after root amputation confirms the bone regeneration observed in Fig 14-18c.

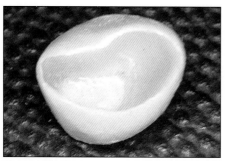

Fig 14-18g The inner aspect of the provisional acrylic resin crown reflects the anatomy of the tooth after a mesiobuccal root amputation. The care evident in this project is important because it translates into the information to construct a permanent crown. (Prosthesis by Dr Howard M. Skurow.)

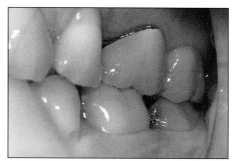

Fig 14-18h Completed crown in place. This represents the postoperative result 10 years after root amputation.

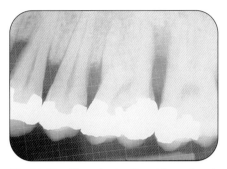

Fig 14-19a There is significant loss of periodontal attachment between the distal root of the maxillary left first molar and the mesial root of the adjacent second molar. It is not possible to locate the buccal and palatal dimensions of bone loss from a two-dimensional radiograph without clinical correlation.

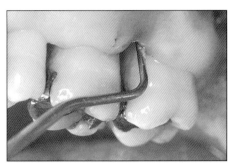

Fig 14-19b The probing depth approaches 10 mm on the buccal surface.

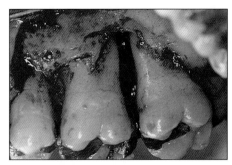

Fig 14-19c The surgical procedure reveals extensive interproximal bone loss involving the distal root of the first molar, the mesial root of the second molar, and both furcations.

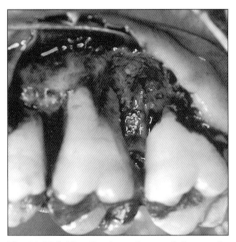

Fig 14-19d The distobuccal root of the maxillary left first molar and the mesiobuccal root of the second molar have been resected. The mesial furcation on the first molar has not been violated, and the distal furcation of the second molar is also intact. The procedure is both investigatory and therapeutic. The interproximal space is inadequate to establish parabolic architecture, and there will be no possibility of cleansing the open proximal furcations. Now is the time to determine the prognosis of both molars. If the remaining furcations are intact and the teeth are stable, it is reasonable to proceed to endodontic therapy.

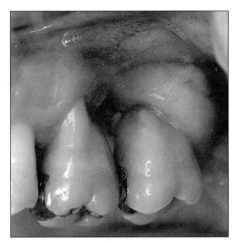

Fig 14-19e Postsurgical result at 6 months. The area has healed nicely, and the embrasure is accessible for plaque removal.

when there is complete loss of the interradicular bone, but it is necessary to perform a root section long before the opening of the remaining furcation, if treatment is to be efficacious and long lasting. If the inner surface of the furcation between the two remaining roots is found to be compromised after one root is removed, the prognosis is significantly reduced because access for cleaning will be severely limited.

The removal of the distobuccal root of the first molar will result in a distal concavity on the mesial root and another concavity between the mesial and palatal roots that will have to be cleansed of plaque. Therefore, if the chief purpose of treatment is to open an embrasure between the two maxillary molars, it will probably be better to remove the mesial root of the second molar because this is wider buccolingually (see Chapter 2 and Figs 14-2 to 14-4). It will be easier to clean this area in a straight-action fashion, rather than by the back-action method behind the prominent mesial root that would have to be exercised following amputation of the distal root. Of course, the embrasure problem can be solved orthodontically, if the position of the teeth allows this (Figs 14-20a and 14-20b). The decision as to which root might be extracted is frequently dictated by furcation invasion or tooth position.

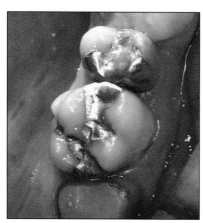

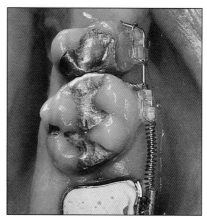

Fig 14-20a The maxillary second molar crown has been lost and the tooth has drifted mesially to touch the first molar and eliminate the embrasure.

Fig 14-20b Orthodontic tooth movement is used to open an embrasure between the molars.

It is necessary to recognize the horizontal level of bone loss on the radiograph. If it measures 7 mm, and the furcation is approximately 5 mm from the CEJ, the clinician can anticipate either a furcation opening or fused roots. In cases of fixed restorative dentistry, it should be noted whether the distal root of the maxillary molar diverges toward the mesial aspect of the second molar or if there is a potential embrasure space apically. If the roots are parallel to one another it is possible that the preparation of both teeth can result in a significant enhancement of the embrasure without orthodontics (see Chapter 2). This can be visualized radiographically.

Vital Root Amputations

There are two reasons to consider vital root amputations for maxillary molars, and both focus on the diagnostic limitations of this area. Surgical procedures are considered to be both investigatory and therapeutic (see Figs 14-17a and 14-17b):

1. The presence of a limited molar embrasure, which makes an accurate furcation probing difficult when the gingival crest is in the area of the cementoenamel junction. The radiograph may be difficult to read, and surgical exposure is necessary to arrive at a decision regarding root resection. If the furcation is not involved or the roots are fused, presurgical endodontics would be a poor decision.

2. The recognition of a furcation involvement in one or two areas of the tooth, where the third furcation seems secure (see Figs 14-19a to 14-19e). Surgical exposure is the only way to be sure that the interradicular inflammatory disease has not resulted in the loss of

bone on the internal surface of the furca between the two remaining roots (Fig 14-21a) and to remove the remaining granulation tissue and to observe the seam of bone and root structure (Fig 14-21b). The removal of a second root might condemn the tooth, and the presumptuous decision to perform presurgical endodontics would be unfair to the patient. It might encourage the clinician to attempt to keep a tooth that should be extracted.

Enough root structure must be exposed so the crown margin will not end in the pulp chamber (see Fig 14-21b). These questions cannot be answered until the root has been amputated; therefore, endodontic therapy is best performed after it is certain that the tooth is saved. Pulp vitality has been demonstrated for up to 10 years after root sectioning by pulp capping rather than by conventional root canal treatment.[43,44] The appropriate time for endodontic treatment is 2 weeks after vital root amputation, when the periodontal surgical wounds have healed. Thermal insulation is provided by the periodontal dressing and the recementation of the provisional crown, if there is one.

Interradicular Periodontal Regeneration

The opportunities for periodontal regeneration are limited for maxillary molars.[21] Regeneration is a possibility when only the buccal furcation is open and the loss of periodontium has not continued between the palatal root and the proximal roots (Figs 14-22a to 14-22h, and 14-23a to 14-23f). This is even more so when there is a buccal wall of bone with an intrabony configuration. Perhaps the most difficult step will be the removal of granulation tissue and root debridement. It is very difficult to use standard

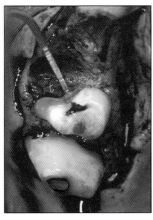

Fig 14-21a After the mesiobuccal root has been removed, the periodontal probe is used to determine whether the internal surface of the furcation between the two remaining roots has been damaged by inflammatory disease.

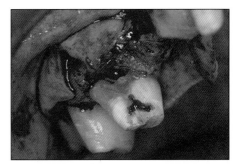

Fig 14-21b It is important to expose enough root structure so that the crown margin will not be placed on the pulp chamber. Additionally, there must be an adequate dimension of tooth structure above bone to prevent violation of the biologic width when the new crown has been placed.

curettes for this procedure because they frequently are larger than the interradicular space, and the use of old, worn instruments can result in the loss of the instrument tip in the furcation (see Fig 14-10). Root preparation can be augmented with small ultrasonic instrumentation, finishing burs, and chemotherapy.[21] It is not crucial to remove all the cementum from the surface because new cementum can form on both old cementum and dentin surfaces (see Chapter 15).

The timing of root sectioning is crucial to the long-term prognosis of the tooth. It is relatively easy to remove a root with complete loss of the supporting structures, but it will be too late if the problem extends to the interradicular periodontium of the remaining two roots (see Figs 14-7 and 14-8). The decision is best made when the furcation is observed to be too deep to allow maintenance of plaque control and there is a fear that it will worsen, as observed surgically. Even perfect osseous resection may not solve such a problem, and careful observation will reveal continued deterioration. The resection of one root may be the best resolution for a deep infrabony pocket when only one furcation is involved (see Figs 14-18a to 14-18h).

Surgical Techniques

A root resection is easily performed on teeth that are prepared for complete-coverage restorations. Surgical access is gained via buccal and palatal flaps; crestal anticipation is used to create the incision line for the palatal flap (Figs 14-24a to 14-24g). It is important to consider the width of the alveolar process when making the determination of how far apically to make the incision. A vertical incision greatly enhances the visibility provided by a palatal flap. The distal

wedge procedure is best performed with concave and convex incisions separated on the distal surface of the last molar by a distance approximating the probing depth on the distal surface of the terminal molar (see Fig 14-24d). The vertical incision at the distobuccal line angle of the distalmost tooth will enable the buccal flap to be positioned at the crest of bone independent of the distal wedge procedure (see Fig 14-24f). The buccal flap of the distal wedge can then be rotated so that there is complete coaption of the tissues, resulting in a flat distal wedge area postsurgically (see Fig 14-24g).

The next surgical step will be to eliminate the collar of tissue that exists around the teeth and expose the seam of bone and tooth structure. Exploration of the furcation with flap reflection provides a true reading as to the depth of furcation involvement. If furcation invasion extends beyond Ricchetti's class IIA (see Chapter 13), it will be impossible to design a restoration that the patient can cleanse, and the tooth preparation should be continued to resect the remaining roots or to extract the tooth.[45] It is frequently necessary to trace the furcation invasion significantly in toward the center of the tooth with tooth preparation before determining invasion in other directions. Once it has been determined that a root is to be removed, then the resection can take place at the expense of that root. This will leave an overhang of tooth structure on the remainder that is removed via odontoplasty (see Figs 14-21a and 14-21b).

It is more difficult to resect a root when the tooth has not been prepared for a provisional crown. Root resection requires a delicate procedure in the presence of a very limited interproximal embrasure between the distobuccal and mesiobuccal roots of approximating maxillary molars. After the surgical flaps are reflected, the furcation openings are located on the buccal and distal (or mesial) surfaces. The tooth structure is then sectioned with a non-crosscutting

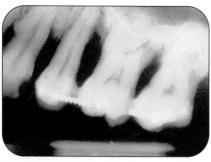 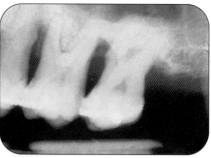

Figs 14-22a and 14-22b There is significant interproximal loss of bone at the maxillary left second premolar and both molars.

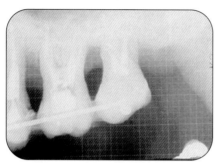 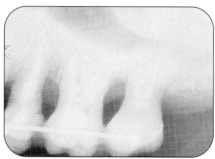

Figs 14-22c and 14-22d The mesial root has been resected from the second molar, and periodontal regeneration procedures, including bone grafts and barrier membranes, have been used to treat the vertical lesions. Note the interproximal regeneration of bone between the teeth.

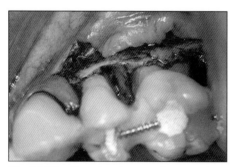

Fig 14-22e Flap elevation reveals severe loss of attachment between the maxillary left premolar and molar as well as between the distal root of the first molar and the second molar.

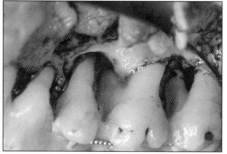

Fig 14-22f The palatal view reveals severe osseous defects; however, these are contained lesions in the apical area. The furcation on the mesial aspect of the first molar is not involved; however, there is furcation involvement on the mesial aspect of the second molar. The mesial root of the second molar was sectioned, and the osseous lesion between the first molar and the premolar was committed to regeneration.

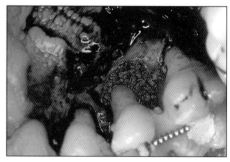

Fig 14-22g A mineralized bone allograft has been placed after degranulation, decortication, and root instrumentation.

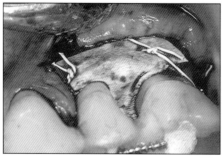

Fig 14-22h An expanded polytetrafluoroethylene interproximal membrane has been placed over the bone graft.

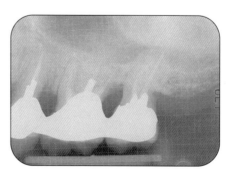

Fig 14-22i Radiograph of the same teeth 5 years after treatment.

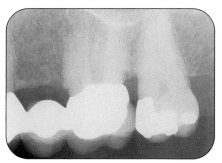

Fig 14-23a The pretreatment radiograph provides no indication of the invasion of the buccal furcation.

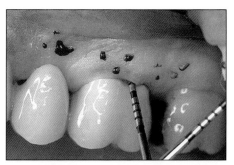

Fig 14-23b A 15-mm probe is in place, showing a 9-mm probing depth associated with the buccal furcation.

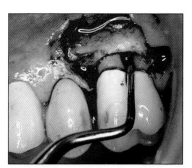

Fig 14-23c A probe shows the presence of a buccal wall of bone with an intrabony configuration.

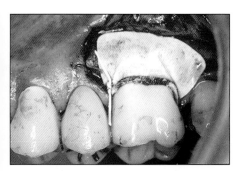

Fig 14-23d An expanded polytetrafluoroethylene membrane is in position, completely covering the buccal furcation.

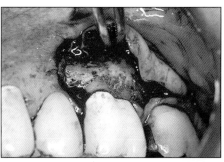

Fig 14-23e Twelve weeks after membrane placement, the membrane is removed and there appears to be complete fill of the buccal furcation.

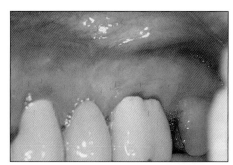

Fig 14-23f The buccal aspect of the first molar is shown 3 months after the membrane has been removed.

fissure bur, apical to the level of the furcations, so as to protect the remaining roots (Figs 14-25a to 14-25c). After the root incision has been completed, the same enamel shaver is used to perform an odontoplasty of the overhanging root trunk and to allow for the delivery of the root without breaking the buccal plate (Figs 14-25d and 14-25e). The instrument of choice is a flat, pointed elevator (see Fig 14-25e). Observation of the extraction socket will reveal a tiny septum of bone on the adjoining tooth that indicates the importance of preserving the buccal plate to provide a contained osseous extraction wound for healing. All remaining granulation tissue is removed, and interdental cratering is eliminated (Fig 14-25f).

The removal of a mesial root is more complicated because the apex usually curves distally, necessitating a path of extraction that collides with the remainder of the tooth (see Figs 14-18a and 14-18b). Great care should be exercised to be sure that the root to be resected has been disconnected from the trunk of the tooth.

Severe loss of proximal bone between maxillary molars may result in the invasion of both proximal furcations (Figs 14-26a to 14-26d, and see 14-19a to 14-19e). If the palatal wall of the interdental crater is reasonably intact and there is no evidence of damage in the mesial furcation of the first molar and the distal furcation of the second molar, the two approximating buccal roots can be extracted. This then provides a view of the interradicular periodontium of the remaining roots. If they are not damaged and the teeth are stable, the periodontal surgery is taken to completion and endodontic therapy is performed 2 weeks later.

It is possible to use only the palatal root of a maxillary molar to retain a tooth, but the opportunities are limited due to prosthetic design complications (Figs 14-27a to 27c, 14-28a, 14-28b, and 14-29a to 14-29d). This technique is limited to stable teeth with long clinical roots for short edentulous spans.[35–40]

All factors considered in root selection for mandibular molars are important for maxillary molars: the state of repair of the tooth; embrasure problems; the pattern of bone loss; and, very importantly, the strategic value of the tooth. The length of the edentulous span and the presence of an opposing tooth are also considerations (see Figs 14-26a to 14-26d).

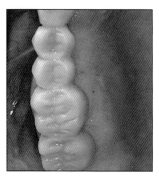

Fig 14-24a A provisional prosthesis is in place prior to periodontal surgery.

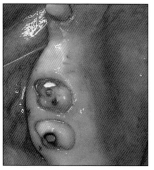

Fig 14-24b The trial restoration has been removed. There are many advantages of placement of the trial restoration, not the least of which is that it allows increased access to the surgical site. Note the perception of health following debridement therapy. It is important not to confuse pink gingiva with periodontal health.

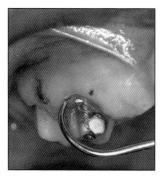

Fig 14-24c A Nabers probe elicits purulent exudate from the buccal furcation.

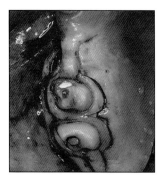

Fig 14-24d The surgical access is gained via buccal and palatal flaps. Crestal anticipation is utilized to create the incision line for the palatal flap. It is critical to consider the width of the alveolar process when making the determination of how far apically to make the incision. The distal wedge procedure has been described as pie shaped; however, concave and convex incisions separated on the distal aspect of the last molar by a distance approximating the probing depth will help considerably in closure.

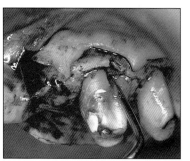

Fig 14-24e A vertical incision enhances the visibility provided by the flaps. A probe is in place to show the vertical component to the furcation lesion. The collar of tissue that exists around the teeth has been removed, and the seam of bone and tooth structure are visible.

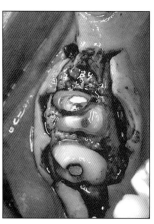

Fig 14-24f The mesiobuccal root has been resected. The plan to remove the mesial root in the absence of the premolars eliminates the need for a mesial wedge.

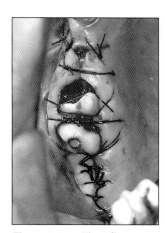

Fig 14-24g The flaps are sutured. The vertical incision of the buccal flap at the distobuccal line angle of the second molar allows the buccal flap to be repositioned for the teeth independently and the distal wedge flaps to close and heal by primary intention.

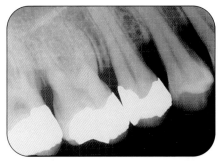

Fig 14-25a There is moderate to advanced loss of attachment on the premolars and advanced loss of periodontal support on the molar teeth. The vertical loss of bone is beyond the level of the furcation.

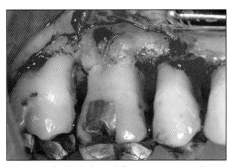

Fig 14-25b Periodontal flap surgery reveals an open distal furcation on the first molar. It is far more difficult to resect a root when the tooth has not been prepared for the provisional crown. Note the divergence of the distobuccal root toward the second molar, limiting the interproximal space apically.

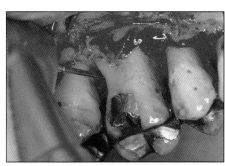

Fig 14-25c The tooth structure is sectioned with a non-crosscutting fissure bur apical to the level of the furcations, to protect the remaining roots.

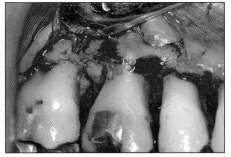

Fig 14-25d The distobuccal root has been resected but has to be elevated without damaging the bony housing. The tooth trunk is reshaped by odontoplasty with the same rotary instrument.

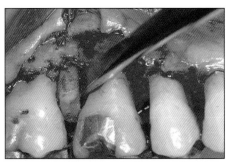

Fig 14-25e After root resection has been completed, the sectioned root is elevated without breaking the buccal plate of bone. The instrument of choice is a flat-ended elevator.

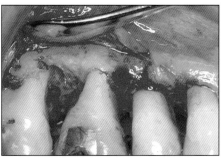

Fig 14-25f Observation of the extraction socket reveals a tiny septum of bone on the mesial surface of the adjacent tooth. This underlines the importance of preserving the buccal plate of bone to provide a contained osseous extraction wound for healing. All remaining degranulation tissue has been removed.

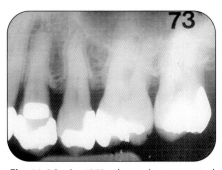

Fig 14-26a In 1973, the patient presented moderate to advanced bone loss in the maxillary left sextant. The patient could not afford to undergo prosthetic rehabilitation and periodontal therapy.

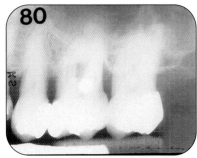

Fig 14-26b The patient returned to the office 7 years later with additional attachment loss associated with the maxillary left first molar. At that time it was deemed necessary to remove the maxillary left first molar and place a four-unit restoration utilizing the mesial and palatal roots of the maxillary left second molar as a distal end abutment.

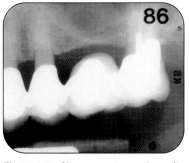

Fig 14-26c Six-year postoperative radiograph (1986).

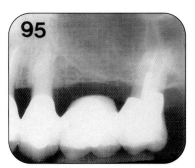

Fig 14-26d Fifteen-year postoperative radiograph (1995). The technique has been successful because the teeth were stable with long clinical roots and there was a short edentulous span.

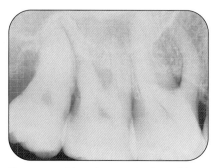

Fig 14-27a There is extensive loss of bone in the furcation and interproximal regions, together with tight embrasures (1971). The third molar is untreatable and requires extraction.

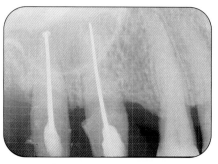

Fig 14-27b Root sectioning of all four buccal roots has been completed, along with endodontic therapy of the palatal roots. Note the size of the palatal roots and the absence of a long edentulous span.

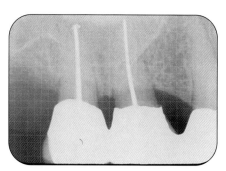

Fig 14-27c Radiograph taken 21 years after surgery. The palatal roots have been successfully retained as abutments for a fixed prosthesis.

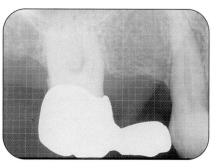

Fig 14-28a This radiograph taken in 1969 shows a cantilever restoration with bone loss in the furcation region.

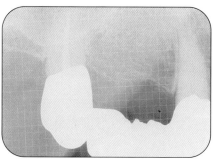

Fig 14-28b Twenty-seven years later, the palatal root is the only posterior abutment as it connects to the canine in the absence of both premolars. This technique is especially useful for treatment of stable teeth with long roots.

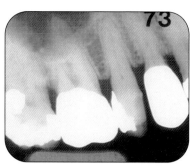

Fig 14-29a The maxillary right posterior teeth demonstrate interproximal bone loss in 1973.

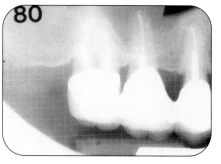

Fig 14-29b Same quadrant with a fixed prosthesis in place (1980). Both buccal roots have been resected from the first molar and the mesiobuccal root has been resected from the second molar.

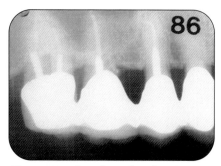

Fig 14-29c A radiograph taken in 1986 reveals no osseous change.

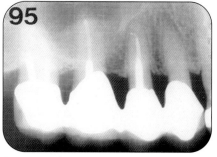

Fig 14-29d A radiograph taken in 1995 reveals long-term stability (22 years) of the periodontium following root resection procedures.

Restorative Considerations

Restorative procedures for sectioned maxillary molars require an approach different from that used for anterior teeth. Sectioned maxillary molars are not in the esthetic zone for most patients, and internalized tooth preparations to provide space for ceramics should be limited to preserve tooth structure. Sometimes the mesial surface of the first molar is an issue for a patient with a broad smile line, but it is most unusual for this to be a factor with second molars. The palatal root is large enough to receive a post and core, but the mesial root resembles the mesial root of the mandibular root and is too fragile. A shallow extension of the palatal post and core can extend into the mesial root to prevent rotation.

Conclusion

The difficulties encountered in treating furcation invasions of maxillary molars should be sufficient to stimulate the clinician to use extensive diagnostics for these teeth. The treatment of an early furcal invasion is more readily provided, and the prognosis is better. Therefore, a probing depth or attachment loss of 5 mm should be taken seriously and result in immediate treatment to prevent a more complicated set of circumstances. Pocket elimination treatment is mandatory, and therefore, the apically repositioned flap is the procedure of choice.

The treatment of the early furcal invasion is less invasive and less costly than treatment of the later problems. It is very important to be responsive to changes in radiographs or in probing depth. Root resection is a strong candidate for treatment of more advanced problems, because the likelihood of proximal furcation regeneration is small.[21]

References

1. Carnevale G, Pontoriero R, Hurgeler M. Management of furcation involvement. Periodontology 2000 1995;9:69.

2. Kalkwarf K, Kadahl WB, Patil KD. Evaluation of furcation region response to periodontal therapy. J Periodontol 1988;59:794–804.

3. Wheeler RC. A Textbook of Dental Anatomy and Physiology. Philadelphia: Saunders, 1968; chap 12.

4. Stambaugh R, Dragoo M, Smith DM, Carasali L. The limitations of subgingival scaling. Int J Periodont Rest Dent 1981;1(5):30–41.

5. Nordland P, Garrett S, Kiger R, Vanooteghem R, Hutchens LH, Egelberg J. The effect of plaque control and root debridement in molar teeth. J Clin Periodontol 1987;14:231–236.

6. Leon LE, Vogel RI. A comparison of the effectiveness of hand scaling and ultrasonic debridement in furcation as evaluated by darkfield microscopy. J Periodontol 1987;58:86–94.

7. Gher ME, Vernino AR. Root morphology—Clinical significance in pathogenesis and treatment of periodontal disease. J Am Dent Assoc 1980;101:627–633.

8. Gher ME, Vernino AR. Root anatomy: A local factor in inflammatory periodontal disease. Int J Periodont Rest Dent 1981;1(5):52–63.

9. Fleischer HC, Mellonig JT, Brayer WK, Gray JL, Barnett JD. Scaling and root planing efficacy in multirooted teeth. J Periodontol 1989;60:402–409.

10. Matia JI, Bissada NF, Maybury JE, Ricchetti P. Efficiency of scaling of the molar furcation area with and without surgical access. Int J Periodont Rest Dent 1986;6(6):24–35.

11. Parashis AO, Anagnou-Vareltzides A, Demetriou N. Calculus removal from multirooted teeth with and without surgical access. II. Comparison between external and furcation surfaces and effect of furcation entrance width. J Clin Periodontol 1993;20:294–298.

12. Svärdström G, Wennström JL. Furcation topography of maxillary and mandibular first molars. J Clin Periodontol 1988;15:271–275.

13. Bower RC. Furcation morphology relative to periodontal treatment: Furcation entrance architecture. J Periodontol 1979;50:23–27.

14. Bower RC. Furcation morphology relative to periodontal treatment: Furcation root surface anatomy. J Periodontol 1979;50:366–374.

15. Bissada NF, Abdelmalek RG. Incidence of cervical enamel projections and its relationship to furcation involvement in Egyptian skulls. J Periodontol 1973;44:583–585.

16. Larato DC. Some anatomical factors related to furcation involvements. J Periodontol 1975;46:608–609.

17. Leib AM, Berdon JK, Sabes WR. Furcation involvements correlated with enamel projections from the cemento-enamel junction. J Periodontol 1967;38:330–334.

18. Grewe JM, Meskin LH, Miller T. Cervical enamel projections: Prevalence, location and extent—With associated periodontal implications. J Periodontol 1965;36:460–465.

19. Masters DH, Hoskins SW. Projection of cervical enamel into molar furcations. J Periodontol 1964;35:49–53.

20. Swan RH, Hurt WC. Cervical enamel projections as an etiologic factor in furcation involvement. J Am Dent Assoc 1976;93:342–345.

21. Pontoriero R, Lindhe J. Guided tissue regeneration in the treatment of degree II furcations in maxillary molars. J Clin Periodontol 1995;22:756–763.

22. Schallhorn R, McClain P. Combined osseous composite grafting, root conditioning and guided tissue regeneration. Int J Periodont Rest Dent 1988;8(4):9–31.

23. McClain P, Schallhorn R. Long-term assessment of combined osseous composite grafting, root conditioning and guided tissue regeneration. Int J Periodont Rest Dent 1993;13(1):9–27.

24. Purisi T. Masters thesis [unpublished]. Boston University School of Graduate Dentistry, 1980.

25. Hamp SE, Nyman S, Lindhe J. Periodontal treatment of multirooted teeth: Results after 5 years. J Clin Periodontol 1975;2:126–135.

26. Hirschfeld L, Wasserman B. A long term survey of tooth loss in 600 treated periodontal patients. J Periodontol 1978;49:225–237.

27. Bjorn AL, Hjort P. Bone loss of furcated mandibular molars: A longitudinal study. J Clin Periodontol 1982;9:402–408.

28. McFall WT. Tooth loss in 100 treated patients with periodontal disease: A long term study. J Periodontol 1982;53:539–549.

29. Goldman MJ, Ross IF, Goteiner D. Effect of periodontal therapy on patients maintained for 15 years or longer: A retrospective study. J Periodontol 1986;57:347–353.

30. Becker W, Berg L, Becker BE. The long term evaluation of periodontal treatment and maintenance in 95 patients. Int J Periodont Rest Dent 1984;4(2):54–71.

31. Ross OF, Thompson RH. A long term study of root retention in the treatment of maxillary molars with furcation involvement. J Periodontol 1978;49:238–244.

32. Martin M, Gantes B, Garrett S, Egelberg J. Treatment of periodontal furcation defects. I. Review of the literature and description of a regenerative surgical technique. J Clin Periodontol 1988;15:227–231.

33. Wang HL, Burgett FC, Shyr Y, Ramfjord S. The influence of molar furcation involvement and mobility of future clinical periodontal attachment loss. J Periodontol 1994;65:25–29.

34. Becker W, Berg L, Becker BE. Untreated periodontal disease: A longitudinal study. J Periodontol 1979;50:234–244.

35. Carnevale G, DiFebo G, Tonelli MP, Marin C, Fuzzi MA. Retrospective analysis of the periodontal-prosthetic treatment of molars with interradicular lesions. Int J Periodont Rest Dent 1991;11:189–205.

36. Langer G, Stein SD, Wagenberg B. An evaluation of root resections: A ten year study. J Periodontol 1981;52:719–722.

37. Klavan B. Clinical observation following root amputation in maxillary molar teeth. J Periodontol 1975;46:1–5.

38. Bergenholtz A. Radectomy of multi-rooted teeth. J Am Dent Assoc 1972;85:870–875.

39. Erpenstein H. A three year study of hemisected molars. J Clin Periodontol 1983;10:1–10.

40. Buhler H. Evaluation of root resected teeth: Results after ten years. J Periodontol 1988;59:805–810.

41. Basten CH-J, Ammons WF Jr, Persson R. Long term evaluation of root resected molars: A retrospective study. Int J Periodont Rest Dent 1996;16:207–219.

42. Blomlöf L, Jansson L, Applegren R, Ehnevid H, Lindskog S. Prognosis and mortality of root-resected molars. Int J Periodont Rest Dent 1997;17:191–201.

43. Haskell T, Stanley H. A review of vital root resection. Int J Periodont Rest Dent 1982;2(6):29–49.

44. Smukler H, Tagger M. Vital root amputation: A clinical and histologic study. J Periodontol 1976;47:324–330.

45. Ricchetti P. A furcation classification based upon pulp chamber: Furcation relationships and vertical radiographic bone loss. Int J Periodont Rest Dent 1982;2(5):51–59.

Periodontal Regeneration: Bone Grafts

James T. Mellonig, DDS, MS

The ideal goal of periodontal therapy is the reconstruction of bone and connective tissue that have been destroyed by the disease process. Bone grafting is one of the therapeutic modalities employed to fulfill this goal. The objectives of this procedure are pocket reduction or elimination; gain in clinical attachment; restoration of lost alveolar bone; and regeneration of a functional attachment apparatus. The first three objectives can be assessed by clinical measurements and radiographs; the fourth can only be determined through histologic analysis. Currently, bone grafting is the only therapy for which there is significant histologic evidence in humans for regeneration of new bone, new cementum, and a new periodontal ligament about tooth surface that was once contaminated by bacterial plaque.[1] This does not imply that periodontal bone graft therapy is uniformly successful, routinely predictable, or always heals with restoration of the entire attachment apparatus. Healing may occasionally occur by a renewed sulcus of significant depth, adherence of a long junctional epithelium to the root surface, adhesion of connective tissue fibers oriented parallel to the root surface, or insertion of connective tissue fibers into new cementum (new attachment).[2]

Definitions

Periodontal regeneration has its own particular terminology. These terms warrant definition to prevent confusion in semantics:

Active bone formation. When osteogenic precursor cells of the graft survive the transplantation process and form new bone.

Allograft. A tissue (bone) graft between individuals of the same species but of nonidentical genetic disposition. An allograft was formerly referred to as a *homograft*.

Alloplast. A synthetic bone graft material; a bone graft substitute.

Attachment apparatus. The cementum, the periodontal ligament, and the alveolar bone.

Autograft. A tissue (bone) graft transferred from one position to a new position in the body of the same individual. Periodontal autografts may be intraoral or extraoral.

Bone fill. The presence of bone tissue within a periodontal osseous defect following therapy.

Graft. Anything (specifically, a piece of bone) inserted into something else so as to become an integral part of the latter.

Implant. To insert or graft a material into intact tissues of a host; implies surgical transfer of nonliving tissue (nonviable bone).

Intraosseous defect. A bone defect within the structure of alveolar bone. An angular bone defect composed of one, two, three, or a combination of bony walls.

New attachment. Formation of new cementum with the insertion of new connective tissue fibers about a tooth root surface previously exposed to bacterial plaque.

Osteoconduction. Process in which the graft acts as a trellis or scaffold over which new host bone can form.

Osteoinduction. Process in which new bone is induced to form through the action of factors contained within the grafted bone, such as proteins or growth factors.

Regeneration. The formation of new bone, new cementum, and periodontal ligament about a tooth root surface previously exposed to bacterial plaque.

Repair. The healing of a wound by tissue that does not fully restore the architecture or the function of the part, ie, scar tissue.

Transplant. To transfer tissue from one part to another as in grafting; implies surgical transfer of living tissue (viable bone).

Xenograft. A tissue (bone) graft between members of differing species, ie, animal to man. A xenograft was formerly referred to as a *heterograft.*

Indications for Periodontal Bone Grafts

The indications for osseous grafts include but are not limited to the following.

Deep Intraosseous Defects

The deeper the defect, the greater amount of bone fill that can be expected; at the same time, the residual defect may be significant. For example, if the osseous defect measures 8 mm in depth and a 75%, or 6-mm, bone fill is achieved, the residual bone defect will be 2 mm. This may require a renewed attempt at grafting, osseous resective therapy, or maintenance of a potentially compromised lesion. On the other hand, a 3-mm defect with the same percentage of bone fill will heal with a residual defect of less than 1 mm.

It is the opinion of many clinicians that the greater the number of osseous walls and the greater the support and containment for the graft material, the greater will be the bone fill. The degree of regeneration in an osseous defect of a given volume and morphology varies directly with the adequacy of the soft tissue cover and with the surface area of the vascularized bony walls lining the defect; it varies inversely with the root surface area.[3] Therefore, a three-wall defect should heal with more bone fill than a two-wall or a one-wall lesion, and a one-wall defect should heal better than a furcation defect. Furthermore, intraosseous defects caused by periodontal abscesses or pulpal pathosis will respond favorably with bone fill without a graft, following appropriate emergency or endodontic therapy.

Tooth Retention

The use of bone grafts may restore functional stability to such a degree as to obviate the need for extraction.

Support for Critical Teeth

Teeth severely weakened by loss of alveolar support can benefit from the use of osseous grafts. This may be the case for an abutment tooth or those teeth that are critical for the preservation of arch integrity.

Bone Defects Associated With Juvenile Periodontitis

These extensive lesions have been reported to respond very favorably to osseous grafting, especially when grafting is combined with an antibiotic, such as tetracycline.[4,5]

Esthetics (Shallow Intraosseous Defects)

The resection of shallow intraosseous defects in the anterior region of the mouth by osteoplasty/ostectomy followed by an apically positioned flap to eliminate the periodontal pocket will result in gingival recession and a long clinical crown. This may be esthetically unacceptable. The use of osseous grafts to reconstruct bone architecture allows placement of the gingival margin as close as possible to its original position. Successful healing will result in minimal apical displacement of the gingival margin.[6]

Furcation Defects

This indication applies mainly to class II furcation defects. Bone grafts, especially if used in conjunction with guided tissue regeneration, have proven to be the therapeutic modality of choice for treating this type of lesion. However, the results are variable.[7,8]

Anatomic Limitations for Other Procedures

The relationship of mandibular molars to the external oblique ridge associated with intraosseous defects presents an anatomic problem that may not be corrected by osseous surgery. Intraosseous defects that closely approximate the maxillary sinus pose a similar problem. Osseous grafting procedures are often necessary to manage such areas.

Other Considerations

The use of bone grafts is also dictated by patient acceptance, economic factors, availability of graft material, case selection, and clinical experience. The therapist's lack of clinical experience often terminates in discouraging results.

Types of Bone Graft Materials

There are several types of periodontal bone graft materials that are, or have been, used in periodontal therapy. These include autografts, allografts, xenografts, and alloplasts. Periodontal autografts are considered to be vital, and all other graft materials are nonvital. Bone is formed in response to graft materials in overlapping phases.

The first wound-healing phase is revascularization. Revascularization is initiated within the first few days following the grafting procedure. Blood vessels originating from the host bone invade the graft. A pore size of 100 to 200 μm is very conducive to vascular invasion. Revascularization is followed by the incorporation of the grafted bone particles by new bone emanating from the host. If the graft material contains vital osteogenic precursor cells that survive the transplantation process, these cells may contribute to new bone formation. The graft may possess inductive proteins that actively stimulate the host to form new bone (osteoinduction), or the graft may simply act passively as a lattice network over which the new host bone forms (osteoconduction).

As the graft is being incorporated, it is gradually resorbed and replaced by new host bone. This process is sometimes referred to as *creeping substitution*. The final phase of healing is bone remodeling. Resorption, replacement, and remodeling take many years. Large allografts may never be fully resorbed and replaced.[9] Most alloplasts do not undergo resorption, replacement, or remodeling. Formation of new bone, new cementum, and a new periodontal ligament has been reported to occur following most types of autograft and allografts but not alloplasts.[1]

Autogenous Bone Grafts

Autogenous bone grafts are believed to be preferable to other types of graft materials because they contain viable cells. These cells, one transplanted, may go on to actively form new bone. Unless an autogenous graft is in close apposition to a vascular supply, it will not survive the transplantation process.[9] Therefore, most autografts function as osteoinductive or osteoconductive agents. The healing sequence of an autogenous periodontal bone graft has been identified as initiation of new bone formation at 7 days, cementogenesis at 21 days, and a new periodontal ligament at 3 months. By 8 months, the graft should be fully incorporated into the host with functionally oriented fibers coursing between bone and cementum.[10] Maturation may take as long as 2 years.

Cortical bone chips, osseous coagulum, bone blend, and intraoral and extraoral cancellous bone and marrow are included in the category of periodontal autograft.

Cortical Bone Chips

The impetus for the modern-day use of periodontal bone grafts can be traced to the work of Nabers and O'Leary.[11] They reported that shavings of cortical bone removed by hand chisels during osteoplasty/ostectomy from sites within the surgical area could be used successfully to effect a coronal increase in bone height. Cortical chips, because of their relatively large particle size and potential for sequestration, were replaced by autogenous osseous coagulum and bone blend techniques. There is evidence of new bone, cementum, and periodontal ligament following this type of graft.[12]

Osseous Coagulum

Intraoral bone, when obtained with high- or low-speed burs and mixed with blood, becomes a coagulum.[13] The rationale for the use of osseous coagulum is the belief that the smaller the particle of the donor bone, the more certain its resorption and replacement with host bone. The disadvantages of this technique were the unknown quantity and quality of the collected bone fragments; the inability to aspirate during the collection process for fear of aspirating graft material; and complications of salivary contamination and bleeding.

Bone Blend

The bone blend technique was devised to overcome the disadvantages of the osseous coagulum technique.[14] Cortical and cancellous bone is procured with a trephine or rongeurs, placed in an amalgam capsule used only for the purpose of blending, and triturated for 10 to 30 seconds to the consistency of a slushy osseous mass. A controlled clinical study showed that the osseous coagulum–bone blend type of graft provided 2.98 mm of coronal growth of new bone, compared with the 0.66 mm of growth that was obtained when open flap debridement was used.[15] A mean bone fill of 75% in 25 defects has also been reported.[16] Regeneration of the periodontium has been documented with osseous coagulum–bone blend type of graft.[17,18]

Intraoral Cancellous Bone and Marrow

Healing extraction sockets, edentulous ridges, mandibular retromolar areas, and the maxillary tuberosity have all been used as sources of intraoral cancellous bone and marrow.[19–22] The most productive source appears to be an 8- to 12-week healing extraction socket. Bone fill in all types of intraosseous and furcation defects has been demonstrated with this material. A mean bone fill of 3.65 mm, with bone fill of up to 12 mm in some defects and more than 50% fill on a predictable basis has been reported.[19,22] Histologic evidence of new bone cementum and periodontal ligament has been provided.[19,20,23]

Extraoral Cancellous Bone and Marrow

It is generally agreed that extraoral cancellous bone and marrow from the iliac crest offer the greatest osteogenic potential. Reports of complete eradication of furcation and interproximal two-wall "crater" defects spurred interest in this material.[7,24] Subsequent reports attested to the efficacy of this material to successfully treat furcations, dehiscences, and intraosseous defects of varying morphology. Mean clinical bone fill of 3.33 mm in 182 defects and 4.36 mm in seven defects has been reported. In addition, a mean bone apposition of 2.54 mm in crestal or zero-wall defects has been documented.[25] New bone, cementum, and periodontal ligament is a result of treatment.[26] However, the root resorption associated with fresh iliac cancellous bone and marrow has limited the use of this material.[27]

Bone Allografts

The need of an allogeneic source or substitute for autogenous bone arose from the need for a supply of donor material to fill multiple or deep bone defects within the same patient and the morbidity accompanying a second surgical site to procure donor bone. There are two types of bone allografts in routine use: mineralized freeze-dried bone allograft and demineralized freeze-dried bone allograft. The terms *decalcified* and *demineralized* are used interchangeably. In addition, allogeneic, autolyzed, antigen-extracted (AAA) bone, demineralized bone powder, demineralized bone matrix, and demineralized bone matrix gelatin can be thought of as synonymous with decalcified freeze-dried bone, although there are differences in the processing of these materials.

Disease transfer is a concern for both the patient and the clinician. There has never been a reported case of disease transfer with mineralized or demineralized freeze-dried bone allograft. The risk of disease transfer with a fresh frozen bone allograft has been calculated to be approximately one in 2 million if the tissue bank uses exclusionary techniques.[28] The risk for disease transfer for freeze-dried bone has been calculated at 1 in 2.8 billion.

These exclusionary techniques may include (1) omission of donors from high-risk groups by medical and social screening—unless reliable information regarding previous hospitalizations, blood transfusions, serious illness, and lifestyle can be acquired, a donor must be regarded as unacceptable; (2) human immunodeficiency virus (HIV) antibody and antigen testing—a positive test excludes the procurement of donor tissue; (3) autopsy to rule out occult disease such as carcinoma; (4) special lymph node studies beyond those usually performed at autopsy—such studies are performed to recognize changes characteristic of early HIV infection and provide another opportunity to exclude individuals with morphologic nodal changes typical of nonspecific infection (eg, bacterial, viral, parasitic, or fungal infection and chronic infection or drug use); (5) blood cultures for bacterial contamination; (6) serologic tests for syphilis and all types of hepatitis; (7) follow-up studies of grafts from the same donor—a significant number of the tissue bank's bone donors may also be donors of vital organs. With the exception of fresh bone allografts, months usually pass between procurement and the clinical use of a processed bone allograft. If a vital organ recipient were to be identified as having HIV or another related illness, the bone from the donor would not be released for clinical use.

In addition, there is evidence that freeze-drying, washing with ethyl alcohol, and demineralization with an acid at low pH, will inactivate the HIV virus.[29–32] Processing a bone allograft contaminated with HIV in this manner has been shown to inactivate HIV, which, under extremely rare circumstances, may go undetected by exclusionary techniques.[33] Immunologic concerns are likewise unfounded because anti-HLA antibodies are not detected in recipients of freeze-dried bone allograft for treatment of periodontal bone defects.[34]

Bone allografts are procured usually within 12 hours of death of a suitable donor. The sequence of processing differs among tissue banks, but usually includes the following steps:

1. Cortical bone is harvested in a sterile manner. This negates the need for a secondary means of sterilization. Long bones are the source for periodontal bone allografts. Cortical bone is the material of choice because it is less antigenic than cancellous bone and contains a greater concentration of inductive proteins.

2. The cortical bone is rough cut to a particle size ranging from 500 μm to 5 mm. This fragmentation increases the efficiency of the defatting and demineralization of the graft.

3. The graft material is then immersed in 100% ethyl alcohol or a similar solvent for 1 hour to remove fat that may inhibit osteogenesis. Furthermore, ethyl alcohol and other defatting agents have virucidal activity. This procedure may be done several times.

4. The cortical bone is ground and sieved to a particle size range of approximately 250 to 750 μm. Particle

sizes within this range have been shown to promote osteogenesis, whereas particle sizes below 125 μm may promote a significant foreign-body giant cell response and are rapidly resorbed.[35]

5. Decalcification with 0.6 or 0.5 N hydrochloric acid removes the calcium, leaves the bone matrix, and exposes the bone-inductive proteins. This step is bypassed if mineralized freeze-dried bone is the desired end product for orthopedic or oral surgical applications where structural stability is necessary.

6. The bone is washed in a sodium phosphate buffer to remove residual acid.

7. The cortical bone is frozen at −80°C for 1 to 2 weeks to interrupt the degradation process. During this time, the results from bacterial cultures, serologic tests, and antibody and antigen assays are analyzed. If contamination is found, the bone is discarded or sterilized by additional methods and so labeled.

Freeze-drying removes more than 95% of the water content from the bone. It preserves three major specimen characteristics: size, solubility, and chemical integrity. Although freeze-drying destroys all cells and the graft is rendered nonviable, it has the advantage of reducing antigenicity and facilitating long-term storage. Vacuum sealing in glass containers protects against contamination and degradation of the graft material while permitting storage at room temperature for an indefinite period of time.

Mineralized Freeze-Dried Bone Allograft

Mineralized freeze-dried bone allograft (FDBA) was introduced to periodontal therapy in 1976.[36] This material is osteoconductive. Although FDBA contains inductive proteins, the polypeptides are sequestered by calcium. This material is resorbed and replaced by host bone very slowly. Freeze-dried bone allograft is the only graft material that has undergone extensive field testing for the treatment of adult periodontitis.[37] Eighty-nine clinicians implanted a total of 997 sites with FDBA alone and 534 sites with FDBA plus autogenous bone (FDBA+A). Sufficient data, as determined by surgical reentry at 6 months, were collected to determine results in 329 defects treated with FDBA alone and in 176 sites treated with FDBA+A. Complete or more than 50% bone fill was obtained in 220 (67%) of sites treated with FDBA and 137 (78%) of the sites treated with with FDBA+A. Significant probing depth reduction occurred in 69% (FDBA) and 79% (FDBA+A) of the sites. Field testing suggested that the combination of FDBA with autogenous bone was a more efficacious treatment than FDBA alone, especially in the treatment of furcation defects.

Altiere et al[38] investigated FDBA sterilized with 3 Mrads of gamma-irradiation and compared it with a nongraft procedure for debridement in 10 paired sites. Both grafted and nongrafted sites demonstrated more than 50% bone fill in 60% of the sites. A composite graft of FDBA and tetracycline in a 4:1 volume ratio has shown promise in the treatment of the osseous defects associated with localized juvenile periodontitis. A study in 12 patients with juvenile periodontitis revealed that bone fill and resolution of the osseous defects are significantly greater in grafted sites than in nongrafted control sites.[5]

Decalcified Freeze-Dried Bone Allograft

Decalcified freeze-dried bone allograft (DFDBA) has been shown to induce new bone formation by osteoinduction (Figs 15-1a to 15-1c).[39,40] The osteogenic potential of DFDBA was compared to that of autogenous bone and FDBA in calvarial defects of guinea pigs. It was concluded that DFDBA is a graft material of high osteogenic potential; the autogenous materials have less osteogenic potential, and FDBA has even less potential.[41,42] This suggests that DFDBA may have clinical application and may be a superior allograft for dental applications. Demineralization with hydrochloric acid exposes the bone-inductive proteins located in the bone matrix. These proteins are collectively referred to as *bone morphogenetic protein* (BMP). They are composed of a group of acidic polypeptides that have been cloned and sequenced.[43] Some of the BMPs are available in human recombinant form for research purposes.

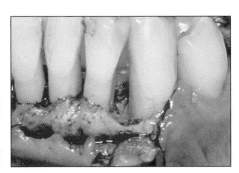

Fig 15-1a Two-wall intraosseous defect on the mesial surface of the mandibular left canine.

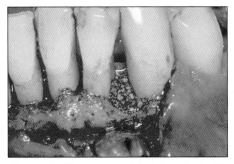

Fig 15-1b The osseous defect is grafted with decalcified freeze-dried bone allograft.

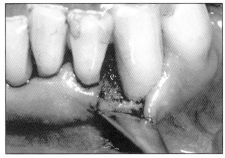

Fig 15-1c Complete bone fill with 1.0 to 2.0 mm of crestal bone apposition is found at the 12-month postsurgery reentry.

Libin et al[44] were the first to report the use of cortical and cancellous DFDBA in humans. The three grafted sites responded with 4 to 10 mm of new bone formation. Cortical DFDBA was evaluated in 27 intraosseous periodontal defects and yielded a mean of 2.4 mm.[45] In six patients, Werbitt[46] showed bone fill ranging from 75% to 95% of the original defect. The radiographic analysis of sites treated with cancellous DFDBA revealed a mean bone fill of 1.38 mm, whereas control sites showed 0.33 mm.[47] The reason for meager bone fill following a graft of DFDBA may lie in the fact that the bone-inductive proteins are located in the bone matrix.[48] Because the mass of bone matrix is lower in cancellous bone than in cortical bone, the yield of new bone could be expected to be lower.[49] Another controlled study found a mean bone fill of 2.6 mm (65% defect fill) in sites treated with cortical DFDBA and 1.3 mm (38%) in sites treated without DFDBA.[6] The single study that directly compared FDBA and DFDBA in human periodontal osseous defects could not determine any statistical difference.[50] This result may be reflective of insufficient inductive proteins in the volume of DFDBA grafted or in the types and depths of the grafted lesions. It was subsequently found that the addition of an inductive protein (BMP-3/Osteogenin) to DFDBA significantly enhances its osteogenic potential.[51]

Xenografts

Xenografts are not acceptable for human use because of their immunogenic properties. Os purum, anorganic bone, and Boplant are some of the xenografts that have been used in the past to treat the bone defects of periodontitis. These materials are usually of a bovine source and are treated by a number of chemical processes to render the graft acceptable for human implantation. The widespread clinical use that followed reports of successful Boplant use resulted in routine rejection and failure.[52] From time to time, xenografts appear on the market, but are subsequently withdrawn.

Alloplasts

A wide variety of alloplastic materials have been suggested for use in periodontal therapy. These include plaster of paris, polymers, calcium carbonates, tricalcium phosphate, crystalline hydroxyapatite, dense hydroxyapatite, porous hydroxyapatite, and bioglass. Some of these materials are resorbable to varying degrees, but most are nonresorbable. Clinical results with alloplastic materials are essentially similar to results obtained with autogenous or allogeneic materials.[53] The choice of material then becomes based more on availability, cost, morbidity, and ease of handling than on clinical superiority. Histologically, sites grafted with autogenous or allogeneic bone heal by regeneration, whereas sites grafted with synthetic materials heal with fibrous encapsulation of the synthetic graft particles. If a clinical objective is regeneration of the periodontium, then the choice of materials is autograft or allograft. If repair is an acceptable objective, then an alloplast will suffice.

Technique for Periodontal Bone Grafting

Periodontal bone grafting is technique sensitive. The feasibility of the procedure is dictated by the level of success to which the clinician aspires. Those procedures demanding total osseous reconstruction, supracrestal bone apposition, or complete bone fill of the defect will have a lower level of success than those accepting partial fill. Although bone grafting may not be completely successful in eliminating the defect, it may convert defects into residual osseous defects that are amenable to regrafting or that may be managed by osseous resective techniques.

Patient Selection

At the minimum, the patient selected for a periodontal bone graft procedure should be in good physical health, have a positive attitude toward therapy, have repeatedly demonstrated an acceptable level of plaque control, and be committed to a periodontal maintenance program. Informed consent should be obtained prior to beginning the procedure.

Defect Selection

Most often, the site selected for a bone graft procedure will present with deep probing depths (greater than 7.0 mm) and bleeding on probing (Fig 15-2a). Clinical attachment loss over time also indicates the need for surgical intervention. The preoperative radiograph will usually confirm the presence of a vertical bone defect, depending on the location of the defect and thickness of the alveolar cortical plates. A minimal amount of gingival recession is a positive factor for successful therapy. The closer the gingival margin is to or above the cementoenamel junction, the more soft tissue there will be to cover the wound. Complete wound closure is considered essential for success. Extensive gingival recession and/or soft tissue cratering are contraindications for bone grafting. Therefore, it may be considered feasible to forego subgingival instrumentation where it is certain that resolution of gingival inflammation will result in soft tissue deformities that might preclude complete wound closure.

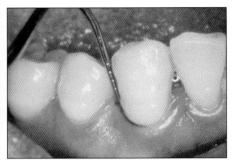

Fig 15-2a Probing depth and attachment loss are measured at 6.0 mm.

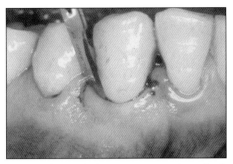

Fig 15-2b A sulcular incision is made on both the facial and lingual aspects to preserve as much soft tissue as possible.

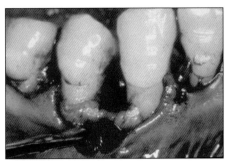

Fig 15-2c The flaps are reflected the minimum distance necessary to gain access to the flaps for debridement and root planing.

Anesthesia

Prior to administration of anesthesia, the patient's mouth is rinsed with chlorhexidine to reduce the oral bioburden. Depending on the surgical site, block or infiltration anesthesia may be used. The local anesthetic should contain a vasoconstrictor because good hemostasis is important for visualization of the defect and the root surface. Excessive bleeding at the graft site has a negative influence on results. An intraligamentary injection is sometimes useful to control bleeding but should be used with caution because the combination of thin papillae and a vasoconstrictor may lead to necrosis.

Graft Procurement and Preparation

If the patient has sufficient donor sites, an intraoral bone autograft is the material of first choice. Autogenous bone can be procured from a healing extraction socket, edentulous ridge, or exostoses. A No. 8 round bur used at slow speed, back-action chisel, rongeurs, or large curettes are instruments that can be used for harvesting the bone, depending on the circumstances. The autogenous bone is placed in a sterile receptacle, such as a Dappen dish, and covered with saline-moistened gauze to prevent dehydration until the defect is prepared for graft insertion.

If the patient does not have sufficient intraoral donor sites, a demineralized freeze-dried bone allograft is the appropriate substitute. The allograft is reconstituted with a solution of 50 mg of tetracycline per mL of sterile water. The rationale is that the addition of an antibiotic will provide a zone of antibacterial activity and have an anticollagenolytic effect during the critical stages of wound healing.[56] The concentration of 50 mg/mL of solution is important because a greater concentration may be toxic to bone-forming cells rather than act as a chemoattractant.

Synthetic grafts are used when neither an autograft nor an allograft is feasible.

Flap Design and Reflection

Sulcular incisions to bone are made on both the facial and lingual aspects (Fig 15-2b). The incisions are carried as far as possible interproximally to preserve the entire interproximal papilla. Gingival thinning techniques are avoided. Maximum tissue conservation and preservation of vascular integrity are the desired outcomes. The flap is extended as far as is necessary to the mesial and distal of the surgical site to gain access for debridement and root planing. Vertical releasing incisions are avoided if possible.

Once the tissues are incised, the interproximal papillae are gently elevated to make sure they are freely movable; this will prevent undue trauma to the flap during reflection (Fig 15-2c). Full-thickness flaps are reflected 2 to 3 mm beyond the alveolar crest. If the flaps are extended beyond the mucogingival junction, some degree of gingival recession can be expected.

Soft Tissue Debridement

After flap reflection, granulation tissue and adherent connective tissue tags are judiciously removed from the inner surface of the flaps (Fig 15-2d). Excessive thinning should be avoided. All granulation tissue, including fibers at the base of the osseous defect, must be removed. Ultrasonic instrumentation is particularly effective in removing tenacious soft tissue. Bleeding within the defect should rapidly subside once all granulation tissue is debrided. If bleeding

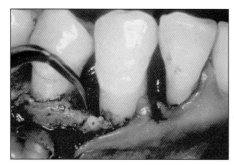

Fig 15-2d All soft tissue is carefully debrided from all aspects of the osseous defect.

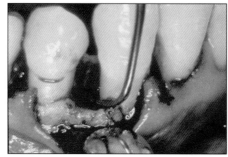

Fig 15-2e Root planing is accomplished to an end point of a clean, smooth root surface. The root surface is then conditioned with citric acid (pH 1) or tetracycline (50 µm/mL).

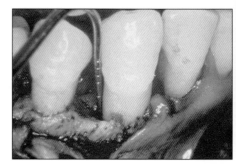

Fig 15-2f The osseous defect measures 4 mm from the alveolar crest to the base of the defect.

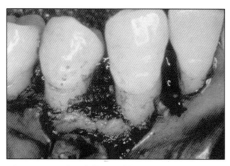

Fig 15-2g The defect is filled to a level slightly above the crest of the osseous defect.

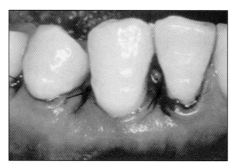

Fig 15-2h A monofilament suture is used to position the flaps so as to obtain complete wound closure.

persists, it can usually be controlled with pressure and saline-moistened gauze or hemostatic agents. If bleeding cannot be controlled, adequate visualization of the root surface cannot be achieved; the success of the procedure will be jeopardized, and an alternate treatment modality should be pursued.

Root Planing

Meticulous removal of all hard accretions, soft deposits, and altered cementum is essential for success (Fig 15-2e). The root surface may first be debrided with ultrasonic instrumentation and then planed with hand instrumentation. An acceptable end point is a root surface that appears white and clean and is smooth to tactile sensation. A fiberoptic light source and magnifying loupes may be used as adjuncts.

Depending on the operator's preference, root surface chemotherapy may now be employed. The tetracycline solution (50 mg/mL) used for the reconstitution of the allograft is now applied to the root surface with a cotton pellet for 3 minutes. The rationale is that demineralization of the root surface will expose intact collagen fibers, remove the smear layer, detoxify the root surface, and provide some antibacterial activity.[55] Citric acid is also frequently used with a similar rationale. The depth of the defect can now be measured (Fig 15-2f).

Intramarrow Penetration

This step may or may not be used, depending on the character of the bone lining the defect. A lining of cancellous bone does not require exposure of the marrow spaces. If the defect is lined by cortical bone, a No. ½ round bur is used to perforate the cortical plate. Theoretically, this should allow the egress and proliferation of undifferentiated mesenchymal cells from the marrow spaces. This may also aid in clot promotion and revascularization of the graft.

Graft Placement

Excess solution (tetracycline, 50 mg/mL) is removed from the graft material by blotting with cotton gauze. The graft is carried to the site with a suitable instrument; a large amalgam carrier is frequently the instrument of choice. The graft material is packed firmly into the defect in a step-by-step fashion until the entire defect is filled with the graft relative to the level of the existing osseous walls. After each increment of graft material is placed, it is blotted with saline-moistened gauze to absorb excessive blood and fluid. A slight overfill approach may be used with the understanding that excessive graft material will impede flap closure (Fig 15-2g).

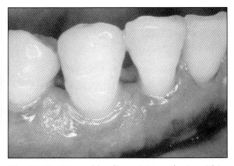

Fig 15-2i Wound healing at 2 weeks is within normal limits; slight soft cratering is noted.

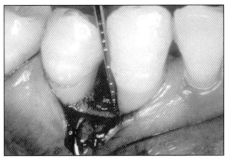

Fig 15-2j Complete bone fill of the osseous defect is revealed at surgical reentry of the defect 1 year postsurgery.

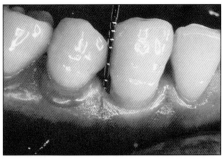

Fig 15-2k Three years posttreatment, the 2.0-mm probing depth has been maintained.

Wound Closure

Every attempt is made to cover the graft site completely with soft tissue (Fig 15-2h). If, after the flaps are replaced, the interdental papillae do not abut, judicious scalloping of the gingival margin on the facial and/or lingual aspects may be necessary to achieve the desired result. If conditions permit, a slight reduction in the width of the interproximal bone on the facial or lingual aspect can also be used to assist in flap closure. Care should be taken not to reduce the bony walls lining the defect.

Suturing

A vertical mattress or interrupted suturing technique is used to close the flaps. Use of a monofilament suturing material is best. Once the wound is sutured, firm finger pressure is applied with gauze moistened in saline to the facial and lingual surfaces of the wound area. This will maximize healing by allowing only a thin blood clot to develop between the tooth and the flap.

Periodontal Dressing

A periodontal dressing is placed to protect the wound from trauma and to act as a stent. Verbal and written postoperative instructions are given to the patient. A mild analgesic, such as a nonsteroidal anti-inflammatory drug, is usually all that is necessary to control postsurgical discomfort. The analgesic is taken at least 4 hours before the commencement of the procedure. Systemic antibiotic coverage is prescribed, with the rationale that it aids in the control of the putative periodontal pathogens. Doxycycline, 100 mg daily for 14 days, starting the day before the procedure, is the usual antibiotic of choice.

Postoperative Management

The patient is seen 7 to 10 days postsurgery for removal of sutures and changing of the dressing. Plaque and loosely adherent debris are gently removed from the site (Fig 15-2i). Irrigation with hydrogen peroxide can be used as an adjunct. The wound is dressed for a second week. The rationale for the second week of dressing is empirical, but the procedure appears to offer additional wound protection and stabilization.

At the second postoperative visit, the dressing is removed and the site is closely inspected. At this time, some soft tissue cratering may be evident. The patient should be reinstructed in plaque control measures for this area. With proper plaque control, the papilla will rebound to its proper physiologic contour. Chlorhexidine rinses should be reinstituted as soon as the final dressing is removed. If the soft tissue crater presents a plaque control problem or persists after 6 months, it is removed via gingivoplasty.

Maintenance

The patient is seen bimonthly for the first 6 months and then every 3 months for as long as the patient remains in the care of the clinician. Rarely are maintenance visits extended beyond the 3-month interval for the bone graft patient. At approximately 6 months postsurgery, the patient may return to the referring dentist to complete any needed restorative procedures. Professionally monitored periodontal maintenance to include reinforcement of plaque control, and other dental care, is mandatory for long-term success (Figs 15-2j and 15-2k).

Advantages and Disadvantages of Bone Graft Therapy

During the course of treatment for the periodontal patient, rational therapy will often involve a series of sequential steps. The first step is to identify the patient's immediate problem. This usually is a determination of the extent and severity of the periodontal disease process. Next, all primary and secondary etiologic factors are identified. Once the etiology is determined, a diagnosis is formulated. Based on the objectives of the clinician for a particular patient, the advantages and disadvantages of all modalities used to treat bone defects are weighed. The proper approach is then selected for the patient.

Advantages of Bone Grafts

1. Regeneration of the attachment apparatus is possible. Reconstruction of lost bone, cementum, and periodontal ligament has been adequately documented with autogenous and allogeneic graft materials.
2. By reconstructing the periodontium, it is possible to reverse the disease process.
3. Increased tooth support, improved function, and enhanced esthetics are concomitant results of successful bone graft therapy.
4. Bone grafts have application for all categories of intraosseous defects and certain furcation defects. This is in contrast to other forms of regenerative therapy.
5. Idealistic therapeutic objectives may be achievable. With the advent of growth factors to augment the osteogenic potential of current or future graft materials, complete disease reversal is a realistic goal.

Disadvantages of Bone Grafts

1. Bone graft therapy involves additional treatment time. Because of graft procurement and/or preparation, as well as placement, the time allotted to the surgical procedure must be lengthened. For the clinician inexperienced in regenerative periodontal therapy, the learning curve and the subsequent increase in treatment time will be significant.
2. Autografts require the removal of host donor tissue. Unless bone can be removed from within the primary surgical site, a secondary surgical site, either extraoral or intraoral, is necessary. The risks of any surgical procedure will apply here as well. In addition, the quantity of intraoral bone to fill multiple or deep defects is often lacking. Root resorption and ankylosis are problems encountered only with fresh iliac cancellous bone and marrow.[56]

3. The availability and added expense of bone allografts are ongoing problems. Patients' and clinicians' fears of disease transfer can be ameliorated by reference to the scientific literature.
4. Additional postoperative care is often necessary with bone graft therapy. This can range from technical problems to management of soft tissue defects associated with wound healing.
5. Bone grafts take a long time to heal. As much as a 2-year postoperative interval may be necessary before there is final radiographic resolution of the defect. Although most patients can receive restorative care 6 months following treatment, partial bone fill or delayed healing may delay needed restorative care.
6. Bone graft therapy is not routinely predictable in the hands of all practitioners. Bone grafts are highly successful for those practitioners who have taken the time and effort to master this technique-sensitive therapy.
7. Bone graft adds greater expense to the therapy. Economic considerations involve the cost of procurement or of the material itself, additional surgical treatment time, and postoperative maintenance treatment.
8. Multistep therapy is sometimes necessary, either to regraft residual osseous defects, where additional bone fill is possible and feasible, or to eliminate the residual osseous defect by resection.

For more than 40 years, bone grafts have been used to treat the osseous defects associated with periodontal disease.[57] This therapy has been shown to be clinically successful when encompassed in a comprehensive care program based on effective daily plaque control by the patient and a professionally supervised periodontal maintenance program. Although other treatment modalities have yielded favorable clinical results over varying intervals of time, only osseous grafting therapy has demonstrated histologic regeneration of lost periodontium consisting of new cementum, alveolar process, and a functionally oriented periodontal ligament in the human (Fig 15-3).

Guided Tissue Regeneration

Case reports and controlled clinical trials have indicated that the placement of a physical barrier between the gingival flap and the root surface enhances the potential for wound healing.[58–61] This procedure is known as *guided tissue regeneration* (GTR). The physical barrier retards apical migration of gingival epithelium, prevents the gingival connective tissue from contacting the root surface, and favors healing from the periodontal ligament.[62] Periodontal ligament cells are capable of migrating only a short distance with or without the placement of a physical barrier.[63] Therefore, the critical role of the physical barrier is to

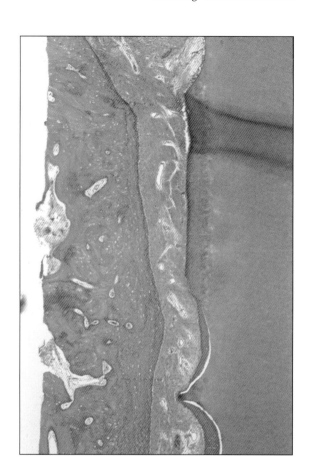

Fig 15-3 Six-month posttreatment human biopsy specimen. The regenerated periodontium is composed of new bone, new cementum, and new periodontal ligament coronal to a root notch placed in a position once occupied by calculus.

create a space into which migrating cells can undergo amplifying cell division and populate the root surface.

Another critical role for the physical barrier is wound stabilization.[64] Stabilization is paramount for periodontal regeneration because it helps to maintain the integrity of a fibrin clot at the tooth-flap interface. In addition, cells from the bone marrow spaces may play a role in guided tissue regeneration. Cells from the endosteal spaces of the alveolar bone can synthesize cementum-like tissue and may migrate from bone into the periodontal ligament spaces.[65]

Guided Tissue Regeneration Alone

Several reports have indicated that treatment of intraosseous defects with the GTR technique using an expanded polytetrafluoroethylene (e-PTFE) physical barrier has resulted in significant bone fill, reduction in probing depth, and gain of clinical attachment.[59,66,67] This has been limited to deep defects composed of three walls or a combination of two and three walls. When compared to open flap debridement for the treatment of mandibular class II furcation defects, GTR yielded greater probing depth reduction, greater gain in horizontal and vertical clinical attachment, and more furcation closure.[61,68] Healing of both intraosseous and furcation defects treated by GTR is by new attachment rather than by regeneration.[58,69]

Mandibular class III furcation defects do not respond as favorably as class II furcation invasions.[70] The size of the furcation defect, as well as the shape of the surrounding alveolar bone, are factors that determine the outcome for the treatment of class III furcation invasion by GTR.[71] In addition, maxillary molar and premolar furcation defects may not respond as favorably as deep intraosseous defects or mandibular class II furcation defects.[72,73]

Bioresorbable membranes, such as polylactic acid with a citric acid ester, polyglactin 910, and collagen, show promise.[74–78] Initial reports indicate that they may have a beneficial effect on the treatment of periodontal bone defects.

Guided Tissue Regeneration With Bone Graft

A number of case reports suggest that the combination of an osseous graft and a physical barrier enhances bone fill and promotes more favorable results in both intraosseous and furcation defects.[79,80] Anderegg et al[8] compared 15 pairs of mandibular class II furcation defects in 15 patients who were treated with DFDBA plus GTR or with an e-PTFE membrane alone. They found both horizontal and vertical bone fill to be more significant with the combined use of the graft and the barrier. Conversely, Wallace et al[81] found that the addition of DFDBA to GTR did not significantly improve any of the clinical measurements, although mean

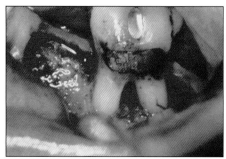

Fig 15-4a Flap reflection revealing short root trunk, cervical caries, and furcation involvement with dehiscence of the mesial and distal roots (From McClain PK, Schallhorn RG.[90] Reprinted with permission.)

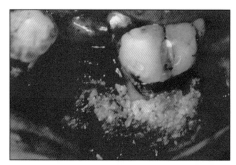

Fig 15-4b After root planing, caries reduction, and citric acid root conditioning, the demineralized freeze-dried bone allograft is placed.

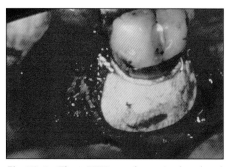

Fig 15-4c The e-PTFE membrane is placed and secured.

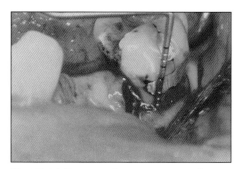

Fig 15-4d Postoperative measurement demonstrating 6.0 to 7.0 mm of bone fill.

measurements tended to be greater for DFDBA plus GTR. Soft tissue closure was noted in two of seven control sites and three of 10 experimental sites in six patients. A similar result was found by Guillimin et al[82] in treating 15 pairs of intraosseous defects either by e-PTFE plus DFDBA or by DFDBA alone. Clinical and surgical measurements suggested a beneficial effect with the use of either technique.[82] Garrett et al,[83] using a graft of DFDBA and dura mater sheets between the replaced surgical flaps and the tooth surfaces, found limited improvement of the treated defects over pretreatment levels.

Technique for Guided Tissue Regeneration

Patient Selection

Patients selected for the GTR procedure should be motivated for a life-long program of oral health, be free of systemic disease, and, in general, fulfill all of those criteria for any regenerative procedure. In addition, patients who are susceptible to infective endocarditis may be excluded from the GTR procedure because membrane exposure during healing may promote a chronic bacteremia. Smoking is also considered a risk factor and should be weighed heavily in the decision-making process.[84]

Defect Selection

Deep intraosseous defects with three walls or two and three walls and mandibular class II furcation defects respond best to the GTR procedure. Other types of intraosseous defects, such as one-wall, combined one and two-wall, and dehiscence defects may benefit from the addition of a bone graft. A bone graft will provide support for the membrane and prevent collapse into the defect. Likewise, furcation defects may benefit from the addition of a bone graft (Figs 15-4a to 15-4d).

Anesthesia

Sufficient anesthesia is provided for patient comfort and for hemostasis. A blood-free environment is essential for visualization of the defect and root planing.

Incision and Flap Reflection

A sulcular incision to bone is performed on the facial and lingual aspects. Full-thickness flaps are atraumatically reflected well beyond the mucogingival junction because the flaps will eventually be coronally positioned. Vertical releasing incisions, when required, should be placed at least one tooth to the mesial and distal of the defect so as not to interfere with the physical barrier.

Wound Debridement and Root Planing

All soft tissue remnants are meticulously removed from the defect. A variety of instruments may be used, but ultrasonic instrumentation is particularly effective in this regard. The roots are planed to an end point at which the root surface is clean and free of all debris. Use of magnifying lenses and a fiberoptic light source is helpful.

Root Surface Chemotherapy

Root surface demineralization with citric acid (pH 1) or a solution of tetracycline in sterile water (50 mg/mL) is believed by some to enhance the GTR technique for reasons previously elucidated. However, several published reports suggest that root surface chemotherapy has no beneficial effect when combined with the GTR procedure.[85,86]

Physical Barrier Placement

Physical barriers come in a variety of sizes and shapes. The proper one is selected for the defect in question. The barrier is placed so that the entire defect is covered and the barrier overlaps the adjacent bone by 2 to 3 mm. It is imperative that the barrier create a space. If the barrier collapses into the defect, little or no regeneration will take place. If collapse of the barrier is perceived, then a bone graft material or some type of support is required. The placement of the graft material and adjunctive procedures are the same as in the bone graft technique. The barrier is sutured firmly in place. This is usually accomplished with a sling-type suturing technique.

Wound Closure

The flaps are coronally positioned so that the gingival margin covers the physical barrier by 2 to 3 mm, if possible. Complete wound closure and coverage of the physical barrier is associated with a greater degree of success.[87] Suturing with nonabsorbable, nonwicking, biocompatible material is recommended. Vertical or horizontal mattress sutures and/or interrupted sutures can be used to obtain primary closure of the flaps. Gentle compression should be applied over the treated area for 2 to 3 minutes to reduce the thickness of the blood clot.

Periodontal Dressing

A periodontal dressing may or may not be used, depending on the operator's preference. Most of the time, it will not be possible to place dressing material because of the coronal flap position. If a dressing is used, it should not compromise blood supply to the flap.

Posttreatment Care

The patient is seen frequently for posttreatment care. Controlling bacterial contamination by mechanical means and/or prophylactic antibiotics is beneficial in promoting success of the GTR procedure. Adjunctive antimicrobial therapy may be imperative when infection has occurred. The physical barrier is removed 6 to 8 weeks after placement. Earlier removal may be necessary if the barrier is prematurely exposed. Use of a chlorhexidine rinse is beneficial during the period of membrane exposure. Once the barrier is removed, the red "rubberlike" connective tissue filling the defect needs to be protected with a protective dressing because this tissue is extremely labile.

Clinical Wound Healing

Four clinical patterns of GTR healing have been identified: rapid, typical, delayed, and adverse.[87] Each of these patterns has distinctive characteristics, although considerable overlap of specific clinical findings occurs among the groups.

Rapid healing is characterized by continuous flap coverage of the physical barrier until its removal 6 to 8 weeks after placement. Surgical dissection is needed to remove the barrier. A bonelike substance is frequently observed adjacent to the barrier. This occurs about 10% of the time and is associated with favorable clinical and radiographic maturation of the site.

The typical healing pattern is the one most observed (75%). This group is characterized by early barrier exposure; relatively easy barrier removal; and a pink, rubberlike appearance or granulation tissue at 6 to 8 weeks that resists gentle probing forces. An additional 2 to 4 weeks is required for keratinization of exposed new tissue. Radiographic evidence of bone fill varies from 3 to 12 months; many sites exhibit favorable maturation at 6 months.

Early clinical and radiographic findings reveal that delayed healing is sluggish compared to the rapid and typical healing. It occurs less than 10% of the time. This group is characterized by early barrier exposure; tissue inflammation external to the barrier with possible bleeding on probing; suppuration with gentle palpation or tissue retraction; easy or premature barrier removal; and immature granulation tissue with minimal or no resistance to probe penetration. With delayed healing, 4 to 8 weeks is required for keratinization of exposed new tissue, and radiographic bone maturation is found 6 to 24 months posttreatment.

Adverse wound healing is associated with failure and occurs less than 10% of the time. It is characterized by a difficult postoperative course (abscess formation); progressive barrier exposure; easy or premature barrier removal; tissue necrosis or loss of tissue height; a variable keratinization period; and gingival recession. Radiographs will show slight improvement to no improvement to regression.

Long-Term Results of Guided Tissue Regeneration

Gottlow et al[889] evaluated 88 sites at 52 teeth with various types of defects treated with e-PTFE barriers alone. Eighty sites gained 2 mm or more and were followed long term. Ninety-one percent of the sites gained more than 2.0 mm, and 68% gained more than 3.0 mm. The results demonstrated that attachment gain can be maintained over periods up to 5 years. Becker and Becker[89] reported on 32 patients with primarily deep three-wall intraosseous defects treated with e-PTFE physical barriers alone and followed for a mean of 4.3 years. There was a significant reduction in probing depth (3.8 mm), gain in clinical attachment (4.2 mm), and increase in gingival recession (–1.2 mm). There was an average defect fill of 4.3 mm. The authors considered these gains to be predictable and maintainable over extended time intervals. McLain and Schallhorn[90] treated 46 furcation defects with DFDBA and an e-PTFE barrier and 16 defects with barrier alone. Ninety-eight percent of the defects treated with graft and barrier and 63% of the defects treated with barrier alone were stable from periods ranging from 53 to 70 months posttreatment. They found that the combined treatment of bone graft and GTR enhanced complete furcation fill in class II and class III furcation defects; complete furcation fill in maxillary defects; the 5-year stability of gains in clinical attachment; the 5-year stability of reduction in horizontal depth of furcations; and the 5-year stability of complete furcation fill. Long-term studies confirm that GTR is a valuable addition to the therapeutic armamentarium.

Future Directions

Bone grafting, GTR, and the combination of GTR and bone graft have been shown to be efficacious for the treatment of periodontal osseous lesions. The mean reconstruction of the periodontal unit appears to be in the mean range of 3 to 4 mm regardless of the type of therapy. Because the ultimate goal of periodontal therapy is complete reversal of the disease process with complete regeneration of the periodontium, additional stimuli to enhance the regenerative process are clearly needed. Polypeptide growth factors may be a partial solution,[91] and current research in this direction is very promising.[92] However, many questions and years of research remain before the ultimate goal may be realized.

References

1. Mellonig JT. Autogenous and allogeneic bone grafts in periodontal therapy. Crit Rev Oral Biol 1992;3:333–352.

2. Stahl SS. Repair potential of the soft tissue-root interface. J Periodontol 1977;48:545–552.

3. Hiatt WH, Schallhorn RG. Intraoral transplants of cancellous bone and marrow in periodontal lesions. J Periodontol 1973;44:194–208.

4. Evans GH, Yukna RA, Sepe WW, Mabry TW, Mayer ET. Effect of various graft materials with tetracycline in localized juvenile periodontitis. J Periodontol 1989;60:491–497.

5. Mabry TR, Yukna RA, Sepe WW. Freeze-dried bone allografts combined with tetracycline in the treatment of juvenile periodontitis. J Periodontol 1985;56:74–81.

6. Mellonig JT. Decalcified freeze-dried bone allograft as an implant material in human periodontal defects. Int J Periodont Rest Dent 1984;4(6):41–55.

7. Schallhorn RG. Eradication of bifurcation defects utilizing frozen autogenous hip marrow implants. J West Soc Periodont Abstr 1968; 15:101–105.

8. Anderegg CR, Martin SJ, Gray J, Mellonig JT, Gher ME. Clinical evaluation of decalcified freeze-dried bone allograft with guided tissue regeneration in the treatment of molar furcation invasions. J Periodontol 1991;62:264–268.

9. Goldberg VM, Stevenson S. Natural history of autografts and allografts. Clin Orthop 1987;225:7–16.

10. Dragoo MR. Clinical and histologic evaluation of autogenous bone grafts. J Periodontol 1972;44:123.

11. Nabers CL, O'Leary TJ. Autogenous bone transplants in the treatment of osseous defects. J Periodontol 1965;36:5–14.

12. Nabers CL, Reed OM, Hammer JE. Gross and histologic evaluation of an autogenous bone graft 57 months postoperatively. J Periodontol 1972;43:702–704.

13. Robinson RE. Osseous coagulum for bone induction. J Periodontol 1969;40:503–510.

14. Diem CR, Bowers GM, Moffitt WC. Bone blending: A technique for bone implantation. J Periodontol 1972;43:295–297.

15. Froum SJ, Ortiz M, Witkins RT, Thaler R, Scopp W, Stahl S. Osseous autografts. III. Comparison of osseous coagulum-bone blend with open curettage. J Periodontol 1976;47:287–294.

16. Froum SJ, Thaler R, Scopp S, Stahl SS. Osseous autografts. I. Clinical response to bone blend or hip marrow grafts. J Periodontol 1975;46:516–521.

17. Froum S, Kosher L, Stahl S. Healing responses of human intraosseous lesions following the use of debridement, grafting and citric acid root treatment. I. Clinical and histologic observations six months postsurgery. J Periodontol 1983;54:67–76.

18. Evans R. Histologic evaluation of an autogenous bone graft. Int J Periodont Rest Dent 1981;2(2):66–79.

19. Hiatt W, Schallhorn R. Intraoral transplants of cancellous bone and marrow in periodontal lesions. J Periodontol 1973;44:194–208.

20. Ross SE, Cohen DW. The fate of a free osseous tissue autograft. A clinical and histologic case report. Periodontics 1968;6:145–151.

21. Soehren SE, VanSwol RL. The healing extraction site: A donor area for periodontal grafting material. J Periodontol 1979;50:128–133.

22. Rosenberg MM. Free osseous tissue autograft as a predictable procedure. J Periodontol 1971;43:195–209.

23. Hawley C, Miller J. A histologic examination of a free osseous autograft. J Periodontol 1975;46:289–293.

24. Schallhorn RG. The use of autogenous hip marrow biopsy implants for bony crater defects. J Periodontol 1968;39:145–147.

25. Schallhorn RG, Hiatt W, Boyce W. Iliac transplants in periodontal therapy. J Periodontol 1970;41:566–580.

26. Dragoo M, Sullivan H. A clinical and histologic evaluation of autogenous iliac bone grafts in humans. Part I. Wound healing 2 to 8 months. J Periodontol 1973;44:599–613.

27. Dragoo M, Sullivan H. A clinical and histologic study of autogenous iliac bone grafts in humans. II. External root resorption. J Periodontol 1973;44:614–625.

28. Buck B, Malinin T, Brown M. Bone transplantation and human immunodeficiency virus (AIDS): An estimate of risk. Clin Orthop 1989;240:129–134.

29. Martin L, McDougal J, Loskoski S. Disinfection and inactivation of the human T lymphocyte virus type III/lymphadenopathy-associated virus. J Infec Dis 1985;152:400–403.

30. Ongradi J, Ceccherini L, Pistello M, Specter S, Bendinelli M. Acid sensitivity of cell-free and cell associated HIV-1: Clinical implications. AIDS Res Hum Retrovirusus 1990;12:1433–1436.

31. Quinnan G, Weiss J, Wittek M. Inactivation of human T-cell lymphotropic virus. Type III by heat chemicals and irradiation. Transfusion 1982;26:481–483.

32. Resnick L, Veren K, Sakahuddin S, Tondreau S, Markham P. Stability and inactivation of HTLV-III/LAV under clinical and laboratory environments. J Am Dent Assoc 1986;255:1987–1991.

33. Mellonig JT, Prewett AB, Moyer MO. Inactivation of HIV in a bone allograft. J Periodontol 1992;63:979–983.

34. Quattlebaum B, Mellonig J, Hansel N. Antigenicity of freeze-dried cortical bone allograft in human periodontal osseous defects. J Periodontol 1988;59:394–397.

35. Mellonig JT, Levey R. The effect of different particle sizes of freeze-dried bone allograft on bone growth. J Dent Res 1984;63(special issue A):222.

36. Mellonig JT, Bowers GM, Bright R, Lawrence J. Clinical evaluation of freeze-dried bone allograft in periodontal osseous defects. J Periodontol 1976;47:125–129.

37. Mellonig JT. Freeze-dried bone allografts in periodontal reconstructive surgery. Dent Clin North Am 1991;35:505–520.

38. Altiere E, Reeve C, Sheridan P. Lymphilized bone allografts in periodontal osseous defects. J Periodontol 1979;50:510–519.

39. Urist MR, Strates B. Bone morphogenetic protein. J Dent Res 1971;50:271–278.

40. Urist MR, Mikulski A, Boyd D. A chemosterilized, antigen-extracted, autodigested, alloimplant for bone banks. Arch Surg 1975;110:416–428.

41. Mellonig J, Bowers G, Baily R. Comparison of bone graft materials. I. New bone formation with autografts and allografts determined by strontium-85. J Periodontol 1981;52:291–296.

42. Mellonig JT, Bowers G, Cotton W. Comparison of bone graft materials. Part II. New bone formation with autografts and allografts. A histological evaluation. J Periodontol 1981;52:297–302.

43. Wozney J, Rosen V, Celeste A, et al. Novel regulators of bone formation: Molecular clones and activities. Science 1988;242:1528–1534.

44. Libin B, Ward H, Fishman L. Decalcified lyophilized bone allografts for use in human periodontal defects. J Periodontol 1975;45:51–56.

45. Quintero G, Mellonig JT, Gambill V. A six month clinical evaluation of decalcified freeze-dried bone allograft in human periodontal defects. J Periodontol 1982;53:726–730.

46. Werbitt M. Decalcified freeze-dried bone allografts: A successful procedure in the reduction of intrabony defects. Int J Periodont Rest Dent 1987;7(5):56–63.

47. Pearson G, Rosen S, Deporter D. Preliminary observations on the usefulness of a decalcified freeze-dried cancellous bone allograft material in periodontal surgery. J Periodontol 1981;52:55–59.

48. Urist MR, Iwata H. Preservation and biodegradation of the morphogenetic property of bone matrix. J Theor Biol 1973;1938:155–167.

49. Urist MR, Jurist J, Dubuc R, Strates B. Quantitation of new bone formation in intramuscular implants of bone matrix in rabbits. Clin Orthop 1970;68:279–293.

50. Rummelhardt J, Mellonig JT, Gray J, Towle H. Comparison of freeze-dried bone allograft in human periodontal osseous defects. J Periodontol 1989;60:655–663.

51. Bowers G, Felton F, Middleton C, et al. Histologic comparison of regeneration in human intrabony defects when osteogenin is combined with demineralized freeze-dried bone allograft and with purified bovine collagen. J Periodontol 1991;62:690–702.

52. Emmings FG. Chemically modified osseous material for the restoration of bone defects. J Periodontol 1974;45:385–390.

53. Yukna RA. Synthetic grafts and regeneration. In: Polson AM (ed). Periodontal Regeneration: Current Status and Directions. Chicago: Quintessence, 1994:103–112.

54. Demirel K, Baer P, McNamara T. Topical application of doxycycline on periodontally involved root surfaces in vitro: Comparative analysis of substantivity on cementum and dentin. J Periodontol 1991;62:312–216.

55. Terranova VP, Franzetti LC, Hic S, et al. A biochemical approach to periodontal regeneration: Tetracycline treatment of dentin promotes fibroblast adhesion and growth. J Periodont Res 1986;21:330–337.

56. Schallhorn RG. Postoperative problems associated with iliac transplants. J Periodontol 1972;43:3–9.

57. Schallhorn RG. Long-term evaluation of osseous grafts in periodontal therapy. Int Dent J 1980;30:101–116.

58. Gottlow J, Nyman S, Lindhe, J, Karring T, Wennström J. New attachment formation in the human periodontium by guided tissue regeneration. Case reports. J Clin Periodontol 1986;13:604–616.

59. Becker W, Becker B, Berg L, Prichard J, Caffesse R, Rosenberg E. New attachment after treatment with root isolation procedures: Report for treated class III and class II furcation and vertical osseous defects. Int J Periodont Rest Dent 1988;8(3):8–23.

60. Pontoriero R, Lindhe J, Nyman S, Karring T, Rosenberg E, Sanavi F. Guided tissue regeneration in degree II furcation involved mandibular molars. J Clin Periodontol 1988;15:247–254.

61. Caffesse R, Smith B, Duff B, Morrison E, Merrill D, Becker W. Class II furcation treated by guided tissue regeneration in humans: Case report. J Periodontol 1990;61:51–54.

62. Minabe M. Critical review of the biologic rationale for guided tissue regeneration. J Periodontol 1991;62:171–179.

63. Aukhil I, Iglhaut J. Periodontal ligament cell kinetics following experimental regenerative procedures. J Clin Periodontol 1988;15:374–382.

64. Haney J, Nilveus R, McMillan P, Wikesjö U. Periodontal repair in dogs: Expanded polytetrafluoroethylene barrier membranes support wound stabilization and enhance bone regeneration. J Periodontol 1993;64:883–890.

65. Melcher A, Cheong T, Cox J. Synthesis of cementum-like tissue in vitro by cells cultured from bone: A light and electron microscopic study. J Periodont Res 1986;21:592–612.

66. Cortellini P, Pini Prato G, Tonetti MS. Periodontal regeneration of human infrabony defects. I. Clinical measures. J Periodontol 1993;64:254–260.

67. Cortellini P, Pini Prato G, Tonetti MS. Periodontal regeneration of human infrabony defects. II. Re-entry procedures and bone measures. J Periodontol 1993;64:261–268.

68. Mellonig J, Seamons B, Gray J, Towle H. Clinical evaluation of guided tissue regeneration in the treatment of grade II molar furcation invasions. Int J Periodont Rest Dent 1994;14:255–271.

69. Stahl S, Froum S. Healing of human suprabony lesions treated with guided tissue regeneration and coronally anchored flaps. J Clin Periodontol 1991;18:69–74.

70. Pontoriero R, Lindhe J, Nyman S, Karring T, Rosenberg E, Sanavi F. Guided tissue regeneration in the treatment of furcation defects in mandibular molars. A clinical study of degree III involvements. J Clin Periodontol 1989;16:170–178.

71. Pontoriero R, Nyman S, Ericsson I, Lindhe J. Guided tissue regeneration in surgically produced furcation defects. J Clin Periodontol 1992;19:159–163.

72. Metzler D, Seamons B, Mellonig J, Gher M, Gray J. Clinical evaluation of guided tissue regeneration in the treatment of maxillary Class II molar furcation invasions. J Periodontol 1991;62:353–360.

73. Proestakis G, Bratthall G, Soderholm G, et al. Guided tissue regeneration in the treatment of infrabony defects on maxillary premolars. A pilot study. J Clin Periodontol 1992;19:766–773.

74. Gottlow J. Guided tissue regeneration using bioresorbable and nonresorbable devices; initial healing and long-term results. J Periodontol 1993;64:1157–1165.

75. Laurell L, Falk H, Fornell J, Johard G, Gottlow J. Clinical use of a bioresorbable matrix barrier in guided tissue regeneration therapy. Case series. J Periodontol 1994;65:967–975.

76. Gager A, Schultz A. Treatment of periodontal defects with an absorbable membrane (Polyglactin 910) with and without osseous grafting: Case reports. J Periodontol 1994;65:1037–1045.

77. Caton J, Greenstein G, Zappa U. Synthetic bioabsorbable barrier for regeneration in human periodontal defects. J Periodontol 1994;65:1037–1045.

78. Wang H, O'Neal R, Thomas C, Shyr Y, MacNeil R. Evaluation of an absorbable collagen membrane in treating Class II furcation defects. J Periodontol 1994;65:1029–1036.

79. Schallhorn R, McClain P. Combined osseous composite grafting, root conditioning, and guided tissue regeneration. Int J Periodont Rest Dent 1988;8(4):8–31.

80. McGuire MK. Reconstruction of bone on facial surfaces: A series of case reports. Int J Periodont Rest Dent 1992;12:133–144.

81. Wallace S, Gellin R, Miller M, Mishkin D. Guided tissue regeneration with and without decalcified freeze-dried bone in mandibular class II furcation invasions. J Periodontol 1994;65:244–254.

82. Guillemin M, Mellonig JT, Brunsvold M, Steffensen B. Healing in periodontal defects treated by decalcified freeze-dried bone allografts in combination with ePTFE membranes. Clinical and SEM analysis. J Clin Periodontol 1993;20:528–536.

83. Garrett S, Loos B, Chamberlain D, Egelberg J. Treatment of intraosseous periodontal defects with a combined adjunctive therapy of citric acid conditioning, bone grafting, and placement of collagenous membranes. J Clin Periodontol 1988;15:383–389.

84. Preber H, Bergstrom J. Effect of cigarette smoking on periodontal healing following surgical therapy. J Clin Periodontol 1990;17:324–328.

85. Handelsman M, Davarpanah M, Celletti R. Guided tissue regeneration with and without citric acid treatment in vertical osseous defects. Int J Periodont Rest Dent 1991;11(5):351–363.

86. Kersten B, Chamberlain A, Khorsandi S, Wikesjö U, Selvig K, Nilveus R. Healing of the intrabony periodontal lesion following root conditioning with citric acid and wound closure including an expanded PTFE membrane. J Clin Periodontol 1992;63:876–882.

87. Schallhorn R, McClain P. Clinical and radiographic healing pattern observations with combined regenerative techniques. Int J Periodont Rest Dent 1994;14:391–403.

88. Gottlow J, Nyman S, Karring T. Maintenance of new attachment gained through guided tissue regeneration. J Clin Periodontol 1992;19:315–317.

89. Becker W, Becker B. Treatment of mandibular 3-wall intrabony defects by flap debridement and expanded polytetrafluoroethylene barrier membrane. Long-term evaluation of 32 treated patients. J Periodontol 1993;64:1138–1144.

90. McClain P, Schallhorn R. Long-term assessment of combined osseous composite grafting, root conditioning, and guided tissue regeneration. Int J Periodont Rest Dent 1993;13(1):9–27.

91. Graves D, Cochran D. Mesenchymal cell growth factors. Crit Rev Oral Biol 1990;1:17–36.

92. Sigurdsson T, Lee M, Kubota K, Turek T, Wozney J, Wikesjö U. Periodontal repair in dogs: Recombinant human bone morphogenetic protein–2 significantly enhances periodontal regeneration. J Periodontol 1995;66:131–138.

CHAPTER 16

Periodontal Regeneration: Clinical Application

Myron Nevins, DDS

The angular bony defect, predominantly associated with the interproximal septa of bone, is a precursor to a further loss of attachment apparatus[1] (Figs 16-1a to 16-1d). The end point of treatment should be an interdental space that can be easily cleaned of plaque by both the patient and the hygienist. To this end, the scope of treatment can include only three options: maintain the defect as is and rely upon patient compliance; reduce the defect by ostectomy; or reduce the defect by regenerating the lost periodontium. Although it is obvious that the third option is preferred, defect morphology may preclude it as an answer.[2]

The definition of *periodontal regeneration* is the formation of new bone, new cementum, and new periodontal ligament to create a new functional attachment apparatus over a pathologically exposed root surface. Regeneration can only be completely ascertained by biopsy of the tooth and supporting structures. Because the opportunities to accomplish this goal are limited, the next most reliable barometer of success is reentering and visualizing the bone (Figs 16-2 and 16-3). Radiographs and probing measurements are important but less meaningful evidence to the clinician.

The nonsurgical approach to an intrabony pocket is presumptuous in light of all records of patient compliance after

Fig 16-1a There is an interdental angular crest toward the distal surface of the first molar. The probing depth is 5 mm. This patient is on a periodontal maintenance program, and the problem was committed to observation, rather than correction, at the request of the patient.

Fig 16-1b Note the extreme radiographic loss of bone in 4 months *(arrow)*. No dentist can be sure which defect will deteriorate and at what time interval.

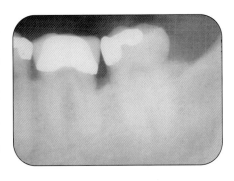

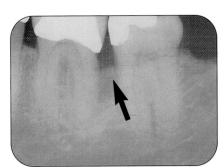

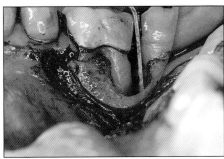

Fig 16-1c There is advanced loss of the interdental bone, extending to the buccal surface of the mandibular first molar.

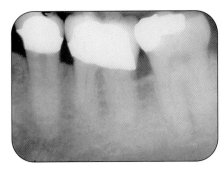

Fig 16-1d A radiograph taken 1 year later reveals that periodontal regeneration surgery has resulted in correction of the defect.

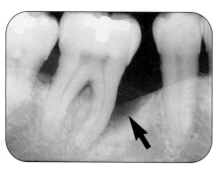

Fig 16-2a The presurgical radiograph reveals an intrabony defect on the mesial surface of the molar *(arrow)* as it approaches the apex. (Courtesy of Dr Richard Evans.)

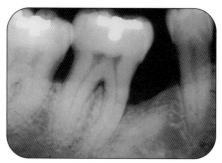

Fig 16-2b The posttreatment (19-month) radiograph indicates that the autogenous graft surgery has been successful.

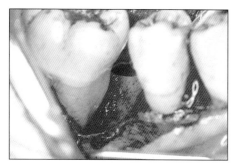

Fig 16-2c The osseous defect is revealed at the time of surgery.

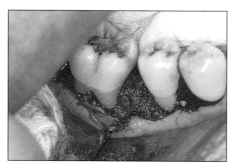

Fig 16-2d The defect is filled with autogenous bone harvested distal to the third molar.

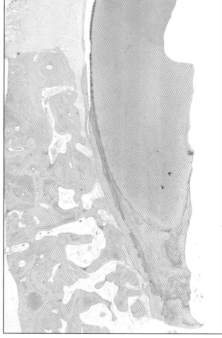

Fig 16-2e The mesial root and its periodontium were removed as a block section 24 months after the regeneration procedure.

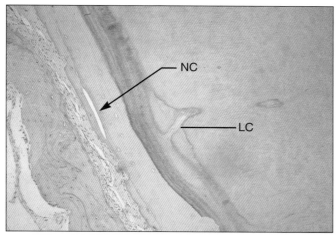

Fig 16-2f Cementum is covering the root surface (NC) and invaginating the lateral canal (LC). A periodontal ligament (PDL) is interspersed between the new bone (NB) and the new cementum (NC).

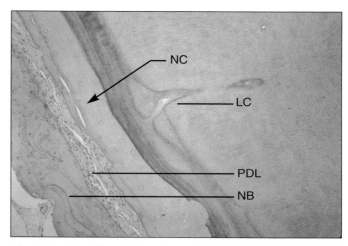

Fig 16-2g This is four serial sections after that in Fig 16-2f. It demonstrates the proximity of the lateral canal from the pulpal tissue to the previous pocket area. The root surface is covered with new cementum (NC).

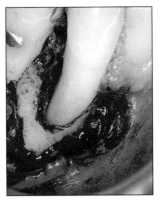

Fig 16-3a There is conspicuous loss of periodontium on the distal surface of the mandibular canine. The deep defect has no buccal wall. Ostectomy is contraindicated because it would jeopardize the adjacent premolar. Most of the defect is a two-wall, or uncontained defect; only the extreme apical portion has three walls. It is not possible to do ostectomy to eliminate all but the contained portion of the defect.

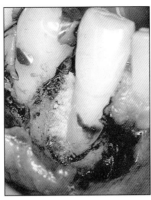

Fig 16-3b An osseous allograft is in place.

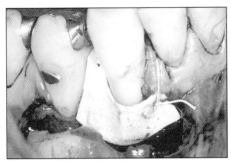

Fig 16-3c An expanded polytetrafluoroethylene membrane (Gore-Tex, WL Gore, Flagstaff, AZ) has been tailored to cover the interproximal space and extends to the buccal surface.

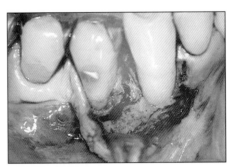

Fig 16-3d The area is reopened 6 years after treatment. The canine is now a serviceable tooth with a regenerated periodontium.

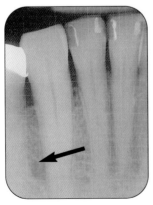

Fig 16-3e The preoperative radiograph demonstrates the intraosseous defect between the canine and first premolar (*arrow*) (1988).

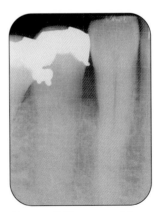

Fig 16-3f The 6-year follow-up radiograph demonstrates resolution of the lesion (1994).

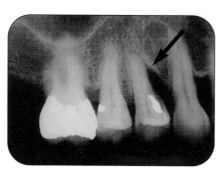

Fig 16-4a There is an osseous defect *(arrow)* on the mesial surface of the maxillary first premolar (1966).

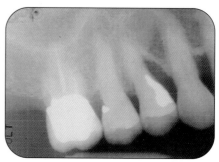

Fig 16-4b The defect has not progressed after 27 years (1994). This is unpredictable therapy because it is not possible to predict which angular defect will result in additional loss of periodontium.

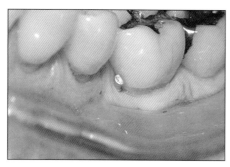

Fig 16-5a A Hirschfeld point demonstrates a severe probing depth in the absence of bleeding. Note the pink gingiva.

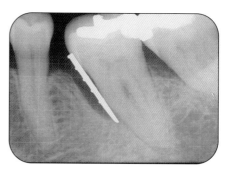

Fig 16-5b The radiograph shows the point in place and a deep, uncontained intraosseous defect on the mesial surface of the mandibular molar.

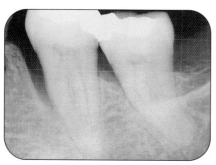

Fig 16-5c The intrabony technique has resulted in regeneration of approximately 25% of the osseous defect. This has not changed the prognosis of the tooth. Neither the hygienist nor the patient will be able to maintain this area.

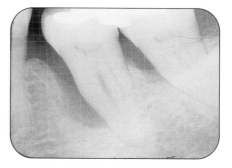

Fig 16-5d This radiograph, made 2 years later, reveals a severe worsening of the problem that resulted in the loss of this tooth.

the conclusion of active treatment.[3–5] Every periodontist has observed untreated deep osseous defects that have not progressed, but it is impossible to predict which patient will be susceptible to further destruction before treatment and long-term observation (Figs 16-4 and 16-5). No retrospective study has demonstrated more than 30% recall compliance after 5 years in a private practice, and it is not possible to predict which patients will cooperate.[6] It is therefore preferable to achieve a definitive result rather than to assume a posture of "wait and see." No one can determine the damage when the patient fails to return.

The most common osseous defects are shallow interdental craters and marginal reverse architecture, for which ostectomy is the most predictable and therefore preferable approach because it results in an interdental septum that is flat mesiodistally and buccolingually.[7] If the depth of the defect precludes pocket elimination by reduction, then use of addition procedures, or perhaps a combination of the two, is more appropriate.[8] The most rewarding resolution of an intrabony defect is the regeneration of the periodontium. Although the initial goal of such treatment is to recoup 100% of lost periodontium, a realistic goal is to convert an untreatable lesion into a treatable defect that can be resolved by ostectomy. Anything less fails to achieve the stated goal that is necessary for predictable long-term success (Figs 16-6a to 16-6g).

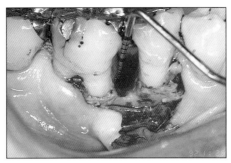

Fig 16-6a There is an intrabony crater between the mandibular second premolar and the first molar. The buccal view seems to indicate that this shallow crater could be reduced by ostectomy.

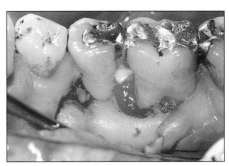

Fig 16-6b The lingual view of the interdental lesion shows that it extends to the lingual surface of the mesial root of the first molar. If this defect were treated by ostectomy, it would take a significant toll on the supporting apparatus of the second premolar. Therefore, every effort should be made to resolve this problem by regenerating the lost periodontium.

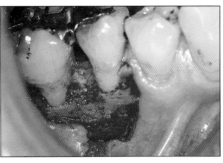

Fig 16-6c A freeze-dried mineralized allograft has been placed in the defect (buccal view).

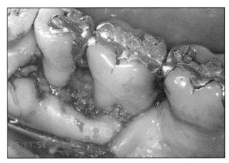

Fig 16-6d A freeze-dried mineralized allograft has been placed in the defect (lingual view).

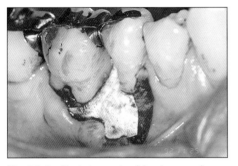

Fig 16-6e An interproximal barrier membrane has been fitted.

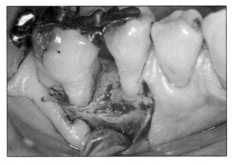

Fig 16-6f One year later, there is no evidence of the interdental crater on the buccal surface.

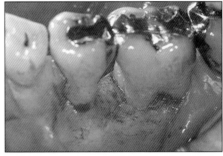

Fig 16-6g There is no evidence of the interdental crater or the circumferential lesion on the mesial root of the first molar. The interdental problem has been resolved.

Treatment Considerations

Surgical Entry and Root Preparation

Surgical entry is accomplished by flap elevation and should extend one full tooth beyond the defect (Figs 16-7a to 16-7i). Vertical incisions provide surgical access and visibility for defect preparation and are rarely not contraindicated by anatomic obstacles. They are best produced with a minor cutback toward the procedure as they proceed apically. It is possible to elevate the intact interproximal tissues from the buccal or lingual aspect when there is a missing tooth or a large interdental space. This procedure provides excellent soft tissue coverage for barrier membranes and reduces the risk of their premature exposure (see Figs 16-17d to 16-17h). It is necessary to remove all infected granulation tissue to gain access to the remaining alveolar process and the osseous defect. This is followed by root preparation by hand and/or ultrasonic debridement to remove all accretions from the surface. Both procedures are tedious in the most apical recesses of the osseous deformity.

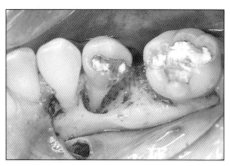

Fig 16-7a The surgical procedure extends one tooth mesially beyond the circumferential intraosseous defect. At that point, there is a vertical incision with a small cutback toward the procedure. All infected granulation tissue has been removed, and the root has been mechanically debrided. Note the natural decortication of the bone structure, allowing communication of the elements in the marrow spaces during healing. This is also true on the mesial surface of the molar.

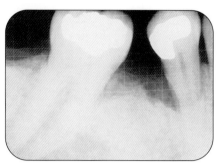

Fig 16-7b Radiographic view of the osseous defect on the premolar and molar. Treatment solely by resection would weaken both teeth.

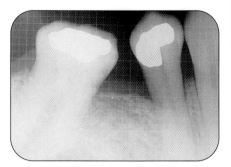

Fig 16-7c Five-year observation of the result of the periodontal regeneration procedure.

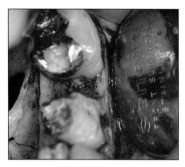

Fig 16-7d There is a deep interproximal osseous crater between the mandibular molars.

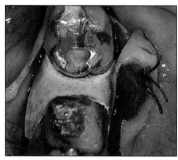

Fig 16-7e An interproximal barrier membrane has been adapted over a bone graft. The surgical incision was made to preserve the interproximal gingiva, which is sutured to the buccal mucosa to improve visibility.

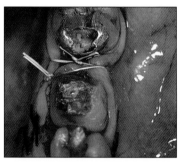

Fig 16-7f The surgical flaps are sutured into position. This incision strategy allows reflection of soft tissue that can then be coapted to provide better coverage of the barrier membrane.

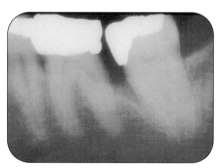

Fig 16-7g The pretreatment radiograph reveals an osseous defect mesial to the mandibular second molar.

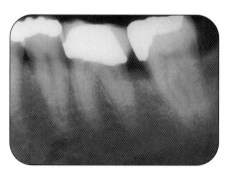

Fig 16-7h The posttreatment radiograph demonstrates resolution of the defect.

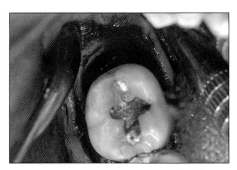

Fig 16-8a An intraosseous three-wall defect is located on the distal surface of the mandibular molar. The bone in this region is very cancellous, and it is unnecessary to decorticate the walls.

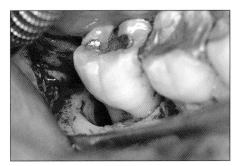

Fig 16-8b The totally contained defect extends to the buccal surface, approaching, but not invading, the furcation. This defect has been treated with a barrier membrane.

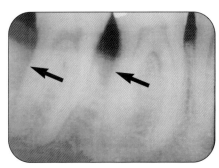

Fig 16-8c The preoperative radiograph demonstrates intraosseous defects on the distal surfaces of both molars (arrows).

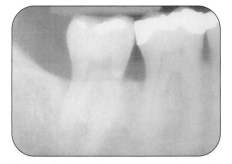

Fig 16-8d The 4-year postoperative radiograph reveals that the intraosseous lesions have been resolved.

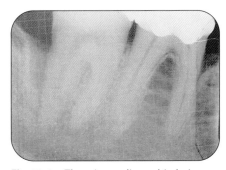

Fig 16-8e There is a radiographic lesion on the distal surface of the distal molar.

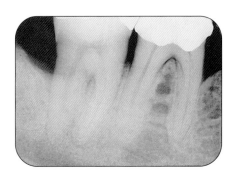

Fig 16-8f A radiograph taken 1 year after treatment reveals that the lesion on the distal surface of the distal molar has been resolved.

Bowers et al[9] demonstrated that periodontal regeneration results in new cellular cementum with Sharpey's fiber attachment on both old cementum and fresh dentin surfaces. This has eliminated the need to remove acellular cementum as a condition to achieving periodontal regeneration. It is unusual to be able to reach those areas most difficult to cleanse with rotary instruments or to control chemotherapeutics at the base of the defect. The use of citric acid has to be debated because it has a pH of 1, and the pH of the blood, bone marrow, and periodontal ligament is 7.4. There is a very real possibility that the process of regeneration could be adversely affected because it occurs at a slightly positive pH.[10] The cell walls of progenitor cells may be altered. To alter the surface of exposed tooth structure in vitro, citric acid requires concentrated contact with the root surface for approximately 5 minutes. To date, animal and human studies demonstrate little or no advantage.[11–13]

Tetracycline has also been advocated for root preparation because of its antibiotic and collagen-promoting properties.[14] Used as a sludge rather than a liquid, its lower pH probably has less possibility of negatively affecting the environment of the progenitor cells. There is some minor evidence that it is useful as an additive to bone grafts.[15]

Some defects present with many open marrow spaces and thus offer the possibility of rapid movement of both vascularity and undifferentiated cells into the defect. A deep defect should be decorticated with either hand instrumentation or a small carbide bur to create communication with the marrow spaces[16] (see Figs 16-7a to 16-7h).

The predictability of the regenerative procedures will vary according to defect selection and how well they are contained in the envelope of bone. Clot stability and protection are paramount and are difficult to attain in less well-contained defects.[17] Stability of mobile teeth would appear to provide an enhanced opportunity for future bone formation during the stages of clot organization and angiogenesis. The complete removal of all infected granulation tissue and accretions on the root surface are extremely important because only one thing can occupy a given space at a given time.

Defect Size and Morphology

At this point, the predictability of the treatment for the periodontal bone defect can best be established. All evidence demonstrates that the most contained defects offer the best predictability for regeneration.[18] If the defect is completely surrounded by bone, all three walls of bone can contribute to populating the exposed root surface with cells that can be considered progenitors for bone formation. Treatment is especially successful when these three-wall defects are encountered in the mandibular posterior area, where the bony housing of the teeth is largely cancellous[19] (Figs 16-8a to 16-8f). The only disadvantage is the infrequency with which they are encountered. Treatment has been successful with the intrabony technique, with the use of a barrier membrane alone, and with autografts or allografts used alone or in combination with a barrier membrane.

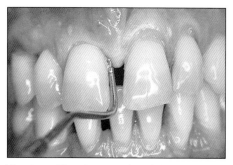

Fig 16-9a There is a periodontal abscess on the mesial surface of the maxillary right central incisor. Note the buccal swelling in the vestibule.

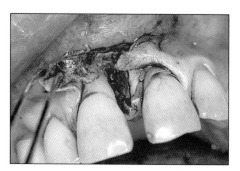

Fig 16-9b The flap has been elevated, and the frenum has been removed. There is evidence of an uncontained two-wall intraosseous defect on the mesial surface of the central incisor.

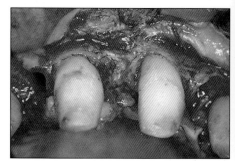

Fig 16-9c The central incisor area is reentered after 6 months, after the teeth were prepared for a provisional fixed restoration. The intraosseous defect has resolved without additional bone therapy. It is necessary to treat acute defects differently from chronic long-standing defects.

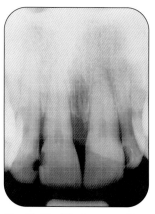

Fig 16-10a The long-standing chronic defect between the maxillary central incisors was treated by open cleanout, similar to the technique shown in Figure 16-9. The error was that this is not an acute defect.

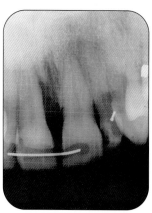

Fig 16-10b The teeth were splinted to improve the patient's comfort, but a radiograph taken 2 years later shows that the intraosseous defect has advanced remarkably on the mesial surface of the right central incisor.

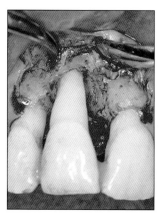

Fig 16-10c Clinical appearance at the time Figure 16-10b was taken. It is now unpredictable to treat this tooth with a regenerative procedure. Intraosseous cleanout alone is not the treatment of choice for a long-standing, uncontained defect.

The intrabony technique of surgical cleanout is very applicable to acute periodontal lesions, where complete regeneration is reported for a variety of defects[20] (Figs 16-9a to 16-9c). When intrabony cleanout is applied to less contained (one- to two-wall) chronic defects, results are less predictable (Figs 16-10a to 16-10c).

The volume of regeneration expected is another variable to be considered in combination with the defect morphology.[2] The contiguous autogenous graft helps to reduce defect size by moving the wall of the defect closer to the tooth[21] (Figs 16-11 and 16-12), while orthodontic tooth movement will alter both defect morphology and size[22] (Figs 16-13a and 16-13b). A combination of approaches is often indicated to resolve clinical problems. The clinician with a varied armamentarium is able to offer a combination of approaches that will address the resolution of many defects that are difficult to treat.

Unfortunately, most defects are a combination of one, two, and three walls, the three-wall portion found at the most apical extent. Some may be treated by just introducing ostectomy to eliminate the less contained portions (one- and two-wall), but most require regenerative treatment of the difficult areas to make a meaningful difference to the periodontal prognosis and to avoid worsening the prognosis of adjacent teeth[23] (see Figs 16-6a to 16-6g).

Successful treatment of less contained defects with intraoral and extraoral bone grafts has been demonstrated for many years[23,24] (Figs 16-14 to 16-16), but it appears that the predictability of the clinical treatment of advanced osseous defects is enhanced by the combined use of a bone graft and a membrane[25,26] (Figs 16-17a to 16-17i). It is not remarkable for some residual lesion to be present after regeneration therapy, and it is necessary to reenter and use ostectomy to eliminate it. It may be that a defect of tooth position

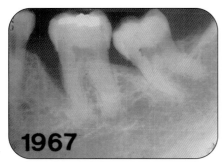

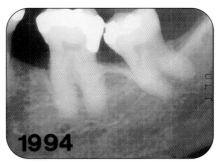

Fig 16-11a Radiograph of an intrabony, uncontained defect that was treated in 1967 with contiguous autogenous graft ("swedging").

Fig 16-11b The same tooth is shown in 1994 after 27 years of clinical observation. Note the resolution of the deep intraosseous lesion.

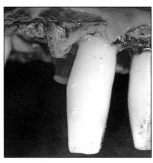

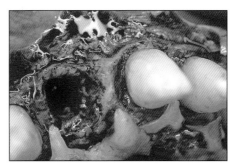

Fig 16-12a There is an uncontained one-wall defect on the mesial surface of the maxillary left central incisor. The right central incisor was extracted.

Fig 16-12b An occlusal view of the defect on the mesial surface of the left central incisor reveals that the defect is too wide and too uncontained to consider treating with an intrabony technique or with a conventional bone graft.

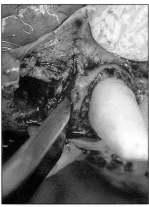

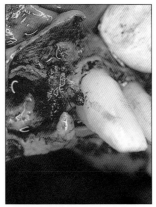

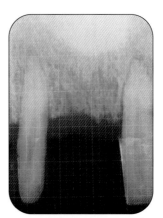

Fig 16-12c A monobevel chisel is used to swedge the bone toward the incisor, thus reducing the distance from the osseous wall to the surface of the tooth. The bone being swedged maintains its attachment to the alveolar process; thus, the blood supply is not challenged.

Fig 16-12d The swedged bone is in contact with the tooth, and the space previously occupied by the chisel is filled with resorbable collagen or bone graft material. This is to prevent the bone from returning to its original position.

Fig 16-12e This area is observed radiographically during healing until the defect made by the chisel is resolved.

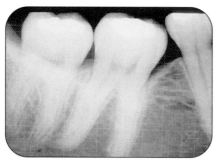

Fig 16-13a The interdental septum will be parallel to the line joining the two approximating cementoenamel junctions when viewed radiographically. This angulated crest is thus relative to the position of the teeth.

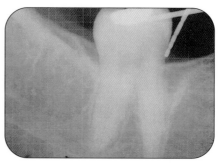

Fig 16-13b Note the radiographic resolution of the defect after extraction of the third molar and correction of the position of the second molar.

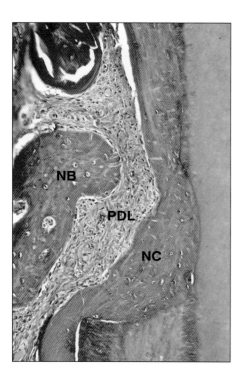

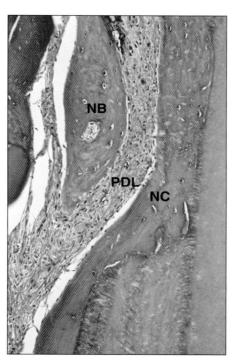

Figs 16-14a and 16-14b Periodontal regeneration after treatment of intraosseous defects with freeze-dried demineralized bone allografts. Note the new cellular cementum covering the notch in the tooth and both the old cementum and the dentinal surface. The new cementum (NC) demonstrates Sharpey's fiber attachment to the periodontal ligament (PDL) and to new bone (NB). (From Bowers and Middleton.[24] Reprinted with permission.)

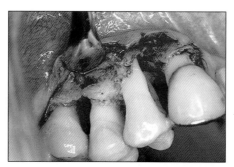

Fig 16-15a There are intraosseous defects on the mesial surface of the first premolar and between the second premolar and the first molar (1970). The mesial defect on the first premolar is an uncontained, mostly one-wall defect with a small three-wall base.

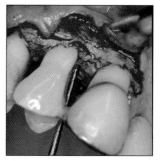

Fig 16-15b The same area is reentered in preparation for a new fixed partial denture (1992). The periodontal regeneration was accomplished with bone harvested from the posterior iliac crest with a trephine. The intraosseous defect has remained corrected for a significant period of time (22 years).

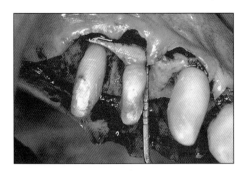

Fig 16-16a Each tooth in the maxillary posterior quadrant has suffered extreme loss of supporting structure (1969). Interdental osseous defects extend to the buccal surface.

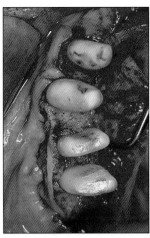

Fig 16-16b An occlusal view demonstrates intraosseous defects involving the canine and both premolars.

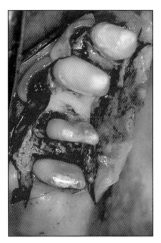

Fig 16-16c A reentry procedure after 1 year reveals the resolution of the intraosseous defects resulting from bone-grafting procedures (an autogenous graft harvested from the maxillary tuberosity) and the healed extraction wound of the first molar.

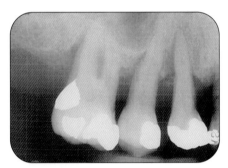

Fig 16-16d The intraosseous lesions are visible in the periapical radiograph.

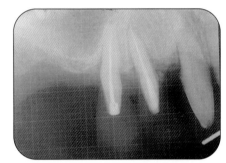

Fig 16-16e The intraosseous defects have been resolved by the use of autogenous bone grafts.

(uneven cementoenamel junctions) has suffered a superimposed inflammatory lesion. Successful regenerative treatment will result in an osseous crest that is parallel to a line connecting the adjacent cementoenamel junctions or to an uneven level that originally demonstrated susceptibility (Figs 16-18 and 16-19). Of course, the purely tooth-position deformity should have been corrected at an earlier time (see Figs 16-13a and 16-13b).

Ankylosis and root resorption are reported to be an infrequent consequence of the use of fresh iliac crest marrow grafts to treat intrabony pockets (Dragoo and Sullivan[27] reported 2.8% and Schallhorn et al[28] reported 5.4%). Pinpoint ankylosis has been noted with the use of osteogenin to induce periodontal regeneration, but no root resorption has been reported with the use of frozen iliac crest marrow grafts in humans or bone morphogenetic protein–2A in dogs to date.[29]

Researchers have extracted teeth in dogs and attempted to reimplant the roots into healed edentulous ridges after root planing and endodontic treatment.[30–32] The experiment resulted in some root resorption and ankylosis, and the researchers concluded that this occurred because the root was in contact with the supporting bone or connective tissue. It is erroneous to relate this conclusion to bone graft therapy where teeth were not extracted and reimplanted.

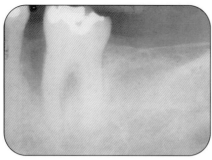

Fig 16-17a A deep vertical osseous defect located on the mesial surface of the molar apparently extends, on the radicular surface, toward the furcation.

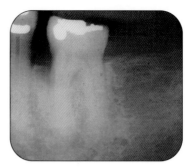

Fig 16-17b Postoperative radiograph.

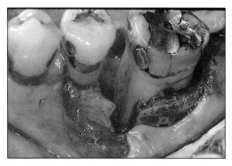

Fig 16-17c The buccal view shows a deep intraosseous defect extending from the premolar apically toward the molar. The buccal wall is absent.

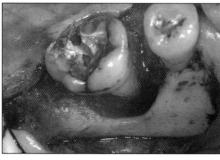

Fig 16-17d The lingual view of the osseous defect shows that it wraps around on the lingual surface to include an early furcation invasion.

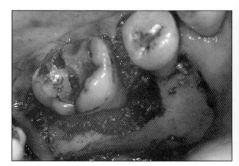

Fig 16-17e The bone defect has been filled with freeze-dried mineralized bone allograft.

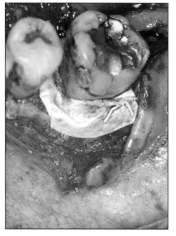

Fig 16-17f A Gore-Tex interproximal membrane has been fitted to cover the buccal and interproximal surfaces of the defect.

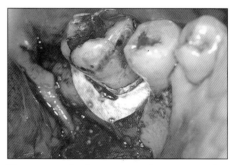

Fig 16-17g The Gore-Tex membrane covers the defect on the lingual surface.

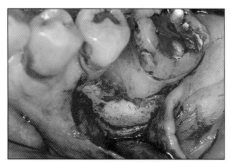

Fig 16-17h At surgical reentry after 1 year (buccal view), most of the defect has been eliminated. The once-untreatable lesion is now easily managed by minor ostectomy and osteoplasty.

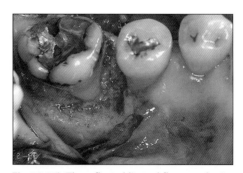

Fig 16-17i The reflected lingual flap reveals virtually a complete fill of the osseous defect.

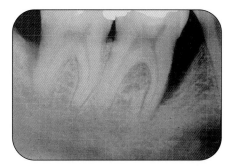

Fig 16-18a There is a deep osseous defect on the mesial surface of the mandibular second molar and an osseous defect on the distal surface of the third molar; the first molar is missing. The remaining molars are at a mesial angle to compensate for the premature loss of the first molar. Therefore, the osseous crest was angular and parallel to a line connecting the cementoenamel junction before inflammatory periodontal disease occurred.

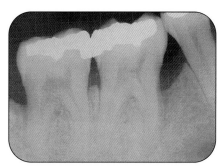

Fig 16-18b Periodontal regeneration has resolved the distal defect and most of the mesial defect. The osseous crest now is parallel to the cementoenamel junctions; this may very well represent the radiographic appearance before an inflammatory defect was superimposed on the angular crest.

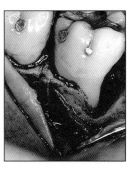

Fig 16-18c The uncontained osseous defect is too advanced for ostectomy. The most predictable treatment for this type of defect is a combination of an osseous graft and a barrier membrane. This photograph correlates to the radiograph in Figure 16-18a.

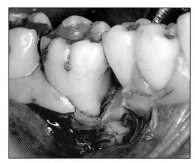

Fig 16-18d Posthealing reentry at 11 months. This view correlates to the postoperative radiograph in Figure 16-18b. At this time, the angular lid will be flattened so this area will not be predisposed to further osseous destruction.

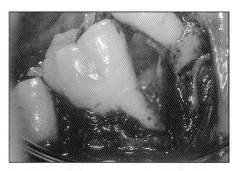

Fig 16-19a A deep, uncontained defect is present on the mesial surface of the mandibular molar.

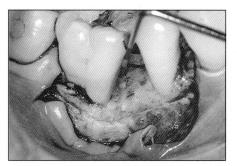

Fig 16-19b The area is reentered 1 year after treatment with a freeze-dried mineralized allograft and a barrier membrane. (Courtesy of Dr Yoshihiro Ono.)

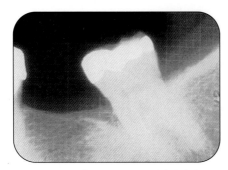

Fig 16-20a There is a mesial infrabony defect that extends to, and includes, the buccal furcation. This tooth is a questionable abutment for a fixed partial denture.

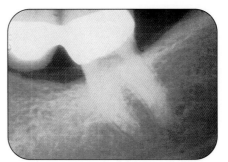

Fig 16-20b Radiograph taken 20 years after construction of the fixed partial denture. The periodontal regeneration has been successful, enabling this tooth to service the dentition as the distal abutment and support for the fixed prosthesis.

Barrier Membranes

Nyman et al[33] used a Millipore filter to achieve regeneration for an intrabony pocket of a mandibular incisor, and thus guided tissue regeneration was recognized as an attainable goal. Their finding was significantly reinforced by Gottlow et al[34] with five more human biopsy specimens. Becker and Becker[35] demonstrated the successful use of guided tissue regeneration to treat three-wall defects.

The use of barrier membranes to treat less contained defects adds another measure of expertise and clinical experience. Both meticulous fitting of the membrane and careful postsurgical monitoring of the patient are essential. Most defects include interproximal areas, and interproximal membranes frequently become exposed.[36] Once exposed, they must be managed by cleansing procedures until removed. If the membrane is mobile, if there is an exudate, or if the margins of the membrane are exposed, it must be removed immediately. This procedure usually requires local anesthetic and careful tissue dissection to preserve the regenerating tissue. The membrane should not be pulled or torn to remove it forcefully.

Conclusion

The newly recognized predictability of periodontal regeneration procedures has helped change dentistry for patients. It offers opportunities to obviate the need for fixed restorative dentistry, just as it can provide abutment teeth with a meaningful prognosis to support restorative dentistry (Figs 16-20a and 16-20b). It is necessary to exercise judgment in selecting defects for these procedures because clinicians will be judged by how frequently they reach their goals.

References

1. Papanou PN, Wennström JL. The angular bony defect as an indicator of further alveolar bone loss. J Clin Periodontol 1991;18:317–322.

2. Steffensen B, Weber HP. Relationship between the radiographic periodontal defect angle and healing after treatment. J Periodontol 1989;60:248–254.

3. Wilson TG, Hale S, Temple R. The results of efforts to improve compliance with supportive periodontal treatment in a private practice. J Periodontol 1993;64:311–314.

4. Badersten A, Nilveus R, Egelberg J. Scores of plaque, bleeding, suppuration and probing depth to predict probing attachment loss. Five years of observations following nonsurgical periodontal therapy. J Clin Periodontol 1990;17:102–107.

5. Claffey A, Nyland K, Kiger R, Garrett S, Egelberg J. Diagnostic predictability of scores of plaque, bleeding, suppuration and probing depth for probing attachment loss. Three and one-half years of observation following initial periodontal therapy. J Clin Periodontol 1990;17:108–114.

6. Wilson T. Compliance: A review of the literature with possible application to periodontics. J Periodontol 1987;58:706–714.

7. Manson JD. Bone morphology and bone loss in periodontal disease. J Clin Periodontol 1976;3:14–22.

8. Ochsenbein C. A primer for osseous surgery. Int J Periodont Rest Dent 1986;6(1):8–47.

9. Bowers GM, Chadroff B, Carnevale R, et al. Histologic evaluation of new attachment apparatus formation in humans. Part III. J Periodontol 1989;60:683–693.

10. Aukhil I, Pettersson E. Effect of citric acid conditioning on fibroblast cell density in periodontal wounds. J Clin Periodontol 1987;14:80–84.

11. Stahl S, Froum S. Human clinical and histological repair responses following the use of citric acid in periodontal therapy. J Periodontol 1977;48:262–266.

12. Marks S, Mehta N. Lack of effect of citric acid treatment of root surfaces on the formation of new connective tissue attachment. J Clin Periodontol 1986;13:109–113.

13. Smith B, Manson WE, Morrison EC, Caffesse RG. The effectiveness of citric acid as an adjunct to surgical re-attachment procedures in humans. J Clin Periodontol 1986;13:701–708.

14. Demirel K, Baer P, McNamara TF. Topical application of doxycycline on periodontally involved root surfaces in vitro: Comparative analysis of substantivity on cementum and dentin. J Periodontol 1991;62:312–316.

15. Masters LB, Mellonig JT, Brunsvold MA, Nummikoski PV. A clinical evaluation of demineralized freeze-dried bone allograft in combination with tetracycline in the treatment of periodontal osseous defects. J Periodontol 1996;67:70–81.

16. Mellonig JT. Decalcified freeze-dried bone allograft as an implant material in human periodontal defects. Int J Periodont Rest Dent 1984;4(6):41–55.

17. Wikesjö UME, Nilveus R. Periodontal repair in dogs: Effect of wound stabilization on healing. J Periodontol 1990;61:719–724.

18. Hiatt WW, Schallhorn RG. Intraoral transplants of cancellous bone and marrow in periodontal lesions. J Periodontol 1973;44:194–208.

19. Becker W, Becker B, Berg L, Samsam C. Clinical and volumetric analysis of three-wall intrabony defects following open flap debridement. J Periodontol 1986;57:277–285.

20. Prichard JF. The etiology, diagnosis and treatment of the intrabony defect. J Periodontol 1967;38:455–465.

21. Ewen SJ. Bone swaging. J Periodontol 1965;36:57–63.

22. Wise RJ, Kramer GM. Predetermination of osseous changes associated with uprighting tipped molars by probing. Int J Periodont Rest Dent 1993;13:69–81.

23. Cortellini P, Bowers G. Periodontal regeneration of intrabony defects: An evidence-based treatment approach. Int J Periodont Rest Dent 1995;15:128–145.

24. Bowers GM, Middleton C. Histologic evaluation of cementogenesis on periodontitis-affected roots in humans. Int J Periodont Rest Dent 1990;10:429–435.

25. McClain PK, Schallhorn RG. Long-term assessment of combined osseous composite grafting, root conditioning, and guided tissue regeneration. Int J Periodont Rest Dent 1993;13:9–27.

26. Machtei E, Schallhorn RG. Successful regeneration of mandibular Class II furcation defects. An evidence-based treatment approach. Int J Periodont Rest Dent 1995;15:146–167.

27. Dragoo M, Sullivan H. A clinical and histologic evaluation of autogenous iliac bone grafts in humans. II. External root resorption. J Periodontol 1973;44:614–625.

28. Schallhorn RG, Hiatt W, Boyce W. Iliac transplants in periodontal therapy. J Periodontol 1970;41:566–580.

29. Bowers GM, Felton F, Middleton C, et al. Histologic comparison of regeneration in human intrabony defects when osteogen is combined with demineralized freeze-dried bone allograft and purified bovine collagen. J Periodontol 1991;62:690–702.

30. Lyman S, Gottlow J, Karring T, Lindhe J. The regenerative potential of the periodontal ligament. An experimental study in the monkey. J Clin Periodontol 1982;9:275–279.

31. Karring T, Nyman S, Lindhe J. Healing following implantation of periodontitis-affected roots into bone tissue. J Clin Periodontol 1980;7:96–105.

32. Nyman S, Karring T, Lindhe J, Planten S. Healing following implantation of periodontitis-affected roots into gingival connective tissue. J Clin Periodontol 1980;7:394–401.

33. Nyman S, Lindhe J, Karring T, Rylander H. New attachment following surgical treatment of human periodontal disease. J Clin Periodontol 1982;9:290–296.

34. Gottlow J, Nyman S, Lindhe J, Karring T, Wennström J. New attachment formation in the human periodontium by guided tissue regeneration. J Clin Periodontol 1986;13:604–616.

35. Becker W, Becker B. Treatment of mandibular three-wall intrabony defects by flap debridement and expanded polytetrafluoroethylene barrier membranes. Long-term evaluation of 32 treated patients. J Periodontol 1993;64:1138–1144.

36. Guillemin MR, Mellonig JT, Brunsvold MA. Healing in periodontal defects treated by decalcified freeze-dried bone allografts in combination with ePTFE membranes. I. Clinical and scanning electron microscopic analysis. J Clin Periodontol 1993;20:528–536.

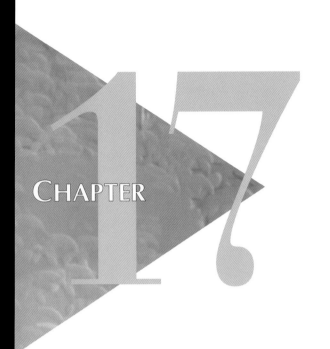

Surgical Complications in Guided Tissue Regeneration

Kevin G. Murphy, DDS, MS

Guided tissue regeneration (GTR) with barrier membranes, such as expanded polytetrafluoroethylene (e-PTFE) membranes, is an accepted treatment modality of periodontal reconstructive surgery.[1] The GTR technique delays apical migration of the gingival epithelium by excluding the gingival connective tissue and allows granulation tissue derived from the periodontal ligament space and osseous tissues to repopulate the space adjacent to the denuded root surface. New connective tissue attachment is often a result of this technique.[2–5]

The postoperative healing after GTR procedures with e-PTFE or resorbable materials is physiologically different from the healing that occurs after replaced flap techniques. Sites treated using GTR procedures also demonstrate distinct clinical healing patterns. In periodontal applications, by 4 weeks of healing, a small portion of the coronal aspect of the e-PTFE membrane is often exposed, and a space lateral to the e-PTFE barrier is created. This space, or "pseudopocket," can be the site of bacterial colonization[6] and abscess formation.[7] In GTR procedures, exposure of the membrane is common and introduces variability to the healing response. In contrast, abscess formation during the healing of conventional replaced flap procedures is rare.[8] Other surgical healing complications have been previously described after use of the GTR technique with the Gore-Tex Periodontal Material (GTPM) (WL Gore, Flagstaff, AZ),[9,10] Gore-Tex Augmentation Material (GTAM) (WL Gore),[11–13] Guidor (Guidor AB, Bensenville, IL),[14] and Vicryl (Johnson & Johnson, Arlington, TX)[15] materials. These include perforation of the flap, abnormal pain, and postoperative swelling.

The postoperative blood supply to the flap in a conventional replaced flap procedure is derived from the base of the flap, the underlying bone, the periodontal ligament space, and newly formed periosteum. Neovascularization of the gingival flap from vessels within the osseous tissues, the periodontal ligament space, and bone-periosteal surface is blocked by GTR membranes in periodontal applications (Fig 17-1). This prevents establishment of critical collateral microvasculature anastomoses[16] necessary for gingival flap survival. Because the healing gingival flap is deprived of this secondary blood supply in a GTR procedure, sloughing or necrosis of a portion of the gingival flap is not rare. Blood perfusion studies have demonstrated that blood flow to the coronal edges of the mucosal flap is significantly decreased after a GTR procedure compared to the blood flow allowed by a replaced flap procedure.[17] This altered neovascularization of the healing flap is fundamental to most of the postoperative complications of GTR.

Many treatment variables may influence the amount of attachment level gained as a result of a GTR procedure. These variables include the preoperative depth of the defect, the use of allografts or autografts, the degree of the furcation involvement, the exposure of the membrane into the oral cavity, and the length of time the membrane remains in the surgical site. If the occurrence of surgical complications affects the efficacy of the treatment, prevention and correction of the complications may result in improved attachment level gains.

This chapter will describe the most common postoperative complications associated with GTR and suggest methods of prevention and treatment. The effect of the postoperative healing complications on wound regeneration subsequent to GTR procedures will also be discussed.

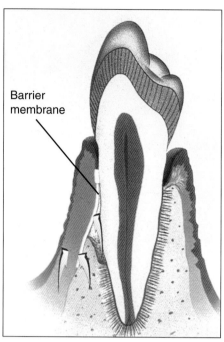

Fig 17-1 Barriers used in GTR procedures exclude neovascularization of the gingival flap from osseous, periosteal, and periodontal ligament sources. The decreased neovascularization of the flap impairs integration of the flap with the coronal edge of the membrane. Recession of the gingival flap and creation of a pseudopocket are likely to develop.

Types of Complications

Periodontal Applications

The following complications have been described for GTR procedures performed in the periodontal environment:

1. *Pain.* An objective assessment of any thermal sensitivity, pain on percussion, or the need for immediate endodontic therapy to alleviate the pain.
2. *Swelling.* A raised area, immediately adjacent to the surgical site, detected by digital examination more than 1 week postoperatively. It is often associated with pain.
3. *Purulence or abscess formation.* Suppuration or the presence of an unclear exudate in the pseudopocket or space external to the membrane (Fig 17-2). The pseudopocket is a space that develops lateral to the membrane during healing as a result of the failure of the membrane to become incorporated into the most coronal aspect of the gingival flap.

4. *Sloughing.* The postoperative reduction or recession of the flap height of greater than 4 mm (Figs 17-3a and 17-3b).
5. *Exophytic tissue.* Rapidly growing granulation tissue that grows past the barrier material. It may bleed spontaneously (Figs 17-4a and 17-4b).
6. *Apical perforation of flap.* An exposure of the membrane through the mucosal flap at the apical border of the membrane (Fig 17-5).

Bone Applications

Postsurgical complications associated with guided bone regeneration (GBR) techniques using GTAM, for bone augmentation alone or in association with implant placement, are similar to those seen in periodontal applications. The most problematic and common complication is soft tissue dehiscence of the mucosal flap. Soft tissue dehiscence usually occurs near a crestal incision site or adjacent to a proximal tooth surface (Fig 17-6). Abscess formation can also occur in areas of small perforations (Fig 17-7).

Frequency of Complications

A retrospective study[10] of 102 sites in 62 patients examined the frequency of complications associated with the use of GTPM (Fig 17-8). Of the previously defined complications, abnormal postoperative pain was the most frequently described complication (16%). Purulence occurred in approximately 11% of the sites. Swelling, sloughing, and the presence of exophytic tissue occurred in approximately 7% of the sites. The coronal aspect of the GTPM became exposed in 87% of sites treated. The average time to exposure was between 2 and 3 weeks (16.2 days) postoperatively. Clinical inflammation of the marginal gingival tissue was used as the determining factor for timing of the GTPM removal; the majority of sites had the material removed between 6 to 8 weeks, with an average time of 52.5 days. In a controlled study in monkeys, Gottlow et al[18] compared the postoperative complications of GTR procedures with GTPM to those with Guidor. They found less recession and inflammation in sites treated with Guidor.

The most common complication reported after GBR procedures is flap dehiscence. The frequency of this complication ranges from 4% to 41% of sites treated and depends heavily on the surgical experience of the clinician.[19–21] The chance of soft tissue dehiscences increases when GBR is done in conjunction with immediate implant placement in extraction sockets.

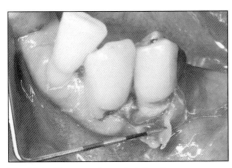

Fig 17-2 The pseudopocket develops as a space lateral to the membrane.

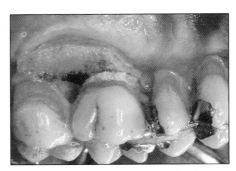

Fig 17-3a Severe postoperative palatal recession with the use of GTPM in a smoker.

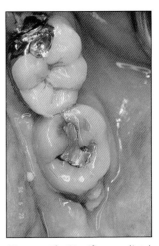

Fig 17-3b Significant distal exposure of Guidor membrane at 4 weeks.

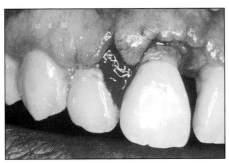

Fig 17-4a The occurrence of exophytic tissue subsequent to a GTR procedure is rare.

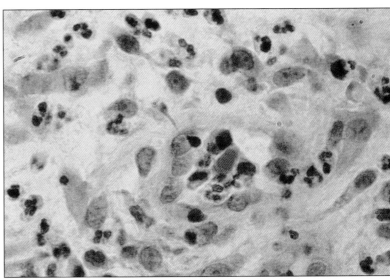

Fig 17-4b A biopsy specimen of exophytic tissue reveals granulation tissue. (Hematoxylin-eosin stain; original magnification × 250.)

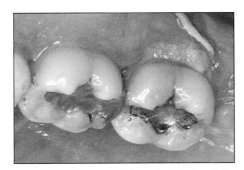

Fig 17-5 Perforation of the apical border of the membrane is most likely to occur in areas where the alveolar mucosa is thin and when the membrane has been inadvertently folded.

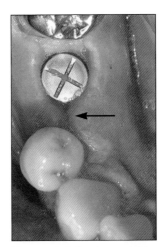

Fig 17-6 Soft tissue dehiscence resulting in exposure of GTAM material is most likely to occur in areas where midcrestal incisions have been made or adjacent to proximal tooth surfaces *(arrow)*.

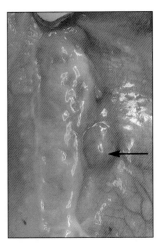

Fig 17-7 Abscess formation can occur in areas with small perforations of the mucosal flap in guided bone regeneration techniques *(arrow)*.

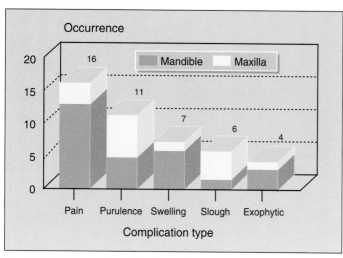

Fig 17-8 Incidence of complications when GTPM is used.

Associations and Treatment of Complications

Pain

Of the sites associated with abnormal pain, the majority are located in mandibular molars; class II and class III furcations represent the most sites with abnormal pain. There is also a strong correlation between the presence of pain and the presence of postoperative swelling.[10] A possible explanation for the associations with pain is that increased attachment loss in the furcal area will involve an increased risk of accessory pulpal canal exposure. The presence of accessory canals in the furcal area has been reported to be as high as 76% in human molars.[22] Patent accessory canals that traverse the cementum and dentin from the furcal periodontal ligament to the pulp appear in 46% of mandibular molars[23] and 59% of all molars.[24] Because of the physical difficulties in gaining access with hand instrumentation, furcal areas often require adjunctive debridement to compensate for incomplete hand instrumentation. The use of chemical root preparation during debridement may contribute to postoperative pulpal inflammation.[25,26] Tetracycline hydrochloride is an acid when mixed with saline and may enter the patent accessory canals in the furcal areas. This will most likely result in pulpal inflammation. Therefore, pain can be expected as a postoperative complication where the furcal involvement is significant and the root preparation has been excessive.

High-speed rotary instrumentation in the furca is also frequently employed to compensate for incomplete hand instrumentation. The use of low-speed rotary instrumentation with finishing burs or diamonds may result in less pulpal damage. Root preparation therapy, whether rotary or chemical, may precipitate pulpal inflammation that results in either a transient pulpitis or pulpal necrosis. Proper preoperative assessment of the pulpal status is critical.

Swelling

The incidence of swelling is disproportionately greater in the mandible than the maxilla. This is possibly related to the increased amount of postsurgical edema normally seen in the mandibular buccal areas as a result of dependent edema. The use of methylprednisilone (Medrol Dospak, Upjohn, Kalamazoo, MI) dramatically decreases the incidence of postoperative swelling in mandibular molar sites. This effect probably occurs as a by-product of the ablation of the swelling and edema, which exert a tensile force on the coronal edge of the healing gingival flap. Therefore, early integration of the flap with the membrane may be facilitated by the use of steroids. The incidence of flap dehiscence in GBR is dramatically reduced when steroids are used. However, steroids are not suggested for routine procedures and should be used discriminately. Proper presurgical evaluation and examination of the patient's medical history are required before administration of this glucocorticoid.

Purulence

When GTPM is used, the average time of the onset of purulence is approximately 6 weeks (44 days) postoperatively.[10] Purulence occurs only at sites that demonstrate material exposure. However, in many sites that demonstrate purulence, associated gingival tissues present with only mild gingival inflammation.

Because only sites that demonstrate material exposure display purulence, the presence of purulence appears to be dependent on the development of the pseudopocket, or gingival space, lateral to the GTPM. Once this pseudopocket is present, purulence is related to the length of time that the material is allowed to remain in place. Given that most GTPM surgical sites will develop material exposure, prevention of purulence is related to timely removal of the material within 4 to 6 weeks. The manufacturer recommends that the material be removed at 4 to 6 weeks, and this guideline is consistent with prevention of the purulence complication. However, removal of material at this recommended interval may decrease the regenerative result if the newly regenerated tissues have not yet fully matured and will not survive intact in the oral environment.[27,28]

Microflora

Bacteriologic studies[10] of purulent or abscessed sites associated with periodontal applications reveal that the morphotypes of the purulent sites are predominantly cocci and nonmotile rods, constituting 46.2% and 49.1% of the flora, respectively. Spirochetes accounted for 1.7% and motile rods accounted for 2.9%. The most common species cultured were *Streptococcus* and *Actinomyces* species. *Prevotella intermedia* and enteric flora were also found. Half of the purulent sites display some form of antibiotic resistance to penicillin, tetracycline, or metronidazole.[10]

Purulent areas respond to home irrigation devices using tap water and the administration of a systemic antibiotic. In the event of abscess formation, amoxicillin with clavulanate potassium (Augmentin, SmithKline Beecham, Pittsburgh, PA), 250 mg, three times daily for 10 days, is prescribed. Augmentin has been suggested[9,10] for treatment of abscessed sites because the clavulanate potassium portion of this drug will render inactive the beta-lactamase enzyme produced by penicillin-resistant microflora. The beta-lactamase enzyme destroys the beta-lactam ring in penicillin, rendering penicillin inactive. If the patient is allergic to penicillin, or if enteric bacteria are cultured, ciprofloxacin hydrochloride (Cipro, Miles, West Haven, CT), 500 g, twice daily for 10 days, is prescribed. A combination of Cipro and metronidazole has been suggested[9,10] as an effective means of treating infections caused by enteric bacteria.[12] Candidal infections in GTPM membranes have also been reported.[29,30] Because of this risk of superinfection, the use of GTR procedures in systemically ill patients or those who require antibiotic premedication for routine dental procedures has to be critically evaluated.

The flora associated with GTPM membranes in abscessed or purulent sites is similar to that of samples in nonabscessed sites. The predominant flora of the purulent sites is *Actinomyces* and *Streptococcus* species. These are usually associated with normal gingival health or gingivitis. It is not known whether this predominant flora is responsible for the gingival inflammation and exudate associated with the purulent sites.

Nalbandian and Tempro[31] demonstrated a similar distribution of *Actinomyces* and *Streptococcus* species on four pieces of GTPM implanted in humans. In a scanning electron microscopy (SEM) study of 20 retrieved pieces of GTPM, Selvig et al[6] described the presence of bacteria on both the inner and outer surfaces of the GTPM, which had been left in place for 4 to 6 weeks. They also morphologically identified the majority of bacteria as cocci and rods. Other SEM studies support these findings; heavy colonization is always found in the open microstructure portion of GTPM (Table 17-1).

In nonpurulent sites, Demolon et al[36] found no significant differences in the flora between patients receiving Augmentin and those receiving no antibiotic after 4 weeks of GTR with GTPM. However, a significant decrease in the clinical signs of inflammation was associated with the use of Augmentin. The timing of the onset of purulence may be related to the gradual deepening of the pseudopocket as the epithelium repopulates the inner surface of the gingival flap. Ciancio et al[38] have demonstrated that the use of systemic doxycycline improves the immediate postoperative health of the gingival tissues and decreases swelling in a GTPM GTR procedure. However, the development of resistant strains of bacteria found in the pseudopocket may be due to the use of doxycycline. Rams et al[39] and Fiehn and Westergaard[40] have both described the development of doxycycline-resistant flora and the emergence of enteric flora after a 3-week course of 100 mg of doxycycline daily.

Sander et al[41] and Frandsen et al[42] have demonstrated that the local application of a metronidazole gel at the time of surgery decreases the amount of microorganisms present during early healing with GTPM GTR procedures. This decrease in flora was not sustained over a 2-week period. At the time of membrane removal, bacterial accumulation was evident on the membranes. However, an increase in attachment levels was seen in metronidazole-treated sites as compared to controls.

Several in vitro studies have examined the ability of microorganisms to adhere to and diffuse through GTR membranes.[43–45] *Streptococcus mutans*, *Actinomyces* species, and *Prevotella melaninogenica* have demonstrated a significant affinity for e-PTFE, polyglactin 910, and collagen membranes. The e-PTFE membrane demonstrates the least affinity for the aforementioned microorganisms and does not degrade over time as do the polyglactin 910 and collagen membranes. The mechanism of bacterial adherence to GTR membranes is not completely understood but seems to be related to the development of glycocalyx biofilm.[46] Unfortunately, the glycocalyx is also a virulent factor associated with the predominant bacteria identified with GTR healing sites, such as *Actinomyces* species and *Streptococcus* species. *Streptococcus* species are the most common cause of bacterial endocarditis related to dental procedures.[47] Simion et al[44] have demonstrated that bacteria can diffuse through occlusive portions of Gore-Tex material by 4 weeks and that, once diffused into the membrane or colonized on nonvital cortical bone, microorganisms demonstrate an increased ability for antibiotic resistance.[41]

In summary, the most predominant flora associated with GTPM membranes are *Actinomyces* and *Streptococcus* species. Periodontal pathogens present frequently; *Prevotella intermedia* has been found to be prevalent in many studies. The greatest biomass is present in the open microstructure portion of the GTPM. Therefore, the open microstructure may actually be a liability to successful regeneration if the gingival flap fails to integrate with it. Because of the large differences in microflora identified in healing GTPM sites, the variability of delayed purulence, and the possibility of antibiotic resistance, the ideal postoperative antibiotic and dosage for a periodontal GTR procedure remains to be determined. However, recommendations for treatment can be made.

Treatment of Purulence

- Irrigate with chlorhexidine rinse
- Decide if membrane removal is appropriate
- Culture the site if the membrane is to be left in place for more than 3 weeks
- Prescribe systemic antibiotics (Augmentin or Cipro)
- Recommend home irrigation with chlorhexidine
- Advise the patient of the situation
- Reassess weekly

Table 17-1 Clinical microbiology of Gore-Tex Periodontal Material (GTPM)

Study	Methods, sites examined	Predominant flora	Potentially pathogenic flora	Effect on regeneration	Comments
Selvig et al[6]	SEM of retrieved GTPM	NA	NA	NA	Heavy colonization in open microstructure.
Selvig et al[32]	SEM of retrieved GTPM and 1-y AL	Cocci, gram-positive rods in coronal third of GTPM	NA	Negative	Heavy colonization had a negative effect, and membrane integration had a positive effect on AL gain.
Mullally et al[29]	Site of failed GTR in diabetic patient	*Candida*	*Candida*	Negative	Patients with uncontrolled diabetes may be prone to superinfection.
Grevstad and Leknes[30]	TEM of retrieved GTPM	Gram-positive cocci invade open microstructure	Spirochetes in apical portion	NA	Flora is more pathogenic in the apical direction.
Tempro and Nalbandian[33]	TEM, anaerobic culture	*Streptococcus* species	*Candidae, Haemophilus*	NA	The thickness of biomass decreases in the apical direction.
Guillemin et al[34]	SEM of interproximal GTPM	Cocci and rods in coronal aspect	Some spirochetes	None	Bacteria seen on both sides of the membrane.
Mombelli et al[35]	Cultivable flora of GTPM and site at 12 wk, AL gains	Gram-positive facultative cocci, *Actinomyces*	*Prevotella intermedia, Prevotella melaninogenica, Porphyromonas gingivalis*	None	Successful gain without antibiotics, if home case is excellent.
Demolon et al[36]	Sequential-healing DNA probes; Augmentin vs no antibiotic	Not described	*Prevotella intermedia, Fusobacterium nucleatum, Bacteroides forsythus*	NA	There was no difference in flora at 4 wk, but the Augmentin group had less inflammation.
Demolon et al[37]	1-y AL of above study	NA	NA	None	There was no difference in bone fill between groups.
Nowzari and Slots[13]	Cultivable flora, DNA probes of GTPM sites, AL gains	Not described	*Fusobacterium* species, *Prevotella intermedia, Peptostreptococcus micros, Campylobacter recta, Porphyromonas gingivalis*	Negative	When less than 10^8 cultivable organisms is present, there is gain of 3 mm or more. When greater amounts of organisms are present, there is less gain.
Murphy[10]	Cultivable flora from abscessed GTPM sites	*Actinomyces* species, *Streptococcus* species	*Prevotella intermedia, Peptostreptococcus micros, Staphylococcus species*	None	Antibiotic resistance is common.

SEM = scanning electron microscopy; TEM = transmission electron microscopy; AL = attachment levels; NA = not applicable.

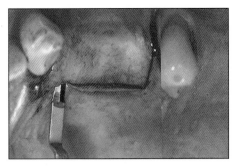

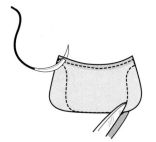

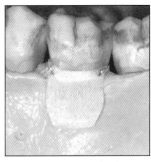

Fig 17-9 When remote incisions are used, they should be beveled. Beveled incisions are used to increase the surface area between the flap margins. The greater the surface area, the better the chance for revascularization of the flap.

Fig 17-10 Trimming of GTPM as shown will facilitate apical positioning of the membrane when interproximal bone heights are high. The open microstructure is more flexible than the occlusive portion of the GTPM. Suturing is done directly through the open microstructure.

Microflora

Less is known about the microbiology of the flora associated with GTAM membranes. Simion et al[11] compared the flora present on GTAM membranes that had experienced partial exposure and those that had remained completely submerged during healing. Bacteria were found on both sides of those membranes that became exposed during healing. *Micrococcus* species, *Staphylococcus*, and *Peptostreptococcus* species were identified. Nowzari and Slots[13] examined the flora from GTAM sites and also found *Peptostreptococcus* species, as well as *Fusobacterium* species, enteric rods, *Staphylococcus*, and yeast.

Exophytic Tissue

The occurrence of exophytic tissue is rare. This reaction usually presents within the first 3 weeks of postoperative healing. These areas are treated by incisional biopsy.

Sloughing of the Gingival Flap and Exposure of the Membrane

Sloughing of the flap is rare in GTR but occurs more frequently in the maxillary arch. The incidence is associated with smoking and poor oral hygiene. The presence of sloughing can be attributed to a decrease in the vascular supply to the flap in the early stages of healing. Sloughing is frequently related to improper flap designs.

In areas normally prone to postsurgical recession, such as palatal surfaces, the use of local anesthetics containing vasoconstrictors should be limited.[48] Nerve block anesthesia is suggested for GTR procedures, and local infiltration with vasoconstrictors should be avoided. Also, the incidence of flap recession appears to be greater in smokers than in nonsmokers.

In periodontal applications, the use of crestal incisions and maintenance of the full thickness of papillae decrease the incidence of flap recession in esthetically sensitive areas. Prevention of exposure of the membrane in periodontal applications depends on two variables: coronal repositioning of the gingival flap and maintenance of the membrane in an apical direction. In GBR, beveled flap edges and remote incisions help to reduce membrane exposure[20] (Fig 17-9).

Releasing the flap from the underlying periosteum will often allow passive coronal repositioning of the gingival flap and decrease the amount of tension applied to the flap during suturing. Therefore, in most GTR procedures, periosteal fenestration or releasing incisions are necessary for predictable healing of the flap.

Positioning the apical portion of the membrane is often difficult if the interproximal bone levels are high. In these situations, if the membrane is sutured through the occlusive microstructure portion, the membrane will often be positioned above the cementoenamel junction. Trimming the lateral borders of the membrane exclusive of the open microstructure portion will result in a configuration resembling an apron. Sling suturing through the flexible open microstructure will allow apical repositioning of the membrane. For integration of the membrane into the flap, the flap should be kept 3 mm above the open microstructure portion of the membrane (Fig 17-10).

Exposure of the membrane in periodontal applications occurs most frequently in interproximal sites. In esthetically sensitive areas, GTR may be contraindicated because of the incidence of postoperative sloughing of the flap. A surgical technique that enhances primary flap coverage over interproximal membranes is described in Figures 17-11a to 17-11f.[49] Early infrabony and supracrestal bone fill is a routine finding when this procedure is used. This success is thought to be related to the maturation of the granulation tissue in a "sealed" environment. Because there is no exposure of the membrane, it can be retrieved

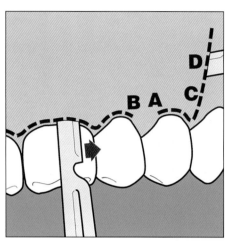

Fig 17-11a Initial buccal incisions. (1) An interproximal defect to be treated by GTR is present between line angles A and B. An intrasulcular or crestal incision is made from the distal to line angle B. (2) An incision is made from the mesial to line angle A. No incision is made between line angles A and B. (3) A vertical incision C is made into the depth of the vestibule. (4) A full-thickness flap is reflected by "tunneling" in a mesial to distal direction, starting from the mesial vertical incision. No effort is made to detach the buccal flap from the interproximal tissue, leaving the buccal flap contiguous with the interproximal tissue. (Figs 17-11a to 17-11f from Murphy.[49] Reprinted with permission.)

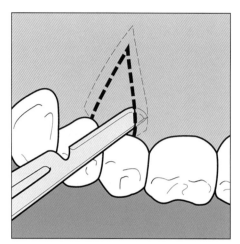

Fig 17-11b Initial palatal incisions. (1) An intrasulcular incision is made from a point two teeth mesial to the defect to the mesiopalatal line angle of the defect. A second intrasulcular incision is made from the distopalatal line angle of the defect to a point two teeth distal to the defect. (2) Two beveled incisions are made from the *palatal* line angles to a common point 7 to 15 mm directly apical to the interproximal defect. The incision results in the formation of a long, thin triangle-shaped wedge of tissue, which has a large surface area. The large surface area enhances early neovascularization of the interproximal tissue.

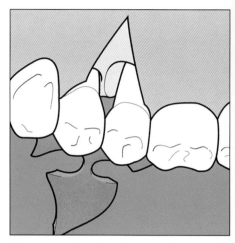

Fig 17-11c Elevation of the papillary triangle (PT). The PT is elevated from the alveolar bone and, along with the isthmus of interproximal tissue, is displaced toward the buccal under the contact area.

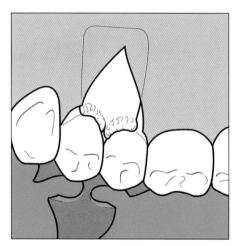

Fig 17-11d Placement of the GTR material under the palatal flap.

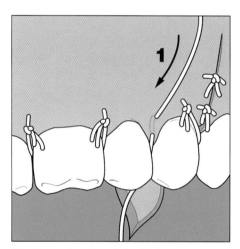

Fig 17-11e Suturing of the PT from the buccal aspect. (1) A modified vertical mattress suture begins the closure procedure.

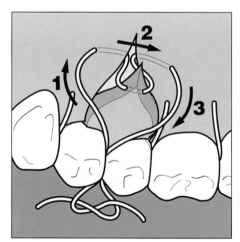

Fig 17-11f Suture 1 continues under the contact and over the PT and engages the palatal flap mesial to the tip of the PT. The suture is then placed through the tip of the PT and exits through the distal aspect of the palatal flap (2). The suture is passed over the PT and under the contact to the buccal. This suture (3) is then tied to the free end of suture 1 on the buccal side.

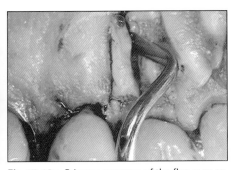

Fig 17-12a Primary coverage of the flap over an interproximal site requires the use of remote incisions. A long, thin triangular wedge of palatal tissue is created. This wedge remains attached to the buccal flap. Keeping this attachment with the buccal flap will create primary coverage interproximally and facilitate neovascularization of the palatal wedge.

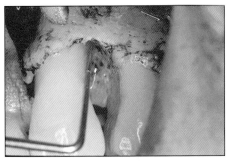

Fig 17-12b Intraoperative view of the intrabony defect.

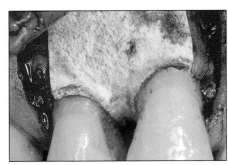

Fig 17-12c GTPM is laid passively over the defect and is not sutured.

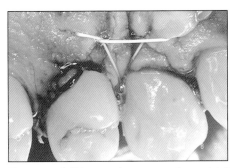

Fig 17-12d Primary closure on the palatal aspect.

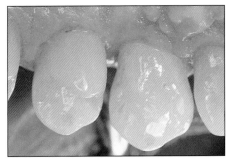

Fig 17-12e Four-month soft tissue healing with the membrane in place. No soft tissue dehiscence is present.

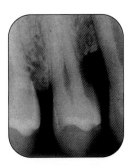
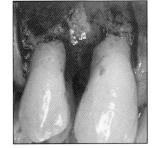

Fig 17-12f Bone fill at 4 months.

at atypically late times. With this technique, the membrane is removed at 4 to 6 months, and the bone healing response is similar to that seen with GBR and GTAM (Figs 17-12a to 17-12f).[49]

Treatment of exposed periodontal sites involves supportive care to the patient until the membrane is removed. Chlorhexidine rinses have been suggested but have never proven to affect regeneration when good mechanical oral hygiene is instituted. A balance has to be achieved between mechanical oral hygiene procedures and disruption of the healing wound in GTR procedures.

The ideal management of exposed GTAM membranes is controversial. Exposure of the membrane results in bacterial contamination,[11,13] which may impair successful regeneration. However, premature removal of the membrane results in significantly decreased regeneration.[50] Some clinicians suggest maintenance of the exposed membrane for 6 to 8 weeks with stringent oral hygiene procedures and chlorhexidine rinses.[20,51] The patient should be assessed weekly. If the exudate associated with membrane no longer remains clear, the membrane should be removed.[20] Alternatively, Valentini et al[52] have suggested replacement of the membrane if it becomes exposed. In a limited series of case reports, they described significant gains in alveolar bone volumes after placement of a second membrane.

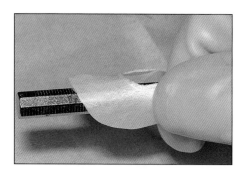

Fig 17-13 To achieve desired shapes, the GTPM membrane is pulled over an instrument handle with a tensile force.

Apical Perforation of the Mucosal Flap

Perforation of the mucosal flap occurs in areas where thin alveolar mucosa is laid over sharp osseous contours. Perforation is related to the tendency of the GTPM material to return to its original shape after the surgical placement of the material. If the GTPM, which is flat in its original contour, is placed over a sharp osseous crest, the GTPM will exert a force on the mucosa in an effort to return to its original shape. This force will often result in perforation of the thin mucosa. Perforation usually occurs between 2 and 5 weeks postoperatively. Prevention of this complication can be achieved by bending or contouring the GTPM under a gentle tensile force into a shape that will lie passively over the bone defect and the sharp contours of the adjacent alveolar bone (Fig 17-13). Inadvertent folding of the apical corners of the GTPM frequently results in mucosal flap perforation. Resorbable membranes are less likely to result in this complication.

Effects of Complications on Regeneration

Periodontal Applications

Only one study has examined the effect of complications of regeneration.[10] Complications have no significant effect on short-term regeneration (Fig 17-14). However, sloughing of the gingival flap decreases the gain in attachment levels. In this study, the data were reviewed to identify whether complications demonstrated a significant association with the use of allografts and later removal of the GTPM. The use of allografts potentiates the gain in vertical attachment levels when the GTPM is left in for a longer period of time (longer than 6 weeks). When the GTPM was left in for shorter periods of time, the benefit of grafting was not apparent. Likewise, the enhancing effect of prolonged

retention of the GTPM was seen only when grafting was employed (Fig 17-15).

Removal of the GTPM 4 to 6 weeks postoperatively will significantly decrease the incidence of purulence as a surgical complication. However, early removal (4 to 6 weeks) of the GTPM may have a negative influence on the amount of regeneration in sites that receive a graft. Tonnetti et al[27] have demonstrated that the ability to achieve soft tissue coverage over the newly regenerated tissue is a strong predictor for long-term maintenance of attachment levels. It can be inferred from these data that the newly regenerated tissue should be allowed to mature in an environment that is protected from microbial invasion and micromovement trauma.

In summary, at this time there are limited data that support the hypothesis that healing complications do not have a significant effect on short-term gain in attachment levels. However, there is evidence that the sloughing of the flap decreases the regenerative result. A synergistic enhancement occurs when allografts are used and the GTPM is retained longer. The removal of the GTPM at 4 to 6 weeks will decrease the incidence of complications but may impair the regenerative process.

Bone Applications

There are two types of complications that dramatically affect regeneration in GBR: membrane exposure by soft tissue dehiscence and membrane displacement or collapse.

Soft Tissue Dehiscence and Membrane Exposure

Membrane exposure in GBR is often associated with compromised bone fill. Clinicians often remove GTAM membranes early (4 to 8 weeks) if exposure occurs. What is unclear is whether the compromised bone fill is a result of inflammation secondary to bacterial invasion[11,13] or the lack of some "protective" barrier function as a result of the early removal of the membrane.[21,50] Both factors probably influence the regenerative result.

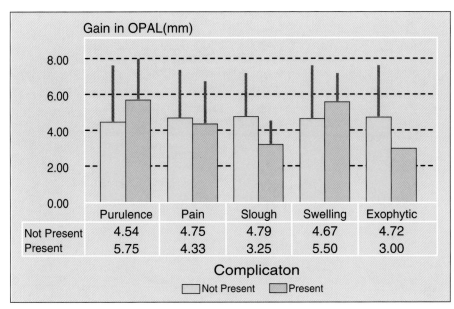

Fig 17-14 Effect of complications on regeneration.

Complicaton	Purulence	Pain	Slough	Swelling	Exophytic
Not Present	4.54	4.75	4.79	4.67	4.72
Present	5.75	4.33	3.25	5.50	3.00

☐ Not Present ☐ Present

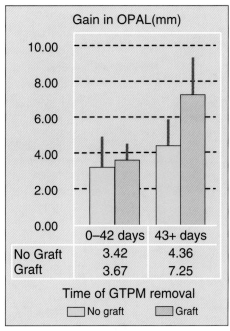

Fig 17-15 Synergistic effect of grafting and delayed removal of GTPM.

Time of GTPM removal	0–42 days	43+ days
No Graft	3.42	4.36
Graft	3.67	7.25

☐ No graft ☐ Graft

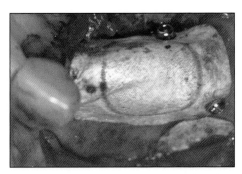 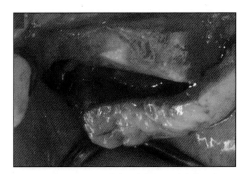

Fig 17-16 Collapse of GTAM because of the failure to support the interior of the defect with a fixed element.

Soft tissue dehiscence does not necessarily imply treatment failure; Shanaman[12] and Mellonig and Triplett[53] have demonstrated good bone fill in flap dehiscent sites. This complication does, however, significantly decrease the predictability of the GBR procedure.[20]

Membrane Displacement or Collapse

Displacement of the GTAM will result in the failure to produce a sufficient volume of regenerated calcified tissues. It is believed that micromovement of the membrane will disturb the periosteal callus formation. Clinically, this often occurs when patients wear mucosa-borne removable appliances during healing. Ideally, all removable appliances should be tooth-supported in patients who are undergoing GBR procedures. If this is unfeasible, the appliance should not be worn for 2 to 3 weeks postoperatively. Thereafter,

soft denture liners should be replaced every 3 weeks and there should be no tissue contact directly over the membrane site. If physical elements, such as bone grafts, pins (Memfix, Straumann, Waldenberg, Switzerland), and titanium-reinforced membranes (WL Gore) are not used, collapse of the membrane is common (Fig 17-16).

Conclusion

Guided tissue regeneration and guided bone regeneration techniques have a unique set of postoperative complications. Most complications can be prevented with modifications of the basic techniques. When complications do occur, treatment failure does not necessarily follow, but the predictability of successful regeneration decreases.

References

1. Mellonig J. Research in Periodontology Committee of The American Academy of Periodontology. Reconstructive Periodontal Surgery. Chicago: American Academy of Periodontology, 1990:3.

2. Nyman S, Lindhe J, Karring TH. New attachment formation in the human periodontium by guided tissue regeneration. J Clin Periodontol 1982;9:290.

3. Gottlow J, Nyman S, Lindhe J, Karring T, Wennström J. New attachment formation in the human periodontium by guided tissue regeneration. J Clin Periodontol 1986;13:604.

4. Becker W, Becker B, Berg C, Prichard J, Caffesse R, Rosenberg E, Gian-Grasso J. Root isolation for new attachment procedures—A surgical and suturing method: Three case reports. J Periodontol 1987;58:819.

5. Stahl SS, Froum S, Tarnow D. Human histologic responses to guided tissue regenerative techniques intrabony lesions. Case reports on 9 sites. J Clin Periodontol 1990;17:191–198.

6. Selvig K, Nilveus R, Kersten B, Khorsandi S. Scanning electron microscopic observation of cell population and bacterial contamination of membranes used for guided tissue regeneration in humans. J Periodontol 1990;61:515–520.

7. Schallhorn RG, McClain PR. Combined osseous composite grafting, root conditioning and guided tissue regeneration. Int J Periodont Rest Dent 1988;8(4):9–31.

8. Curtis JW, McLain JB, Hutchinson RA. The incidence and severity of complication and pain following periodontal surgery. J Periodontol 1985;56:597–601.

9. Murphy KG. Incidence of postoperative complications with the GTR technique. Presented at the Annual Meeting of the American Academy of Periodontology, San Diego, 1988.

10. Murphy KG. Incidence, characterization and effect of postoperative surgical complications using Gore-Tex periodontal material. Part I. Incidence and characterization of complications. Int J Periodont Rest Dent 1995;15:363–375.

11. Simion M, Baldoni M, Rossi P, Zaffe D. A comparative study of the effectiveness of e-PTFE membranes with and without early exposure during the healing period. Int J Periodont Rest Dent 1994; 14:167–180.

12. Shanaman R. A retrospective study of 237 sites treated consecutively with guided tissue regeneration. Int J Periodont Rest Dent 1994;14:293–301.

13. Nowzari H, Slots J. Microorganisms in polytetrafluoroethylene barrier membranes for guided tissue regeneration. J Clin Periodontol 1994;21:203–210.

14. Laurell L, Falk H, Fornell J, Johard G, Gottlow J. Clinical use of a bioresorbable matrix barrier in guided tissue regeneration therapy. Case series. J Periodontol 1994;65:967–975.

15. Laurell L, Gottlow J, Rylander H, Lundgren D, Rask M, Norlindth B. Gingival response to GTR therapy in monkeys using two bioresorbable devices. J Dent Res 1993;72:824.

16. Selliseth NJ, Selvig KA. The vasculature of the periodontal ligament: A scanning electron microscopic study using corrosion casts in the rat. J Periodontol 1994;65:1079–1087.

17. Zanetta-Barbosa D, Klinge B, Svensson H. Laser Doppler flowmetry of blood perfusion in mucoperiosteal flaps covering membranes in bone augmentation and implant procedures. A pilot study in dogs. Clin Oral Implants Res 1993;4:35–38.

18. Gottlow J, Laurell L, Rylander H, Lundgren D, Rudolfsson I, Nyman S. Treatment of infrabony defects in monkeys with bioresorbable and non-resorbable GTR devices. J Dent Res 1993;72:823.

19. Buser D, Bragger U, Lang NP, Nyman S. Regeneration and enlargement of jaw bone using guided tissue regeneration. Clin Oral Implants Res 1990;1:22.

20. Buser D, Dula K, Hirt HP, Berthold H. Localized ridge augmentation using guided bone regeneration. In: Buser D, Dahlin C, Schenk R (eds). Guided Bone Regeneration in Implant Dentistry. Chicago: Quintessence, 1994.

21. Lang NP, Hammerle CHF, Bragger U, Lehmann B, Nyman SR. Guided tissue regeneration in jawbone defects prior to implant placement. Clin Oral Implants Res 1994;5:92–97.

22. Burch JG, Hulen S. A study of the presence of accessory foramina and the topography of molar furcations. Oral Surg Oral Med Oral Pathol 1974;38:451.

23. Vertucci F, Williams RG. Furcation canals in the human mandibular first molar. Oral Surg Oral Med Oral Pathol 1974;38:303.

24. Lowman JV, Burke RS, Pellen GV. Patent accessory canals: Incidence in molar furcation region. Oral Surg Oral Med Oral Pathol 1973;36:580.

25. Berg JO, Blomlöf L, Lindskog S. Cellular reactions in pulpal and periodontal tissues after periodontal wound debridement. J Clin Periodontol 1990;17:165–173.

26. Vojinovic O, Nyborg H, Brännström M. Acid treatment of cavities under resin fillings: Bacterial growth in dentinal tubules and pulpal reactions. J Dent Res 1973;52:1189–1193.

27. Tonetti MS, Pini-Prato G, Cortellini P. Periodontal regeneration of human periodontal intrabony defects. IV. Determinants of healing response. J Periodontol 1993;64:934–940.

28. Murphy KG. Incidence, characterization and effect of postoperative surgical complications using Gore-Tex periodontal material. Part II. Effect of complications on regeneration. Int J Periodont Rest Dent 1995;15:549–561.

29. Mullally BH, Linden GJ, Napier SS. Candidal infection as a complication of barrier membrane placement in a diabetic patient. J Ir Dent Assoc 1993;39:86–88.

30. Grevstad HJ, Leknes KN. Ultrastructure of plaque associated with polytetrafluoroethylene (PTFE) membranes used for guided tissue regeneration. J Clin Periodontol 1993;20:193–198.

31. Nalbandian J, Tempro PJ. Microbial plaque polytetrafluoroethylene membranes [abstract]. J Dent Res 1991;70 (special issue):536.

32. Selvig KA, Kersten BG, Chamberlain ADH, Wikesjö UME, Nilveus RE. Regenerative surgery of intrabony periodontal defects using ePTFE barrier membranes: Scanning electron microscopic evaluation of retrieved membranes versus clinical healing. J Periodontol 1992;63:974–978.

33. Tempro PT, Nalbandian J. Colonization of retrieved polytetrafluoroethylene membranes: Morphological and microbiological observations. J Periodontol 1993;64:162–168.

34. Guillemin MR, Mellonig JT, Brunsvold MA. Healing in periodontal defects treated by decalcified freeze-dried bone allografts in combination with ePTFE membranes. I. Clinical and scanning electron microscope analysis. J Clin Periodontol 1993;20:528–536.

35. Mombelli A, Lang N, Nyman S. Isolation of periodontal species after guided tissue regeneration. J Periodontol 1993;64:1171–1175.

36. Demolon IA, Persson GR, Moncla BJ, Johnson RH, Ammons WF. Effects of antibiotic treatment on clinical conditions and bacterial growth with guided tissue regeneration. J Periodontol 1993; 64:609–616.

37. Demolon IA, Persson GR, Ammons WF, Johnson RH. Effects of antibiotic treatment on clinical conditions with guided tissue regeneration: One year results. J Periodontol 1994;65:713–717.

38. Ciancio S, Mather M, Kazmierczak M. Effectiveness of systemic antibiotics in a barrier method of periodontal regeneration [abstract]. J Dent Res 1990;69(special issue):165.

39. Rams TE, Babalola OO, Slots J. Subgingival occurrence of enteric rods, yeasts and staphylococci after systemic doxycycline therapy. Oral Microbiol Immunol 1990;5:166–168.

40. Fiehn N-E, Westergaard J. Doxycycline-resistant bacteria in periodontally diseased individuals after systemic doxycycline therapy and in healthy individuals. Oral Microbiol Immunol 1990;5:219–222.

41. Sander L, Frandsen EVG, Arnbjerg D, Warrer K, Karring T. Effect of local metronidazole application on periodontal healing following guided tissue regeneration. Clinical findings. J Periodontol 1994; 65:914–920.

42. Frandsen EVG, Sander L, Arnbjerg D, Theilade E. Effect of local metronidazole application on periodontal healing following guided tissue regeneration. Microbiological findings. J Periodontol 1994; 65:921–928.

43. Wang HL, Yuan K, Burgett F, Shyr Y, Syed S. Adherence of oral microorganisms to guided tissue membranes: An in vitro study. J Periodontol 1994;65:211–218.

44. Simion M, Trisi P, Maglione M, Piattelli A. A preliminary report on a method for studying the permeability of expanded polytetrafluoroethylene membrane to bacteria in vitro: A scanning electron microscopic and histological study. J Periodontol 1994;65:755–761.

45. Webb LX, Holman J, de Araujo B, Zaccaro DJ, Gordon ES. Antibiotic resistance to staphylococci adherent to cortical bone. J Orthop Trauma 1994;8:28–33.

46. Passariello C, et al. Periodontal regeneration procedures may induce colonization by glycocalyx-producing bacteria. Med Microbiol Immunol 1991;180:67–72.

47. Ullman RF, Miller SJ, Strampfer MJ, Cunha BA. *Streptococcus mutans* endocarditis: Reports of three cases and reviews of the literature. Heart Lung 1988;17:209–212.

48. Beckerly JM. The use of laser Doppler flowmetry to monitor the effect of local anesthetics on human gingival blood flow [abstract]. J Periodontol 1994;65:976.

49. Murphy KG. Interproximal tissue maintenance in GTR procedures. Int J Periodont Rest Dent 1996;16:463–477.

50. Leckholm U, Becker W, Dahlin C, Becker B, Donath K, Morrison E. The role of early versus late removal of GTAM membranes on bone formation at oral implants placed into immediate extraction sockets. An experimental study in dogs. Clin Oral Implants Res 1993;4:121–129.

51. Jovanovic SA, Spiekermann H, Richter EJ, Koseoglu M. Guided tissue regeneration around titanium dental implants. In: Laney WR, Tolman DE (eds). Tissue Integration in Oral, Orthopedic, & Maxillofacial Reconstruction: Proceedings of the Second International Congress on Tissue Integration in Oral, Orthopedic, and Maxillofacial Reconstruction. Chicago: Quintessence, 1992:208–215.

52. Valentini P, Abensur D, Missika P. Membrane exposure during bone regeneration before implant placement: Management and results. A report of two cases. J Oral Implantol 1993;19:364–368.

53. Mellonig JT, Triplett RG. Guided tissue regeneration to facilitate ideal prosthetic placement of implants. Int J Periodont Rest Dent 1993;13:108.

CHAPTER 18

Mucogingival Surgery: The Rationale and Long-Term Results

Myron Nevins, DDS
Emil G. Cappetta, DMD

Periodontal defects that transcend the mucogingival junction have been of concern to clinicians for generations.[1,2] Pocket elimination by resective techniques tended to yield marginal tissues consisting of minimal dimensions of keratinized tissue or alveolar mucosa (Fig 18-1). The difficult maintenance of such marginal tissues in humans resulted in the development of contemporary mucogingival surgery. Early investigators thought the alveolar mucosa too fragile to be able to withstand the physiologic forces of mastication and oral hygiene procedures.[1–4] This loose areolar connective tissue is less fibrous, unkeratinized, and more vascular than the keratinized attached gingiva. The vasculature is of particular significance, in that

the spread of the inflammatory lesion occurs perivascularly.[5,6] Many patients have an acceptable periodontium in spite of a minimal zone of keratinized gingiva (Fig 18-2).

Rationale for Mucogingival Surgery

The design of the most formidable soft tissue fortress would include a large dimension of naturally occurring keratinized tissue that is tightly adherent to teeth placed properly in the alveolar process with a deep vestibular fornix (Fig 18-3). When the marginal tissues begin to cleft, however, the

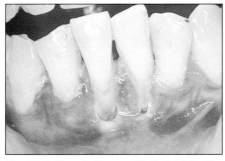

Fig 18-1 The shallow vestibule inhibits the access for cleaning. The central incisors have lost attachment to the point that extraction is necessary. It is realistic to learn from mistakes and to provide adequate zones of keratinized tissue for the adjacent teeth that will serve as abutments for a fixed partial denture.

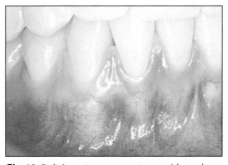

Fig 18-2 It is not necessary to consider enlarging the dimension of attached gingiva in the absence of disease or restorative dentistry that engages the gingival sulcus.

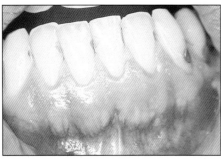

Fig 18-3 This mandibular anterior dentition exhibits a large zone of keratinized attached gingiva, a high alveolar process, and a deep vestibule. Measurements indicate that a good portion of the keratinized gingiva is attached at the level of the alveolar process.

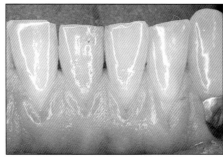

Fig 18-4 In this mandibular anterior dentition, a large zone of attached gingiva has been disrupted by gingival clefting. The entities of the biologic width begin at the most apical level of the cleft.

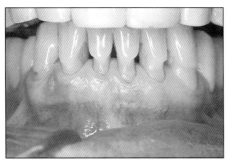

Fig 18-5a The treatment of gingival clefts by excisional surgery will result in periodontal health, but the teeth suffer from tooth wear due to cleansing over a period of years.

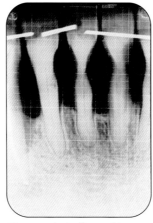

Fig 18-5b Radiographic evidence of tooth abrasion after many years of interproximal instrumentation and enthusiastic oral hygiene.

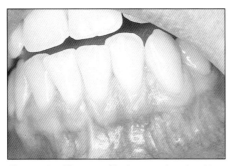

Fig 18-6a The mandibular anterior dentition exhibits clefting.

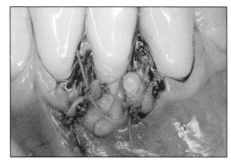

Fig 18-6b An alternative to excision of the gingival tissue is the double papilla procedure. The interproximal connective tissues are left intact as partial-thickness papilla flaps are brought into approximation with each other.

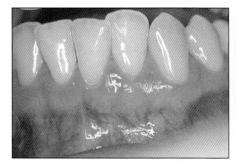

Fig 18-6c The gingival units are stable 27 years after surgery.

clinician must consider treatment alternatives to correct the problem (Fig 18-4). Excision of the surrounding tissues may result in a healthy periodontium but could lead to pathologic wear of the roots (Figs 18-5a and 18-5b). The result could be a deficiency of attached gingiva; therefore, it would be more prudent to attempt to reconstruct the damaged tissues by a gingival enhancement procedure (Figs 18-6a to 18-6c).

Anatomic considerations, in the form of frenum attachments, shallow vestibules, and discrepancies in the tooth size–alveolar process size ratio, further complicate mucogingival decisions (Figs 18-7 and 18-8). As early as 1939, Hershfeld associated the frenum with gingival recession, pocket formation, and a possible role in the etiology of gingivitis.[1] Its location is particularly precarious when found

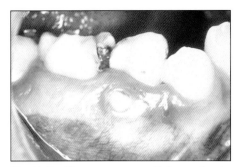

Fig 18-7a The permanent tooth is erupting in buccal version. (Figs 18-7a to 18-7c courtesy of Dr Gianpaolo Pini Prato.)

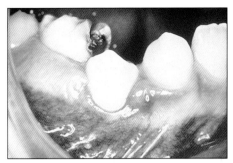

Fig 18-7b The primary tooth has exfoliated, and there is very little attached gingiva available for the erupting permanent tooth.

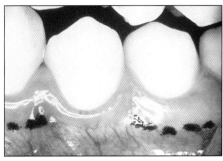

Fig 18-7c The tooth has erupted completely, but the small band of keratinized gingiva evident from the initial eruption continues to be present.

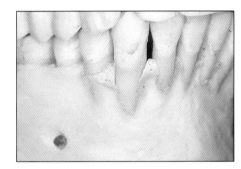

Fig 18-8 Prominent roots are frequently a reflection of a discrepancy between tooth size and the size of the alveolar process.

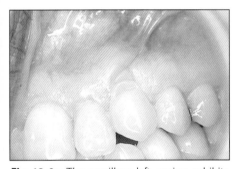

Fig 18-9a The maxillary left canine exhibits recession of the gingival tissues, abrasion on the labial surface of the root, and a gingival cleft running obliquely to meet the frenum.

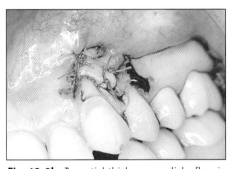

Fig 18-9b A partial-thickness pedicle flap is moved mesially to create an adequate dimension of attached gingiva on the buccal surface of the canine.

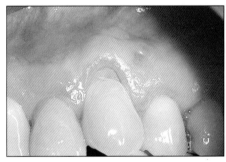

Fig 18-9c Clinical examination 23 years postoperatively reveals a good dimension of attached gingiva that has been enhanced by some "creeping attachment." The frenum concern has been eliminated.

near the gingival margin, where it can exert a mechanical pull that is evidenced by blanching of the tissues or can be an esthetic scar. The frenum must be addressed when it is associated with periodontal irregularities and must be carefully considered as a threat to long-term periodontal health, especially when superimposed on a shallow vestibule (Figs 18-9 to 18-12).

A shallow vestibule is an impediment to oral cleansing procedures for most patients.[7] It demands greater dexterity and more time from the patient and is likely to be a factor in reduced compliance (Figs 18-13a to 18-13d). Bohannon measured the success of vestibular-deepening procedures with small metal pellets and radiographic analysis, but the procedures of the era were no match for today's mucogingival armamentarium.[2] In fact, the pouch and pushback and stripping procedures depended on denudation of bone and were of questionable use to resolve mucogingival problems in the presence of anatomic limitations. The shortcomings of these procedures ushered in an era of wound-healing investigations that demonstrated the value of flaps to protect the vulnerable marginal bone and avoid further complications.[1] A partial-thickness apically repositioned flap that allows periosteum to be exposed is still used on occasion by some clinicians, but in the presence of minimal keratinized tissue and a prominent root, it has the potential to produce unwanted gingival recession.

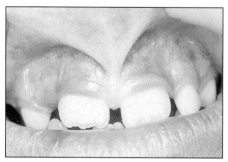

Fig 18-10 The frenum attachment blanches when the lip is pulled. This is not responsible for the diastemata, however, which will not close until the permanent canines erupt.

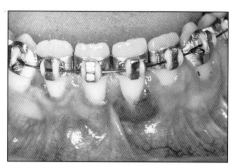

Fig 18-11 The erythematous tissue adjacent to this mandibular anterior frenum is of greater concern than the blanching in Fig 18-10.

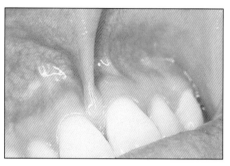

Fig 18-12a There is only 1 mm of keratinized tissue where the frenum attaches to the gingival margin. This can only cover the sulcus and obviously cannot be attached to the tooth and the alveolar process. There is a small loss of tissue at the tip of the interdental papilla.

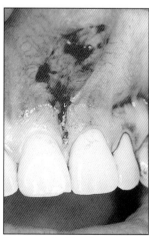

Fig 18-12b The frenum has been removed.

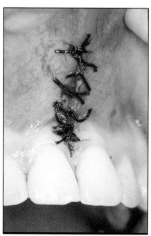

Fig 18-12c The wound has been sutured so that all but the most incisal aspect will heal by primary intention.

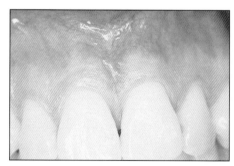

Fig 18-12d The wound is completely healed. The most incisal portion healed by secondary intention and is scar tissue. This has even less vascularization than attached gingiva.

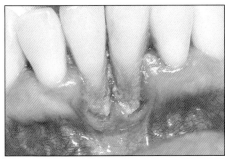

Fig 18-13a The mandibular incisors are particularly difficult for this patient to cleanse. There is a small dimension of keratinized attached gingiva, a high frenum attachment, and a minimum vestibule.

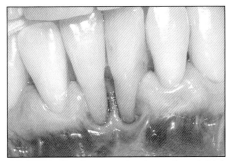

Fig 18-13b The examination after initial debridement reveals a dramatic improvement by the patient in the removal of plaque. In spite of this, the patient continues to struggle with the mandibular central incisors.

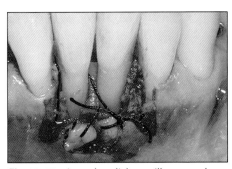

Fig 18-13c Lateral pedicle papillae procedures transpose partial-thickness tissue from the central and lateral incisor area to the labial surface of the central incisors. The papilla between the central incisors remains intact.

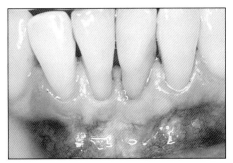

Fig 18-13d Twenty years postoperatively, the dimension of attached gingiva is intact.

In the wound healing of a denudation procedure or a split-flap procedure, the wound fills with granulations from the periodontal ligament (PDL), endosteal spaces of bone, retained periosteum, and the neighboring gingiva and mucosa.[1] The PDL, like the connective tissue of the gingiva, has the ability to induce keratinization. Thus, it seems as if the greater the contribution of the PDL in the wound-healing process, the greater the amount of tissue with the ability to induce keratinization and the greater the chance of increased gingival width.

Gingival clefting and recession were once attributed to occlusal trauma (by Stillman) but later recognized as sequelae to prominent roots and gingival inflammation.[1] The gingival cleft is an invagination of the oral and sulcular epithelium that chokes off the connective tissue corium and results in pathologic root exposure. Histologic observation quickly ends thoughts that this problem can be predictably resolved with curettage (Figs 18-14a to 18-14c). Such mucogingival problems are not necessarily self-limiting and are correctable with a good long-term prognosis.

The wisdom of enhancing the zone of attached gingiva for establishment and maintenance of periodontal health has been debated for more than 20 years (Figs 18-15a and 18-15b). Clinicians are concerned that an inadequate zone of gingiva makes the patient susceptible to gingival recession, attachment loss, and frenum pull, as they become less resistant to the spread of inflammation.[4,7] Contemporary periodontal literature has established the rationale to deepen the vestibular fornix, to create "adequate" zones of keratinized tissue, and reverse the loss of radicular periodontium via reattachment procedures that recreate an esthetic periodontium[7] (Figs 18-16a to 18-16d). It is important first to correct superficial periodontal inflammatory problems before attempting to diagnose a mucogingival problem and to determine the need for correction (Figs 18-17a and 18-17b).

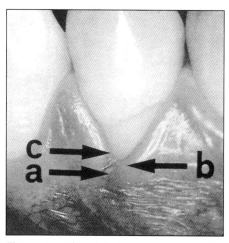

Fig 18-14a This clefted mandibular premolar will be extracted for orthodontic reasons. (Figs 18-14a to 18-14c courtesy of Dr Gianpaolo Pini Prato.)

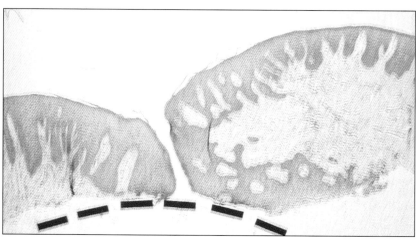

Fig 18-14b Site c on Fig 18-14a. The total epithelial invagination results in a gingival cleft. It is not possible to remove the epithelium and conserve the connective tissue by curettage procedures.

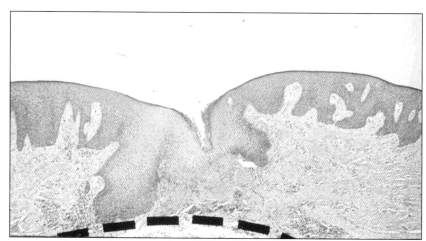

Fig 18-14c Site a on Fig 18-14a. The epithelial invagination is less complete as the cleft extends apically.

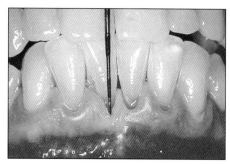

Fig 18-15a Gingival cleft. (Figs 18-15a and 18-15b courtesy of Dr Richard Wilson.)

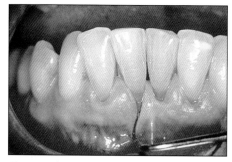

Fig 18-15b Untreated mucogingival defect 18 months later. It is unsettling to explain the apical migration of the marginal gingiva if it results in recession that is an esthetic and functional problem.

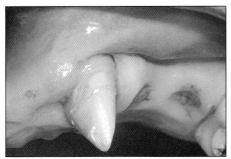

Fig 18-16a There is no zone of keratinized attached gingiva and no vestibule. It is important to create an adequate dimension of tissue to prevent recession at the finish line of the proposed restoration and a vestibule to enable the patient to use the necessary tools for debridement. The maxillary canine area extends into the canine fossa, providing the space for the creation of a new vestibule.

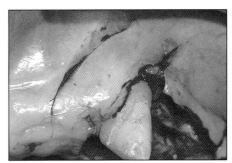

Fig 18-16b A laterally positioned flap is selected rather than a free gingival graft because it will afford the opportunity to have the vestibule lined by mature tissue. It is not necessary to be concerned with the postsurgical maintenance of the vestibule. The base of the pedicle is at the recipient site to alleviate tension when the pedicle graft is sutured in place.

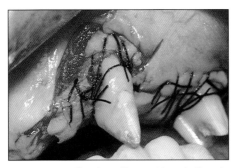

Fig 18-16c The laterally positioned flap is sutured in place.

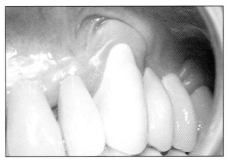

Fig 18-16d The finished restoration. There is an adequate zone of keratinized attached gingiva and enough room for the placement of a toothbrush to remove plaque.

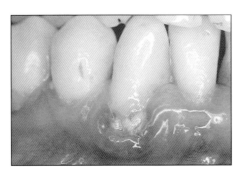

Fig 18-17a The gingival tissues of the mandibular canine are extremely inflamed, making it difficult to discern the mucogingival junction. It is necessary to remove the debris and teach the patient to cleanse this area before assessing the quantity of the keratinized attached gingiva.

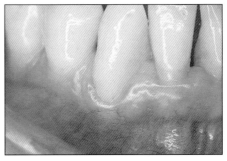

Fig 18-17b The same tissues are shown 2 weeks after debridement therapy. It is now possible to delineate the mucogingival junction and to determine the adequacy of the zone of attached gingiva.

Gingival Enhancement

It has been postulated that the dentogingival fiber complex may act as a barrier to increased apical formation of plaque.[8,9] It is suggested that there are too few fibroblasts in alveolar mucosa to set up a fibrous defense to the advancing inflammatory exudate.

Kramer[10] offered a biologic rationale for mucogingival surgery that suggests that the topography of the periodontium can preclude or deter the inception and progression of the inflammatory process. The gingival fiber connection to the tooth offers an impediment to the spread of inflammation and further destruction of the periodontium. The quality of the attachment is reduced when there is a small zone of attached gingiva that cannot accommodate sufficient gingival fibers, which are the most reliable naturally occurring defense structure. Goldman[1] postulated that the destruction of these fibers is necessary before the epithelium can migrate apically along the root. The gingiva has more dense connective tissue fibers and less vasculature and thus is proposed as a better deterrent to the initiation and progression of the inflammatory process.[5,7,10]

Gingival width varies among patients and can vary within the same patient.[11,12] Lang and Löe, in a 6-week study,[13] concluded that all sites with less than 2 mm of gingiva exhibit persistent clinical signs of inflammation. They suggested that 2 mm of gingiva, 1 mm of which is attached, is the adequate amount of gingival tissue to maintain health. This, together with the clinical impressions of others, was interpreted to mean that, if the gingival zone is less than 2 mm, surgical intervention is indicated.

Stoner examined 1,000 children and noted an increased likelihood of recession in those areas that had a minimal zone of gingiva. Beardmore[15] proposed that the strength of the gingival adaptation to the tooth is the result of a mechanical barrier mediated by the tonicity of the connective fibers and that this lessens the intrasulcular accumulation of plaque and debris. In addition, inflammation can be caused by trauma (wounding). Acute trauma, which is sudden and violent (hand instrumentation, rotary instrumentation, retraction cord, rubber dam, impression making, casting try-in, or cementation), or chronic trauma, which includes injuries sustained over time (toothbrush trauma and oral habits), have the potential to cause tissue inflammation.[16]

Some have designated these gingival enhancement procedures as unnecessary, but corrective endeavors must enlist the maintenance of the result as a factor of long-range success. Becker et al[17] documented that patients who participate in organized maintenance programs outperform those who are not compliant. It has been demonstrated that no more than 30% of periodontal patients cooperate with a planned periodicity of recall visits. These humbling accounts, combined with limits placed on the number of hygienists that can be employed to accommodate the needs of patients, severely hamper the likelihood of plaque-free dentitions. Added to this dilemma is the inescapable fact that the human race is composed of creatures of habit. Clinicians strive to create new habits, but the behavioral stability of plaque control disciplines is very fragile. Not many patients are "champions" in plaque removal; changes in domestic situations, employment, health, finances, and habits can and do affect patients' performances.[16,18]

There are studies that question the concept of enhancing the zone of attached gingiva for maintenance of periodontal health.[2,11,19–31] They conclude that minimal dimensions of attached gingiva are sufficient in a plaque-free environment, but it is unlikely that the population of private patients exists in this plaque-free state. As a group, these critics avoid the issue of restorative margins in or at the gingival sulcus. Although it is frequently acceptable to maintain a minimal zone of keratinized tissue on the radicular surface of an intact tooth (see Fig 18-2), the rules change when a complete-coverage restoration is contemplated. The unintentional insults and irritation associated with restorative endeavors such as tooth preparation, impression making, casting try-ins, partial denture design, and delivery of the final restoration mandate a more secure periodontium.[7,16] Furthermore, these studies are frequently difficult to interpret in terms of patients' needs.

It is necessary to question the use of dental students as subjects for short-term trials of clinical significance. Will this be a reliable test of patient compliance? It is also necessary to determine a meaningful time frame before reaching conclusions, and, if animals are used as subjects, they should be selected on a basis of similarity to the human model.

Miyasato et al[20] studied the mandibular premolars of 16 dental students or faculty for only 24 days. The "minimal" bands of keratinized tissue had no attached gingiva, while the "appreciable" zone of attached gingiva had a mean of 1.1 mm of attached gingiva. If 1.1 mm was the mean in a group considered to have appreciable gingiva, then there were those in that group who had less than 1 mm. It is questionable whether this is truly representative of a zone of adequate attached gingiva. This study was too short to be important in private practice.

Hangorsky treated 34 patients and found an inverse relationship between the zone of attached gingiva and probing depth. In the nongrafted sites, a decreased zone of attached gingiva corresponded to an increase in gingival recession and the loss of attachment. They proposed that an increased zone of attached gingiva acts as a barrier to the spread of inflammation and thus prevents the apical migration of the junctional epithelium. They interpreted the data as showing no difference in periodontal health with or without attached gingiva. There was no clinical documentation (clinical photographs) for the reader to judge clinical performance, and a high percentage of cases included in the "long-range results" were, in fact, less than 2 years old.

Kisch et al[23] completed a 5-year study of only 20 patients and found unattached and mobile gingiva to be prone to recession.

Salkin et al[24] reported a 4-year study performed on 39 dental students with no frenal complications or restorations near the gingival margin. Ten sites revealed a slight decrease in the amount of keratinized tissue. Not every area with minimal keratinized tissue will result in recession or attachment loss, but how does a clinician predict which sites in clinical practice will become problematic?

The studies by Wennström and Lindhe[28-31] were performed on dogs and introduced anatomic questions. Inflammatory periodontal disease in these animals does not result in pocket formation, but in attachment loss and recession, and the applicability of findings and results in dogs to the studies of gingival recession in man have been questioned.[32] The researchers had to create zones of inadequate keratinized tissue and this artificially created "lack of keratinized tissue" may not be applicable to the human situation.

In a later dog study, in which strips of metal were attached to the tooth surface in the presence of an inadequate width of keratinized gingiva, inflammatory reactions were almost always accompanied by a loss of gingival tissue. The findings of this study suggested that, in sites with a narrow zone of keratinized tissue, subgingival plaque formation in the presence of a subgingival restoration may result in recession of the gingival margin. The conclusion is in agreement with findings of similar microscopic studies (reported by Ericsson and Lindhe[33] and Waerhaug[8,34]) and with clinical findings (reported by Silness[35,36] and Valderhaug[37]). This observation corroborates data reported from another model experiment in the rat[38] that suggested that recession involves a localized inflammatory process and leads to proliferation of both junctional and oral epithelia into the site of connective tissue destruction. Proliferation of the epithelial cells can manifest as gingival recession.

De Trey and Bernimoulin[21] treated 12 patients with submarginal soft tissue grafts over a 6-week period and reported a decrease in the quantity of gingiva in the nongrafted sites. Although they concluded that this was due to an increased level of oral hygiene, it might indicate that patients with good oral hygiene showed signs of gingival recession. It was concluded that it is acceptable to augment the zone of keratinized attached gingiva if inflammation and/or recession persists after debridement therapy and a

period of observation. This is a dangerous posture for a clinician who is evaluating and treating a periodontium to accept restorative dentistry. It also is remarkably difficult to have the patient return multiple times for observation, and it is naive to believe that this routinely occurs in private practices.

The studies by Dorfman et al[25,26] and Kennedy et al[27] provide a worthwhile opportunity to study the relationship of attached gingiva to periodontal health over a significant time frame. The study did not evaluate the frenum, orthodontic intervention, or the placement of restorative margins in proximity to the gingival margins, but was extended long enough (7 years) to allow a comparison of compliant and noncompliant patients. This is very pertinent, considering that no study to date demonstrates 40% periodontal maintenance 5 years after completion of periodontal treatment.

Their 1985 publication[27] reported a decrease in plaque and inflammation at both grafted sites and nongrafted control sites but a significantly greater reduction in inflammation at the grafted sites. The grafted areas exhibited a reduction in recession and a gain in clinical attachment compared to nongrafted areas. Some sites worsened, even under controlled conditions, and were grafted. In those patients who followed a maintenance routine, the nongrafted sites showed no recession or further loss of attachment over a period of 6 years. Those who discontinued participation in the study showed further recession on the nongrafted side, unlike the grafted group, which did not show further recession.

This is a critical problem that deserves special attention in private practice patients, who frequently drift away from periodontal maintenance programs for unanticipated reasons. This is especially true for patients referred for prescription surgery. It is unlikely that the population of private patients exists in a plaque-free state. It is also important to note that increased recession has been recorded on clean teeth.[39-41]

Other factors that support the need for the resolution of mucogingival problems include the difficulties in cleaning areas of recession and the association of tooth wear with further recession. It has been observed that areas of buccal recession in subjects with a high standard of oral hygiene are susceptible to additional apical displacement of the gingival margin.[41] It has also been demonstrated that it is hard to remove plaque in isolated areas of gingival recession.[40]

Wilson[18] studied the natural history of mucogingival defects in patients in his private practice and noticed that untreated sites demonstrated marginal tissue recession and attachment loss between recall visits in patients who exhibited good oral hygiene. Alveolar mucosa margins were easily irritated, and patients may temporarily decrease or eliminate brushing in these areas, which results in inflammation and recession.

Orthodontics

Publications to date concerning the relationship between orthodontics and an adequate zone of attached keratinized tissue are numerous and controversial. The relationship of orthodontics to gingival recession presents three concerns (see Chapter 19):

1. The presence of an inadequate zone of attached keratinized tissue
2. The direction in which teeth are being repositioned
3. The control of gingival inflammation during orthodontic tooth movement

If recession occurs during tooth movement, root coverage can be attained at that time; however, the predictability is much higher for a graft placed on a bleeding bed of periosteum than for a graft placed on a larger surface area of denuded root. The probability of recession during tooth movement is sufficiently high to justify gingival augmentation when the dimension of gingiva is inadequate.[3] Wennström[2] stated that a periodontium with an alveolar dehiscence is susceptible to recession, especially when there is a thin gingival cover over the bone/dehiscence.

The dentist should consider prophylactic grafting before orthodontic intervention when the presence of an adequate zone of keratinized tissue is questionable.[3]

Objectives of Mucogingival Surgery

1. To eliminate pockets that transverse the mucogingival junction
2. To create an adequate zone of attached gingiva, especially when restorative margins will approach the gingiva
3. To correct gingival recession by root coverage techniques
4. To relieve the pull of frena and muscle attachments on the gingival margin
5. To correct deformities of edentulous ridges
6. To permit access to the underlying alveolar process and correction of osseous deformities when there is sufficient or insufficient attached gingiva
7. To deepen a shallow vestibule
8. To assist in orthodontic therapy, eg, uncovering an impacted tooth and positioning gingiva onto the facial aspect of a canine

The 1989 World Workshop on Clinical Periodontics recognized the following mucogingival procedures[3]:

1. Lateral sliding flap
2. Free gingival graft
3. Pedicle graft
4. Coronally positioned graft
5. Double papilla flap
6. Semilunar positioned flap
7. Connective tissue graft
8. Edentulous ridge augmentation

The category of *soft tissue grafts* includes the epithelialized free masticatory gingival graft, as well as the free de-epithelialized connective tissue graft, placed on periosteum and not covered by a flap or placed under the flap (subepithelialized connective tissue graft).

Nabers[43] and Friedman and Levine[44] are recognized as early contributors to the concept of mucogingival surgery. Their procedures repositioned the gingiva, the alveolar mucosa, and the vestibule, so that there would not be a shallowing of the vestibule because the flap was composed of mature tissue. Thus, when moved apically, the tissues would not change their spatial relationship (see Figs 18-16a to 18-16d). This procedure is routinely used when there is sufficient keratinized tissue, but it is detached, and when there are osseous defects that are best treated by ostectomy and osteoplasty.

Perhaps the major disappointment with this procedure experienced by the clinician is the occlusal displacement of the flap during suturing and healing. The first solution to this problem was to perform a secondary procedure to resect the tissue that had moved occlusally, but this reduced the dimension of gingiva. The partial-thickness apically repositioned flap solved this problem by allowing the flap to be sutured to the underlying periosteal cover of the bone.[45] The partial-thickness dissection created a flap of even thickness that would fit over the parabolic architecture of the osseous structures.

In 1956, Grupe and Warren[46] introduced the laterally repositioned flap to create gingiva and cover a root that was previously exposed. The following years introduced the double papilla graft, the pedicle graft, and the pedicle papilla graft, all of which used adjacent gingiva to correct mucogingival defects. These were followed by the free gingival autograft[47] to first create gingiva and then to predictably cover denuded roots. Examples of each technique and their indications will be discussed in Chapters 20 to 25.

References

1. Corn H. Reconstructive mucogingival surgery. In: Goldman HM, Cohen DW (eds). Periodontal Therapy, ed 6. St Louis: Mosby, 1980:795–943.

2. Wennström JW. Mucogingival surgery. In: Lang NP, Karring T (eds). Proceedings of the 1st European Workshop on Periodontology. II. London: Quintessence, 1994:193–209.

3. Nevins M, Becker W, Kornman K. Proceedings of the World Workshop in Clinical Periodontics. Chicago: American Academy of Periodontology, 1989:VII-1–VII-21.

4. Friedman N, Levine HL. Mucogingival surgery: Current status. J Periodontol 1964;35:5.

5. Weinmann J. Progress of gingival inflammation into the supporting structures of the teeth. J Periodontol 1941;12:71.

6. Ruben MP, Smukler H, Schulman SM, Kon S, Bloom A. Healing of periodontal surgical wounds. In: Goldman HM, Cohen DW (eds). Periodontal Therapy, ed 6. St Louis: Mosby, 1980:640–754.

7. Nevins M. Attached gingiva—Mucogingival therapy and restorative therapy. Int J Periodont Rest Dent 1986;6(4):9.

8. Waerhaug J. Healing of the dento-epithelial junction following subgingival plaque control. II. As observed on extracted teeth. J Periodontol 1978;49:119.

9. Miller PD Jr. A classification of marginal tissue recession. Int J Periodont Rest Dent 1985;5(2):9.

10. Kramer GM. Rationale of periodontal therapy. In: Goldman H, Cohen DW (eds). Periodontal Therapy, ed 6. St Louis: Mosby, 1950:378–402.

11. Hangorsky U, Bissada F. Clinical assessment of free gingival graft effectiveness on the maintenance of periodontal health. J Clin Periodontol 1980;51:274.

12. Bowers GM. Study of the width of attached gingiva. J Periodontol 1963;34:201.

13. Lang NP, Löe H. The relationship between the width of keratinized gingiva and gingival health. J Periodontol 1972;43:623.

14. Stoner JE, Mazdyasna S. Gingival recession in the lower incisor region of 15 year old subjects. J Periodontol 1980;51:74.

15. Beardmore HD. The tonus of the marginal gingiva. J Dent Res 1961;40:706.

16. Wilson RD, Maynard JG. Intracrevicular restorative dentistry. Int J Periodont Rest Dent 1981;1(4):35.

17. Becker W, Berg L, Becker BE. The long term evaluation of periodontal treatment and maintenance in 95 patients. Int J Periodont Rest Dent 1984;4(2):55.

18. Wilson R. Marginal tissue recession in general practice: A preliminary study. Int J Periodont Rest Dent 1983;3(1):41.

19. Wennström JW, Lindhe J, Nyman S. Role of keratinized gingiva for gingival health: Clinical and histologic study of normal and regenerated gingival tissue in dogs. J Clin Periodont 1981;8:311.

20. Miyasato M, Crigger M, Egelberg J. Gingival condition in areas of minimal and appreciable width of keratinized gingiva. J Clin Periodontol 1977;4:200.

21. de Trey E, Bernimoulin JP. Influence of free gingival grafts on the health of marginal gingiva. J Clin Periodontol 1980;7:381.

22. Schoo WH, van der Velden U. Marginal soft tissue recessions without attached gingiva: A 5 year longitudinal study. J Periodontol Res, 1985;20:209–211.

23. Kisch J, Badersten A, Egelberg J. Longitudinal observation of "unattached" mobile gingival areas. J Clin Periodontol 1986;13:131.

24. Salkin LM, Freedman AL, Stein MD, Bassiouny NA. A longitudinal study of untreated mucogingival defects. J Periodontol 1987;58:164.

25. Dorfman HS, Kennedy JE, Bird WC. Longitudinal evaluation of free autogenous gingival grafts. J Clin Periodontol 1980;7:316.

26. Dorfman HS, Kennedy JE, Bird WC. Longitudinal evaluation of free autogenous gingival grafts—A four year report. J Clin Periodontol 1980;7:316–324.

27. Kennedy JE, et al. A longitudinal evaluation of varying widths of attached gingiva. J Clin Periodontol 1985;12:667.

28. Wennström JL, Lindhe J. The role of keratinized gingiva and plaque associated gingivitis in dogs. J Clin Periodontol 1982;9:75.

29. Wennström JL, Lindhe J. Regeneration of gingiva following surgical excision: A clinical study. J Clin Periodontol 1983;10:287.

30. Wennström JL, Lindhe J. Role of attached gingiva for maintenance of periodontal health. J Clin Periodontol 1983;2:206.

31. Wennström JL, Lindhe J. Lack of association between width of attached gingiva and a development of soft tissue recession: A five year longitudinal study. J Clin Periodontol 1987;14:181.

32. Hall WS. The present status of soft tissue grafting. J Periodontol 1977;48:587.

33. Ericsson I, Lindhe J. Recession in sites with inadequate width of keratinized gingiva: Experimental study in the dog. J Clin Periodontol 1984;11:94.

34. Waerhaug J. Tissue reactions around artificial crowns. J Periodontol 1953;54:172.

35. Silness J. Periodontal conditions in patients treated with dental bridge. II. The influence of full and partial crowns on plaque accumulation, development of gingivitis and pocket formation. J Periodont Res 1970;5:219.

36. Silness J. Fixed prosthodontics and periodontal health. Dent Clin North Am 1980;24:317.

37. Valderhaug J. Oral hygiene in a group of supervised patients with fixed prostheses. J Periodontol 1977;48:221.

38. Baker D, Seymour G. The possible pathogenesis of gingival recession: A histologic study of induced recession in the rat. J Clin Periodontol 1976;3:208.

39. O'Leary TJ, Drake RB, Jividen GF, Allen MF. The incidence of recession in young males. Relationship to gingival and plaque scores. Periodontics 1968;6:109.

40. Smuckler H, et al. Gingival recession and plaque control. Compend Contin Educ Dent 1987;8:194.

41. Serino G, Wennström JL, Lindhe J, Enroth L. The prevalence and distribution of gingival recession in subjects with high standards of oral hygiene. J Clin Periodontol 1994;21:57.

42. Wennström JL. Mucogingival therapy. Ann Periodontol 1996; 1:67–701.

43. Nabers CL. Repositioning the attached gingiva. J Periodontol 1954;25:38.

44. Friedman N, Levine HL. Mucogingival surgery. Dent Clin North Am 1994;63:

45. Kramer GM, Nevins M, Kohn JD. The utilization of periosteal suturing in periodontal surgical procedures. J Periodontol 1970;457–462.

46. Grupe H, Warren R. Repair of gingival defects by sliding flap operations. J Periodontol 1956;27:92.

47. Nabers JM. Free gingival grafts. Periodontics 1966;4:243.

Mucogingival Considerations for the Adolescent Patient

J. Gary Maynard, Jr., DDS

The periodontium of the pediatric patient is constantly changing and provides for the astute clinician a dynamic model for study and evaluation of the developing dentition and periodontium. The control of inflammation has been emphasized as the essential ingredient in providing an environment for the maintenance of a healthy periodontium. However, lack of inflammation in the pediatric dentition is rarely observed because of the inconsistency of plaque control in this age group.

The mucogingival complex is easily observed and readily evaluated in the developing periodontium. The observant clinician can study the influence of tooth position, relative thickness of the periodontium, frenulum tension, tooth movement, and the lack of plaque control on the developing mucogingival complex. The recession observed in the adult can so often be prevented through its early diagnosis in the pediatric patient. Although predictable techniques are available for root coverage, no treatment technique is as predictable as the prevention of the problem.

Definition of Mucogingival Problems

Mucogingival problems may be defined as developmental and acquired aberrations in the morphology, the position, and/or the amount of gingiva surrounding teeth. These defects may be observed throughout the dentition on both the facial and lingual surfaces of anterior and posterior teeth, but tend to be most prevalent in canine and maxillary first molar areas, as well as in areas of tooth malposition. What factors influence the amount and position of the gingiva around a tooth? What factors might be observed that can be considered to place the patient at risk of developing recession?[1]

Development of Mucogingival Problems in the Adolescent Patient

Eruption Pattern

A tooth that erupts in labioversion or is forced in a labial direction by tongue pressure, crowded intercanine space, and/or lateral incisor pressure most likely would exhibit minimal keratinized tissue and reduced osseous support at its facial aspect. A wide zone of keratinized tissue and a thick bony plate would be present at the lingual aspect of the tooth. The gingival margin would be more coronal on the lingual aspect than on the labial aspect. The converse would be true for lingually positioned teeth (Figs 19-1a and 19-1b).

If a tooth is in a labially prominent position and has no keratinized tissue, the mucosal marginal tissue will *not* become keratinized tissue with time and function. In addition, if a tooth is in a labially prominent position and has a minimal width of keratinized tissue, there may be no further increase in the apicocoronal dimension of the gingival tissue.

Similar problems are observed on the rotated incisor. Orthodontic correction of the rotated tooth without consideration of the mucogingival problem may result in further "stripping" of the facial soft tissue attachment.

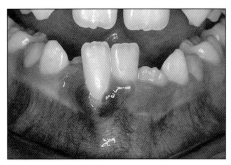

Fig 19-1a Mandibular left central incisor erupted in a labially prominent position. There is approximately 1 mm of keratinized tissue at its labial aspects. Marginal gingivitis is apparent. A mucogingival problem already exists in this 7-year-old patient. Further loss of attachment and/or keratinized tissue and root exposure are possible if treatment is not afforded.

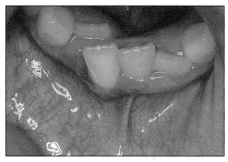

Fig 19-1b Occlusal view demonstrating the labial position of the mandibular left central incisor.

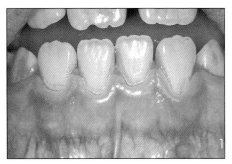

Fig 19-2 Clinical representation of the ideal dimension of keratinized tissue and bone.

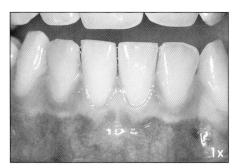

Fig 19-3 Clinical representation of thin keratinized tissue over an alveolar process of normal labiolingual width.

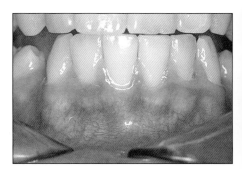

Fig 19-4 Clinical representation of the ideal dimension of keratinized tissue over a narrow alveolar process.

Thickness of the Periodontium

The thickness of the periodontium has a significant effect on mucogingival problems. There are four possibilities:

Type I. Normal or "ideal" dimension of keratinized tissue and normal or ideal labiolingual width of the alveolar process. Clinically, the width of keratinized tissue is 3 to 5 mm, and palpation reveals a relatively thick periodontium (Fig 19-2). A sufficient dimension of attached gingiva separates the "retractable" free gingival margin from the mobile alveolar mucosa.

Type II. Thinner keratinized tissue and normal labiolingual width of the alveolar process. Figure 19-3 demonstrates a minimal amount (less than 2 mm) of keratinized tissue over the facial aspect of the teeth. The subjacent bone, when palpated, seems reasonably thick.

Type III. Normal or ideal dimension of keratinized tissue and thin labiolingual width of the alveolar process. This is observed clinically as normal keratinized tissue width, but the bone is thin and the roots can be palpated (Fig 19-4).

Type IV. Thin keratinized tissue (less than 2 mm) and thin labiolingual dimension of the underlying bone (Fig 19-5a). With this tissue situation (Fig 19-5b), there is potential for recession in the presence of poor plaque control and local trauma as the patient matures. The gingiva tends to be thin labiolingually, favoring its through-and-through loss with inflammation.

The ideal periodontium may well endure. The type II periodontium likewise may survive. The type III periodontium frequently may mislead the family dentist, and the orthodontist must be especially attentive because labial tooth movement may result in attachment loss via the bony

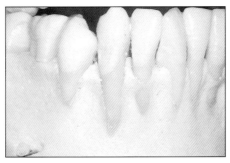

Fig 19-5a Thin dimension of labiolingual bone.

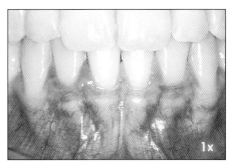

Fig 19-5b Clinical representation of thin keratinized tissue over a narrow alveolar process.

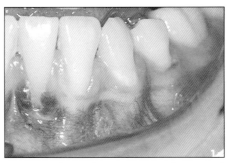

Fig 19-6 Gingival recession at the central incisor area, resulting from predisposing factors of thin bone and overlying soft tissue, exacerbated by plaque-induced inflammation and/or trauma.

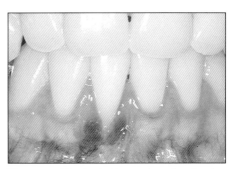

Fig 19-7 Marginal tissue that is alveolar mucosa and is located at or apical to the cementoenamel junction.

septum. The type IV periodontium should generate the most concern, and the patient must be considered at risk for mucogingival problems.

These predisposing factors, modified by plaque-induced inflammation and/or trauma (eg, toothbrushing, cervical restoration, crown margins, toothpicks), may with time result in gingival recession (Fig 19-6). Hall[2] has expressed a logical and clear hypothesis:

1. Teeth that erupt in prominence (are malpositioned) are likely to have inadequate attached gingiva and dehiscences or fenestrations.
2. The gingiva of prominent teeth is prone to recession.
3. Such prominent teeth erupt at or near the mucogingival junction and do not bring bone with them as they erupt "off" basal bone.
4. Inadequate attached gingiva and dehiscences (or thin alveolar bone) may predispose a tooth to recession with inflammation and wounding. In the absence of disease, recession may not occur despite the predisposition.

Rationale for Mucogingival Therapy in the Adolescent Patient[3]

When Is Gingival Augmentation Necessary?

Nonorthodontic Pediatric Patients

Eversion of the marginal tissues. When the marginal tissue is alveolar mucosa and is located at or near the cementoenamel junction, and when frenulum manipulation causes movement or eversion of the marginal tissue, augmentation of attached gingiva is necessary (Fig 19-7). The attached gingiva provides a keratinized or parakeratinized epithelium with underlying attached connective tissue, separating the retractable free gingival margin from the mobile alveolar mucosa. Without this barrier of attached tissue, the muscles of expression and the mobility of the lip and cheek may cause movement or eversion of the free gingival tissue.

Lang and Löe implied that such movement facilitates plaque accumulation and microbial movement into the gingival crevice.[4] Blanching of the tissues occurs when the frenulum has been activated. This has been considered a diagnostic method for determining the need for gingival augmentation. The blanching may be present when the tissue is adequately attached and is not necessarily an indication for gingival augmentation. Such blanching may represent transient reduction of the blood supply to the tissues. However, marginal movement with eversion is more threatening to long-term periodontal health. Adequate plaque debridement is difficult, if not impossible, when eversion of the marginal tissue is observed.

Root exposure. Exposure of the cementum surface creates several problems that are generally observed only by the parent and clinician. However, with time they may become of equal importance to the developing and maturing pediatric patient. The following are some of these problems:

1. *Fear of tooth loss.* This is rarely expressed by the pediatric patient, but is a frequent concern of the parent. Having noted recession in their own mouths and having heard tales of teeth extracted from the mouths of friends and relatives, parents are often alarmed to see areas of recession and root exposure in their own children. In many instances, treatment of such problems is sought by the parent; the therapist must first reassure the parent that loss of the tooth is not imminent.

2. *Cosmetic considerations.* Root exposure in the pediatric patient frequently is a cause for embarrassment. The patient is often self-conscious and becomes anxious about being different from his or her peers. The parent frequently exhibits extreme concern and requests immediate correction of the problem by the dentist. The psychological impact on the patient of "being different" because of having longer teeth cannot be ignored.

3. *Root sensitivity.* The pulp chamber and root canal are significantly larger in the pediatric permanent dentition than in the more mature adult tooth. In the pediatric patient, root exposure frequently creates a more noticeable response to thermal and external stimuli than is observed in the adult with similar root exposure. As a result of the marked response to thermal and external (eg, brushing) stimuli, the pediatric patient frequently avoids brushing the sensitive sites. This lack of good hygiene leads to plaque accumulation and to increased gingival inflammation.

Progressive recession. Most investigators and clinicians agree that a gingival graft should be performed if documentation substantiates progressive attachment loss and recession of the marginal tissue.[5–7] DeTrey and Bernimoulin[5] suggest, "If gingival recession and inflamma-

tion are present despite good oral hygiene measures and if, after an observation period of several months, the recession continues to develop or progress, then a free gingival graft may be indicated to stabilize the level and amount of attached gingiva."

However, the question of at what point documentation should begin has not been properly addressed. For example, Fig 19-8a shows a patient with no root exposure, no attached gingiva, and an associated frenulum pull in the area of the mandibular central incisor. It was decided to monitor the patient. Figure 19-8b shows the same site 4 months later. There is now root exposure, no attached gingiva, frenulum eversion, and plaque accumulation. If the patient is examined for the first time as is observed in Fig 19-8b, would it be advisable for the therapist to wait until additional attachment is lost before recommending a surgical procedure, or should the gingiva be immediately augmented to stop the recession? How long should the clinician monitor before making such a recommendation?

In the pediatric or young adult patient, once the marginal tissue recedes apical to the cementoenamel junction, there is no attached gingiva or minimal keratinized tissue, and a frenulum pull is present, a gingival graft should be recommended. The relationships of the existing attached gingival margin, alveolar mucosa margin, and width of the bone to the cementoenamel junction should be the dictating factors, not the monitoring of attachment levels over long periods of time.

Orthodontic Pediatric Patients

The patient presenting for orthodontic treatment may show sites with minimal keratinized tissue or no attached gingiva and with thin or absent labial bone. Generally, these problems may be seen in patients who demonstrate the following:

1. Labially prominent teeth (see Fig 19-8b)
2. Rotated labially prominent teeth (Fig 19-9a)
3. Anticipated labial movement or lingual tipping (Figs 19-10a and 19-10c)
4. Distal movement of a tooth with a thin periodontium into a narrow labial or lingual edentulous area (Figs 19-11a to 19-11c)

Labially prominent teeth. Teeth that erupt in a labially prominent position will usually have a thin labial plate with or without fenestrations or dehiscences in the bone. The soft tissue margin will be more apically positioned than that of the adjacent teeth. This creates inconsistent marginal tissues with increased potential for accumulation of bacterial plaque (see Fig 19-8b). The apical or coronal, as well as the labial or lingual dimension of the keratinized tissue, will be smaller than normal because of the labially prominent position of the tooth. Lingual movement of this tooth will not increase the width or thickness of the attached gingiva if none is present prior to movement.[8–10]

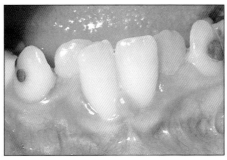

Fig 19-8a Labially prominent mandibular incisors. The probe traverses the mucogingival junction; therefore, there is no attached gingiva and no overt root exposure.

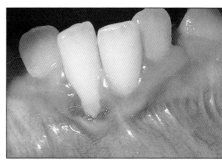

Fig 19-8b Same site 4 months later. Three mm of root exposure and marginal inflammation. How long should such a patient be monitored before gingival augmentation is recommended?

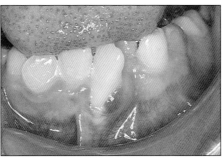

Fig 19-9a Rotated mandibular incisors with no attached tissue in a 6-year-old child. The frenulum attachment creates tensional stress with obvious marginal inflammation.

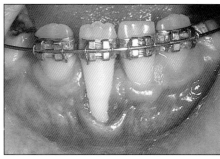

Fig 19-9b Recession associated with orthodontic correction of rotated and labially prominent incisors. When such recession occurs during or after orthodontic therapy, a patient may become litigious.

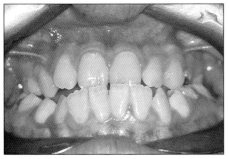

Fig 19-10a Class III malocclusion in a 16-year-old patient. Note the crowded mandibular incisors and relative thinness of the periodontium.

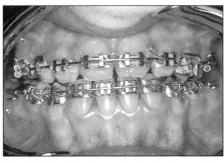

Fig 19-10b Class III malocclusion treated by labial tilting of the maxillary incisors and lingual tilting of the mandibular incisal edges. Note the further thinning of labial tissue. Root surfaces moved labially as incisal edges moved lingually.

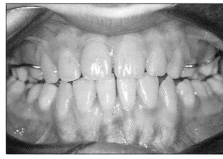

Fig 19-10c Postorthodontic view with appliances removed. Note the recession, the thin periodontium, and the prominent root position of the mandibular left central incisor.

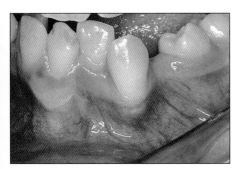

Fig 19-11a Labially prominent canine with thin periodontium. The tooth is to be retracted distally into a narrower, labiolingual edentulous area.

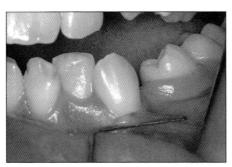

Fig 19-11b Total absence of attached gingiva.

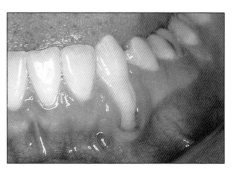

Fig 19-11c Labially prominent canine with thin periodontium and no attached gingiva that has been moved distally into a narrow labiolingual edentulous area. The result is recession and apical migration of the attachment level.

Orthodontic appliances may significantly impede efforts at hygiene because the dentogingival junction is anatomically compromised. Further recession and attachment loss may result during tooth movement in association with the plaque-induced inflammatory process.

Rotated and labially prominent teeth. Prior to retraction of a rotated labially prominent tooth, space must be created within the arch. Once the tooth is retracted in a lingual direction, it may then be rotated with less chance of marginal tissue recession. In an effort to reduce treatment time, the orthodontist may elect to correct the rotation as the tooth is retracted lingually. If this is attempted, the facial prominence of the tooth will be moved outside of the labiolingual dimension of the periodontium (bone and soft tissue), and stripping of the periodontium will be observed (see Fig 19-9b). Augmentation of the soft tissue with a gingival graft prior to orthodontic therapy will supplement the labial tissue dimension and minimize the loss of labial attachment and stripping.

Labial movement or lingual tipping. Orthodontic therapy is an art as well as a science. Total control of each tooth during movement may not be as exact as the clinician might think. Inadvertent labial movement of a precariously positioned incisor or an incisor with a thin periodontium may result in facial stripping of the tissue.

To correct a Class III malocclusion, the maxillary incisors are frequently tipped labially and the mandibular incisors are tipped lingually. In a thin periodontium, this tipping may create labial movement of the roots of the mandibular incisors, resulting in stripping (see Figs 19-10a to 19-10c). Class II elastics are frequently used to stabilize the position of the teeth in the Class II malocclusion. The elastics move the entire mandibular arch in an anterior direction, thereby moving the mandibular incisors labially. In the thin periodontium, this excessive movement may cause facial recession and attachment loss.

Distal movement. A tooth with a thin periodontium is often moved distally into a narrower, labiolingual edentulous area. Frequently, the first premolars are removed as part of preparation for orthodontic therapy. Too often after extraction of the premolars, the labial and lingual plates of bone are compressed, decreasing the labiolingual dimension of the edentulous ridge. The compression also reduces the labiolingual width of the masticatory mucosa. If a canine with a thin periodontium erupts into a prominent labial position, movement of this tooth into a narrow edentulous ridge will result in facial attachment loss and stripping (see Figs 19-11a to 19-11c). An adequate width of attached gingiva on this canine would minimize the occurrence of the recession.

Labially prominent teeth with no keratinized tissue. If a tooth is labially prominent and has no keratinized tissue, the marginal tissue will not become keratinized with movement. Furthermore, the potential for recession during orthodontic movement in these patients is far greater than

if they had a sufficient quantity of keratinized tissue. Coatoam et al[10] stated, "Teeth lacking in any keratinized tissue prior to orthodontic treatment will not form any new keratinized tissue during the course of the orthodontic therapy." Teeth with 0.0 mm of keratinized gingiva at the start of therapy ended up with 0.0 mm of keratinized gingiva and were associated with clefts 27% of the time.

Clinicians frequently will state that moving a tooth lingually will increase the width of attached gingiva.[11] If a patient starts out with keratinized tissue over the facial surface of a tooth, and the tooth is moved lingually and extruded, then an increase in the width of keratinized tissue may be expected. However, lingual movement alone or movement in any other direction in the absence of keratinized tissue will not predictably increase the width of keratinized tissue (Figs 19-12a and 19-12b).

The reason that some clinicians claim lingual movement results in a change in width of keratinized tissue may relate to a change in the appearance of the tissue from its original appearance when the tooth was in a labially prominent position. When a tooth is prominent in the arch, all of the labial tissue resembles alveolar mucosa (Fig 19-13a). Once that same tooth is moved or erupts into a more lingual position, the tension of the soft tissues is relieved. The tissue acquires the normal clinical appearance of stippling and attached gingiva (Fig 19-13b). Because the tissue was stretched when the tooth was prominent, it was thought to be alveolar mucosa.

To make the proper evaluation and diagnosis the clinician must first determine the location of the mucogingival junction. This is accomplished by placing a blunt instrument in an apical direction. The tissue is then "jiggled" or "rotated" coronally. This will locate the mucogingival junction, and the amount of keratinized tissue can then be determined even though it appears to be alveolar mucosa. Clinicians who state that there is an increase in keratinized tissue and attached gingiva following lingual movements are not closely evaluating the tissue and particularly the location of the mucogingival junction prior to tooth movement. In such cases there probably was keratinized tissue prior to movement, although it initially resembled alveolar mucosa.

During or After Orthodontics in the Pediatric Patient

If the loss of attachment results in root exposure, a concern might be expressed by the patient or parent. Throughout tooth movement, evaluation of the integrity of the periodontium is a responsibility of the general dentist and the orthodontist. Failure to be aware of the state of the periodontium may create an embarrassing and a potentially legal consequence for the irresponsible therapist. If, following orthodontic therapy, a functional occlusion and cosmetically acceptable result are accomplished, but incisors or canines are "stripped out," treatment has not been successful. A gingival graft procedure should have been suggested and effected between the onset of tooth eruption

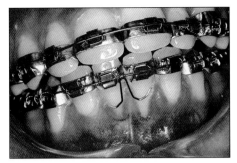

Fig 19-12a Labially prominent tooth with no attached gingiva and keratinized tissue is intentionally moved lingually.

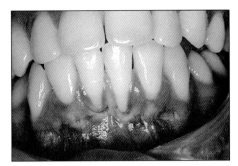

Fig 19-12b Same patient after completion of orthodontics. There has been no increase in the width of attached gingiva or keratinized tissue.

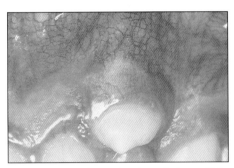

Fig 19-13a Tooth erupting through tissue. This type of eruption creates tremendous tension or stretching, thereby causing keratinized tissue to resemble alveolar mucosa.

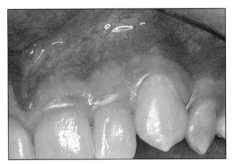

Fig 19-13b Once the tooth has erupted and is in more lingual position, there is less tension on the tissue. It resembles the normal clinical appearance of stippled, keratinized tissue.

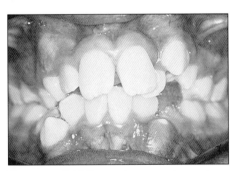

Fig 19-14a Labially prominent erupting canines. (Figs 19-14a and b courtesy of Dr Kent Palcanis.)

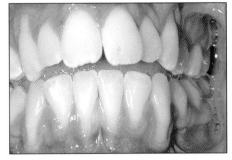

Fig 19-14b Same patient 6 years later following completion of orthodontics. Note the severe recession on the canines. Between the time of eruption of the canines and the completion of orthodontic therapy, a close evaluation of the periodontium should have been accomplished and possible augmentation with a gingival graft should have been recommended.

(Fig 19-14a) and the completion of orthodontic therapy (Fig 19-14b).

If the thin periodontium and/or labially prominent or rotated tooth with minimal or no keratinized tissue withstands orthodontic therapy without recession, a successful orthodontic and periodontal case ensues. However, if recession develops during or after orthodontic therapy (see Figs 19-6, 19-7, 19-10c, and 19-12b), a patient may become litigious. Hall[12] states:

"If a prophylactic graft is not done, recession may never occur, but, if it does occur, the current seemingly small chance of *totally* covering the exposed root must be understood by the patient.... As the legal doctrine of informed consent spreads, the need to fully discuss the pros and cons of grafting to prevent or correct recession relating to inadequate attached gingiva has become increasingly obvious.... If recession which might have been prevented occurs and damage in the legal sense occurs, that is malpractice and may result in a monetary reward."

Coatoam et al[10] and Matter[7] support the concept that consideration should be given to the quantity and quality of gingiva prior to orthodontic movement.

Excessive Stress on the Periodontium

The stress placed on the thin periodontium during orthodontic therapy may be more demanding than that periodontium can tolerate. In the adolescent with a thin periodontium, bone fenestrations and/or dehiscences are most likely present beneath the very thin overlying soft tissue. Repeated episodes of marginal tissue trauma can result from tooth movement or from plaque-induced inflammation, which is caused by improper hygiene when orthodontic appliances are present. These combined factors may result in excessive stress on the fragile periodontium; in this type of periodontium, it is difficult to prevent recession from occurring. Clinical observations and experience imply that a thicker periodontium will withstand the stress of orthodontic movement more favorably than will a thin periodontium. Stoner and Mazdyasna[13] reported that, as the width of keratinized tissue decreases, the percentage of teeth with recession increases and that when incisors have 1 mm or less of keratinized tissue there is a statistically significant increase in recession.

Technical Therapeutic Considerations

In the experience of the author, it is much easier and more predictable to graft masticatory mucosa prior to a loss of attachment and recession than to try to repair a defect after it develops. If the pediatric patient demonstrates the potential or predisposition for recession because of any of the previously mentioned reasons, it is much more efficacious to perform a predictably successful graft procedure and thus be assured that initial recession or further recession will not occur than to attempt to cover up any root surface that might be exposed later. In recent years, numerous researchers have achieved excellent results in covering exposed root surfaces with gingival grafts.[14-40] However, many periodontists have found these to be technique-sensitive procedures with substantially less predictability than the literature would indicate. Placement of a graft in a patient predisposed to recession will predictably prevent apically directed recession and root exposure. This finding has been demonstrated repeatedly during the author's 29 years of clinical experience. Figures 19-15a to 19-15d show one such 27-year result.

Increasing the width of keratinized tissue with a graft has the potential to increase the attachment level, whereas leaving a minimal width of keratinized tissue with no attached gingiva will, at best, only maintain the status quo. Creeping attachment was reported in the periodontal literature years ago.[41] Its basis and predictability of occurrence have not been clarified. Clinical findings demonstrate a reduction in marginal tissue recession and gain in attachment after placement of a gingival graft.[15,42-45] The gain in attachment probably results from the creeping phenomenon. Figures 19-16a and 19-16b demonstrate a case in which grafts were placed over the central incisors and gain in attachment occurred. Dorfman et al[46] reported a significant reduction in marginal tissue recession and gain in attachment after the placement of a graft.

Objective of Dental Therapy

Maintaining the dentition in a state of optimum function, esthetics, comfort, and health should be the goal of every therapist. The preservation of the dentogingival unit at or near the cementoenamel junction will contribute substantially to fulfilling that goal. If breakdown of the gingiva and attachment apparatus is observed in the pediatric dentition, then a weakness in the periodontium that most likely will result in progressive breakdown may exist. The abnormalities previously described are not necessarily self-limiting and will most likely only become more destructive, leading to eventual loss of hard and soft tissue attachment. Augmentation with an autogenous gingival graft will support the dentogingival unit, increase its resistance to additional breakdown, and in many instances reconstruct the lost segment of the periodontium. For periodontal recessions to develop, loss of the underlying labial alveolar bone must occur along with destruction of the supra-alveolar connective tissue fibers and apically directed migration of the junctional epithelium.

In the majority of patients who demonstrate gingival recession, the alveolar plates of bone are absent or extremely thin. This may be caused by genetic or developmental aberrations, eg, the resorption and remodeling of the labial plate of bone attending the eruption of a tooth through its alveolar housing. Placement of an autogenous gingival graft with its components of dense connective tissue and overlying parakeratinized or keratinized epithelium provides the best available means of reconstructing the area of recession and serves as a protective barrier against further tissue loss. Recession will most likely not occur if there is adequate bone over the facial and lingual tooth surface. In this situation, recession may not occur, even when there is inadequate or no keratinized and attached gingiva. However, if there is no bone, thin bone, dehiscence, or fenestration, and the overlying soft tissue is thin and there is no dense attached gingiva and keratinized tissue, then recession may occur if "wounding" results.[2] The gingival graft serves as a therapeutic bandage over a genetically or developmentally aberrant deficiency.

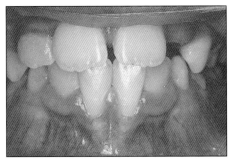

Fig 19-15a Eversion of the marginal tissue, produced by a combination of a labially prominent central incisor, an absence of keratinized tissue or attached gingiva, tissue that is apical to the cementoenamel junction, and frenulum manipulation.

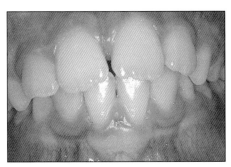

Fig 19-15b Same patient 1 year after augmentation.

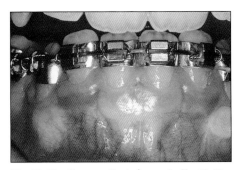

Fig 19-15c Same patient shown in Fig 19-15a during orthodontic therapy 5 years after graft placement.

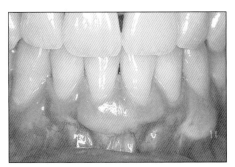

Fig 19-15d Same patient 26 years after graft placement. Firm attachment of the gingival graft is detected. Numerous cases of this type could be presented to demonstrate the stability of gingival grafts during orthodontic therapy in the years following graft placement.

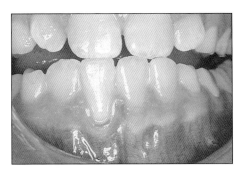

Fig 19-16a Eight-year-old patient with no attached gingiva on the labially prominent erupted central incisors. A gingival graft was placed over the facial aspect of both central incisors.

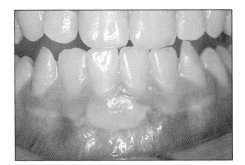

Fig 19-16b Same patient following completion of orthodontic therapy. An increase in attachment has occurred on the mandibular central incisors, possibly as a result of creeping attachment.

Why Is Gingival Augmentation Necessary in the Pediatric Patient?

Susceptibility to Inflammatory Periodontal Disease

Most of the studies on the necessity for keratinized tissue support the concept that, in the absence of bacterial plaque, there seems to be no minimal requirement for the width of keratinized tissue (viz, gingiva) needed to maintain periodontal health. It is difficult to dispute such evidence. A plaque-free mouth would be free of all dental diseases; however, such a mouth is rarely seen, especially in the pediatric patient. Gingivitis is prevalent in the pediatric patient population.[47,48] Parfitt[48] reported a 90% incidence of gingivitis in a study of a young population. Wade[49] and Powell[50] reported an 80% incidence of gingivitis in 11- to 13-year-old patients.

Inconsistent gingival margins accumulate more plaque than do gingival margins that are consistent with those of adjacent teeth. Pediatric patients have difficulty brushing and maintaining a plaque-free mouth under the best of conditions; if an inconsistent gingival margin is present, noticeable buildup of plaque occurs and inflammation results, with attachment loss at the site. Plaque-free dentitions are rarely observed in the pediatric patient. Isolated areas of recession complicate the hygiene efforts and compromise the clinician's ability to fulfill the objective expressed by Powell and McEniery[51]: "When isolated gingival recession occurs in relation to mandibular central incisors in young children, the most important aim would be to control plaque and inflammation." No one could disagree with this objective; however, it is not realistic.

Powell and McEniery report that when children with localized recession were seen every 2 weeks for professional cleaning and supervised brushing for 2 years, 12% demonstrated additional breakdown and recession.[50] When a group of 18 pediatric patients was seen every 2 weeks for 2 years for supervised toothbrushing, 44% demonstrated additional deterioration. Even with optimum professional and supportive plaque control, the pediatric patient with localized gingival recession may be susceptible to further tissue destruction. The pediatric patient is going through a time when he or she is experiencing "his or her most serious gingival disease."[52] Recommending the "control of plaque" to prevent recession in the absence of keratinized tissue or for the tooth with localized gingival recession is only giving lip service to preventing a potentially progressive disorder from causing further breakdown.

Risk of Recession

Coatoam et al,[10] in a study relating to gingival recession, demonstrated that 28% of the sites had increased recession following orthodontic therapy. It is important to compare the frequency of the risk of recession with the reliability of a procedure to prevent recession from occurring. Kennedy[53] suggested that 28% is a reasonable estimation of the frequency at which recession might occur in children who are undergoing labial orthodontic tooth movement of mandibular anterior teeth. On the other hand, in 72% recession will not occur. The practitioner cannot reliably differentiate which patient would be in the 28% at risk and which would be in the remaining "no recession" group. Therefore, every preorthodontic patient should be considered at risk, and gingival augmentation should be a clinical consideration. Grafting prior to orthodontic therapy in a patient with a thin periodontium should be considered by all practitioners. It is less traumatic and highly predictable, resulting in a sure tissue attachment to the tooth that has the potential to reduce the risk of soft tissue recession during orthodontic therapy. The augmentation should be considered therapeutic.

Techniques for Gingival Augmentation

For technique demonstration, a case has been selected that encompasses the following concerns: eversion of the marginal tissue; minimal keratinized tissue; no attached gingiva; and thin underlying bone (or absence of bone) at the mandibular central incisors in a preorthodontic patient (Fig 19-17a).

Bed Preparation

Outline incisions are made in the mucosa around the mandibular central incisors. A No. 15C Bard-Parker blade is used to carry out a partial-thickness dissection of the frenulum, alveolar mucosa, and the area of minimal width of keratinized tissue following the outlined incisions. The flap is apically positioned. Tissue scissors may be used to make sure the bed is free of loose mucosa, exposing the periosteum. The partial-thickness flap is then sutured to the periosteum at the base of the dissection and the vestibule. Suturing is performed with a needle holder and P2 needle on plain gut suture. The dimensions of the prepared bed are determined with a periodontal probe to ascertain the size of the graft to be applied to the site (Fig 19-17b and 19-17c).

Donor Site

The palatal masticatory mucosa in the area of the first and second molars is palpated. The thickness of the mucosa should be ascertained prior to dissection of the donor tissue. Frequently exostoses with thin overlying soft tissue are observed in this area, precluding procurement of a suitable graft. The measured dimensions are outlined with the No. 15C Bard-Parker blade. A 1.5- to 2.0-mm thickness of

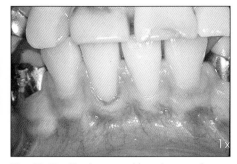

Fig 19-17a Twelve-year-old patient undergoing orthodontic therapy. Keratinized tissue is minimal. The probe traverses the mucogingival junction. Manipulation of the frenulum causes eversion of the marginal tissue on the facial aspect of the mandibular incisors. The right central incisor has 1 mm of root exposure.

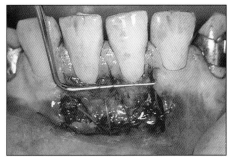
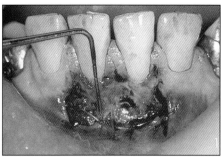

Figs 19-17b and 19-17c Measurement of the size of the tissue bed for placement of an autogenous gingival graft.

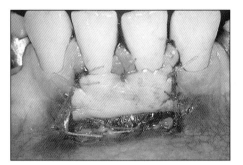

Fig 19-17d Donor tissue is placed on the prepared bed and sutured at the mesial and distal corners.

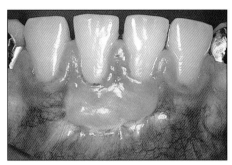

Fig 19-17e Changes occurring during tooth movement are monitored.

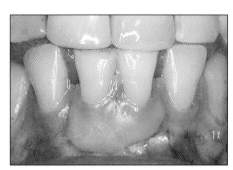

Fig 19-17f Appearance 21 years after placement of graft. Note the stability of the grafted tissues.

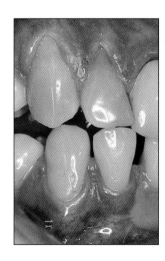

Fig 19-17g Recession has occurred on the maxillary right lateral incisor and canine and the mandibular left canine, but stability and "creepage" of marginal tissue over the cementoenamel junction are observed on the mandibular central incisors.

masticatory mucosa is removed gingerly and smoothly from the palatal area. Uniformity in thickness and smoothness of the underlying surface and freedom from adipose tissue are the desirable features of the donor tissue. Close inspection of the tissue for these qualities is fundamental to the successful integration of the graft.

Graft Suturing

The donor tissue is placed on the prepared bed and sutured with the P2 plain gut suture. Sutures are recommended at the mesial and distal corners (Fig 19-17d). Suspensory sutures directed apically or coronally and mesially or distally will provide additional stabilization to the graft, if necessary.

Postoperative Care and Instructions

Placement of a periodontal dressing over both the grafted and donor sites is recommended. This provides protection to both areas and minimizes postoperative discomfort. The pediatric patient is usually advised to keep the tongue away from the surgical sites and to avoid mastication with the anterior teeth to prevent dislodgment of the dressing material and injury to the graft. An ice pack should be applied to the recipient area externally for 24 hours (on 15 minutes and off 15 minutes).

Postoperative discomfort is managed with acetaminophen with codeine, 30 mg (Tylenol 2), in tablet or elixir form, every 3 to 4 hours for pain. The patient is seen in 7 to 10 days; the dressing removed and the area polished, and postoperative instructions are provided. A soft bristle brush is given to the patient, and the patient is instructed not to floss. Teeth should be carefully brushed to the margin of the grafted tissue, but care should be taken not to traumatize the healing tissue. Patients are usually examined again in 3 weeks for reevaluation and then every 4 to 6 months thereafter for documentation and monitoring of the result (Figs 19-17e and 19-17f).

In this patient, 21 years later, recession of the marginal tissue has occurred at the maxillary right canine and lateral incisor and mandibular left canine (see Fig 19-17g). Stability is apparent at the mandibular incisors (see Fig 19-17f).

References

1. Maynard JG, Wilson RD. Diagnosis and management of mucogingival problems in children. Dent Clin North Am 1980;24:683.

2. Hall B. Pure Mucogingival Problems: Etiology, Treatment, and Prevention. Chicago: Quintessence, 1984:58.

3. Maynard JG. The rationale for mucogingival therapy in the child and adolescent. Int J Periodont Rest Dent 1987;7(1):37–51.

4. Lang NP, Löe H. The relationship between the width of keratinized gingiva and gingival health. J Periodontol 1972;43:623.

5. DeTrey E, Bernimoulin JP. Influence of free gingival grafts on the health of the marginal gingiva. J Clin Periodontol 1980;7:381.

6. Dorfman HS, Kennedy JE, Bird WC. Longitudinal evaluation of free autogenous gingival grafts. J Clin Periodontol 1980;7:316.

7. Matter J. Free gingival grafts for the treatment of gingival recession: A review of some techniques. J Clin Periodontol 1982;9:103.

8. Ochsenbein C, Maynard JG. The problem of attached gingiva in children. J Dent Child 1974;41:263.

9. Maynard JG, Ochsenbein C. Mucogingival problems: Prevalence and therapy in children. J Periodontol 1975;46:543.

10. Coatoam G, Behrenta R, Bissada N. The width of keratinized gingiva during orthodontic treatment. Its significance and impact on periodontal states. J Periodontol 1981;52:307.

11. Boyd RL. Mucogingival considerations and their relationship to orthodontics. J Periodontol 1978;49:67.

12. Hall WB. The current status of mucogingival problems and their therapy. J Periodontol 1981;52:569.

13. Stoner JE, Mazdyasna S. Gingival recession in the lower incisor region of 15-year-old subjects. J Periodontol 1980;51:74.

14. Grupe H, Warren R. Repair of gingival defects by a sliding flap operation. J Periodontol 1956;27:92.

15. Bernimoulin JP, Luscher B, Muhlemann HR. Coronally repositioned periodontal flap. J Clin Periodontol 1975;2:1.

16. Maynard JG. Coronal positioning of a previously placed autogenous gingival graft. J Periodontol 1977;48:151.

17. Langer B, Calagna LJ. The subepithelial connective tissue graft. A new approach to the enhancement of anterior cosmetics. Int J Periodont Rest Dent 1982;2(2):22–34.

18. Miller PD. Root coverage using a free soft tissue autograft following citric acid application. I. Technique. Int J Periodont Rest Dent 1982;2(1):65–70.

19. Corn H, Marks MH. Gingival grafting for deep-wide recession—a status report. Part I. Rationale, case section and root preparation. Compend Contin Educ Dent 1983;4:167.

20. Corn H, Marks MH. Gingival grafting for deep-wide recession—a status report. Part II. Surgical procedures. Compend Contin Educ Dent 1983;4:167.

21. Holbrook T, Ochsenbein C. Complete coverage of denuded root surface with a one-stage gingival graft. Int J Periodont Rest Dent 1983;3(3):9–27.

22. Miller PD. Root coverage using a free soft tissue autograft following citric acid application. II. Treatment of the carious root. Int J Periodont Rest Dent 1983;3(5):39–51.

23. Raetzke PB. Covering localized areas of root exposure employing the envelope technique. J Periodontol 1985;56:397–402.

24. Langer B, Langer L. Subepithelial connective tissue graft technique for root coverage. J Periodontol 1985;56:715–720.

25. Tarnow DP. Semilunar coronally repositioned flap. J Clin Periodontol 1986;3:182–185.

26. Nelson SW. The subpedicle connective tissue graft—A bilaminar reconstructive procedure for the coverage of denuded root surfaces. J Periodontol 1987;58:95–192.

27. Miller PD. Root coverage with the free gingival graft. J Periodontol 1987;58:674–681.

28. Allen E, Miller P. Coronal positioning of existing gingiva, short term results in the treatment of shallow marginal tissue recession. J Periodontol 1989;60:316–319.

29. Borghetti A, Gardella J. Thick gingival autograft for the coverage of gingival recession: A clinical evaluation. Int J Periodont Rest Dent 1990;10:217–230.

30. Tolmie PN, Rubins RP, Buch GS, Vagianos V, Lanz JC. The predictability of root coverage by way of free gingival autografts and citric acid application. An evaluation by multiple clinicians. Int J Periodont Rest Dent 1991;11:261–271.

31. Pini Prato GP, Tinti C, Cortellini P, Magnani C, Clauser C. Periodontal regeneration therapy with coverage of previously restored root surfaces. Case reports. Int J Periodont Rest Dent 1992; 12:450–461.

32. Harris RJ. The connective tissue and partial-thickness double pedicle graft: A predictable method of obtaining root coverage. J Periodontol 1992;63:477–486.

33. Tinti C, Vincenzi G, Cortellini P, Pini Prato GP, Clauser C. Guided tissue regeneration in the treatment of human facial recession. A twelve-case report. J Periodontol 1992;63:554–560.

34. Pini Prato GP, Tinti C, Vincenzi G, Magnani C, Cortellini P, Clauser C. Guided tissue regeneration versus mucogingival surgery in the treatment of human buccal recession. J Periodontol 1992;63:919–928.

35. Schanaman RH. Gingival augmentation using guided tissue regeneration. Two case reports. Int J Periodont Rest Dent 1993;13(4):373–377.

36. Pini Prato GP, Clauser C, Cortellini P. Guided tissue regeneration and free gingival graft for the management of buccal recession. A case report. Int J Periodont Rest Dent 1993;13(4):487–493.

37. Jahnke PV, Sandifer JB, Gher ME, Gray JL, Richardson CA. Thick free gingival and connective tissue autografts for root coverage. J Periodontol 1993;64:315–322.

38. Cortellini P, Clauser C, Pini Prato GP. Histologic assessment of new attachment following the treatment of a human buccal recession by means of a guided tissue regeneration procedure. J Periodontol 1993;64:387–391.

39. Bruno J. Connective tissue graft technique assuring wide root coverage. Int J Periodont Rest Dent 1994;14:127–137.

40. Harris R. The connective tissue with partial thickness double pedicle graft: The results of 100 consecutively treated defects. J Periodontol 1994;65:448–461.

41. Goldman HM, et al. Periodontal Therapy, ed 3. St Louis: Mosby, 1964:560.

42. Ward VJ. A clinical assessment of the use of the free gingival graft for correcting localized recession associated with frenulum pull. J Periodontol 1974;45:78–83.

43. Matter J, Cimansoni G. Creeping attachment after free gingival grafts. J Periodontol 1976;47:574–579.

44. Yukna RA, Tow HD, Caroll PB, Vernino AR, Bright RW. Comparative clinical evaluation of freeze-dried skin allografts and autogenous gingival grafts in humans. J Clin Periodontol 1977;4:191–199.

45. Bell LA, Valluzzo TA, Garnick JJ, Pennel BM. The presence of "creeping attachment" in human gingiva. J Periodontol 1978;49:513–517.

46. Dorfman HS, Kennedy JE, Bird WC. Longitudinal evaluation of free autogenous gingival grafts. A four year report. J Periodontol 1982;53:349–352.

47. Marshall-Day DC, Stephens RG, Quigley LF. Periodontal disease: Prevalence and incidence. J Periodontol 1955;26:185.

48. Parfitt GJ. Five year longitudinal study of the gingival condition of a group of children in England. J Periodontol 1957;28:26.

49. Wade AB. An epidemiological study of periodontal disease in British and Draqi children. Paradontopathies (Geneva) 1966;18:19.

50. Powell RN. The Rx of periodontal disease in children. Br Dent J 1966;120:351.

51. Powell RN, McEniery TM. A longitudinal study of isolated gingival recession in the mandibular central incisor region on children aged 6–8 years. J Clin Periodontol 1982;9:357.

52. Vanarsdall RL. Management of the child and adolescent periodontium before and during orthodontic treatment. In: Richardson ER (ed). Periodontal Disease in Children and Adolescents: State of the Art. Nashville, TN: Meharry Medical College, 1971:131.

53. Kennedy J. Gingival augmentation/mucogingival surgery. Plenary session. In: Nevins M, Becker W, Kornman K (eds). Proceedings of the World Workshop in Clinical Periodontics. Chicago: American Academy of Periodontology, 1989:VII–21.

CHAPTER 20

The Biologic Width: Preventing Postsurgical Recession

Myron Nevins, DDS
Emil G. Cappetta, DMD

The principles of the biologic width date to the observation of necroscopy materials by Gargiulo et al[1] in 1961. The study included different stages of tooth eruption and the relationship of the hard and soft tissues of the periodontium to the tooth surface (Fig 20-1).

An examination of the histologic components of the periodontium shows that the alveolar crest is covered by the supracrestal fiber complex, the junctional epithelium, and the gingival sulcus. The supracrestal fibers insert into the first 1 mm of cementum occlusal to the osseous crest by means of Sharpey's fibers. The next 1 mm of cementum is populated by the junctional epithelium, the gingival sulcus beginning at its occlusalmost position. The depth of a healthy sulcus varies, depending on the position of a tooth in its alveolar housing and the quality of the soft tissue, but it is unlikely to be less than 1 mm. A large tooth in a thin alveolar process will usually have less crevicular depth than a small tooth in a wide periodontium.

The *biologic width*, as adapted to clinical strategy, is the sum of the supracrestal fibers, the junctional epithelium, and the gingival sulcus and has a proposed minimal dimension of 3 mm. Because it is impossible to have a smaller distance from the alveolar crest to the gingival margin, the gingival margin cannot recede unless there is new damage to the alveolar crest (see Fig 20-1).

This hypothesis was adapted as a means of planning for a stable postsurgical result at the time of periodontal surgery. It specifically offers the opportunity to address two difficult clinical problems:

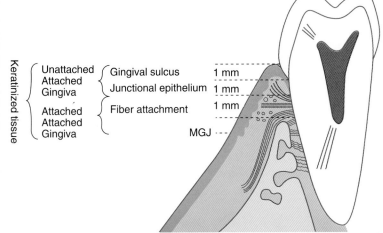

Fig 20-1 This diagram illustrates those entities that must be considered when the biologic width is evaluated for a particular surface of a tooth. It denotes the difference between keratinized tissues that can be considered attached and those that are not attached to the tooth and are thus less formidable barriers to insults from restorative dentistry. It is valuable to place the periodontal probe on the outer surface of the tissue desired for a clinically healthy periodontium that will resist the insults of restorative dentistry.

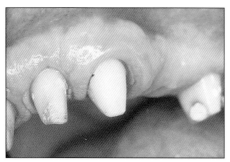

Fig 20-2a A fixed partial denture is being reviewed for compliance with periodontal health before being cemented. The gingiva has been injured by the tooth preparation, the provisional prosthesis, the impression technique, and the casting adjustment procedures. The technician was not able to read the dies accurately but was obligated to demarcate the finish line. He therefore erred on the side of extending apically below the gingival crest to avoid an exposed crown margin. This tissue was detached and probably will not remain stable in height or offer soft tissue protection for the underlying alveolar process.

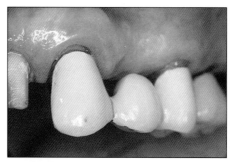

Fig 20-2b The prosthesis is seated so that the interproximal margin extends 1.5 mm below the tissue margin. The buccal margin has not yet reached the gingiva.

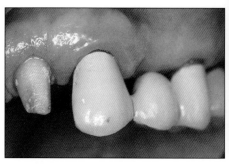

Fig 20-2c The prosthesis is further seated so that the buccal margin is in contact with the gingival margin. This places the interproximal margin of the restoration farther subgingivally.

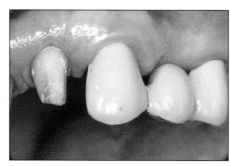

Fig 20-2d The prosthesis is now completely seated. The buccal gold collar is no longer visible, but the interproximal margin extends 4 to 5 mm below the gingival crest. It is difficult to imagine achieving complete removal of cement, let alone an intact soft tissue attachment to the tooth. This is the wrong depth to contemplate for placement of the intracrevicular margin. No margin should be placed this far subgingivally.

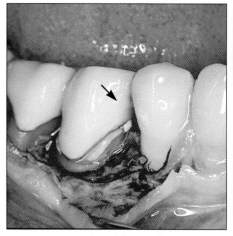

Fig 20-3 A periodontal flap is reflected to eliminate interproximal pocketing. Note the retained cement years after the permanent cementation of a complete-coverage restoration.

1. Recession after the final prosthesis is constructed
2. Reduction of the possibility of recurrent caries by providing an elongated clinical crown for the retainer

If, in fact, the healed dimension of the periodontium from osseous crest to gingival margin is the minimal measurement, prosthetic intervention will not result in gingival recession unless it disengages the supracrestal fiber connection to the root. Because neither the sulcus nor the crevicular epithelium is vascular, bleeding is an indication that the rotary instrument has engaged the gingival corium and perhaps destroyed the Sharpey's fiber connection. This would result in apical proliferation of the epithelium and offset the mechanism that would prevent recession.

The Intracrevicular Margin

The first proposal is that no restorative margin be placed subgingivally and that all margins be supragingival. Subgingival margins have been associated with greater plaque accumulation, inflammation, bacterial shifts, and mechanical irritation (Figs 20-2 and 20-3). The clinical alternative is the intracrevicular margin, which is the benchmark of the integration of periodontics and prosthetic dentistry (Figs 20-4a and 20-4b).

The clinical definition of *intracrevicular*,[2–4] when referring to the gingival margin of a dental restoration, is placement in that space bounded by the tooth and the sulcular epithelium without infringing on the junctional epithelium. This is not to be confused with the *subgingival* placement of the restorative margin, which frequently is defined only as disappearing from sight below the gingival crest. The sulcus is very limited in depth in a healthy untreated or healthy treated periodontium. It will probably be only 1 to 3 mm in depth, and it is very difficult to maneuver in this limited space. It is not easy to propose this marginal placement unless there is strong evidence of the likelihood that the position of the gingival margin is stable over an extended period of time (Figs 20-5a to 20-5l).

The most challenging aspect of the complete-coverage restoration is the placement of the intracrevicular margin. The complexity of the basic steps necessary to routinely construct and deliver this restoration without damaging a

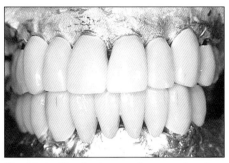

Fig 20-4a The final restorations are placed on the articulator before delivery to the patient. Note the small gingival metallic margin that will be placed in the intracrevicular position.

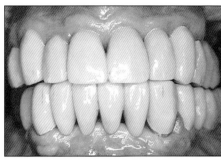

Fig 20-4b The metal margins barely extend into the sulcus when the prostheses are delivered to the patient. This documents that the prosthesis extends no farther than 1 mm into the sulcus and therefore is not a threat to the connective tissue attachment to the tooth.

healthy periodontium gives credence to its detractors, who proclaim the wisdom of placing a supragingival margin for the complete crown. All clinicians and members of academia comprehend that it would be preferable to avoid the gingival sulcus with any restorative endeavor.[2,5–11]

There are, however, daily clinical situations that tend to transform this debate from the esoteric to the pragmatic. The following are considerations[2]:

1. *Esthetics.* Patients are aware that a more refined esthetic result can be achieved where neither the restorative margin nor the root structure is in evidence. This is particularly true in the esthetic zone.

2. *Replacement restorations.* The exposure and refinement of a preexisting tooth preparation to replace existing dental restorations frequently necessitates periodontal surgery to create sound tooth structure on which to finish the new tooth preparation (Figs 20-6a to 20-6i). This is particularly important on the interproximal surface when principles of "extension for prevention" have resulted in the subgingival placement of alloys. It is also necessary when a previous crown preparation extends beyond the gingival sulcus and cannot be captured with routine impression techniques. Periodontal surgical procedures result in additional clinical crown length but do not always preclude the extension of the preparation beyond the sulcus. This is especially true for a molar on which the separation of the roots (furcations) is only 3 to 5 mm from the cementoenamel junction (Figs 20-7a to 20-7c). It is of paramount importance when there is a long edentulous span extending to a single abutment.

3. *Mechanical and technical retention.* There are times when the clinician strives for each millimeter of tooth structure because of preexisting damage to the

coronal tooth structure, to or below the osseous margin (see Figs 20-7a and 20-7b).

4. *Root caries.* Even with the advent and recognition of the beneficial use of fluoride, root caries remains a concern. This problem can be devastating when it involves a strategic abutment tooth, and extending the restoration to the gingival sulcus in a dentition showing prior evidence of root caries is justified (see Fig 20-7a).

5. *Severe cervical abrasion.* It is necessary to end the restoration on sound tooth structure apical to the damaged area. Tooth preparation should be preceded by a crown exposure procedure (Figs 20-8a and 20-8b).

6. *Root sensitivity.* All clinicians have encountered patients with root sensitivity; fortunately, it is a short-lived problem.

Avoiding Disruption of the Biologic Width

It has been hypothesized that it is necessary to disrupt the sulcular epithelium and/or the junctional epithelium to establish an inflammatory lesion in the gingival corium and fiber apparatus that will result in permanent bone loss. If one considers this hypothesis in reverse, it would not be possible to conceptualize the gingival margin moving apically when the flap margin has been placed at the crest of bone, allowing the formation of the minimal dimension of the three entities as befits the individual tooth, unless the crest of bone moved apically (Figs 20-9a to 20-9c). This would require an injury to the soft tissue that would leave the alveolar crest vulnerable to an inflammatory lesion.

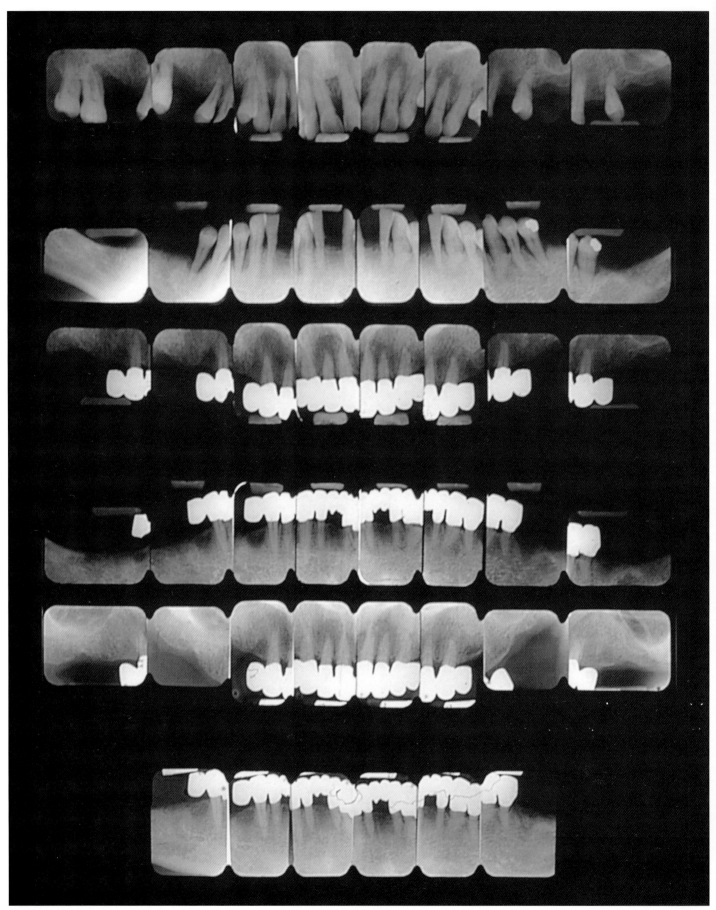

Fig 20-5a *(top)* Original full-mouth radiographic survey (1968). *(middle)* The 1969 full-mouth radiographic survey offers a guideline as to the original radiographic relationship of the restorative margins to the interproximal crest of bone. *(bottom)* The 1995 full-mouth radiographic survey demonstrates that all abutment teeth remain from 1969 and that there is no measurable loss of supporting bone.

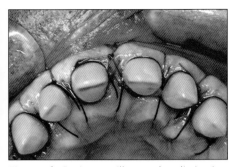

Fig 20-5b During maxillary pocket elimination surgery, a buccal partial-thickness flap and a palatal flap were utilized; the flap margins were apically repositioned to the osseous crests.

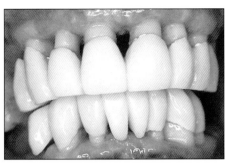

Fig 20-5c Appearance 4 weeks after pocket elimination. The provisional prostheses are not extended to the gingival margin until approximately 8 to 10 weeks after surgery.

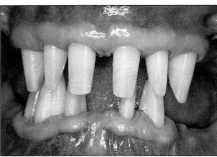

Fig 20-5d Appearance of the final tooth preparation and periodontal soft tissues. The dentition was restored with acrylic resin and gold restorations in 1968. The margins of the tooth preparations are of the feather-edged variety.

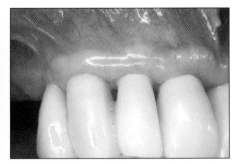

Fig 20-5e The provisional restoration has been relined and replaced at the final tooth preparation.

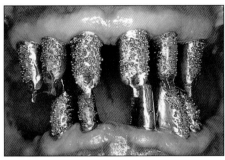

Fig 20-5f The periodontal tissues continue to remain in a state of health at the time the castings are fitted to the tooth preparations. This reflects the care that has been exercised during the restorative procedures.

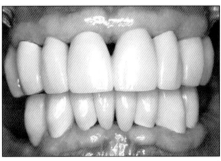

Fig 20-5g The final prostheses are cemented into place. Note the harmony between the periodontium and the restoration. (Prostheses constructed by Dr Howard M. Skurow.)

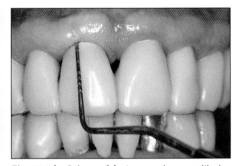

Fig 20-5h A loss of facing on the mandibular incisor provided an opportunity to examine the patient 18 years after treatment. The marginal relationship is approximately the same as it was when the fixed partial dentures were delivered. This reflects the surgical management, the care of the manipulation of the periodontium during the construction of the prostheses, and the care exercised by the patient.

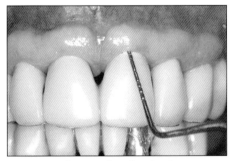

Fig 20-5i The periodontal probe demonstrates that, 18 years after treatment, the gingival margin is intact spatially and biologically. The patient's cooperation with debridement procedures has contributed significantly to the result.

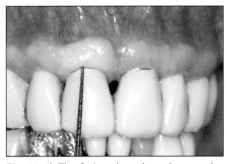

Fig 20-5j The facings have been lost on the mandibular right incisors (1994). There is no recession on the maxillary incisors, although a margin of acrylic resin has been lost on the left central incisor.

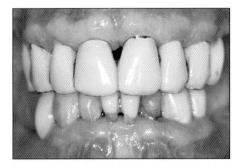

Fig 20-5k The facings have been replaced with resin composite.

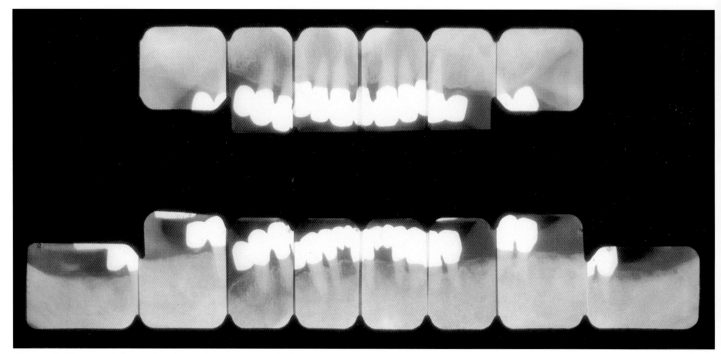

Fig 20-5l The 1994 full-mouth radiographic survey reveals the same bony profile when the restorative margins are used as parameters. The restorations have been in place for 24 years.

Tooth Preparation Procedures

The potential to insult the periodontium is great when a complete-crown restoration is performed. First it is necessary to prepare the tooth with a rotary instrument revolving at greater than 200,000 rpm. There is an obvious possibility of damaging the soft tissues, but the restorative dentist must minimize this factor. Underpreparation of the tooth should be avoided because an underprepared tooth inevitably results in an overcontoured crown. This is not meant to provide a license for the indiscriminate violation of the dental pulp because it is not necessary to encounter prophylactic endodontics to create the proper space for the restoration.

Apical overextension of the tooth preparation is the most common cause of damage to the junctional epithelium and the supra-alveolar connective tissue fibers.[3] Cementation of a final restoration with an apical overextension of the margin is a permanent violation of that territory which normally houses the dentogingival unit and results in increased plaque accumulation, inflammation, apical migration of the junctional epithelium, and pocket formation (see Fig 20-3). If injury occurs on the facial aspect of a tooth with thin dimensions of both keratinized attached gingiva and underlying bone, the result may be the loss of facial attachment and eventual gingival recession (Fig 20-10).

In summary, if the clinician does not disrupt the junctional epithelium or the gingival fiber apparatus, there should be no change in the level of the alveolar crest, and the gingival margin will not migrate apically (recede). The more probable result of minor irritations during mechanical endeavors will be gingival hyperplasia, which can be easily corrected (Fig 20-11). If recession can be eliminated during and following the restorative procedure, a major problem in the construction of a cosmetically acceptable restoration can be avoided.

Periodontal Surgical Procedures

The application of the biologic width hypothesis to the healing of the periodontium requires unique precision in the periodontal surgical procedure. Because it is not possible to predict the exact minimal dimension of healing for a specific tooth in its housing, it is arrogant to arbitrarily position the flap anywhere but the osseous crest when the periodontium is being prepared for a fixed restoration. The postsurgical visits and compliance of the patient are critical to the timely sequencing of treatment to protect the healing of the surgical wound and to provide an optimal result for the completion of the restorative effort.

Restorative Procedures

It is mandatory for the same precision to be exercised by the periodontist, the restorative dentist, and the patient. It is, therefore, of integral importance to the maintenance of a healthy periodontium that no restorative effort violate the junctional epithelium or connective tissue fiber apparatus. This priority establishes that the most apical extent of the complete-coverage restorations must not exceed the depth of the sulcus, although it is not possible for the clinician to identify the most coronal extent of the junctional epithelium when preparing a tooth (Figs 20-12a to 20-12m).

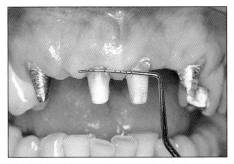

Fig 20-6a The maxillary central incisors are different lengths before surgery. The maxillary right canine demonstrates damaged tooth structure near or at the buccal gingiva. The maxillary left canine has detached buccal gingiva, and there is insufficient sound tooth structure to receive the final margin.

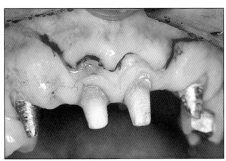

Fig 20-6b A partial-thickness buccal flap is elevated with a long bevel. Note the root fenestration on the surface of the right central incisor, indicating that the bone height is similar for both teeth.

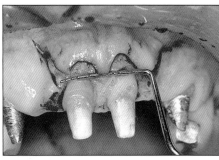

Fig 20-6c The detached tissue has been excised, revealing that the central incisor tooth preparations will be of equal length. The bone is covered with periosteum.

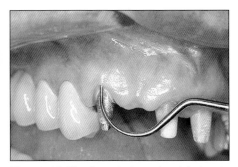

Fig 20-6d The buccal tissue is pink but is detached from the root surface of the canine and can be probed without bleeding.

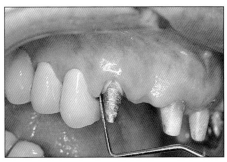

Fig 20-6e There is a periodontal pocket between the maxillary right canine and first premolar.

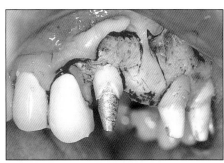

Fig 20-6f The buccal flap is elevated with a mesial vertical incision that will allow it to be rotated apically. Ostectomy is performed to create a flat interdental crest. Note the loss of attachment under the pink tissue of the buccal surface.

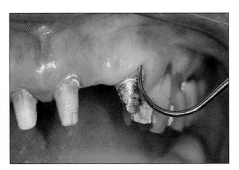

Fig 20-6g The pink buccal tissue on the maxillary left canine is detached beyond the mucogingival junction.

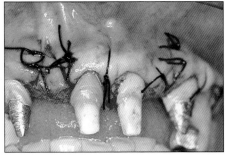

Fig 20-6h Three separate surgical procedures were performed to allow independent repositioning of the buccal flaps at the osseous crest. The central incisors will be of equal length.

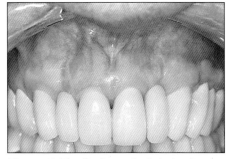

Fig 20-6i The fixed prosthesis is in place 12 years later. There is no recession of the buccal gingiva on any abutment.

The goal of establishing a finish line for a tooth preparation is based on the retention of the retainer and the provision of adequate space for the restorative cosmetic materials. Therefore, it is necessary to select the proper method of tooth preparation as required by the challenge at hand. Although shoulder and/or chamfer preparations are necessary to accommodate the cosmetic material of a restoration, there is usually no apparent reason for more than minimal extension of perhaps 0.5 to 1 mm below the gingival crest. There is some question whether any restorative margin that extends more than 1 mm into a healthy gingival crevice, even if totally confined within that crevice, can be adequately cleaned by the patient. This, then, can serve as a first guide in tooth preparation that will be helpful in respecting the boundaries of the crevice. When elongated posterior teeth are restored, the cosmetic material is not as critical, and the space for it can be provided for in the design of the casting, rather than in the tooth preparation. Therefore, a full shoulder or deep chamfer tooth preparation is usually not necessary for elongated posterior teeth.[2]

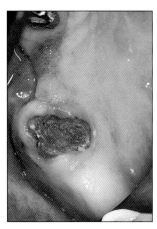

Fig 20-7a This molar is strategic as a potential abutment because it is the only posterior tooth in this quadrant. Crown-lengthening procedures will be challenging because of the limited tooth structure available from the cervical line of the maxillary molar to the opening of the furcations.

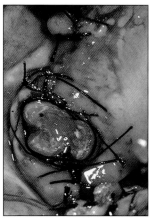

Fig 20-7b The same tooth after periodontal surgery. There is now sufficient tooth structure to proceed with the restoration. The surgical procedure consisted of one palatal flap and three buccal flaps. The distal wedge was separated on the buccal aspect via a vertical incision to allow independent suspension of the radicular flap at the osseous crest, while the buccal portion of the wedge could be rotated to allow complete coaption of the distal tissues and primary healing. The mesial wedge was treated the same as the distal wedge.

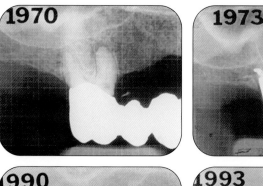
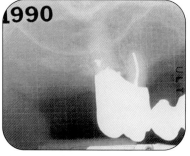
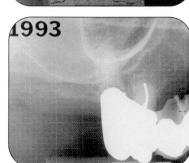

Fig 20-7c This patient presented for treatment in 1970, and the 1973 radiograph exhibits the new fixed prosthesis. It is still present in the 1993 radiograph 20 years later.

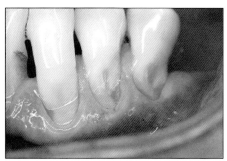

Fig 20-8a As a result of cervical abrasion, there is no place to finish the mandibular abutment tooth preparations on the buccal surface of the canine and premolars. Crown-lengthening periodontal surgery, together with mucogingival surgery, should be performed before the final restorations are completed.

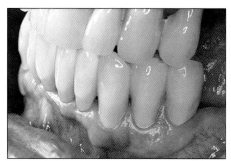

Fig 20-8b The same area is shown 21 years after placement of the permanent crowns. Even teeth that have demonstrated exaggerated gingival recession respond to surgical correction that is based on the principle of biologic width.

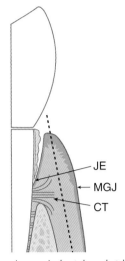

Fig 20-9a There is a periodontal pocket before periodontal surgery. Mucogingival junction (MGJ); junctional epithelium (JE); connective tissue attachment (CT).

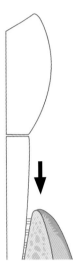

Fig 20-9b The flap margin has been sutured to place at the level of the alveolar crest, allowing the entities of the biologic width to form at their minimal dimension.

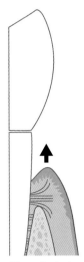

Fig 20-9c The gingival margin has moved coronally to account for I mm of connective tissue attachment, I mm of functional epithelium, and a minimal gingival sulcus. Gingival recession will not occur unless the supracrestal fibers or the alveolar crest is damaged iatrogenically.

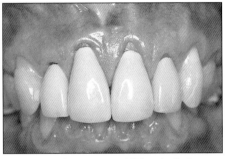

Fig 20-10 The patient exhibits gingival recession on the maxillary central incisors after the crowns are cemented in place.

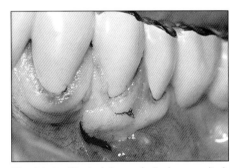

Fig 20-11 Gingival hyperplasia has resulted from insulting the periodontium during the process of achieving complete-coverage restorations. This area was treated surgically in accordance with the principles of biologic width, and the healed gingival margin was in position at the minimal dimension from the osseous crest. Recession would only occur if the attachment of the gingival fibers to the cementum were destroyed.

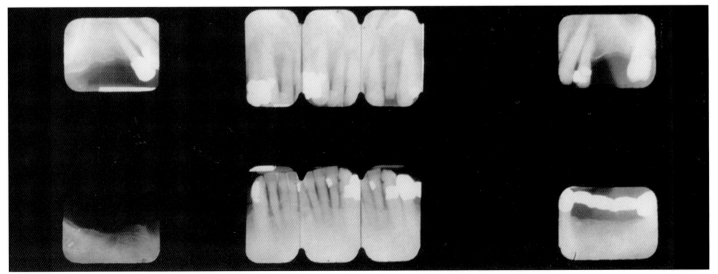

Fig 20-12a A full-mouth radiographic survey was taken in 1968 at the onset of treatment.

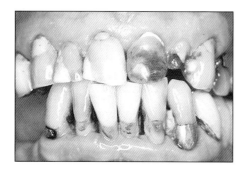

Fig 20-12b The patient presented with a damaged periodontium and an extensive need for restorative surgery. Note the complete lack of centric occlusion on the right side but the absence of posterior bite collapse. The existing restorations or dental caries extend to or below the gingival margin on each tooth. This complicates the presurgical tooth preparations.

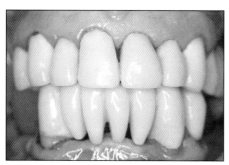

Fig 20-12c The provisional restorations are in place.

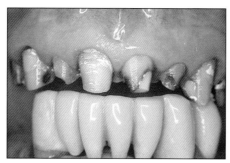

Fig 20-12d The provisional maxillary restoration has been removed at the time of periodontal surgery. There is a need for adequate sound tooth structure, as well as periodontal pocket elimination.

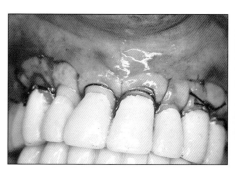

Fig 20-12e The provisional prosthesis is replaced following surgery. Note the additional tooth structure available after pocket elimination surgery.

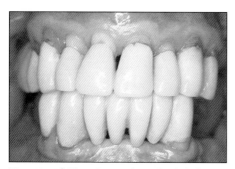

Fig 20-12f The tissues have healed for 10 weeks. It is now time for the patient to return to the restorative dentist to continue with the restorative effort, including the final tooth preparations, impressions, casting try-ins, etc, that are necessary to finish the prosthesis.

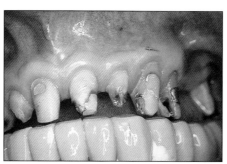

Fig 20-12g The day of insertion of the new permanent prosthesis. The tissue was nicked over the maxillary left canine during the removal of the provisional bridge. Note the form and the state of health of the interproximal tissues. Proximal probing measurements are minimal.

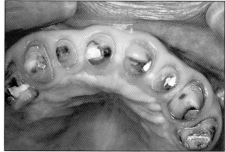

Fig 20-12h Occlusal view of the interproximal tissues on the day of insertion of the new permanent prosthesis. All restorative manipulations have been accomplished without endangering the soft tissue attachment to the tooth. It is conceivable that exquisite care can result in the maintenance of the soft tissue attachments after the final fixed partial denture is in place without further damage to the remaining osseous structure.

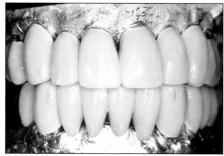

Fig 20-12i The final restorations are placed on the articulator before delivery. Note the small metallic gingival margins that will be placed intracrevicularly.

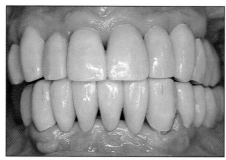

Fig 20-12j The final restorations are in place. The minimal gold margins extend into the gingival crevice. (Prostheses constructed by Dr Howard M. Skurow.)

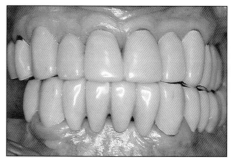

Fig 20-12k Restorations 12 years later. Note the integrity of all the gingival margins, as well as the state of health of the interproximal tissues.

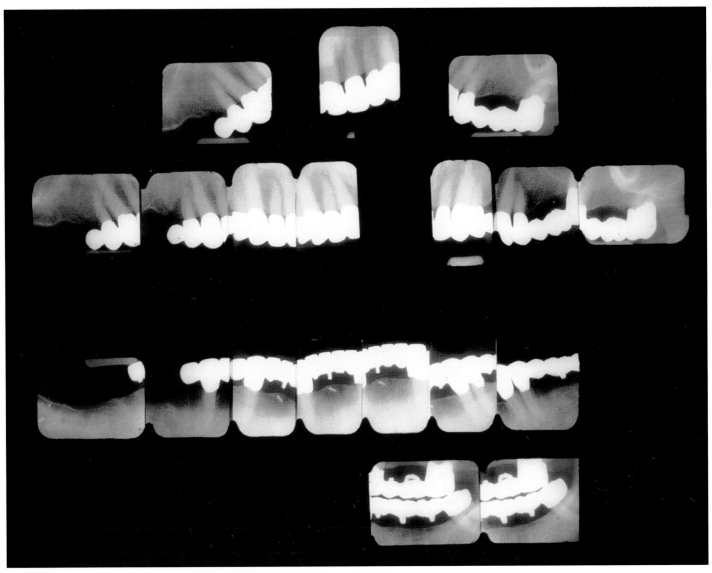

Fig 20-12l Full-mouth radiographic survey at the conclusion of treatment in 1969.

There is frequently a disparity between the apical extents of a restoration interproximally and radicularly. The parabolic architecture of the anterior area, with its narrow alveolar process, is more severe than that of the posterior area, where the alveolar process widens to accommodate the larger root surfaces. Interestingly, this anterior disparity approaches the same 3 mm as the minimal biologic width. Inexperienced clinicians may mistakenly extend the tooth preparation on all surfaces to the same circumferential depth, and this is likely to violate the interproximal soft tissue attachments of the periodontium (Figs 20-13a and 20-13b). It is imperative not to commit this error because it results in the extension of the interproximal margin too far subgingivally (Fig 20-14).

It is not important which impression technique is used. It is important to respect the fragility of the junctional epithelium and the attachment of the supracrestal fibers and to be careful not to disrupt them. It is necessary to be cognizant of the advantages and disadvantages of each technique and to be able to select and apply the methodology best suited to the problem at hand.

After the impression is secured and the die is constructed, the next critical step is the demarcation of the finish line. This is referred to generally as "ditching the die" and can be most precise only when accomplished by the person who prepared the tooth. It is not possible to extend a casting too far apically if the die is properly ditched. This, then, precludes damage to the soft tissue attachment apparatus when a casting or the framework for a fixed partial denture is fitted in place. It should also establish the finish line in an area that is accessible to allow the removal of excess cement after the permanent restoration is cemented in place. When the restorative margin extends too far subgingivally, excess cement may be retained on its margin (see Fig 20-3).

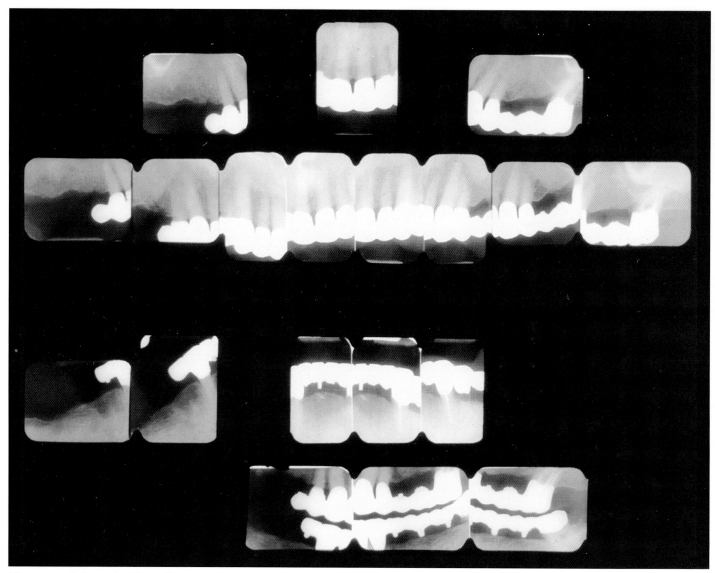

Fig 20-12m Full-mouth radiographic survey 12 years later, with the prostheses in place. There has been no loss of teeth, and the level of the osseous crests appears to be the same if the crown margins are used as fixed reference points.

Amalgam Alloy Restorations

Numerous studies have reported a high percentage of alloy restorations with overhangs and faulty margins that allow abundant plaque retention, resulting in gingival inflammation.[3] Others[12] believe that an overhanging restoration is associated with the excessive loss of adjacent marginal bone.[3] Wilson and Maynard[3] noted the smoothness of the amalgam margin in the gingival crevices as an important factor in preventing gingivitis and periodontitis.

The placement of the matrix band to contain the restorative material is another consideration because this band should not be forced so far apically that it cuts into the junctional epithelium and the gingival corium. A gingival wedge may cause supplemental damage to the underlying connective tissue as well. Damage to the connective tissue fiber system can result in increased crevicular depth and the loss of the interdental papilla with lateral food impaction.

The contacting surface between a new alloy restoration and its approximating tooth is critical to success. It is important that irregularities in the old adjacent restorations be smooth so as to develop a properly contoured contact area and prevent food impaction or shredding of dental floss and gingival impingement.[3]

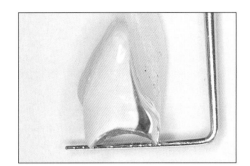

Fig 20-13a The buccal and palatal aprons of an incisor crown extend almost 3 mm further apically than the interproximal margins.

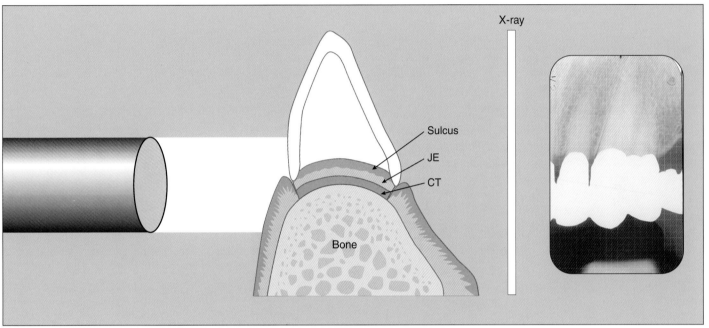

Fig 20-13b The level of the alveolar support can be measured radiographically relative to the apical extent of the restorative margin. A dental radiograph reduces the three-dimensional tooth and periodontium to two dimensions and projects the buccal crown margin to be at approximately the same height as the alveolar process, if the principle of biologic width has been used in surgery. The buccal crown apron serves as a valuable reference point for the level of the crest of bone. The difference in apical extension of crown margins on the radicular and interproximal surfaces is about 2 to 3 mm and therefore equal to the minimal clinical biologic width with the intracrevicular placement of the margin. Junctional epithelium (JE), connective tissue (CT). (From Nevins.[2] Reprinted with permission.)

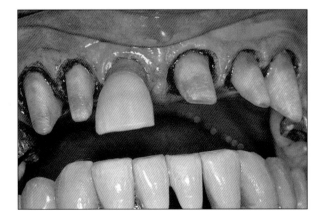

Fig 20-14 The tooth preparation has extended too far apically. Ideally, there should be no bleeding because there are no blood vessels in the gingival crevice or the epithelium. This means that tooth preparation has entered and disrupted the gingival fiber apparatus. This can allow apical migration of the epithelium.

Periodontal Evaluation

The validity of the intracrevicular placement of the gingival margin requires the tracking of patients for an extended period of time and the observation of two factors. The first and easiest to assay is the level of the gingival margin. The premise of the biologic width allows for little or no apical migration because it would be necessary for the level of the alveolar crest to move apically to accommodate recession. This can be observed clinically (see Fig 20-5). The second factor is the level of the alveolar crest. It is always important to protect and preserve the remaining alveolar housing. This can be measured radiographically relative to the apical extent of the restorative margin.

The radiograph is a two-dimensional reduction of the three-dimensional teeth and periodontium. The buccal apron, therefore, is projected as being at the same height as the interproximal bone, although it projects further apically. This serves as a valuable reference point for the level of the crest of bone (see Fig 20-13b) in dentitions with fixed prostheses.

Conclusion

It is necessary to emphasize that the periodontium would fare better if no restorative margin approached the gingiva. However, intracrevicular margins cannot be avoided, for previously explained reasons. Therefore, it is mandatory to adhere to the principles stated in this chapter to avoid insult to the supporting structures.

References

1. Gargiulo AW, Wentz FM, Orban BJ. Dimensions and relations of the dentogingival junction in humans. J Periodontol 1961;32:261.

2. Nevins M, Skurow HM. The intracrevicular restorative margin, the biologic width, and maintenance of the gingival margin. Int J Periodont Rest Dent 1984;4(3):31.

3. Wilson RD, Maynard JG. Intracrevicular restorative dentistry. Int J Periodont Rest Dent 1982;1(4):35.

4. Maynard JG, Wilson RD. Physiologic dimensions of the periodontium fundamental to successful restorative dentistry. J Periodontol 1979;50:170–174.

5. de Waal M, Castellucci G. The importance of the restorative margin placement to the biologic width and periodontal health. Part I. Int J Periodont Rest Dent 1993;13(5):461.

6. Waerhaug J. Tissue reactions around artificial crowns. J Periodontol 1983;54:172.

7. Silness J. Fixed prosthetics and periodontal health. Dent Clin North Am 1980;24.

8. Newcombe GM. The relationship between the location of sublingual crown margins and gingival inflammation. J Periodontol 1974;45:151.

9. Flores de Jacoby L, Zafiropaulous G, Ciancio S. The effect of crown margin location on plaque and periodontal health. Int J Periodont Rest Dent 1989;9(3):197.

10. Donnenfeld W. Therapeutic end points in periodontal therapy. Int J Periodont Rest Dent 1981;1(4):51.

11. Parma-Benfenati S, Fugazzatto P, Ruben M. The effect of restorative margins on the postsurgical development and nature of the periodontium. Part I. Int J Periodont Rest Dent 1985;5(6):31.

12. Hakkarainen K, Ainamo J. Influence of overhanging posterior tooth restorations on alveolar bone height in adults. J Clin Periodontol 1980;7:114–120.

CHAPTER 21

The Biologic Width:
Crown Lengthening

Sergio De Paoli, DDS
Myron Nevins, DDS
Emil G. Cappetta, DMD

The prognosis of a complete-coverage restoration relates to the tooth preparation that it fits and to the state of health of the periodontium that supports it. The placement of the margin of the tooth preparation and its interaction with the gingiva is the most important interaction of periodontics and restorative dentistry.[1]

One dogma established for long-term success is that every new crown margin should end on sound tooth structure.[1–3] There are everyday clinical situations that challenge this statement, including caries, fractured teeth, perforations from operative dentistry (posts), and root resorption. A short clinical crown preparation is likely to allow the retainer to loosen because of lack of retention. This is especially true when it is adjacent to an edentulous area and can result in recurrent caries (Figs 21-1a and 21-1b). In an effort to offset this, the tooth is prepared substantially below the gingival margin, and this results in destruction of the soft tissue attachment apparatus and eventual damage to supporting bone.

Apical overextension of tooth preparation is a common cause of damage to the sulcular epithelium, the junctional epithelium, and the supra-alveolar connective tissue fibers (Figs 21-2a to 21-2c). Cementation of final restorations with an apical overextension of the margin is a permanent violation of that territory that normally houses the dentogingival unit. The insult results in increased plaque accumulation, inflammation, and pocket formation. If injury occurs on the facial aspect of a tooth with thin dimensions of both keratinized attached gingiva and underlying bone, the result may be loss of facial attachment and eventual

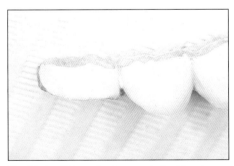

Fig 21-1a This patient presented with a loose fixed prosthesis. The occlusal-gingival length of the crown is inadequate.

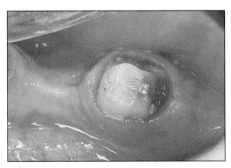

Fig 21-1b Removal of the restoration reveals a soft tissue crater. There is insufficient tooth structure available, and the crown margin extends too far subgingivally. Note the recurrent caries on the distal surface.

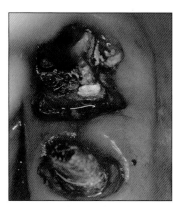

Fig 21-2a The interdental papilla between the two abutments is hyperplastic. No restoration should be placed permanently until this is corrected because the excess tissue will interfere with the fit and the soft tissue is unlikely to be healthy. Note the blunting and separation of the buccal and lingual aspects of the papilla and the red hyperplastic tissue in the sulcular area. Apical overextension of the tooth preparation results in damage to the sulcular epithelium, junctional epithelium, and supraalveolar connective tissue fibers.

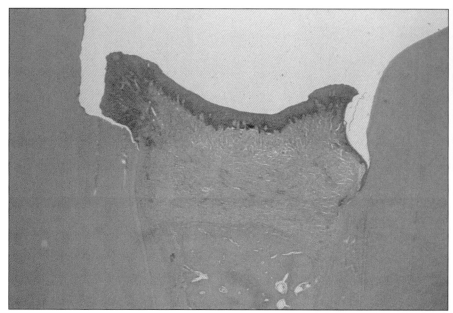

Fig 21-2b Histologic observation of an interdental papilla between two teeth with subgingival preparations. The crowns do not fit properly on the shoulders of the tooth preparations due to gingival hyperplasia.

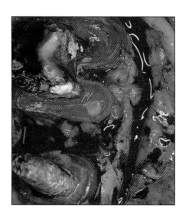

Fig 21-2c Reflection of the buccal flap reveals overzealous tooth preparation. The shoulders were covered with gingiva in Fig 21-2a.

gingival recession. If injury occurs on the interproximal surface, apical migration of the dentogingival attachment and infrabony pocket formation is possible.

There are two corrective procedures that result in significant elongation of the clinical crown: surgical crown lengthening and forced eruption of a tooth.

Surgical Crown Lengthening

Surgical crown lengthening allows the placement of the restorative margin on sound tooth structure without violating the biologic width and causing permanent damage to the periodontium. A crown-lengthening procedure can be accomplished by mucogingival surgery alone in the presence of soft tissue pocketing. In these cases, alveolar bone will remain covered by periosteum, and this demonstrates that bone structure was not reduced (Figs 21-3a and 21-3b).

However, most crown-lengthening procedures require some ostectomy to expose sound tooth structure (Figs 21-4a to 21-4c). It is difficult to make the commitment to remove bone, and the vital question becomes quantitative. The interproximal surfaces present greater difficulty in tooth preparation, control of soft tissue hyperplasia in concert with restorative dentistry procedures, and patient compliance with cleanliness. It is also important to consider the size of the interproximal embrasure and the relationship of the tooth and the alveolar process.[1,3] A small embrasure and a small tooth in a large periodontium both tend to result in a deeper sulcus with a creeping attachment.

The presurgical plan should designate the distance from the osseous crest to the margin of sound tooth structure to be provided on all surfaces of the tooth (Figs 21-5a to 21-5d). The amount of sound supraosseous tooth structure required for placement of a restorative margin varies from 4 to 5.5 mm.[1,4] This decision involves the size of the embrasure, the position of the tooth, and the biologic width hypothesis.

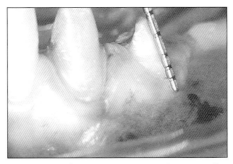

Fig 21-3a The previous restorations on the mandibular premolars extended apically beyond the crest of the interdental papilla and resulted in a lack of sound supragingival tooth structure for the margin of the provisional crowns.

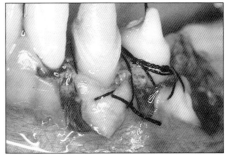

Fig 21-3b Periodontal surgery aimed at the resolution of the mucogingival problems has resulted in a significant increase in supragingival tooth structure. Note that the alveolar bone is covered by periosteum, demonstrating that bone structure was not removed to accomplish this result. This surgical procedure has simultaneously corrected the mucogingival and tooth length problems.

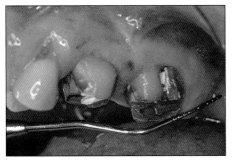

Fig 21-4a The provisional restorations have been removed, revealing short clinical crowns, especially on the distal surface where the soft tissue is at the level of the occlusal surface.

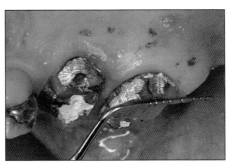

Fig 21-4b Palatal view of Fig 21-4a. Note the level of the tissue on the distal surface. It is necessary to perform crown-lengthening surgery to allow a distal apron on the crown for this tooth. The alternatives would be to construct a four-fifths crown with no distal apron or to place the apron 5 to 6 mm subgingivally and not be able to remove the excess cement.

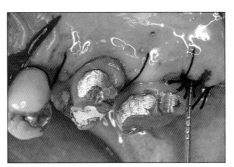

Fig 21-4c Palatal view after surgery. There is now 6 mm of tooth preparation available on the distal surface. In addition, sound tooth structure is available beyond the inadequate margins of the old alloys on the palatal and interproximal surfaces. This is especially important in the areas of the interproximal furcations and allows for improved embrasures.

Whether the biologic width is defined as a combination of the gingival sulcular depth, the junctional epithelial attachment, and the length of the supra-alveolar connective tissue/fiber attachment, or as the junctional epithelium plus the supra-alveolar connective tissue/fiber attachment, is irrelevant to the discussion of intracrevicular marginal placement (Figs 21-5 and 21-6). The intracrevicular margin placed into the sulcus must not violate the junctional epithelium or the fiber attachment apparatus. The sulcus is limited in depth in a healthy treated or healthy untreated periodontium and will probably be only 1 to 3 mm. It is very difficult to maneuver in this limited space (see Figs 21-5d to 21-5h).

These entities occupy approximately at least 3 mm supracrestally. The first 1 mm occlusal to the alveolar crest is occupied by supracrestal fibers that insert into the cementum via Sharpey's fiber attachment. The next occlusal 1 mm of cementum is covered by the junctional epithelium. The depth of the sulcus is relative to the position of the tooth in the alveolar housing but is unlikely to be less than 1 mm in depth. The minimal combined sum of the sulcus, junctional epithelium, and the supracrestal fibers is thus estimated to be at a minimum of 3 mm supracrestally (see Fig 21-6).

If ostectomy is concluded prematurely, and only 3 mm of exposure is accomplished, the postsurgical result will provide little sound tooth structure. Indeed, one study measured the actual amount of tooth elongation and compared it to the presurgical "textbook" goal of 3 mm. Researchers concluded that sufficient crown exposure was not routinely achieved during surgical crown-lengthening procedures.[5] This underscores the necessity of evaluating each clinical situation individually as it relates to each tooth surface, periodontal anatomy, and planned position of the restorative margin. The advantages of performing some tooth preparation during osseous surgery are the development of an optimal emergence profile, the removal of bacterial contaminants, the elimination of root concavities and undercuts, and the improvement in the area of root proximity by enhancing embrasure space. These alterations enhance tooth contours and aid in performance of plaque control.[6,7]

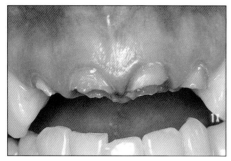

Fig 21-5a The clinical crown length is inadequate to retain new restorations.

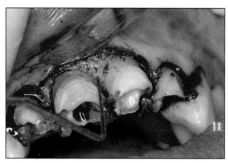

Fig 21-5b The buccal and palatal flaps are reflected. Ostectomy is performed to provide 5 mm of sound tooth structure.

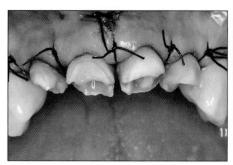

Fig 21-5c The partial-thickness flaps are secured with periosteal suturing techniques.

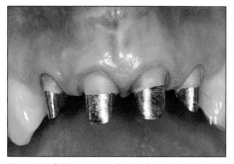

Fig 21-5d The surgical site has healed with barely enough sound tooth structure to end the tooth preparations for new crowns. Cast post and cores have been cemented.

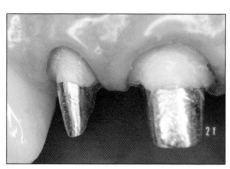

Fig 21-5e Note the healthy interdental papilla and the final intracrevicular tooth preparation between the right incisors.

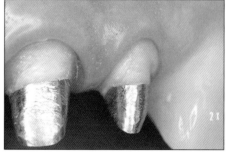

Fig 21-5f Note the healthy interdental papilla and the final intracrevicular tooth preparation between the left incisors.

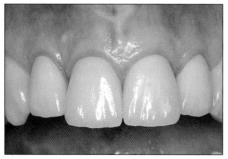

Fig 21-5g The four incisor crowns are in place. The margins fit properly and do not extend beyond the sulcus.

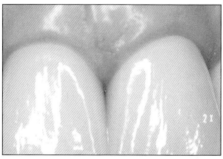

Fig 21-5h Note the healthy interdental papilla between the central incisors.

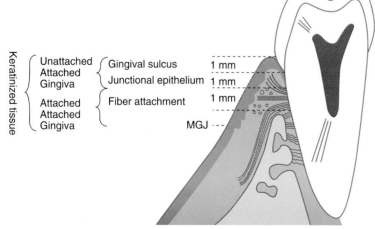

Fig 21-6 The keratinized gingiva is divided into that part that is firmly attached and the more occlusal portion that covers the gingival sulcus and the junctional epithelium and is not physically attached to the tooth. The first 1 mm of root structure supracrestal to the alveolar process is occupied by the gingival fiber apparatus. The next 1 mm is covered by the junctional epithelium. The next 1 mm is covered by the free gingival margin, forming the sulcus. Therefore, if only 3 mm of tooth structure is exposed beyond the osseous crest, the healed result will yield little or no clinical crown in most instances. This is particularly true interproximally.

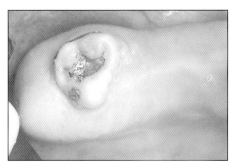

Fig 21-7a A crown-lengthening procedure is required for an isolated maxillary molar. The case was not provisionalized, because the edentulous span was too long and the provisional prosthesis would be prone to breakage. Multirooted teeth are always a special problem for crown-lengthening procedures, because the separation of the roots is usually less than 5 mm from the cementoenamel junction.

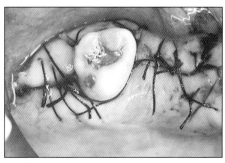

Fig 21-7b The crown-lengthening procedure has yielded additional tooth structure to construct a well-fitted provisional prosthesis.

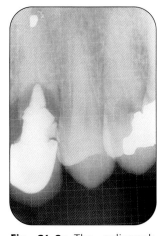

Fig 21-8a The radiograph demonstrates severe damage to the tooth structure on this maxillary canine.

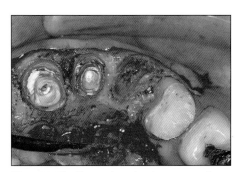

Fig 21-8b Crown-lengthening procedures would damage the adjacent teeth and lessen their prognosis. It is important to identify clinical problems that cannot be reasonably resolved. Crown-lengthening ostectomy would remove an excessive amount of bone from the adjacent teeth.

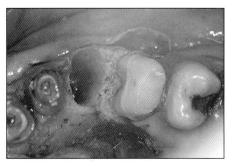

Fig 21-8c Extraction was the best treatment. Crown lengthening can only be successful if the clinical root has sufficient length to provide a secure prognosis.

It is important to note that the final tooth preparation must occur after 6 to 8 weeks of healing. Internalized tooth preparation should not be performed during surgery because it is impossible to predict the exact level of the future, healed gingiva.

Multirooted teeth pose a special problem in crown-lengthening procedures because the separation of the roots (furcation) is usually less than 5 mm from the cemento-enamel junction (Figs 21-7a and 21-7b). Therefore, unless the roots are fused or have long trunks, there is the possibility of opening the furcation to meet the goal of ending the restorative margin on sound tooth structure. This may result in a root resection or extraction rather than crown lengthening if the area is limited to one surface of the tooth.

Another consideration is the need for crown lengthening when there is damage to the tooth that is so far apical that treatment will ultimately worsen the prognosis of adjacent teeth. It is important to identify a clinical problem that cannot be reasonably resolved. Extraction may be the best treatment (Figs 21-8a to 21-8c).

When evaluating a tooth for a crown-lengthening procedure, clinicians must consider these important factors[1,2]:

1. Root anatomy (length and form)
2. Health of the dentogingival unit
3. Loss of mesiodistal space (embrasures)
4. Esthetic concerns, as esthetics may mandate alternative crown lengthening (forced eruption) and/or rapid extrusion or a combination of surgical and mechanical crown lengthening
5. Endodontic status of the tooth
6. Importance of the tooth
7. Apical extent of fracture, caries, or perforation
8. Level of the alveolar crest
9. Interproximal apical extent of old restorations
10. Crown-root ratio, presurgery and postsurgery

Crown lengthening can only be successful if the clinical root has significant length. Ideally, 5 mm of tooth structure must be exposed above the alveolus (see Fig 21-5b). This

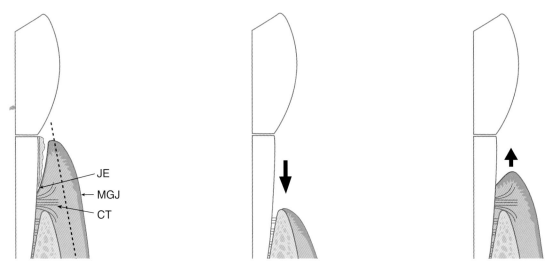

Fig 21-9 Crown-lengthening procedures should expose 5 mm of tooth structure above the alveolar crest. This accounts for the dimensions of the supracrestal fibers (1 mm), the junctional epithelium (1 mm), and the sulcus (1 mm). If 3 mm of tooth structure is exposed, the crest of the papilla could conceivably cover all of the root that was exposed. Mucogingival junction (MGJ); junctional epithelium (JE); connective tissue (CT).

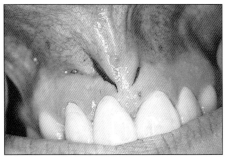

Fig 21-10a The provisional fixed restoration is in place. The right central incisor pontic has been relieved to accommodate the frenum.

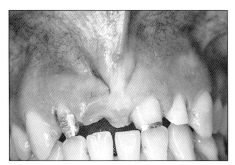

Fig 21-10b The dentist and the laboratory technician have inappropriately allowed the frenum and the poor ridge anatomy to dictate the shape of the pontic. Sound tooth structure is needed on the proximal surfaces of the abutment teeth for margin placement.

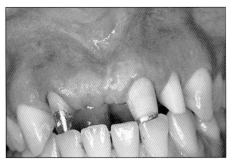

Fig 21-10c Periodontal surgery has eliminated the frenum, corrected the edentulous ridge to receive a bullet-shaped pontic that is easily cleansed, and provided sound tooth structure to accommodate the new restorative margin.

accounts for the dimensions of the supracrestal fibers (1 mm), the junctional epithelium (1 mm), and the sulcus (1 mm). If only 3 mm of tooth structure is exposed, the crest of the papilla could conceivably cover all of the root that was exposed. If the total clinical root measures only 8 or 10 mm, it would be mobile and of little value if substantial bone is removed (Fig 21-9). It is important for the therapist to consider the status of the proposed abutment tooth and whether it would be possible to place the restorative margin on sound tooth structure.

Often the problem in development of the biologic width is superimposed on a mucogingival problem, such as a frenum (Figs 21-10a to 21-10c) or minimal dimension of keratinized tissue. This situation will result in a very demanding clinical procedure that may require a multistage approach or perhaps multisurgical techniques, ie, a variety of flaps in a very small area. This may require several vertical incisions, one for each tooth; that is, instead of one buccal flap there may be independent flaps so that each tooth can have its own solution (Figs 21-11 and 21-12).

Inadequate crown length is frequently coupled with the problem of a limited quantity of gingiva. Assuming there must always be a gingival sulcus, the first 1 mm of keratinized gingiva can only correspond to the sulcus. The junctional epithelium occupies the second 1 mm apically, and therefore the second 1 mm of keratinized gingiva corresponds to the junctional epithelium when there is a 1 mm sulcus. The junctional epithelium has been shown to be a dynamic entity, ever changing, interfacing with the tooth via hemidesmosomes. Even with the most ideal situation, the first 2 mm of keratinized gingiva can be categorized as unattached gingiva when a restoration that involves the gingival sulcus and crown lengthening is contemplated. The next 1 mm represents the entity of the biologic width that is known as the connective tissue fiber apparatus, which is mediated by Sharpey's fibers, ie, the supra-alveolar connective tissue fibers that extend into the cemental surface of the root, and is actually attached gingiva. It is possible that mucogingival surgery alone can resolve the crown-lengthening procedure (see Fig 21-3). Attached gingiva can be

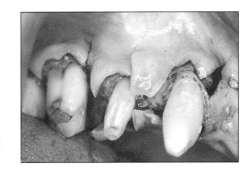

Fig 21-11 Very demanding clinical procedures may require multisurgical techniques, ie, a variety of flaps in a very small area. Several vertical incisions are used to resolve the mucogingival problems, as well as attain crown lengthening.

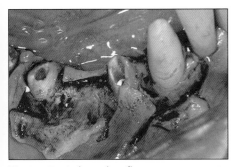

Fig 21-12a Independent flaps are necessary to address individual problems for each tooth. One buccal flap may not offer the opportunity to provide crown lengthening and mucogingival solutions simultaneously.

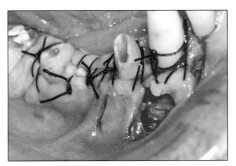

Fig 21-12b The flaps are sutured in place with periosteal suturing techniques on the buccal surface.

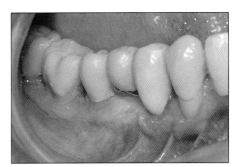

Fig 21-12c The healed result of the multisurgical procedure is satisfactory.

provided by pedicle or free graft procedures. The grafting procedure provides to the recipient site[8] the dense connective tissue that appears to induce keratinization, a process determined by genetics.

In summary, the authors agree with Maynard and Wilson,[9,10] who say that 5 mm of keratinized tissue is the appropriate dimension required for intracrevicular restorative dentistry. This would satisfy the requirement of 2 mm of free gingiva (1 mm for crevicular epithelium and 1 mm for junctional epithelium) and 3 mm of attached gingiva. With less than 3 mm of keratinized gingiva there is probably very little actual attachment to deter an inflammatory lesion and withstand the trauma from restorative procedures.[1,3,11] It is imperative that an adequate dimension of keratinized tissue in the *attached* form be present when the intracrevicular placement of a restorative margin is considered.

Tissue thickness in a buccolingual dimension is also an important consideration.[11–14] The clinician should not take for granted that an adequate dimension of tissue in a vertical dimension necessarily indicates that the tissue is attached and can tolerate intracrevicular restorative procedures. Tissue thickness can be determined by probing. If a

probe is visible through the free gingiva even though the superficial aspect of that margin is keratinized, it is questionable whether that gingiva can serve as a *locus minoris resistentia* to developing recession in the presence of plaque, toothbrush trauma, or a subgingival margin.

Crown lengthening can be used effectively to increase the length of clinical crowns in the patient with a "gummy" smile (Figs 21-13a to 21-13g). This surgery may be possible with only a buccal flap and preservation of the interdental papillae when it is performed for mechanical and esthetic reasons in the absence of disease. It also can be effective to recreate teeth of an acceptable length after extreme wear, such as in bruxism (Figs 21-14a to 21-14h). Because most patients require some ostectomy, the classic procedure requires an apically repositioned buccal flap together with a palatal or lingual flap. These flaps are best performed with vertical incisions to provide ease of access and repositioning to the desired level. It is preferable to incise a partial-thickness flap both to control the flap thickness and for exact positioning at the osseous crest via periosteal suturing. If the flap is positioned haphazardly, the hypothesis of a biologic width loses its importance as a factor of predictability.

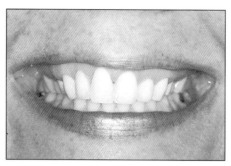

Fig 21-13a The patient's chief complaint was that her teeth "looked too short." This patient has a "gummy" smile with lateral incisors, premolars, and canines that are too short.

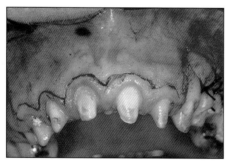

Fig 21-13b The flap design will reposition the buccal flap and preserve the interdental papilla.

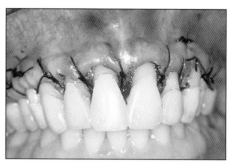

Fig 21-13c The flap is sutured in place and the provisional prosthesis is recemented.

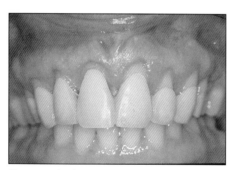

Fig 21-13d The provisional prosthesis in place 6 weeks after surgery and before relining procedures.

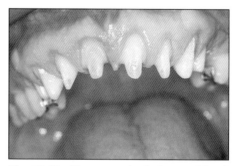

Fig 21-13e The removal of the provisional restoration reveals intact interdental papilla and maxillary anterior teeth of an appropriate length.

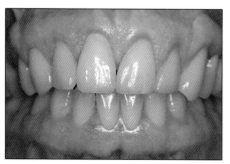

Fig 21-13f The final prosthesis provides the proper harmony of the length and width of the anterior teeth. (Final prosthesis by Dr Kenneth Malament.)

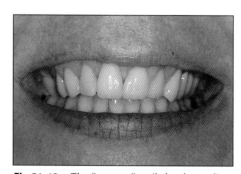

Fig 21-13g The "gummy" smile has been eliminated when the patient smiles.

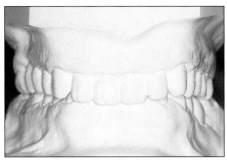

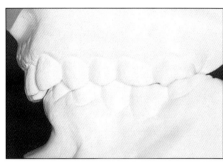

Fig 21-14a The anterior deep overbite, restored by a ceramometal fixed partial denture, has resulted in an esthetic problem. The patient's chief complaint is the short mandibular anterior teeth.

Fig 21-14b Lateral view of the deep vertical overbite.

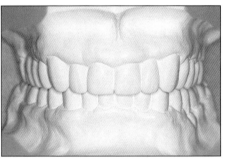

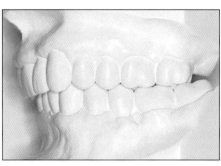

Fig 21-14c The new finished prosthesis has eliminated the deep vertical overbite and provided mandibular incisors that are pleasing to the patient.

Fig 21-14d The lateral view provides a contrast to Fig 21-14b. There is room for the mandibular anterior teeth.

Fig 21-14e On presentation for treatment, the patient has a deep vertical overbite. Crown-lengthening surgery placed the new gingival line 5 mm apically for both the maxillary and mandibular anterior teeth. The badly worn posterior occlusion was returned to its estimated vertical dimension of occlusion, first with a removable posterior occlusal appliance and then in the provisional restorations. Approximately 1 mm was added to the occlusal surface. This translated into 3 mm of anterior space. The combination of distance provided by crown-lengthening procedures and restoration of occlusal vertical dimension offered sufficient space to construct normal-length mandibular anterior teeth.

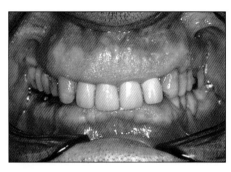

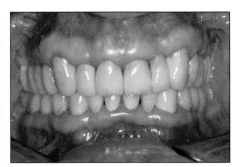

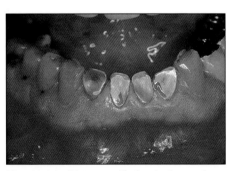

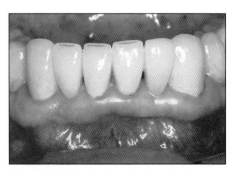

Fig 21-14f The final prosthesis, with appropriately sized anterior teeth, is in place. (Prosthesis constructed by Dr Charles Arnold.)

Fig 21-14g The mandibular incisors show extreme wear and offer minimal clinical crown structure.

Fig 21-14h The final prosthesis includes mandibular incisors that satisfy the patient's desire to show teeth.

327

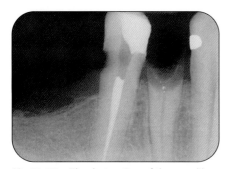

Fig 21-15a The destruction of the mandibular first premolar coronal tooth structure is severe.

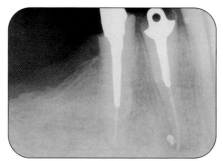

Fig 21-15b Endodontic therapy has been completed, and a post has been placed to allow the insertion of an elastic, which will be connected to a wire to force eruption of this tooth.

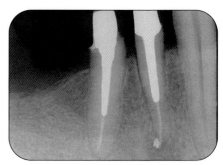

Fig 21-15c After completion of the forced eruption process, ostectomy is performed on the first bicuspid and does not affect the adjacent teeth.

Forced Eruption

An alternative to surgical crown lengthening is the forced eruption of a tooth or root so that ostectomy would only be performed on the tooth that requires the crown lengthening and not affect the adjacent teeth (Figs 21-15a to 21-15c). This may be the preferred solution in the maxillary anterior area, where it is advantageous to avoid ostectomy for adjacent teeth. Papillae will be preserved, and esthetic complications are avoided. The same situation would apply in the case of the maxillary first premolar, where osseous resection to expose additional tooth structure on a canine or second premolar could damage the furcation of the first premolar.

The presence of adjacent teeth has to be taken into consideration when the technique of crown lengthening is selected. If a tooth requires 360 degrees of crown lengthening, it will be easier if there are no adjacent teeth. However, when crown lengthening is required and there are adjacent teeth, the necessary ostectomy will affect adjacent teeth (see Figs 21-8a to 21-8c).

The limitations of forced eruption are found in time expenditure, financial commitment, and the difficulty of grasping the root without causing further structural damage. It is very valuable for the treatment of a fractured maxillary anterior tooth because it obviates the need to disturb the interdental papillae.

References

1. Nevins M, Skurow H. The intracrevicular restorative margin, the biologic width and the maintenance of the gingival margin. Int J Periodont Rest Dent 1984;4(3):31.

2. de Waal H, et al. The importance of restorative margin placement to the biologic width in periodontal health. Part I. Int J Periodont Rest Dent 1981;1(1):9.

3. Nevins M. Interproximal periodontal disease—The embrasure as an etiologic factor. Int J Periodont Rest Dent 1982;2(6):9.

4. Wagenberg BD, Langer B, Eshow R. Exposing adequate tooth structure for restorative dentistry. Int J Periodont Rest Dent 1989;9(5):323.

5. Herrero F, Yukna R. Clinical comparison of desired vs. actual amount of surgical crown lengthening. J Periodontol 1995;66:568.

6. Ross SE, Gargiulo A. The surgical management of the restorative alveolar interface. Int J Periodont Rest Dent 1982;2(3):9.

7. Carnevale GF, Sterrantino S, DiFebo G. Soft and hard tissue wound healing following tooth preparation to the alveolar crest. Int J Periodont Rest Dent 1983;3(6):37.

8. Karring T, Lang NP, Löe H. Role of connective tissue in determining epithelial specificity. J Dent Res 1972;51:1301.

9. Maynard JG, Wilson RD. Physiologic dimensions of the periodontium fundamental to successful restorative dentistry. J Periodontol 1979;50:170–174.

10. Wilson RD, Maynard JG. Intracrevicular restorative dentistry. Int J Periodont Rest Dent 1981;1(4):35.

11. Kramer GM. Rationale of periodontal therapy. In: Goldman HM, Cohen DW (eds). Periodontal Therapy, ed 6. St Louis: Mosby, 1980;378–402.

12. Stetler KJ, Bissada N. Significance of the width of the keratinized gingiva on the periodontal status of teeth with submarginal restorations. J Periodontol 1984;11:95.

13. Ericsson I, Lindhe J. Recession in sites with width of the keratinized gingiva: An experimental study in the dog. J Clin Periodontol 1984;11:95.

14. Wennström JL. Mucogingival surgery. In: Lang NP, Karring T (eds). Proceedings of the First European Workshop on Periodontology. II. London: Quintessence 1994;193–209.

Surgical Preparation of the Edentulous Ridge to Receive a Pontic

Myron Nevins, DDS
Emil G. Cappetta, DMD

This chapter will address the construction of an optimal soft tissue edentulous ridge for pontic placement. The reconstruction of the alveolar process to receive dental implants is discussed elsewhere, but not every patient is a candidate for implant treatment.

The correction of a damaged edentulous ridge serves the purposes of improving esthetics, resolving phonetic dysfunction, and enhancing the patient's ability to perform oral hygiene measures. There are many irregularities that are treated with a removable partial denture because the buccal flange hides them from view and the dentist is unsure of the reconstructive possibilities (Figs 22-1a and 22-2). The surgical intervention should permit pontics and crowns of an appropriate length that is harmonious with the entire arch form. It allows bullet-shaped pontics, which improve accessibility for plaque removal, to be constructed rather than thick or ridge lap designs, which compromise oral hygiene measures.

Edentulous ridge correction frequently has been performed after the extraction wounds heal, but is a more rewarding experience if there is an opportunity to plan for a simultaneous procedure. Although the list of possible etiologies for ridge damage is endless, those that occur most frequently are related to advanced periodontal disease, endodontic failure, and trauma. The creation of an ideal edentulous ridge is best performed at the moment of extraction, before resorption of additional supporting bone occurs.[1] If teeth are already missing when the patient

presents for treatment, reconstruction is possible and will usually improve the prosthesis.

It is necessary to address the issue of color. Previous failure of apicoectomy may result in both soft and hard tissue tattoos that will not permit the construction of a fixed prosthesis, even if there is no need to enhance the size of the ridge (see Fig 22-1b). The tattoo can be completely removed, and the area can be covered with an epithelialized free graft to allow the elimination of the flange of the removable partial denture (Figs 22-1c to 22-1e). A connective tissue graft is most agreeable because of the color match, but may not provide the volume of tissue that is needed.

Many esthetic problems concerning edentulous ridges and pontic design can be corrected by superficial repair. Color uniformity is no problem if the adjacent soft tissues are adjusted in a lateral dimension to correct the deformity with or without the use of grafted tissue (Figs 22-2a to 22-2e).

Long-standing concavities where teeth were lost and the buccal plate was missing or destroyed with a traumatic extraction are difficult to correct. It is necessary to resort to grafting of soft tissue to reconstruct the form necessary for a cleansable and esthetic result (Figs 22-3a and 22-3b). It will be necessary to harvest a thick section of collagen or to double the tissue on itself to achieve enough expansion of the volume. It is not important if the graft is partially epithelialized because this tissue will be desquamated during healing.

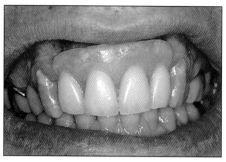

Fig 22-1a The buccal flange of the existing removable partial denture masks the presence of an amalgam tattoo. The patient will not consider a fixed prosthesis until the "black area" is removed.

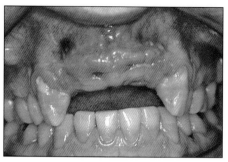

Fig 22-1b An amalgam tattoo has resulted from previous apicoectomies.

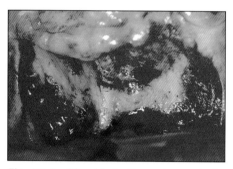

Fig 22-1c The black tissue is surgically removed and the bed is prepared.

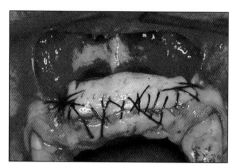

Fig 22-1d An epithelialized free graft is utilized as an onlay graft.

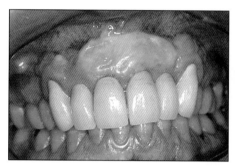

Fig 22-1e Two-year postoperative result with the fixed prosthesis in place. (Final prosthesis constructed by Dr Charles Arnold.)

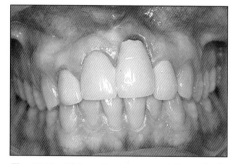

Fig 22-2a This patient presented for esthetic correction. The maxillary left central incisor had a history of trauma followed by endodontic therapy and crown construction. Note the variance in crown length of the maxillary incisors.

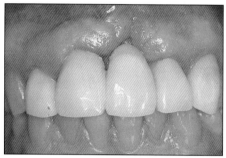

Fig 22-2b The provisional restoration is in place 2 months after the extraction. Note the vertical concavity of the ridge above the pontic.

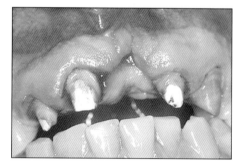

Fig 22-2c The edentulous ridge is visible after the provisional restoration was removed to gain surgical access.

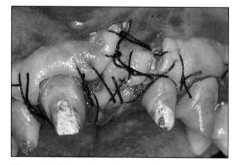

Fig 22-2d Periodontal surgical reconstruction of the edentulous ridge. The surgical access created the opportunity for definitive management of the deformed extraction site. A soft tissue pedicle was moved mesially from the proximal surface of the left lateral incisor and combined with soft tissue that was excised from the palate. The two flaps are coapted by bringing two connective tissue surfaces together.

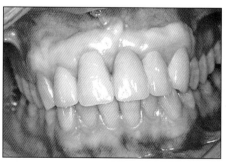

Fig 22-2e The final restoration is in place. Note the improved symmetry that has been established for the maxillary incisors. (Final prosthesis constructed by Dr Howard M. Skurow.)

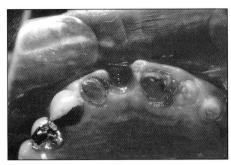

Fig 22-3a Severe damage to the edentulous ridge has occurred during a traumatic extraction. It is difficult to correct this ridge deformity after the extraction wound has healed.

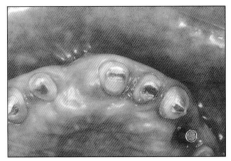

Fig 22-3b Soft tissue has been grafted to reconstruct the edentulous ridge to be cleansable and esthetic. (Courtesy of Dr Yoshihiro Ono.)

Classification of Ridge Defects

Seibert[2] offered a classification of edentulous ridge deformities that describes most volumetric changes but avoids the topic of subtraction when there is excess tissue that interferes with pontic construction. Ridge defects can be classified into three general categories[2]:

1. Class I. Buccolingual loss of tissue with normal ridge height in an apicocoronal dimension
2. Class II. Apicocoronal loss of tissue with normal ridge width in a buccolingual dimension
3. Class III. Combination buccolingual and apicocoronal loss of tissue, resulting in loss of normal height and width

Simultaneous Approach to Ridge Reconstruction and Tooth Extraction

The simultaneous approach to ridge enhancement can be planned efficiently if the tooth to be extracted is still in place (Fig 22-4a). Tooth replacement in the form of a resin-bonded prosthesis or a removable partial denture should be considered so that there will be no edentulous period. The extraction vault requires complete debridement of granulation tissue before the volume of grafting material that is necessary is assessed.

A single tooth almost always can be corrected with a connective tissue graft that is harvested so that it will be a volumetric match (Figs 22-4b and 22-4c). It is made stationary by the use of resorbable sutures before the residual soft tissue flaps are closed over the graft (Fig 22-4d). The edentulous ridge is now close to its final form because little dimensional change is anticipated. The final prosthesis can be constructed after a wait of 3 months (Figs 22-4e to 22-4g). This surgery becomes far more complex when the ridge is reconstructed for the placement of a dental implant (Figs 22-5a to 22-5f).

The management of the simultaneous extraction of multiple teeth and combined buccopalatal and apicocoronal enhancement requires a sequential series of events that is systematically organized. The deformity produced in a healed mature ridge will be directly related to the volume of space previously occupied by the roots of teeth and the loss of alveolar process. The success of the reconstructive treatment will depend on an accurate assessment of this volume and the ability to replace it so as to restore the damaged ridge to the ideal size to accommodate pontics for the prosthesis.

The sequence of events involved in simultaneously treating a complicated ridge and gaining significant enhancement is often critical to success. Presurgical treatment planning begins with an assessment of the quantity of soft tissue available for grafting. Because a considerable amount is needed, palpation of the palate should be replaced with local anesthesia and needle probing to determine the possibility of harvesting connective tissue with a minimum of epithelium and the anterior and posterior extents of the procedure.

It is then important to plan the provisional prosthesis to replace the teeth to be extracted. A removable partial denture that is completely tooth supported is one possibility, although a fixed provisional prosthesis is preferred to avoid impingement on the palatal donor sites. This is an intricate process for both the periodontist and restorative dentist. The proposed abutment teeth are first prepared, and an impression is made to construct the prosthesis. The laboratory will estimate the pontic size, but it probably will have to be adjusted at delivery. The prepared teeth are then provisionalized (Figs 22-6a to 22-6c) before the patient is appointed for extraction or grafting.

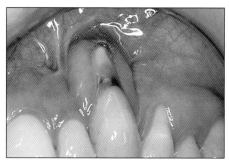

Fig 22-4a There is extreme loss of periodontium on the buccal surface of the maxillary left canine. The tooth will be extracted and the area will receive a simultaneous connective tissue graft.

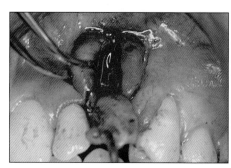

Fig 22-4b The extraction vault requires complete degranulation, and the volume of tissue necessary for grafting is ascertained.

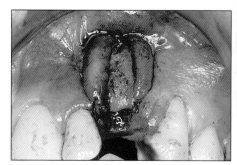

Fig 22-4c The connective tissue graft is placed.

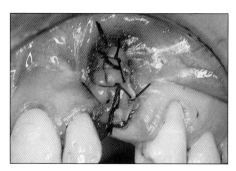

Fig 22-4d The connective tissue graft is sutured in place with resorbable sutures. The flaps are sutured with silk sutures over the connective tissue graft.

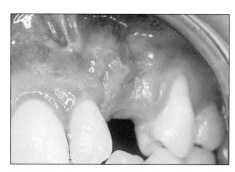

Fig 22-4e Appearance of the tissue 2 months postsurgery.

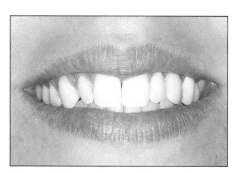

Fig 22-4f The canine area is inconspicuous at the high-lip position of the smile line.

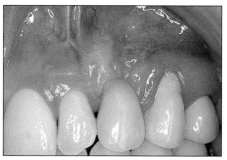

Fig 22-4g The final prosthesis consists of two premolar crowns and a canine cantilever. (Final prosthesis constructed by Dr John Machell.)

The teeth are extracted at the time of the ridge augmentation procedure. The level of difficulty of the procedure is influenced by the accuracy of both the tooth preparation and the prosthesis construction because the provisional prosthesis will be totally supported by the prepared abutments. Buccal and lingual flaps are elevated for the surgical extraction to help preserve any remaining alveolus and to provide access for complete removal of granulation tissue (Fig 22-6d). Approximately 30% of the remaining buccal plate is lost to resorption in the first 30 days after extraction when no regenerative procedure is performed.[1] The extraction sockets are filled with a biocompatible material (allograft or alloplast) to reduce the volume of soft tissue needed to complete the procedure.

Connective tissue grafts are preferred to avoid large open areas of healing at the donor sites (Fig 22-6e). They are oriented to cover the extraction site from the buccal to the palatal aspects. They are first sutured to the palatal flap with resorbable sutures. Then the buccal flap is dissected apically, deep into the vestibule, permitting its advancement to cover the grafted tissue. It may be necessary to take a graft from both sides of the palate if a large procedure is executed. The buccal flap is then sutured to the palatal flap, and the edentulous ridge has been enhanced vertically and horizontally (Fig 22-6f).

The gain of structure can be observed by fitting the provisional restoration in place after the extractions and before the enhancement procedures (see Fig 22-6d). This presents a

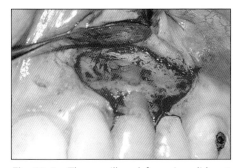

Fig 22-5a The maxillary left canine did not respond to endodontic treatment or to four apicoectomies. The patient preferred implant placement to a traditional fixed prosthesis. An immediate implant was contraindicated, but a staged approach was used.

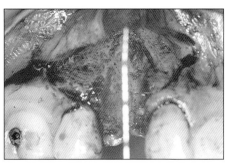

Fig 22-5b The extraction vault demonstrates no buccal wall of bone.

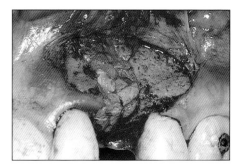

Fig 22-5c Bone, harvested from the posterior iliac crest with a trephine, is placed in the extraction vault.

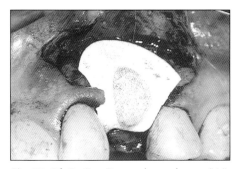

Fig 22-5d A Gore-Tex oval membrane (WL Gore, Flagstaff, AZ) is placed over the graft.

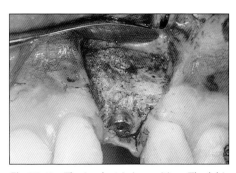

Fig 22-5e The implant is in position. The labial plate of bone has been regenerated.

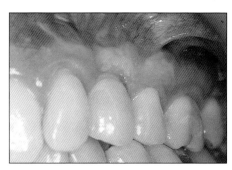

Fig 22-5f The final crown is in place and functions in occlusion. (Final crown constructed by Dr Janice Conrad.)

sobering sight for those who incorrectly would use implants to replace these teeth, and demonstrates the sheer volume of space that has been occupied by the grafts. This appearance can then be compared to the replacement of the provisional prosthesis after treatment (Figs 22-6g and 22-6h).

The optimal end goal of these procedures is the construction of a smooth edentulous ridge when pontics are constructed, to allow pleasing esthetics and phonetics, as well as easy cleansing. Color match is no issue for any type of inlay surgery, because the flap is composed of mature tissue whether the procedure is a complete pouch or a wedge, a variation of the pouch procedure in which the pouch is not closed. Color is an issue with onlay grafting. A gingival graft is taken from the palatal donor site or tuberosity region in a pie-shaped configuration and positioned like a wedge into the pouch opening, increasing the amount of buccolingual augmentation at the crest of the ridge. It is immaterial whether there is a collar of epithelial tissue. The authors concur with Seibert's assessment that densely collagenized connective tissue is slowly resorbed and replaced with a similar volume of new connective tissue.[3–5]

Treatment of Existing Ridge Defects

The procedures available to reconstruct the damaged edentulous ridge with soft tissue are[3–6]:

1. De-epithelialized connective tissue pedicle graft
2. Pouch procedures for subepithelial grafts or subconnective grafts
3. Wedge and inlay graft procedures
4. Onlay grafts

The treatment goals for the inlay type of procedure are:

1. To provide color stability.
2. To treat Seibert class I defects.
3. To treat Seibert class III defects.
4. To provide simultaneous extraction and enhancement treatment.
5. To take advantage of the excellent survival rate and stability of size of gingival grafting procedures.

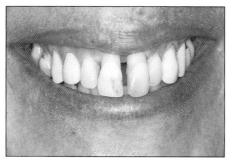

Fig 22-6a The patient is disenchanted with the appearance of her teeth.

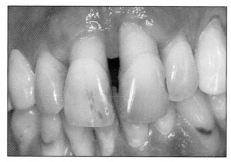

Fig 22-6b The maxillary central incisors are long and demonstrate supereruption and a large diastema.

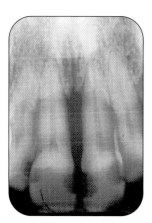 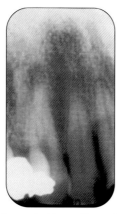 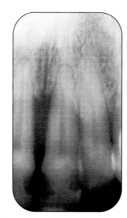 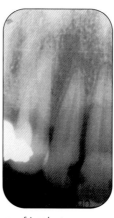 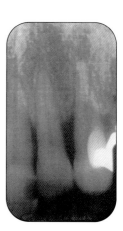

Fig 22-6c Radiographs reveal the vertical loss of bone that will preclude the esthetic use of implants.

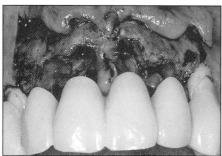

Fig 22-6d The maxillary canines and first premolars were prepared, impressions were taken, and the canines and first premolars received provisional crowns. The dental laboratory then constructed an eight-unit provisional prosthesis. This allowed the extraction of the four hopeless incisors and the simultaneous reconstruction of the edentulous ridge at the time the provisional restoration was delivered. Note the vertical discrepancy between the level of the remaining alveolus and the pontics.

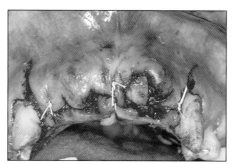

Fig 22-6e The connective tissue grafts are sutured in place with resorbable sutures. The first sutures to close the flaps over the grafts are in place.

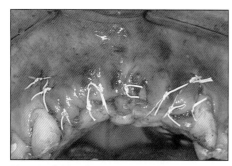

Fig 22-6f The flaps are sutured in place over the grafts.

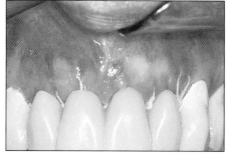

Fig 22-6g The provisional prosthesis is in place after surgery.

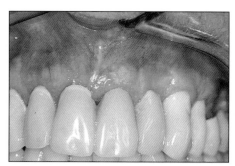

Fig 22-6h The ridge is completely healed.

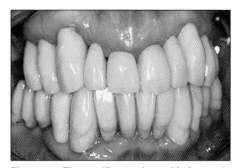

Fig 22-7a The maxillary and mandibular provisional restorations are shown after surgical procedures to eliminate pockets and prosthetic relining of the provisional trial restorations. There is an obvious disparity between the length of the maxillary incisors and canines that cannot be corrected because of the edentulous ridge.

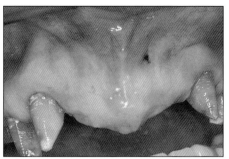

Fig 22-7b The maxillary provisional restoration has been removed to gain surgical access to the edentulous ridge. The vertical position of this ridge interferes with the apical extension of the incisor pontics.

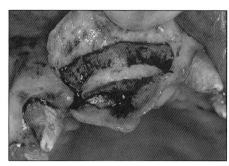

Fig 22-7c Flap elevation exposes the bone crest that needs to be modified.

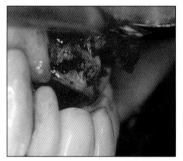

Fig 22-7d While the provisional restoration is in place, the gingiva is elevated to demonstrate the proximity of the remaining premaxilla to the pontics. The provisional prosthesis is used to guide the removal of bone and predict the size of the final pontics.

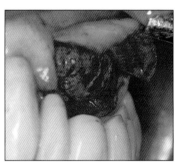

Fig 22-7e The bone crest is relieved to allow apical extension of the pontics and esthetic harmony of the prosthesis.

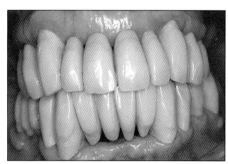

Fig 22-7f The maxillary provisional restoration has been redesigned to achieve the proper length-width ratio of the teeth. The entire occlusocervical length of the maxillary arch has been reduced to improve the crown-root ratio of the maxillary prosthesis. (Prosthesis constructed by Dr Howard M. Skurow.)

The treatment goals for the onlay type of procedure are:

1. To provide color correction (tattoos or pigmentation).
2. To treat Seibert class II defects.
3. To treat the patient with staged events if enough correction is not gained with the first surgery. (Many patients are discouraged by multiple surgical entries.)

Onlay grafts are thick gingival grafts, and the amount of apicocoronal success will depend on the amount of connective tissue that survives the procedure. They require abundant blood supply and rapid revascularization. These procedures are frequently multistage procedures.

It is possible that the correction of the edentulous ridge would best be accomplished by *subtraction* rather than addition. An example of the indications for such a procedure is found in periodontal-prosthesis cases in which there are long clinical crowns for abutment teeth but residual edentulous ridge remains in the anterior region (Figs 22-7a to 22-7c). The presence of the residual premaxilla prevents the

apical extension of the pontics and results in very short incisors and long canines. This scenario is found in Angle malocclusion class II, division I, dentitions. The provisional prosthesis can be used at the time of surgery to guide the removal of bone and predict the size of the final pontics (Figs 22-7c to 22-7f).

Anterior edentulous ridge defects can result from developmental defects, such as cleft lip, cleft ridge and/or palate, and cysts. They are difficult to treat and require an individualized treatment regimen.

The deformity resulting from a cleft makes it very difficult to construct a pontic that will fulfill the objectives of phonetics, esthetics, and cleanliness (Figs 22-8a and 22-8b). It is also precarious to design and execute surgical flaps because of scar tissue from previous surgery. However, the concept of correction fits with the inlay type of procedure and is complemented by guided tissue regeneration. The cleft itself is first covered with a thick connective tissue graft that is sutured to fixed tissue with resorbable sutures

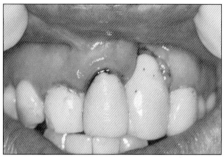

Fig 22-8a A fixed partial denture was constructed so that the maxillary left central incisor pontic covered a deformed edentulous ridge that resulted from a congenital cleft ridge.

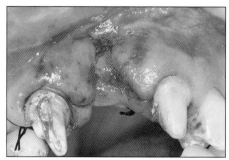

Fig 22-8b An oral-antral communication presents functional problems for the patient.

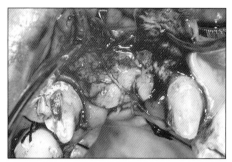

Fig 22-8c The cleft is first covered by a thick connective tissue graft sutured to fixed tissue with resorbable sutures.

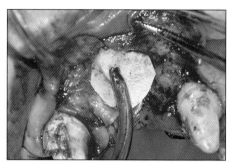

Fig 22-8d The graft is covered with Gore-Tex augmentation membrane.

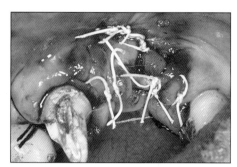

Fig 22-8e The entire assembly is covered by the surgical flaps.

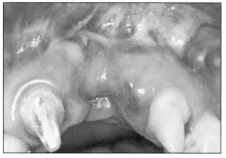

Fig 22-8f The reconstructed edentulous ridge is now appropriate for pontic construction. The cleft and the oral-antral communication have been eliminated.

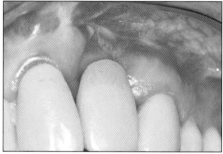

Fig 22-8g The permanent restoration is in place. There is esthetic improvement, and the patient has benefited greatly from the closure of the oral-antral fistula. (Prosthesis constructed by Dr Kenneth Malament.)

(Fig 22-8c). The graft is then covered with an expanded polytetrafluoroethylene augmentation membrane, and the assembly is covered with the surgical flaps (Figs 22-8d and 22-8e). The reconstructed edentulous ridge is then appropriate for pontic construction (Fig 22-8f). An obvious benefit of this procedure is the closure of the oral-antral fistula (Figs 22-8f and 22-8g).

Developmental cysts that involve supernumerary teeth may persist after these teeth are surgically removed (Fig 22-9a). It is possible to determine the etiology only if reasonable records are available, but it is necessary to make this determination to distinguish the background of the radiographic radiolucency (Fig 22-9b). Treatment requires surgical entry and elimination of the diseased granulation tissue and exudate (Figs 22-9c and 22-9d). The area is reconstructed using the techniques of guided bone regeneration (Figs 22-9c to 22-9g). The comparison of computerized tomograms taken before and after treatment (2 years) revealed a remarkable radiographic change (Figs 22-9h and 22-9i). There was no further exudate on clinical examination.

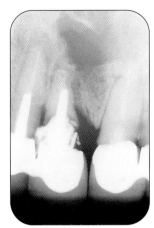

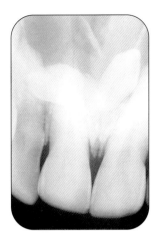

Fig 22-9a A large radiolucency is present apical to the central incisors.

Fig 22-9b A radiograph made many years before Fig 22-9a reveals a developmental cyst that involved the presence of supernumerary teeth. This cyst persisted after the supernumerary teeth had been surgically removed.

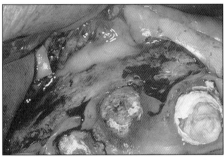

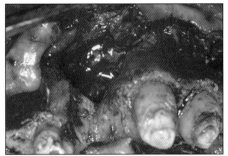

Fig 22-9c Surgical entry via a buccal flap reveals the presence of diseased granulation tissue and purulent exudate.

Fig 22-9d The defect has been degranulated. It extends superiorly to the membrane of the nasal cavities.

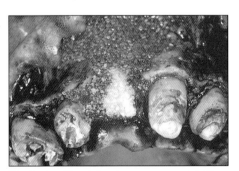

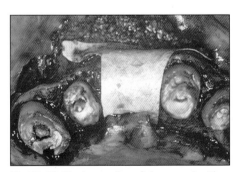

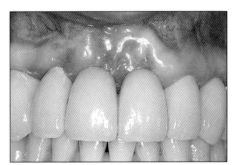

Fig 22-9e The defect is reconstructed with a bone allograft augmentation.

Fig 22-9f The bone allograft is covered with a Gore-Tex augmentation membrane.

Fig 22-9g The final prosthesis is in place 2 years after the reconstruction of the edentulous ridge. (Prosthesis constructed by Dr John Machell.)

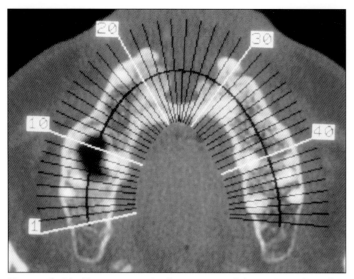

Fig 22-9h Maxillary computerized tomogram of the patient taken after construction of the processed acrylic resin trial restoration. The large radiolucent area indicates that there is complete destruction of the buccal plate and no bone remaining buccal to the incisive canal.

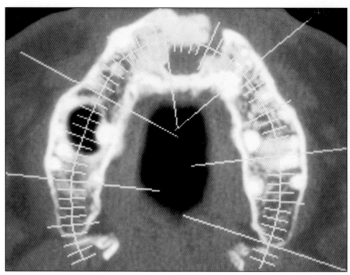

Fig 22-9i Maxillary computerized tomogram taken 18 months after the guided bone regeneration procedure. The buccal plate has almost been replaced.

Conclusion

It is essential to return to the original premise of reconstructing the damaged edentulous ridge, regardless of the etiology. Esthetic correction is usually the driving force behind these procedures, and the optimal result will yield a pontic that is in harmony with the adjacent natural dentition.[7] The need for these procedures is paramount in patients with high lip lines. Phonetic improvement and cleansability are significant benefits to the patient.

The clinician must treat each malformed edentulous area with individual consideration. It is unnecessary to attempt to categorize the deformities or their corrections beyond understanding the indications for and advantages of the corrective procedures.

References

1. Carlsson GE, Thilander H, Hedegard G. Histologic changes in the upper alveolar process after extractions with or without insertion of an immediate full denture. Acta Odontol Scand 1967;25:1–31.

2. Seibert J. Presented at the D. Walter Cohen Periodontal Symposium, Philadelphia, 21 June 1989.

3. Seibert J. Reconstruction of the partially edentulous ridge: Gateway to improved prosthetics and superior aesthetics. Prac Periodontics Aesthet Dent 1993;5:47–55.

4. Siebert J. Ridge augmentation to enhance aesthetics in fixed prosthetic treatment. Compend Contin Educ Dent 1991;12:548.

5. Garber DA. The edentulous ridge and fixed prosthodontics. Compend Contin Educ Dent 1981;2:212.

6. Seibert J, Salama H. Alveolar ridge preservation and reconstruction. Periodontology 2000 1996;11:69–84.

7. Wennström JL. Mucogingival therapy. Ann Periodontol 1996; 1:671–701.

An Overview of Mucogingival Surgery to Cover the Exposed Root Surface

Myron Nevins, DDS
Emil G. Cappetta, DMD

The surgical armamentarium designed to increase the gingival dimension is used to reverse the effects of gingival recession by providing coverage for the exposed root surface. Although the histologic attachment of root coverage continues to be somewhat controversial, patient satisfaction and esthetic improvement are not debatable. Root coverage is routinely attainable and meets the needs and demands of both patients and practitioners. Root coverage procedures are indicated to correct areas of localized or generalized soft tissue recession that are an esthetic problem; to resolve root sensitivity; and to treat shallow areas of root structure loss.[1,2]

There are four surgical methods proposed to cover exposed root structure and correct areas of gingival recession:

1. Pedicle grafts
2. Epithelialized free gingival autografts
3. Connective tissue autografts
4. Guided tissue regeneration with membranes

To date there is human biopsy evidence of a connective tissue attachment to new cementum on the exposed tooth surface for both guided tissue regeneration and the traditional free graft procedures[3,4] (Figs 23-1 and 23-2). There is every reason to assume that the same data will emerge for the connective tissue procedure.

Causes of Gingival Recession

The following conditions are predisposing factors[2-5] to gingival recession:

1. Minimal attached gingiva (buccolingual and/or apico-coronal dimension)
2. Frenum pull
3. Tooth malposition (Tooth position relates to the position of the tooth in the alveolus. The alveolar dehiscence or fenestration with resultant thin bony housing provides a thin gingival cover and is susceptible to recession.)

Precipitating factors[2,6] are:

1. Inflammation related to plaque.
2. Improper brushing that abrades and lacerates the tissue through chronic wounding.
3. Iatrogenic dental care, including tooth preparation, margin placement, impression making, etc (acute wounding).

Maynard theorizes that the periodontal anatomy may predispose certain individuals to gingival recession (see Chapter 19).

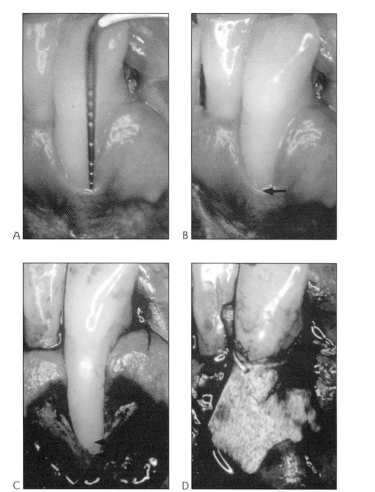

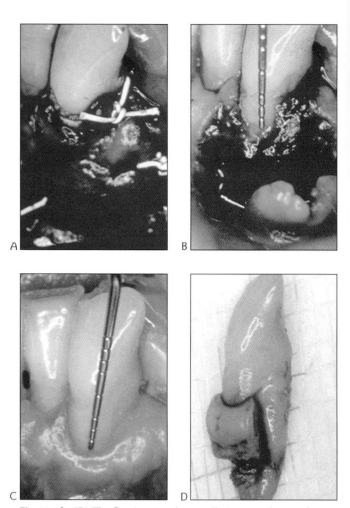

Fig 23-1a (A) An 8-mm recession is present on the mandibular left lateral incisor. (B) Location of the coronal notch at the level of the gingival margin *(arrow)*. (C) The flap is reflected. Levels of the coronal notch *(arrow)* and the most apical level of instrumentation *(arrow)* correspond to the bone crest. (D) A bent membrane is positioned to reach the cementoenamel junction. (Figs 23-1a to 23-1c from Cortellini et al.[3] Reprinted with permission.)

Fig 23-1b (A) The flap is sutured coronally to cover the membrane. (B) Reentry procedure, 4 weeks later; after reflection of the flap, the level of newly formed tissue is assessed with a probe. (C) Residual recession 5 months after reentry. Notice the keratinized tissue width. (D) The tooth has been extracted with buccal tissues.

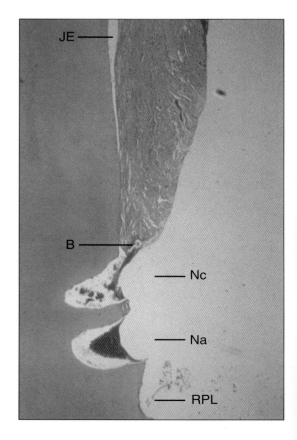

Fig 23-1c Vertical buccolingual section of the extracted tooth with part of the buccal tissues. (Hematoxylin-eosin stain; original magnification × 8.) Note the root coverage; the coronal notch (Nc) represents the baseline level of the gingival margin. The landmarks are the most apical extension of the junctional epithelium (JE), the crestal bone level (B), the coronal notch (Nc), the apical notch (Na), and the most apical extension of instrumented root surface (RPL).

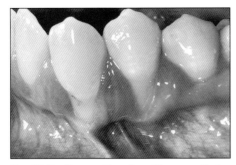

Fig 23-2a Preoperative view. The mandibular left first premolar exhibits 6.0 mm of recession. The facial probing depth is approximately 2.0 mm on both teeth. There is no attached gingiva on either tooth. (Figs 23-2a to 23-2f from Pasquinelli.[4] Reprinted with permission.)

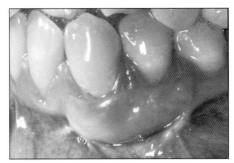

Fig 23-2b Appearance 10 weeks after placement of the graft. The first premolar exhibits 5.0 mm of gingiva and the canine exhibits 6.0 mm of gingiva. Root coverage is to within 0.5 mm of the cementoenamel junction on each tooth. The facial probing depth is approximately 1.0 mm.

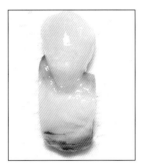

Fig 23-2c First premolar removed in block section 10.5 months after the root coverage procedure.

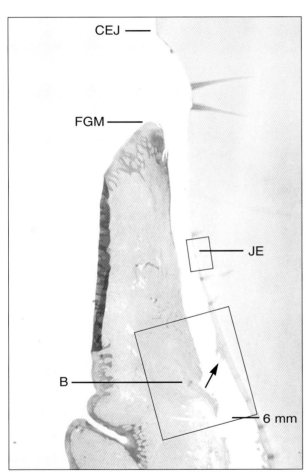

Fig 23-2d Vertical midfacial buccolingual section of the first premolar and the facial soft tissues. The area between the cementoenamel junction (CEJ) and the point marked 6.0 mm is the original extent of recession. There was a 0.4-mm vertical shift between the tissues as a result of processing. Artifactual separation of the soft tissue from the root during processing *(arrow)*. Free gingival margin (FGM); apical extent of junctional epithelium (JE); bone (B). The areas enclosed by squares are shown at greater magnification in Figs 23-2e and 23-2f. (Hematoxylin-eosin staining; original magnification × 4.)

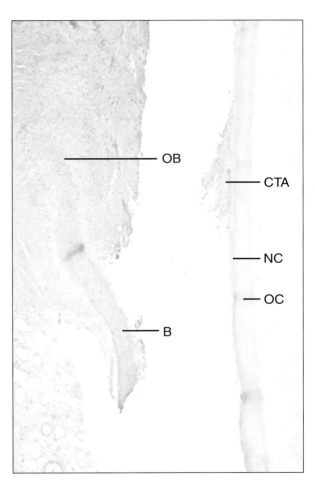

Fig 23-2e New bone growth (B); osteoblasts (OB); old cementum (OC); new cementum (NC); connective tissue attachment (CTA). (Hematoxylin-eosin staining; original magnification × 16.)

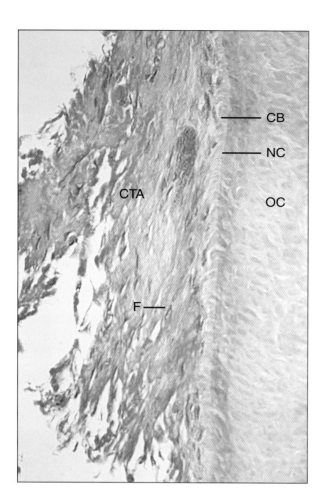

Fig 23-2f Fibrous connective tissue attachment (CTA), consisting of dense collagen with spindle-shaped fibroblasts (F) inserting into new cementum (NC) and old cementum (OC). Cementoblasts (CB) with nuclei parallel to the root surface. (Hematoxylin-eosin staining; original magnification × 100.)

Classification of Gingival Recession

In 1985, Miller[7] described four categories for recession-type defects.

1. Class I. Marginal tissue recession that has *not* extended to the mucogingival junction. There is *no* loss of interdental bone or soft tissue.
2. Class II. Marginal tissue recession that extends to or beyond the mucogingival junction. There is *no* loss of interdental bone or soft tissue.
3. Class III. Marginal tissue recession that extends to or beyond the mucogingival junction. There is loss of interdental bone, and the interdental soft tissue is apical to the cementoenamel junction (CEJ) but remains coronal to the apical extent of the marginal tissue recession.
4. Class IV. Marginal tissue recession that extends beyond the mucogingival junction. There is a loss of interdental bone and soft tissue to a level corresponding to the apical extent of the marginal tissue recession.

The amount of root coverage that can be achieved, regardless of the procedure used, is limited by the height of the adjacent papilla. Miller stated that complete root coverage can be achieved in class I and class II recession defects. Partial coverage may be expected in the type of recession represented by classes III and IV.[5]

Laterally Positioned Pedicle Graft (Rotational Flap)

This procedure, first described by Grupe and Warren[8,9] and modified by numerous clinicians over the years,[10–13] retains the vascularity of the graft by its pedicle design. It has been used as a full-thickness procedure and as a partial-thickness procedure to avoid recession at the donor site, with and without a soft tissue graft at the donor site. Other modifications include treatment of the root with citric acid,[14] and covering subepithelial connective tissue grafts in a "bilaminar procedure."[15,16]

The lateral sliding pedicle graft can be used to increase gingival dimension and for root coverage (Figs 23-3a to 23-3e) and is best used for treatment of localized areas of recession. The advantages are excellent color and texture match and the fact that the pedicle graft retains its blood supply. Evidence to date indicates an expected success rate of approximately 70%.[1]

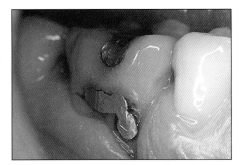

Fig 23-3a The mandibular molar exhibits a gingival cleft that transcends the mucogingival junction.

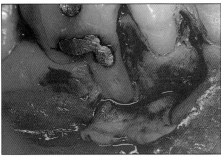

Fig 23-3b A laterally repositioned flap has been mobilized from the second premolar with the base of the pedicle at the recipient site. The goal of the procedure is to create an adequate zone of attached gingiva and to cover the exposed root.

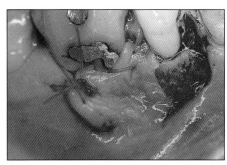

Fig 23-3c The pedicle flap is sutured in place.

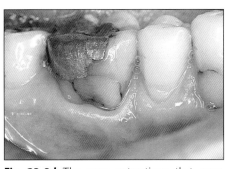

Fig 23-3d The new restorations that were placed after the surgery are in need of replacement after 6 years.

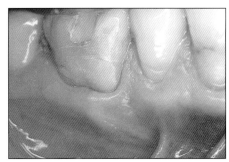

Fig 23-3e The restorations have continually been replaced as years have passed, but the gingiva created by the lateral flap procedure has remained.

The procedure should not be used under the following conditions:

1. When there is insufficient adequate donor tissue
2. When there is a shallow vestibule
3. When high frenum attachments are present
4. When there are multiple adjacent recessions
5. When recession will occur at the donor site as a result of the procedure

It is recommended that the width of the pedicle be three times the width of the root area to be covered, at least 3 mm of gingiva in an apicocoronal direction, and adequate thickness in the donor site.[17] It is best to place the base of the pedicle at the recipient site to alleviate tension on the flap because this will greatly facilitate suturing for all such procedures (see Fig 23-3c).

Coronally Positioned Pedicle Graft (Advanced Flap Without Rotation or Lateral Movement)

The coronally positioned flap by itself offers the obvious advantages of a single surgical site and a successful match of color and contour. However, its indications are limited, and there is debate as to its efficacy.[1,2] It has been suggested that it be applied to treat shallow areas of recession (class I) where 3 mm of keratinized tissue is present.[5,17–19] Harris et al[18] utilized inlaid margins as part of the surgical design to provide a butt joint and an inlay for the pedicle (coronally positioned) graft. Their study reported complete root coverage in cases with less than 3 mm of gingiva and suggested that 3 mm may not be the minimum requirement.

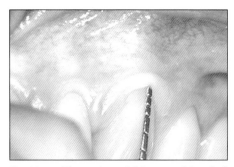

Fig 23-4a The canine exhibits a small band of unattached keratinized gingiva and 2 mm of gingival recession.

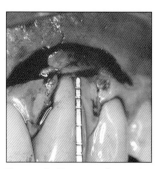

Fig 23-4b Two mm of recession have occurred.

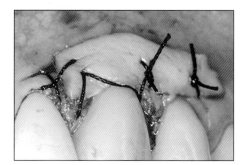

Fig 23-4c An epithelialized gingival graft is sutured in place. It is necessary to extend apically beyond the level of recession to cover a bed of periosteum and to extend to the interdental areas.

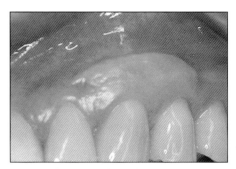

Fig 23-4d The tooth exhibits no recession I year after surgery. The blend of color is most satisfactory.

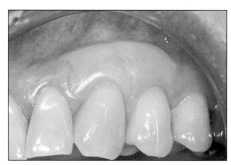

Fig 23-4e Twenty-two years after surgery, the original goals of surgery continue to be successfully maintained.

Combined Technique

The combined technique of following the free gingival graft with a coronally positioned flap seems to be more predictable. Either a gingival graft is placed simultaneously with the coronally positioned flap, or a gingival graft is placed and the entire complex is moved coronally at a second surgical procedure. This procedure surgically resembles a pedicle graft, and the amount of root coverage achieved is usually similar to that achieved with either a two-stage procedure or a single pedicle graft.[20–22]

The coronally positioned flap is a more predictable procedure when combined with the prior placement of a free gingival graft than when used alone.[1] There are esthetic concerns associated with this procedure because with a free gingival graft as the first procedure there may be problems with color match. Studies have reported the percentage of root coverage obtained with coronally positioned pedicle grafts to vary from 50% to 100%, with an average of 64% to 65% of root coverage attained.[1,23]

Epithelialized Free Gingival Graft

The free gingival graft is a versatile, widely used, and very predictable pure mucogingival surgical procedure. It is utilized to increase the zone of attached gingiva around teeth and implants. It is used alone (Figs 23-4a to 24-4e) or in combination with a coronally positioned pedicle graft or a laterally positioned pedicle graft for root coverage.[21,24] It has been placed on periosteum, as well as on perforated or nonperforated bone.[25–27] Many early efforts placed the graft subgingivally, with an incision at the mucogingival junction, resulting in a poor color match.[28] When the incision is placed at the level of the CEJ, the graft can be sutured to the papilla coronally and to the periosteum apically, improving root coverage, reducing shrinkage, and providing an excellent color match.[29] (Figs 23-5a to 23-5c).

This procedure has been used successfully for many years. The contemporary development began in the 1960s.[30] Sullivan and Atkins[31] discussed the concept of "bridging" and the need for plasmatic circulation and

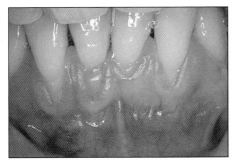

Fig 23-5a There is a minimal zone of keratinized attached gingiva. The root exposure is further compromised by surface abrasion.

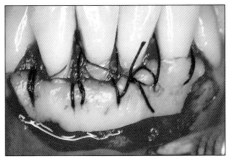

Fig 23-5b The graft is placed approximately at the level of the cementoenamel junction and is sutured to the papillae coronally.

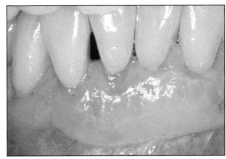

Fig 23-5c Twenty-seven years after surgery, there is excellent color match and the mandibular left incisor roots are completely covered.

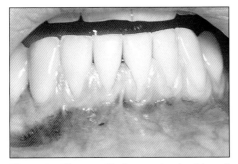

Fig 23-6a The mandibular anterior dentition of a 19-year-old woman exhibits incisal wear and the clefting of the mandibular left incisors with root exposure.

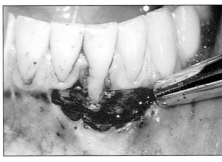

Fig 23-6b The periodontal surgical procedure in process reveals the loss of the labial plate of bone on the mandibular left central incisor.

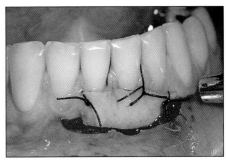

Fig 23-6c A free gingival autograft has been placed on the labial surface of both mandibular left incisors and the right central incisor. The gingival cuff on the other teeth was removed before the graft was positioned.

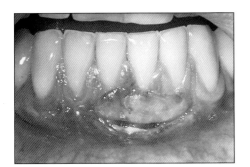

Fig 23-6d The sutures are removed after 1 week.

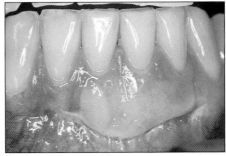

Fig 23-6e The 1-year postoperative appearance indicates total root coverage, an excellent color match, and a deepened vestibule that allows better access for cleansing.

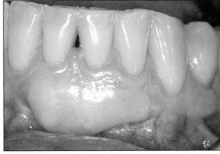

Fig 23-6f Clinical examination 22 years after treatment reveals that the gingival tissues completely cover the labial surface of the incisors up to the cementoenamel junction. No effort has been made to alter the incisal edges or the occlusal function of these teeth; in spite of this, a successful regeneration of the gingival unit has occurred. This eliminates occlusion as an etiologic factor in the clefting of these mandibular anterior teeth.

suggested that this technique would best be limited to narrow areas of recession. Despite favorable reports[32,33] of root coverage in the treatment of deep-wide recession defects, the inability of the gingival graft to predictably cover exposed roots led clinicians to advocate limiting its use to creating an adequate dimension of attached gingiva.[34] Some thought it would not enhance root coverage where recession had occurred earlier except by "creeping attachment."[35]

The tide of opinion shifted toward predictability with the publications of Miller,[36] Corn and Marks,[37] and Holbrook and Oschenbein[38] (Figs 23-6a to 23-6f). Miller showed that the depth and width of the root exposure is not the overriding consideration in obtaining root coverage, as once was believed. He also reported 100% root coverage in 87% (incidence) of deep-wide recession defects and 100% root coverage in 100% of the shallow-narrow recession

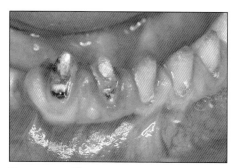

Fig 23-7a There is minimal keratinized attached gingiva on the buccal surface and a limited vestibule.

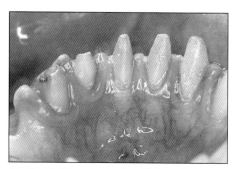

Fig 23-7b There is also insufficient gingiva on the lingual surface for a fixed prosthesis to be constructed.

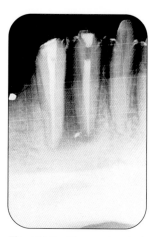

Fig 23-7c The perioapical radiograph demonstrates advanced loss of bone between the lateral incisor and canine.

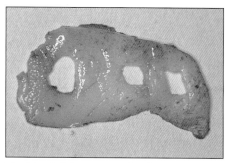

Fig 23-7d A large gingival graft has been harvested from the edentulous maxilla.

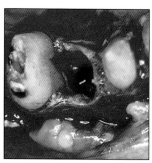

Fig 23-7e The lateral incisor extraction wound reveals an interdental crater on the mesial surface of the canine.

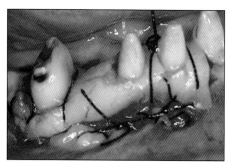

Fig 23-7f The graft is sutured in place (buccal view).

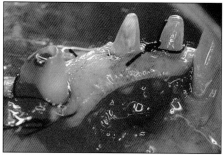

Fig 23-7g The graft is sutured in place (lingual view).

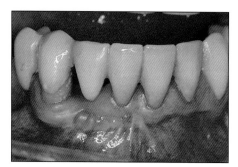

Fig 23-7h Surgical result (buccal surface).

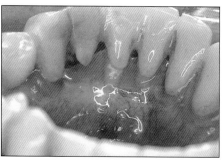

Fig 23-7i Surgical result (lingual surface).

defects. Corn and Marks[37] underscored the importance of proper surgical technique, preparation of the recipient site, and root preparation. They also discussed the importance of the preoperative position of the interdental soft and hard tissues and tooth position.

Other researchers have demonstrated that the success achieved with this procedure could be replicated by many clinicians. Holbrook and Oschenbein[38] reported root coverage of 95.6% when the initial recession defect was less than 3 mm, 80.6% when the recession defect was 4 to 5 mm, and 76.6% when the lesion was greater than 5 mm. This represents a 44% incidence of 100% root coverage.

Borghetti and Gardella[39] demonstrated a mean root coverage of 85.2%, ranging from 1.8 to 4.4 mm, with 100% root coverage in 18 class I and class II defects. The report indicated that the degree of coverage was better for narrow recessions (94.7%) than for wide recessions (71.2%).

Tolmie et al[40] reported a mean root coverage of 86.2% in class I and class II defects; the incidence of complete root coverage was 72.8% (100% root coverage in 75 of 103 sites). They also stressed the importance of making a distinction between mean root coverage and the incidence of 100% root coverage in reports of root coverage, because there are instances when 100% root coverage is not attained and the incidence of partial root coverage is high.

Bertrand et al[41] reported 70% overall root coverage after utilizing thick 1.5- to 2-mm gingival grafts.

The final proof that this procedure has the potential to form a new connective tissue attachment to the tooth was provided by Pasquinelli.[3] A mandibular premolar that was previously treated successfully with a gingival autograft was extracted to provide space for orthodontic therapy. The human biopsy specimen demonstrated a connective tissue attachment of the graft to the previously exposed root surface (see Figs 23-2d to 23-2f).

The first histologic study of the healing of free gingival grafts reported bridging or union of new capillaries with the original vessels of the graft.[30] This establishment and maintenance of plasmatic circulation between the recipient connective tissue bed and the free graft during the initial phase of healing is critical to cover denuded roots.[31] Rapid revascularization can be established early by butt jointing against the capillary network of the interdental papilla.[42]

Other factors[4,5] that influence graft survival and ability to cover roots are:

1. Graft thickness (approximately 1.5 mm to 2 mm is recommended)
2. Suturing techniques
3. Entrapment of a blood clot between the graft and the root, as well as the adjacent soft tissue recipient bed
4. Mechanical root preparation (scaling and root planing)
5. Flattening of the root surface with scaling and root planing or rotary instrumentation

6. Chemical root conditioning (citric acid and tetracycline)

The free gingival graft is routinely used to increase the band of attached gingiva for single teeth, as well as groups of teeth, with a high predictability. There is a superior source of donor tissue than there is for pedicle grafts (Fig 23-7).

The following are contraindications for the use of the free gingival graft procedure alone for root coverage:

1. A perceptible mismatch in color between the donor site and the gingiva adjacent to the recipient site
2. A lack of thick donor tissue; the recommended thickness is a minimum of 1.5 mm
3. A class III or class IV recession defect
4. A root surface of excessive mesiodistal width coupled with interproximal tissue that is too narrow to support the blood supply

The goal of the free autogenous gingival graft for root coverage is the restoration of the marginal tissue to the level of the CEJ with attachment to the previously exposed root surface.

Free Connective Tissue Grafts (Nonepithelialized Connective Tissue Grafts)

Becker and Becker[43] concluded that this procedure should not be recommended for the treatment of recession, although it is a highly predictable procedure for gingival augmentation. The connective tissue can be harvested from under the palatal flap simultaneously with pocket surgery. The disadvantage of this procedure is that it is not always possible to obtain an adequate thickness of donor tissue. The main advantage is the availability of keratinized tissue for teeth with the need for additional gingiva and the rapid, uneventful healing period.[44]

Subepithelial Connective Tissue Grafts

The subepithelial connective tissue graft was introduced by Langer et al[45–47] as an extension of the subepithelial graft employed to correct ridge concavities. The procedure takes advantage of a double blood supply: that of the gingival flap that covers the graft and that of the recipient bed, including the adjacent papilla (Figs 23-8 and 23-9). The technique was later modified and combined with a coronally positioned flap to treat root recession defects. With this technique, connective tissue is placed under the flap, allowing better color

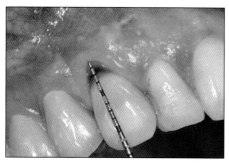

Fig 23-8a The maxillary left canine is an esthetic problem. There is recession that was compounded by root discoloration and early caries.

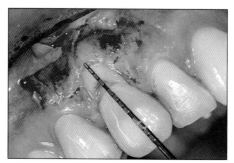

Fig 23-8b A gingival flap has been elevated to prepare the buccal surface of the tooth and the adjoining periodontium to receive a connective tissue graft. The buccal loss of bone is significantly more than is supposed from observing the gingival margin. The root surface is strenuously planed to achieve hard surface.

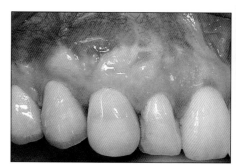

Fig 23-8c The result of treatment with a subepithelial connective tissue graft is excellent.

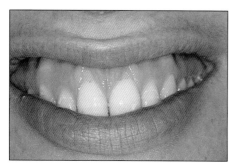

Fig 23-9a This patient is concerned about the esthetics of the central incisors. The root exposure is accentuated by her short upper lip.

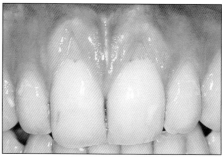

Fig 23-9b The deep clefts on the labial surface of the maxillary central incisors extend almost to the mucogingival junction.

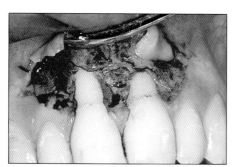

Fig 23-9c A buccal flap is elevated with vertical incisions that are designed to avoid the tissue of the lateral incisors. There is no need to risk the loss of attachment on additional teeth. Note the size of the roots that need to be covered. The interdental tissue is kept intact.

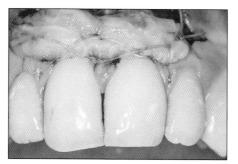

Fig 23-9d A large connective tissue graft is sutured in place with resorbable gut sutures. It is of proper size to extend apically and laterally to cover the exposed tissue beds.

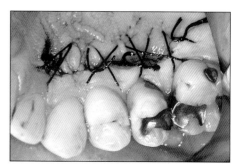

Fig 23-9e The donor site will heal by primary intention.

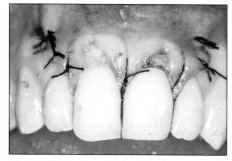

Fig 23-9f The buccal flap has been sutured over the connective tissue graft, providing another source of nourishment.

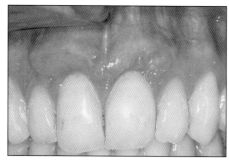

Fig 23-9g The surgical result is excellent at 1 year. The esthetic problem has been resolved. There is minimal probing depth.

as the native tissue covers the connective tissue. In the original technique, a 2-mm band of epithelium is retained at the graft margin to improve the handling quality.

Variations of the original technique and their efficacy have been reported. Nelson[15] described using laterally positioned full-thickness pedicle grafts and double papilla grafts in the same manner as the partial-thickness flap was utilized in the Langer approach. He[15] reported 88% root coverage of advanced recessions and 100% root coverage in 62% of treated sites.

Harris[48] used partial-thickness lateral (double papilla) pedicle grafts to cover connective tissue grafts and reported 100% root coverage 89% of the time; there was a mean of 97.7% root coverage of the class I and class II recession defects.

Jahnke et al[49] compared thick free gingival grafts to subepithelial connective tissue grafts to see which technique would result in more predictable root coverage of Miller class I and class II recession defects. They reported 100% root coverage in five of nine sites (56%) that received the subepithelial graft and only one of nine sites (11%) treated with the free gingival graft. The mean percentage of root coverage was 80% for the subepithelial connective graft and 43% for the free gingival graft.

Raetzke[50] placed the connective tissue graft into a previously created envelope; the epithelium was retained on the graft only where it would cover the exposed root surface. He reported excellent healing and esthetic results for deep-wide recession defects; attained 100% root coverage in 42% of sites (five sites) and 60% to 80% coverage in the remaining seven sites.

Levine[51] used the principles of the Langer technique for grafts with no epithelial collar and reported 97% root coverage, on average, in 21 sites.

Bouchard[52] compared the connective tissue graft with and without the epithelial collar. He suggested that the group without the epithelial collar gave a better esthetic result.

Borghetti[53] reported on the use of the connective graft placed under a double papilla full-thickness flap, as in the Nelson technique. He achieved a mean root coverage of 70.9% in the treatment of class I, class II, and class III recession defects. Of the 15 sites treated, nine were maxillary canines, a tooth that presents a difficult challenge because of its root prominence. Connective tissue grafts placed beneath the alveolar mucosa do not induce the alveolar mucosa to become keratinized tissue. There may be a distinct advantage to complete coverage of the connective tissue graft because it offers additional blood supply and possibly a better esthetic result.

Cohen[54] used a "piggy-back" technique, in which connective grafts were placed one on top of the other to correct the ridge deformity and cover the root recession defect simultaneously.

Allen[55] demonstrated that his modification in the design of the envelope procedure was applicable to multiple adjacent areas of recession. Complete root coverage (100%) was achieved at 14 (61%) of 23 sites. Of the remaining sites, five had 75% root coverage and four showed a range of 20% to 67%. He reported an average root coverage of 84% for all sites.

Bruno[56] reported another variation of the technique (see Chapter 24). This procedure has several advantages:

1. It is predictable for obtaining root coverage.
2. The technique results in good gingival color match, and there is minimal likelihood that keloids will appear.
3. The palatal donor site is less prone to bleeding, and healing is easier than with the epithelialized graft.
4. The double blood supply created in this approach is advantageous.
5. The surgeon's ability to control the thickness is greater than is possible with the free autogenous gingival graft.
6. This procedure can be combined with other procedures in which flap design calls for the dissection and discarding of gingival connective tissue.

The indications are similar to those for epithelialized free gingival grafts. The major contraindication to this surgical approach is the inability to harvest an adequate thickness of donor material. This is particularly true in patients with Class II, division II, malocclusion who present with a square arch.

Langer and coworkers[45–47,57] believed that the following are indications for this procedure:

1. A lack of adequate donor tissue for a lateral sliding flap
2. The presence of root recessions
3. The presence of isolated wide recessions
4. The presence of multiple root recessions and a minimal zone of attached gingiva requiring augmentation
5. The presence of recession adjacent to an edentulous area requiring ridge augmentation
6. The presence of recession in an area where esthetics is of great concern
7. McGuire showed that the technique can be used on previously restored root surfaces[58]

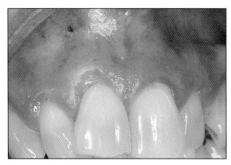

Fig 23-10a This patient was concerned about the gingival recession on the maxillary left central incisor.

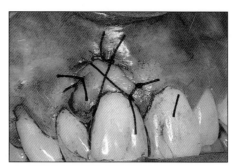

Fig 23-10b A semilunar coronally positioned flap is used to cover the exposed root surface.

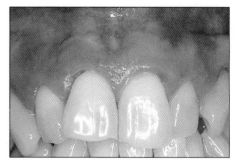

Fig 23-10c The clinical observation 1 year after surgery reveals coverage of the exposed root and gingival symmetry.

Semilunar Coronally Positioned Flap (Advanced Flap)

The semilunar coronally positioned flap is a variation of the coronally positioned flaps of Sumner[22] and Bernimoulin et al[20]; in this modification, a free gingival graft is not utilized in the procedure prior to grafting (Figs 23-10a to 23-10c). An incision with a semilunar form is made at the mucogingival junction or apical to it, and a partial-thickness flap is raised by inserting a blade intrasulcularly and filleting a flap free over the root; the flap is still attached at both lateral borders to the adjacent papilla. The flap is moved coronally to cover the exposed root and held firmly in place with or without sutures.[59] Pollack[60] reported the combination of a submarginal gingival graft and a retained gingival collar, which was, in essence, a semilunar coronally positioned flap (retained collar) simultaneously supported by a submarginal graft.

Guidelines for Successful Root Coverage

Miller[5] provided guidelines for successful root coverage:

1. There should be no root sensitivity.
2. The gingival margin should be at the CEJ after treatment of class I or II defects.
3. There should be a sulcus of 2 mm or less.
4. There should be no bleeding on probing.
5. There should be a good color match.
6. There should be an adequate dimension of gingiva.

Miller[61] reported several factors to be associated with *incomplete* root coverage:

1. Improper classification
2. Inadequate root planing
3. Failure to use root conditioning
4. Improper preparation of the recipient site
5. Inadequate size of the interdental papilla at the recipient site
6. Improper preparation of the donor tissue
7. Inadequate graft thickness
8. Improperly prepared donor tissue
9. Dehydration of donor tissue
10. Failure to stabilize the graft
11. Inadequate adaptation or suturing of the graft
12. Excess or prolonged pressure
13. Failure to reduce prior inflammation
14. Trauma during healing
15. Smoking of 10 or more cigarettes a day

Smoking is believed to constrict blood vessels and therefore to restrict blood flow. However, some studies have indicated that smoking is not a factor in whether root coverage is obtainable.[40,48]

Biomodification of the Root

Miller[5] cited the following as reasons why new attachment is difficult if not impossible to attain on previously exposed root surfaces:

1. An increase in mineral content
2. A decrease in the organic component of cementum
3. The retention of toxins and enzymes
4. Antigen antibody reactions to foreign bacterial proteins
5. The loss of stimulating capacity for cementogenesis

Many clinicians believe that these speculations are factual and propose root biomodification as an integral part of root coverage therapeutics. Root biomodification can be accomplished mechanically or chemically.

Biomodification of the Root

Mechanical Means

- Scaling and root planing (hand curettes and ultrasonic instrumentation)
- Rotary instruments

Chemical Means[5,62,63]

Citric Acid

- Demineralizes an overmineralized root surface.
- Widens the orifice of dentinal tubules to allow cementum to fill these blunderbuss openings, within these orifices (eg, cementum pins).
- Exposes collagen fibrils in the root surface to splice with collagen fibrils of grafts or flaps.
- May remove the smear layer (debris).
- Has no pulpal consequences (minimal microns are affected).
- Has not been associated with root resorption in humans.
- Removes endotoxin and demineralizes calculus.
- Accelerates cementogenesis and allows collagen adhesion.

Tetracycline

- Demineralizes an overmineralized root surface.
- Has a lingering antibacterial effect.
- Has a collagen-stabilizing effect, ie, anticollagenolytic.
- Promotes fibroblast adhesion and growth.

The acidic conditioning of the root surfaces is controversial because success has been reported with and without it.[1,64,65] Theoretically, root surface demineralization could play an important role in regeneration. The periodontally diseased root seems not to favor regeneration because of its surface characteristics. Demineralization does change the surface character of the root surface, which can influence wound healing and provide potentially greater attachment of fibroblasts. The root surface conditioning may regulate the adsorption of plasma proteins, enhance adhesion of the blood clot, and stimulate deposition of collagen against the root surface.[62]

Some studies have concluded that there is no advantage to the use of citric acid and have suggested that it is root planing that removes the endotoxin from the root surface and not the acidic conditioning.[1,64,65] The application of citric acid after root planing and curettage may allow connective reattachment by exposing collagen fibrils, which may splice with new fibrils that form during the healing process. This phenomenon may increase the possibility of fibrous connective reattachment.

The authors believe that this question is unanswered and suggest that each clinician make an individual decision regarding the use of chemical biomodification of the root surface.

Guided Tissue Regeneration

Recent technical advances available to treat gingival recession and cover the denuded root include guided tissue regeneration (Figs 23-11a to 23-11g). Human biopsy specimens have demonstrated a connective tissue attachment to the root, but the procedure is technique sensitive and reserved for the treatment of a single-tooth recession. The technique is discussed in detail in Chapter 25. Ricci[66] compared the use of GTR and subepithelial connective tissue grafts to treat areas of gingival recession and concluded that root coverage was similar with both methods. There was more clinical attachment with GTR as measured by probing.

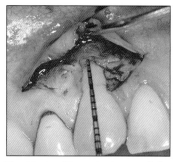

Fig 23-11a There is 5 mm of denuded root surface on the buccal surface of the maxillary right canine.

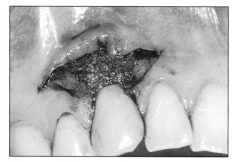

Fig 23-11b The exposed root is covered with freeze-dried bone allograft to provide space for guided tissue regeneration.

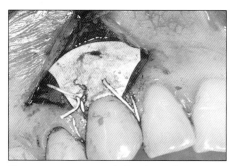

Fig 23-11c An expanded polytetrafluoroethylene barrier membrane is fitted to cover the canine. The membrane extends to the cementoenamel junction.

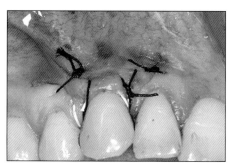

Fig 23-11d The flap is sutured over the membrane.

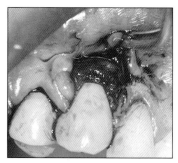

Fig 23-11e The membrane is removed after 5 weeks. The root surface is covered with connective tissue that appears to be attached to the root.

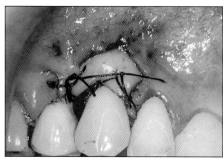

Fig 23-11f To augment the yield of attached gingiva, a free gingival graft is placed after removal of the membrane.

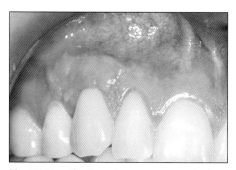

Fig 23-11g The two-stage surgery results in a good dimension of keratinized attached gingiva that does not probe more than 1 mm.

References

1. Hall WB. Gingival augmentation/mucogingival surgery. In: Nevins M, Becker W, Kornman K (eds). Proceedings of the World Workshop in Clinical Periodontics. Chicago: American Academy of Periodontology, 1989:VII-1–VII-21.

2. Wennström JL. Mucogingival Therapy. Ann Periodont 1996; 1:671–701.

3. Cortellini P, Clauser C, Pini Prato GT. Histologic assessment of new attachment following the treatment of a human buccal recession by means of a guided tissue regeneration procedure. J Periodontol 1993;64:387.

4. Pasquinelli KL. The histology of new attachment utilizing a thick, autogenous soft tissue graft in the area of deep recession: A case report. Int J Periodont Rest Dent 1995;15:248.

5. Miller PD. Root coverage grafting for regeneration and aesthetics. Periodontology 2000 1993;1:118.

6. Wilson R. Marginal tissue recession in general practice: A preliminary study. Int J Periodont Rest Dent 1985;5(2):9.

7. Miller PD Jr. A classification of marginal tissue recession. Int J Periodont Rest Dent 1985;5(2):9.

8. Grupe H, Warren R. Repair of gingival defects by sliding flap operation. J Periodontol 1956;27:92.

9. Grupe H. Modified technique for the sliding flap operation. J Periodontol 1966;37:491.

10. Cohen DW, Ross S. The double papilla repositioned flap in periodontal therapy. J Periodontol 1968;39:65.

11. Caffesse RG, Guinard EA. Treatment of localized gingival recession. Part I. Lateral sliding flap. J Periodontol 1978;49:351.

12. Caffesse RG, Guinard EA. Treatment of localized gingival recession. Part IV. Results after three years. J Periodontol 1980;51:167.

13. Guinard EA, Caffesse RG. Treatment of localized gingival recession. Part III. Comparison of results obtained with lateral sliding and coronally repositioned flaps. J Periodontol 1978;49:457.

14. Shiloah J. The clinical effects of citric acid and laterally positioned pedicle grafts in the treatment of denuded root surfaces: A pilot study. J Periodontol 1980;51:652.

15. Nelson SW. The subepithelial connective tissue graft. A bilaminar reconstructive procedure for the coverage of denuded root surfaces. J Periodontol 1987;58:95.

16. Harris RJ. The connective tissue and partial thickness double pedicle graft: The predictable method of obtaining root coverage. J Periodontol 1992;63:5.

17. Allen ET, Miller PD. Coronal positioning of existing gingiva: Short-term results in the treatment of shallow marginal tissue recession. J Periodontol 1989;60:316.

18. Harris RJ, Harris AW. The coronally positioned pedicle graft with inlaid margins: The predictable method of obtaining root coverage of shallow defects. Int J Periodont Rest Dent 1994;14(3):229.

19. Allen EP. Pedicle flaps, gingival grafts and connective tissue grafts in aesthetic treatment of gingival recession. Pract Periodont Aesthet Dent 1993;5:29.

20. Bernimoulin JP, Lüscher B, Mühlemann HR. Coronally repositioned periodontal flap. J Clin Periodontol 1975;2:1.

21. Maynard JG. Coronal repositioning of the previously placed autogenous gingival graft. J Periodontol 1977;48:151.

22. Sumner CF. Surgical repair of recession on the maxillary cuspid: Incisal repositioning of the gingival tissues. J Periodontol 1969;40:119.

23. Wennstrom J. Proceedings of the First European Workshop on Periodontology. Chicago: Quintessence, 1994.

24. Laney JB, et al. A comparison of two techniques for obtaining root coverage. J Periodontol 1992;63:1.

25. Dordick B, Coslet JG, Seibert JS. Clinical evaluation of free autogenous gingival grafts placed on alveolar bone. Part I. Clinical predictability. J Periodontol 1976;47:559.

26. Bissada NF, Sears SB. Quantitative assessment of free gingival grafts with and without periosteum and osseous perforation. J Periodontol 1978;49:15.

27. James WC, McFall WT Jr, Burkes E. Placement of free gingival grafts on denuded alveolar bone. Part II. Microscopic observations. J Periodontol 1978;49:291.

28. Sullivan HP, Atkins JH. Free autogenous gingival grafts. I. Principles of successive grafting. Periodontics 1968;6;121.

29. Pennell BM, Tabor JC, King KO, Towner JD, Fritz BO, Higgason JD. Free masticatory mucosal graft. J Periodontol 1969;40:162.

30. Gargiulo A, Arrocha R. Histochemical evaluation of free gingival grafts. Periodontics 1967;5:285.

31. Sullivan HP, Atkins JH. Free autogenous gingival grafts. II. Principles of successive grafting. Periodontics 1968;6:152.

32. Livingston HL. Total coverage of denuded root surfaces with a free gingival autograft. A case report. J Periodontol 1975;46:209.

33. Mlinek SH, Smuckler H, Buchner H. The use of free gingival graft for the coverage of denuded roots. J Periodontol 1973;44:248.

34. Rateitschak K, Egli U, Fringelli G. Recession: A four year longitudinal study after free gingival graft. J Periodontol 1979;6:158.

35. Matter J. Creeping attachment of free gingival grafts: A five year follow-up study. J Periodontol 1981;51:681.

36. Miller PD. Root coverage using a free soft tissue autograft following citric acid application. Part III. A successful and predictable procedure in areas of deep wide recession. Int J Periodont Rest Dent 1985;5(2):15.

37. Corn H, Marks M. Gingival grafting for deep wide recession: A status report. I. Rationale, case selection and root preparation. Compend Contin Educ Dent 1983;4:53.

38. Holbrook T, Oschenbein C. Complete coverage of denuded root surfaces with a one stage gingival graft. Int J Periodont Rest Dent 1983;3(3):8.

39. Borghetti A, Gardella J. Thick gingival autograft for the coverage of gingival recession: A clinical evaluation. Int J Periodont Rest Dent 1990;10:217.

40. Tolmie E, Reubens RP, Buck GS, Vaganos V, Lanz JC. The predictability of root coverage by way of free gingival autografts and citric acid application: An evaluation by multiple clinicians. Int J Periodont Rest Dent 1991;11(4):261.

41. Bertrand PM, Dunlap RM. Coverage of deep, wide gingival clefts with free gingival autografts: Root planing with and without citric acid demineralization. Int J Periodont Rest Dent 1988;8(1):65.

42. Miller PD Jr. Root coverage using a free soft tissue autograft following citric acid application. Part I. Technique. Int J Periodont Rest Dent 1982;2(1):65.

43. Becker BE, Becker W. The use of connective tissue autografts for treatment of mucogingival problems. Int J Periodont Rest Dent 1986;6(1):88.

44. Edel A. Clinical evaluation of free connective tissue grafts used to increase the width of keratinized gingiva. J Clin Periodontol 1974;1:185.

45. Langer B, Calagna LJ. Subepithelial graft to correct ridge concavities. J Prosthet Dent 1980;44:363.

46. Langer B, Langer L. Subepithelial connective tissue graft technique for root coverage. J Periodontol 1983;56:175.

47. Langer B, Calagna LJ. The subepithelial connective tissue graft: A new approach to the enhancement of anterior cosmetics. Int J Periodont Rest Dent 1982;2(2):23.

48. Harris RJ. The connective tissue and partial thickness double pedicle graft: The results of 100 consecutively treated cases. J Periodontol 1994;65:488.

49. Jahnke P, Sandifer JB, Gher M, Gray J, Richardson AC. Thick, free gingival and connective tissue autografts in root coverage. J Periodontol 1993;64:315.

50. Raetzke P. Covering localized areas of root exposure employing the "envelope" technique. J Periodontol 1985;56:397.

51. Levine RA. Subepithelial connective tissue grafts for root coverage. Compend Contin Educ Dent 1991;12:568.

52. Bouchard P, Etienne D, Duhayoun JP, Nilvéus R. Subepithelial connective tissue grafts in the treatment of gingival recessions: A comparative study of two procedures. J Periodontol 1994;65:929.

53. Borghetti A. Thick gingival autograft for the coverage of gingival recession: A clinical evaluation. Int J Periodont Rest Dent 1990;10(3):217.

54. Cohen ES. Ridge augmentation utilizing the subepithelial connective tissue graft: A case report. Pract Periodont Aesthet Dent 1994;6:47.

55. Allen AL. The use of a supraperiosteal envelope and soft tissue grafting for root coverage. I. Rationale and technique. Int J Periodont Rest Dent 1994;14(3):217.

56. Bruno JF. Connective tissue graft techniques. Assuring wide root coverage. Int J Periodont Rest Dent 1994;14:127–137.

57. Langer L. Enhancing cosmetics through regenerative periodontal procedures. Compend Contin Educ Dent 1994;(supp 18):S699.

58. McGuire MK. Soft tissue augmentation on previously restored root surfaces. Int J Periodont Rest Dent 1996;16:571–581.

59. Tarnow DP. Semilunar coronally repositioned flap. J Clin Periodontol 1986;13:182.

60. Pollack RB. Root coverage using submarginal free mucosal grafts in conjunction with a retained gingival collar. XI. Compend Contin Educ Dent 1990;11(3):160–164.

61. Miller PD Jr. Root coverage with the free gingival graft: Factors associated with incomplete coverage. J Periodontol 1987;58:674.

62. Lowenguth RA, Bleiden TM. Periodontal regeneration: Root surface demineralization. Periodontology 2000 1993;1:54.

63. Terranova VP, Franzetti LC, Hic S. A biochemical approach to periodontal regeneration: Tetracycline treatment of dentin promotes fibroblast adhesion and growth. J Periodont Rest 1986;21:330.

64. Oles RD, Ibbott CG, Laverty WH. Effects of citric acid treatment on pedicle flap coverage of localized recession. J Periodontol 1985;55:259–261.

65. Stahl SS, Froum SJ. Human clinical and histologic repair response following use of citric acid in periodontal therapy. J Periodontol 1977;48:261–266.

66. Ricci G, Silvestri M, Tinti C, Rasperini G. A clinical/statistical comparison between the subpedicle connective tissue graft method and the guided tissue regeneration technique in root coverage. Int J Periodont Rest Dent 1996;16(6):539–545.

CHAPTER 24

The Subepithelial Connective Tissue Graft for Achieving Root Coverage

Gary M. Reiser, DDS
John F. Bruno, DDS, MS

For years, attempts to cover areas of deep-wide gingival recession were met with frustration. Miller,[1] in 1985, classified marginal tissue recession by combining the four classifications of Sullivan and Atkins[2] into his first two classifications and then adding a third and a fourth classification. He indicated that the presence of interdental bone loss, soft tissue loss, or extruded teeth make it impossible to place a free gingival graft at the cementoenamel junction (CEJ), making it impossible to obtain complete root coverage. In a series of articles[3-5] on the free soft tissue graft, Miller demonstrated successful root coverage for his class I (shallow-narrow and shallow-wide) and class II (deep-narrow and deep-wide) recessions.

Before Miller introduced his classification,[1] Langer and Calagna,[6] in 1980, described a subepithelial connective tissue graft technique to correct ridge concavities. This was followed by the benchmark article by Langer and Langer,[7] in 1985, describing a subepithelial connective tissue graft technique for root coverage. They indicated that their technique had "the advantage of a closer color blend of the graft with the adjacent tissue avoiding the 'keloid' healing present with free gingival grafts."[7] In 1994, Bruno[8] described modifications of the original Langer and Langer technique. The modified technique and its indications will be discussed in this chapter.

Technique

Preparation of the Recipient Site

The use of a local anesthetic with a vasoconstrictor limits the blood supply in the injected area. To avoid compromising the blood supply, a mandibular or mental block is given in the mandible. In the maxilla, attempts are made not to inject into the immediate graft site. Interpapillary injections are kept to a minimum.

The initial horizontal right-angle incision is made into the adjacent interdental papillae at, or slightly coronal to, the CEJ of the tooth with an exposed root surface (Figs 24-1a and 24-1b). A butt joint is provided. Care is taken not to make the papillary incisions more than 1 mm in depth, in order to preserve papillary blood supply. The epithelium of the retained papillae is left undisturbed.

A partial-thickness flap is created by sharp dissection (Fig 24-1c). The dissection is carefully accomplished to prevent perforation of the flap. The mesiodistal length of the incision is extended to provide easy access to the denuded root, because vertical incisions are not used. The incision is extended apically, well beyond the mucogingival junction,

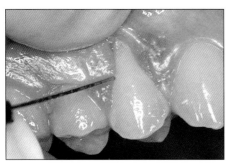

Fig 24-1a The initial horizontal right-angle incision is made into the papillae with a surgical blade.

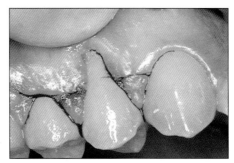

Fig 24-1b The initial incision is made at, or coronal to, the CEJ of the tooth with the exposed root surface.

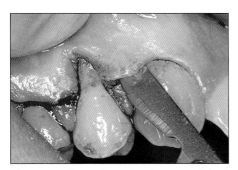

Fig 24-1c Sharp dissection is accomplished with a No. 15 surgical blade to create a partial-thickness flap.

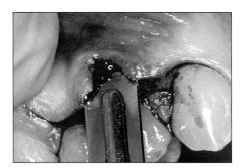

Fig 24-1d The incision is extended apically into the mucobuccal fold, well beyond the mucogingival junction.

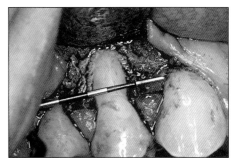

Fig 24-1e A periodontal probe is used to measure the approximate length of the donor tissue that will be required for the recipient site. Note the extent of the hidden recession.

into the mucobuccal fold (Fig 24-1d). In the mandibular premolar area, the mental foramen should be palpated first to avoid violation of the neurovascular bundle (see Fig 24-5a). Sharp tissue scissors may be used in an attempt to remove the crevicular epithelium from the overlying flap.

The exposed root is meticulously planed with curettes. At times, it may be desirable to use finishing burs as well. Definitive reduction of the facial root convexity is not necessary.

Following root planing, the root is treated with tetracycline hydrochloride in a concentration of 250 mg mixed in 5 mL of sterile water. The solution is applied to the root surface for 2 to 3 minutes with cotton pellets or cotton applicators. Tetracycline solution is applied to the root to provide antibiotic medicament; to inhibit collagenase; to remove the smear layer from the root surface; and to open the dentinal tubules to expose collagen fibers. The authors recommend that tetracycline solution be applied to the root surface in all subepithelial connective graft procedures, including those roots that demonstrate abrasions and caries.

Once the root has been treated, the approximate mesiodistal width necessary for the graft is measured with a periodontal probe (Fig 24-1e).

Excision of the Donor Tissue

The groove in which the greater palatal artery and nerve transgress is palpated to determine its location and thus avoid violation of the neurovascular bundle.[9] After local anesthesia is obtained, needle soundings can be accomplished to determine the thickness of the palatal tissue. The first incision on the palate is made perpendicular to the long axis of the teeth, approximately 2 to 3 mm apical to the gingival margin of the maxillary teeth (Fig 24-2a), to avoid sloughing of the palatal tissue in this area. The mesiodistal length of the incision is determined by the length of the graft that is necessary for the recipient site; however, it can be limited by the palatal anatomy.[9]

The second incision is made parallel to the long axis of the teeth, 1 to 2 mm apical to the first incision, depending on the thickness of the graft that is required (Fig 24-2b). The incision is carried far enough apically to provide a sufficient height of connective tissue to cover the denuded root and the adjacent periosteum of the recipient site without violating the neurovascular bundle (Figs 24-2b to 24-2d). A small periosteal elevator is used to raise a full-thickness periosteal connective tissue graft (Fig 24-2e).

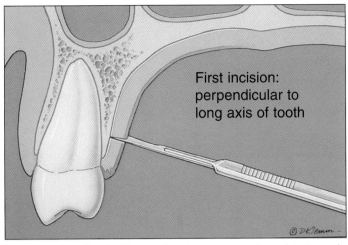

Fig 24-2a The first incision at the donor site on the palate is made approximately 2 to 3 mm apical to the gingival margins of the teeth.

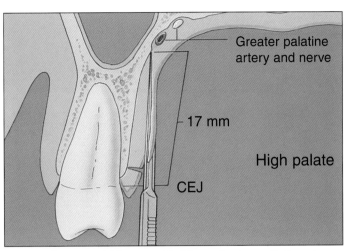

Figs 24-2b to 24-2d The second incision at the donor site is made parallel to the long axis of the tooth, 1 to 2 mm apical to the first incision. The more apical the incision, the thicker the donor tissue will be. The extent of the apical incision is determined by the height of the palate.

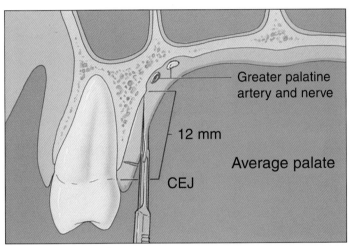

Fig 24-2c Average palate.

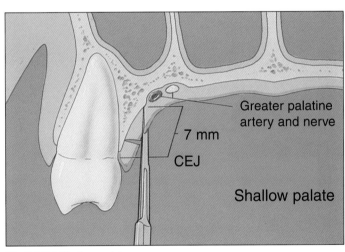

Fig 24-2d Shallow palate.

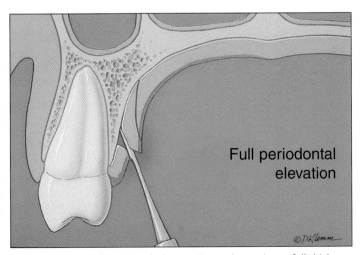

Fig 24-2e A small periosteal elevator is used to raise a full-thickness connective tissue flap.

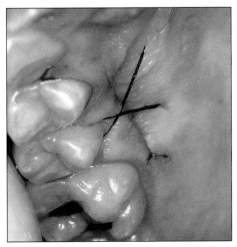

Fig 24-2f The palatal wound is approximated with a crossed horizontal suspension suture.

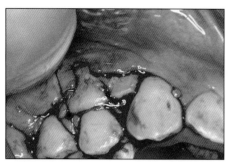

Fig 24-3a The donor connective tissue is stabilized with interrupted sutures. In this case, a 1-mm band of epithelium is retained at the coronal margin of the graft.

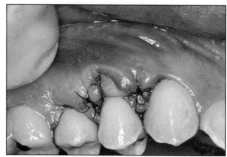

Fig 24-3b The overlying partial-thickness flap is replaced with interrupted sutures into the papillae. Note the lack of keratinized tissue on the overlying flap and the significant portion of the connective tissue graft that has not been covered.

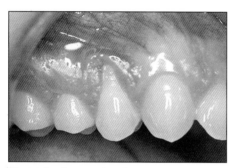

Fig 24-3c Preoperative view.

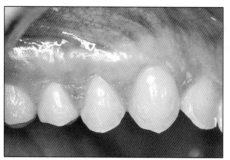

Fig 24-3d Two-month postoperative view. Note the successful result despite the lack of keratinized tissue and the exposure of a portion of the connective tissue graft at the time of surgery.

The donor tissue is removed from the palate, as atraumatically as possible, with the periosteal elevator. The tissue is not removed with tissue pliers, a hemostat, or any other instrument that could compress or injure the donor tissue. The graft is removed with a wet sponge under finger pressure. Vertical incisions may be necessary at the mesial and distal extent of the graft beneath the masticatory mucosa to facilitate removal of the connective tissue. With an FS-2 needle, 4-0 silk suture material is used in a crossed horizontal suspension suture or interrupted sutures to approximate the wound on the palate (Fig 24-2f).

Once the donor tissue is removed and placed on a sterile gauze pad, the 1- to 2-mm band of epithelium at the coronal aspect of the tissue may be removed, but it is usually retained. At that time, the length and thickness of the graft can be modified with a surgical blade. Excess fatty and glandular tissue should be removed.

Grafting to the Recipient Site

The donor connective tissue is secured to the papillae with interrupted sutures with 6-0 monofilament pliabilized nylon used with a (PC-3) conventional cutting needle or 5-0 chromic gut used with a (CE-2) needle (Fig 24-3a). It is important that the graft tissue be closely adapted at the recipient site to prevent the formation of blood clots between the graft tissue and the underlying recipient site. The overlying partial-thickness flap is then replaced over the donor tissue, and interrupted sutures are placed in the mesial and distal papillae, so that the flap covers as much of the donor tissue as possible (Fig 24-3b). No attempt is made to cover the donor tissue completely. A periodontal dressing is placed over the recipient site; however, the donor site may be left uncovered.

Postoperative medications include chlorhexidine rinse, twice daily; oral tetracycline, 250 mg, three times daily for 7 days; oral nonsteroidal anti-inflammatory drug, four times daily for 4 to 5 days; narcotic or non-narcotic analgesics, as needed; ice pack application; and head elevation during sleep for the first 2 nights.

The dressing and sutures are removed 7 days postoperatively. At that time, the patient is advised to continue use of the chlorhexidine rinse and instructed to cleanse the graft site with a cotton swab saturated with chlorhexidine for an additional 2 to 3 weeks, depending on the rate of healing.

Figure 24-3c demonstrates a recipient site preoperatively. Figure 24-3d shows the same area 2 months postoperatively.

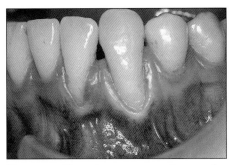 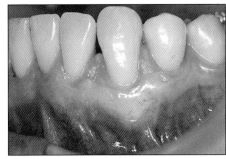

Fig 24-4a There is severe recession on the mandibular left lateral incisor and canine and almost a complete lack of keratinized tissue.

Fig 24-4b Thirteen months postoperatively, it is difficult to determine that a graft procedure has been performed in this area. Note the amount of root coverage obtained.

Factors Affecting the Surgical Result

It is imperative that the initial horizontal right-angle incision into the papillae be made at the CEJ, or slightly coronal to the CEJ because this incision level is the determining factor in achieving complete root coverage. The healed gingival margin of the graft cannot achieve a level coronal to the level of the papillary incisions. To provide easy access, the horizontal incision must be made an adequate distance mesially and distally from the tooth being treated because vertical incisions are not utilized.

Vertical incisions are not made because they would compromise the blood supply of the overlying tissue[10] and result in cicatricial lines. It can be postulated that vertical incisions greatly reduce blood circulation at the graft site. The lack of vertical incisions also decreases the patient's discomfort during the healing process and promotes more rapid healing.

The significant blood supply for the donor tissue must be obtained laterally and apically because the graft survives even though the overlying tissue frequently does not completely cover the connective tissue graft. The retention of the periosteal bed, as well as the vascular periosteum on the donor tissue, likely increase both early fluid exchange and the potential for a more expeditious reestablishment of circulation to the graft. As a result of the excellent blood supply provided, the incomplete coverage of the connective tissue by the overlying tissue at the recipient site apparently is not detrimental to the amount of root coverage that is obtained (see Figs 24-3c and 24-3d).

Often a thick graft is required to cover a wide denuded area to decrease the possibility that the donor tissue will undergo complete necrosis. When a thick graft is utilized, a gingivoplasty may be necessary to enhance esthetics to satisfy the patient. The decision as to whether or not to provide gingivoplasty is typically delayed for at least 2 to 3 months to allow ample healing and graft shrinkage.

Avoiding the use of vertical incisions into the masticatory mucosa at the palatal donor site increases the difficulty of the procedure and does not apparently improve the clinical results. Nevertheless, the absence of vertical incisions minimizes the postoperative sequelae at the donor site and promotes more rapid healing; therefore, the use of vertical incisions at the donor site is not recommended.

The use of small suturing needles permits suturing into very small papillae. Larger, less sharp needles macerate small papillae and make suturing impossible. The use of surgical magnification and a fiberoptic headlight may increase the surgeon's ability to gain optimal results from this procedure.

The keratinized epithelium that results from a subepithelial connective tissue graft appears to corroborate the finding of Karrin et al[11] that the specificity of the gingival epithelium is determined by the underlying connective tissue.

Indications and Benefits

1. This procedure, when employed in the manner described, uniformly covers areas of wide root denudation to fulfill functional and esthetic requirements (Figs 24-4 and 24-5).
2. Failing and esthetically unacceptable root restorations can be removed and subepithelial connective tissue grafts can be used to cover the previously restored root areas (Figs 24-6a and 24-6b).
3. Areas of root abrasion and root sensitivity can be eliminated (Figs 24-7 and 24-8).
4. Multiple areas of recession can be eliminated (Figs 24-7a and 24-7b).
5. Root coverage can be accomplished before or after restorative procedures (Figs 24-5, 24-8, and 24-9).
6. Following removal of caries, the exposed root can be covered (Figs 24-10a to 24-10c).

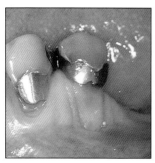

Fig 24-5a Wide recession is demonstrated on the facial aspect of the mandibular left second premolar. Note the complete lack of keratinized tissue. In this region it is important to palpate the mental foramen.

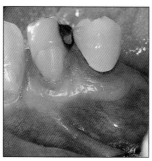

Fig 24-5b The same area, 6 months postoperatively, demonstrates a substantial increase in keratinized tissue. The keratinized tissue allowed the preparation of a final crown while providing a consistent gingival margin.

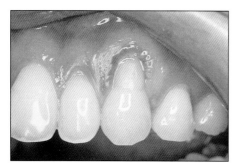

Fig 24-6a A maxillary left canine with a large class V resin composite restoration exhibits severe marginal inflammation.

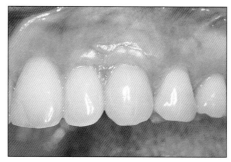

Fig 24-6b The same canine, 14 months postoperatively, exhibits complete root coverage to the CEJ. The resin composite restoration was completely removed prior to the graft procedure.

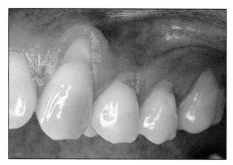

Fig 24-7a Extensive root exposure involves the maxillary left canine and premolars.

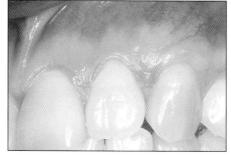

Fig 24-7b The root coverage obtained is shown 3 years postoperatively.

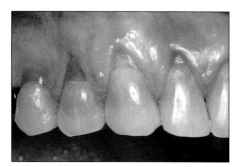

Fig 24-8a Root exposure is present on the right canine and premolars. Both right and left maxillary canines and premolars are to be treated. Note the tetracycline staining. Both sides of the palate can be utilized, if necessary, during the same procedure. If the same side of the palate is to be used again as a donor site, 6 months of healing time is required before reentry for adequate tissue bulk to form.

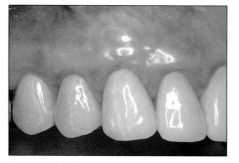

Fig 24-8b The root coverage obtained is shown 1 year postoperatively, following the placement of indirect porcelain veneers. The graft procedures were provided before the placement of the veneers. Complete tissue root coverage facilitated the restorative procedures by eliminating the need for root bonding of the veneers.

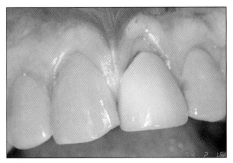

Fig 24-9a The maxillary left central incisor has an exposed crown margin and gingival recession.

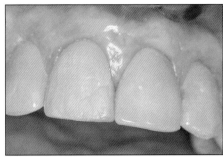

Fig 24-9b The tooth is shown I year postoperatively with a provisional acrylic resin crown in place. The old crown margin was used as a reference for graft margin placement, because the incisogingival dimension of the crown was compatible with that of the adjacent central incisor.

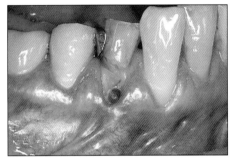

Fig 24-10a The mandibular right first premolar demonstrates severe recession, abrasion, caries, and a complete lack of keratinized tissue.

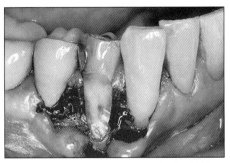

Fig 24-10b At the time of surgery, the hidden dehiscence is exposed. The root has been planed with finishing burs and curettes. Caries has been completely removed.

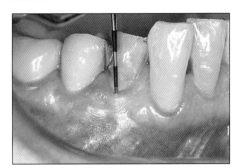

Fig 24-10c One year postoperatively, a probe reveals 2 mm of sulcular depth. Note the complete root coverage and the blanching of the tissue, indicating forceful probing. The gingival margin of the grafted tooth is more coronal than the gingival margins of the adjacent teeth.

Most frequently, a subepithelial connective tissue graft procedure is provided for root coverage of a denuded root with or without root abrasion, erosion, or root caries or following the removal of an existing root restoration. At times, a connective tissue graft is accomplished to cover the exposed margin of a crown or root restoration. The treatment plan frequently requires a subepithelial connective tissue graft to be provided in conjunction with a restorative procedure. The graft procedure may be rendered before or after the placement of a restoration. The exact sequence of therapy is dictated by the specific clinical requirements.

Sequencing With Restorative Procedures

Category 1

The subepithelial connective tissue graft is provided prior to the restoration of single or multiple areas of recession when porcelain veneers and/or complete crowns will be placed. Root coverage grafting prior to veneer placement can eliminate the difficult task of bonding to cementum. Root coverage grafting prior to crown placement enables the clinician to control the incisogingival dimension of the crown and to make crown height compatible with the height of the adjacent teeth.

Frequently, little or no keratinized tissue is associated with these areas of recession. In denuded root situations in which the bleaching of teeth is required, the subepithelial connective tissue graft should be provided prior to bleaching. This sequence of treatment will reduce the possibility of bleaching-induced root sensitivity. Often it is necessary to provide a subepithelial connective tissue graft prior to orthodontic treatment if there is a preexisting dehiscence or lack of keratinized tissue.

Category 2

There are clinical situations in which the subepithelial connective tissue graft procedure follows the restorative procedure. These situations include restorative procedures that involve the clinical crown but do not traverse the CEJ. The subepithelial connective tissue graft is provided subsequent to a class V restoration involving the crown and root of a tooth. This enables the restorative dentist to reestablish the CEJ with the gingival margin of the restoration. The graft can then be placed so that its gingival margin is compatible with the restored CEJ.

To satisfy esthetic requirements, the subepithelial connective tissue graft may be utilized to cover exposed crown margins and exposed implant abutments.

Typically, postoperative sequelae at the donor site are minimal when the subepithelial connective tissue graft is provided; postoperative palatal discomfort is frequently encountered when the free gingival graft is performed.

Both the subepithelial connective tissue graft and the free gingival graft result in increased quantities of keratinized tissue.

Comparison to the Free Gingival Graft

Because the free gingival graft has enjoyed extensive use for more than 25 years, it is appropriate to compare the subepithelial connective tissue graft and the free gingival graft (Table 24-1). The subepithelial connective tissue graft provides predictable root coverage to treat wide and deep root recessions, multiple root incisions, root abrasions, root caries, previously restored roots, and areas in which crown margins on root surfaces have become exposed and require masking. The free gingival graft does not provide predictable root coverage in any of these situations.

Esthetically, the subepithelial connective tissue graft not only provides the potential for root coverage but also creates tissue that is unscarred and that blends extremely well with surrounding tissues. Frequently the graft becomes undetectable as healing progresses. Color, form, and keloid formation are problematic when the free gingival graft is provided.

Comparison to the Guided Tissue Regeneration Procedure

The subepithelial connective tissue graft and the guided tissue regeneration procedure are both used to provide root coverage and both are recent therapeutic innovations. A comparison between the two procedures is necessary so that the clinician can determine when the utilization of each procedure is appropriate (Table 24-2).

The subepithelial connective tissue graft is successfully used to treat both single- and multiple-tooth recessions, whereas the application of the guided tissue regeneration procedure is usually restricted to single-tooth recession.

The subepithelial connective tissue graft also offers the advantage of utilizing autogenous tissue, while the guided tissue regeneration treatment requires the use of a synthetic barrier membrane. The utilization of a synthetic membrane increases the risk of postoperative problems if an exposed membrane becomes infected. Additionally, removal of the

Table 24-1 Comparison of the subepithelial connective tissue graft and the free gingival graft

Characteristic	Subepithelial connective tissue graft	Free gingival graft
Provides predictable root coverage[12]	Yes	No
Provides predictable root coverage for multiple recessions	Yes	No
Provides predictable root coverage for abrasions	Yes	No
Provides predictable root coverage once caries is eliminated	Yes	No
Provides predictable root coverage for previously restored areas	Yes	No
Provides predictable root coverage for restored margins	Yes	No
Esthetic results:		
Graft blends well with surrounding tissue (form and color)	Yes	No
Keloid formation is avoided	Yes	No
It is difficult to detect that a procedure was provided	Yes	No
Typically results in minimal postoperative sequelae at donor site	Yes	No
Periodontal dressing unnecessary at donor site	Yes	No
Results in increased keratinized tissue	Yes	Yes

Table 24-2 Comparison of the subepithelial connective tissue graft and the guided tissue regeneration procedure

Subepithelial connective tissue graft	Guided tissue regeneration
Is used to treat single- and multiple-tooth recessions	Application usually is restricted to single-tooth recessions
Utilizes autogenous tissue	Utilizes synthetic barrier membrane
Results in minimal risk of postoperative infection	Results in increased risk of postoperative infection because of presence of synthetic barrier membrane
Requires no barrier membrane that will have to be removed	Requires procedure to remove barrier membrane (if nonresorbable)
Incurs no additional cost for autogenous donor tissue	Incurs additional cost for commercially produced barrier membrane
Initially requires two surgical sites	Initially requires one surgical site
Is not used for recession where there is an adjacent interproximal bony defect	Is used for single-tooth recession where there is an adjacent interproximal bony defect
Has superior esthetic results	Has variable esthetic results
Results in increased keratinized tissue	Results in increased keratinized tissue
Apparently results in a connective tissue attachment to the root surface[13]	Apparently results in a connective tissue attachment to the root surface[14]

nonresorbable barrier membrane requires a second surgery. Additional cost is associated with the use of a commercially produced membrane, whereas the subepithelial connective tissue graft procedure carries no such cost. However, the subepithelial connective tissue graft requires a second surgical site to procure the donor tissue.

The second surgical site is not required at the time of the grafting procedure when the guided tissue regeneration procedure is utilized. However, the guided tissue regeneration procedure often requires a second-stage free gingival graft at the time of membrane removal, to protect the delicate tissue that has formed on the root surface. If the subepithelial connective tissue graft procedure requires a second-stage surgical procedure, it is typically in the form of gingivoplasty. Once the clinician becomes comfortable with placing a relatively thin graft (approximately 1.5 mm in width), the need for gingivoplasty is significantly reduced, to 20% to 25% of the subepithelial connective tissue graft cases. Cases requiring gingivoplasty are typically those deep-wide recessions that require placement of thick donor tissue at the recipient site, to prevent loss of the graft.

The guided tissue regeneration procedure is primarily used when single-tooth recessions occur adjacent to interproximal bony defects. This combination of problems is a contraindication for the use of the subepithelial connective graft. The guided tissue regeneration procedure is also an option when the clinician encounters a shallow palatal vault. The anatomy of such a palate can create problems for the inexperienced surgeon because the neurovascular bundle is proximal (7 mm) to the gingival margin (see Figs 24-2b to 24-2d).

In general, the subepithelial connective tissue graft provides superior esthetic results, while the guided tissue regeneration procedure provides variable esthetic results. Both procedures result in increased keratinized tissue. Indications are that both procedures provide a connective tissue attachment to the root surface.[13,14]

Discussion

Gingival recession related to periodontal disease or developmental problems can result in root sensitivity, root caries, and esthetically unacceptable root exposures. Consequently, root restorations are frequently performed. These restorations often complicate, rather than resolve, the problems created by exposed roots.

Prior to the efforts of Langer and Langer,[7] Miller,[1,3–5] and others, root coverage was not addressed adequately in periodontal therapy. Minimal consideration was given to providing the patient with improved esthetics. Recently, significant regenerative techniques have been developed to better meet the needs of the patient.

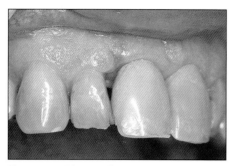

Fig 24-11a The maxillary right central and lateral incisor papilla is substantially damaged by long-standing periodontal disease. Provisional acrylic resin crowns have been placed on both central incisor teeth.

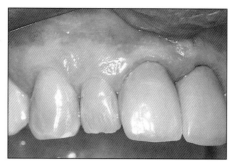

Fig 24-11b Restoration of the papilla has been accomplished by a modification of the subepithelial connective tissue graft. New central incisor crowns have been placed.

The subepithelial connective tissue graft continues to find expanded use. This technique is now being explored as a method of restoring lost papillae (Figs 24-11a and 24-11b). Ridge augmentation utilizing the subepithelial connective tissue graft technique has now become more sophisticated, resulting in highly acceptable esthetics. Amalgam tattoos can be eliminated with this technique so that all discoloration is removed to meet esthetic requirements. This procedure can also be used to cover exposed crown margins and exposed implant abutments, eliminating the need to replace existing crowns. The versatility of this procedure continues to be explored.

Conclusion

The belief exists that periodontal surgery frequently disfigures a patient by exposing root surfaces, resulting in a cosmetically unacceptable smile line. Sensitivity and caries occur concomitantly with root exposure. This paradigm and the perception that periodontal therapy is directed solely at disease control, with little concern for esthetics, are fallacious.

This chapter describes a predictable procedure of providing root coverage for areas of wide denudation in the maxilla and the mandible. This procedure addresses the esthetic needs and requirements of both the patient and the dentist. The procedure is indicative of the advances that are being made in regenerative periodontal therapy.

References

1. Miller PD Jr. A classification of marginal tissue recession. Int J Periodont Rest Dent 1985;5(2):5–9.

2. Sullivan HC, Atkins JH. Free autogenous gingival grafts. III. Utilization of grafts in the treatment of gingival recession. Periodontics 1968;6:152–160.

3. Miller PD Jr. Root coverage using a free soft tissue autograft following citric acid application. I. Technique. Int J Periodont Rest Dent 1982;2(1):65–70.

4. Miller PD Jr. Root coverage using a free soft tissue autograft following citric acid application. II. Treatment of the carious root. Int J Periodont Rest Dent 1983;3(5):38–57.

5. Miller PD Jr. Root coverage using the free soft tissue autograft following citric acid application. III. A successful and predictable procedure in areas of deep-wide recession. Int J Periodont Rest Dent 1985;5(2):15–37.

6. Langer B, Calagna L. Subepithelial graft to correct ridge concavities. J Prosthet Dent 1980;44:363–367.

7. Langer B, Langer L. Subepithelial connective tissue graft technique for root coverage. J Periodontol 1985;56:715–720.

8. Bruno J. Connective tissue graft technique assuring wide root coverage. Int J Periodont Rest Dent 1994;14:127–137.

9. Reiser GM, Bruno JF, Mahan PE, Larkin LH. The subepithelial connective tissue graft palatal donor site: Anatomic considerations for surgeons. Int J Periodont Rest Dent 1996;16(2):131–138.

10. Fedi P. Periodontic Syllabus. Philadelphia: Lea & Febiger, 1985;90.

11. Karring T, Lang NP, Löe H. Role of gingival connective tissue in determining epithelial differentiation. J Periodont Res 1974;10:1–11.

12. Jahnke PV, et al. Thick free gingival and connective tissue autografts for root coverage. J Periodontol 1993;64:318–322.

13. Langer B. Reporting on Dr. Gary M. Reiser's histologic assessment of new attachment following the treatment of a human buccal recession by means of a subepithelial connective tissue graft procedure. Presented at the American Academy of Periodontology Annual Meeting, San Francisco, Sept 1994.

14. Cortellini P, Clauser C, Pini Prato GP. Histologic assessment of new attachment following the treatment of the human buccal recession by means of a guided tissue regeneration procedure. J Periodontol 1993;5:387–391.

Guided Tissue Regeneration in the Treatment of Facial Recession

Stefano Parma-Benfenati, MD, DDS, MScD
Carlo Tinti, MD, DDS

The periodontal literature describes several surgical procedures that were designed to achieve the therapeutic goal of covering exposed root surfaces with gingiva. The laterally positioned flap was one of the first procedures described to attain gingival coverage on denuded roots.[1] Variations of this procedure have been reported in several articles.[2–4] In 1963, Bjorn[5] reported the first free gingival graft. Nabers[6] subsequently reported on the use of a free gingival graft to increase the band of keratinized gingiva.

The past 20 years have seen an explosion of interest in mucogingival surgery, accompanied by variations in surgical techniques to treat various mucogingival problems. Clinical trials measuring the root coverage achieved with mucogingival procedures have produced varying results. The percentage of root coverage reported has varied from 43% to 97%. This wide variation in results may be related to case selection, surgical technique, root conditioning, and evaluation methods.[7–13] Although the clinical results of these studies are encouraging in terms of root coverage, to date, most of the procedures heal by a long junctional epithelium.

The ultimate goal of periodontal therapy is to restore the supporting tissues lost as a consequence of inflammatory periodontal disease. The objective of regenerative procedures is the formation of a new connective tissue attachment to a thoroughly debrided, previously diseased or denuded root surface, preferably with the regrowth of alveolar bone. Guided tissue regeneration (GTR) appears to accomplish this goal. The biologic principle of GTR was initially developed to attain new attachment in various types of periodontal osseous lesions.[14–19] It has been emphasized that the outcome of the GTR surgical procedure is dependent on the morphologic features of the defect, such as configuration and size of the residual bony walls, the residual periodontal ligament, and the quantity of keratinized gingiva, although its use frequently results in minimal gingival recession.[3] To date, histologic examination of human biopsy specimens has confirmed the possibility of achieving new attachment and, in many cases, new bone formation.[14,16,20]

The provision of space is critical for bone regeneration in GTR procedures. It is necessary to create and maintain a sufficient space in which an adequate blood clot can be stabilized; this defines the maximum volume that can be regenerated.[21–33] Non–space-making defects are more prone to membrane collapse. This is especially true when gingival recessions, dehiscences, or fenestration-type bony defects are treated or when no bony envelope is available for membrane support. If there is no naturally occurring provision for space maintenance, it is important to create sufficient space for retention and stabilization of the blood clot. The clot must be protected from mechanical injury and from an invasion by connective tissue or epithelium. New tissue, with included formative cells, derived from the periodontal ligament must preferentially be allowed to occupy the space if new attachment is to occur.

To create and maintain space and to prevent collapse of the barrier membrane, various filling materials, such as hydroxyapatite,[8,34] fibronectin,[35,36] and demineralized freeze-dried bone allograft,[6,37,38] have been employed.

Tinti and Vincenzi[39] proposed the use of expanded polytetrafluoroethylene (e-PTFE) membranes for the treatment of human gingival recessions. They prepared the root surface with rotary instruments in an effort to obtain a concave shape that would allow sufficient space for regenerative tissues to form beneath the membrane. After 3 years of observation, the treated teeth showed no signs of pulpal pathosis. The technique provided limited space for regeneration; the roots, however, were covered with gingival tissue. Their work produced exciting and encouraging treatment potentials.

In a later study, Tinti and Vincenzi[40] introduced a clinical variation of membrane adaptation. The variation allows the surgeon to increase the convexity of the e-PTFE membrane. A single e-PTFE suture is placed through the membrane in a manner designed to provide curvature to the membrane. The curvature can be adjusted by increasing or decreasing the tension on the suture. The concave surface of the membrane is adjusted over the root surface. The suture that adjusts the concavity of the membrane must be placed apical to the defect's bony margin. This avoids interference with the newly regenerated tissue when the membrane is removed. The membrane is then positioned on the prepared area of the root surface, so as to cover the cementoenamel junction, and is held in place by means of a sling e-PTFE suture.

In a clinical report of 12 cases followed for 6 months, it was demonstrated that facial recession can be treated successfully with membrane-augmented mucogingival surgery.[41] Some root coverage and clinical attachment gain were achieved in addition to a reduction of probing depth; the tissues demonstrated clinical health.

Pini Prato et al[42] treated recession defects and compared the GTR technique to conventional mucogingival surgery. They described a trapezoidal full–split thickness flap design, in which the base was raised beyond the mucogingival junction. The exposed root surface was thoroughly planed and intentionally prepared to a concave shape. The flap was displaced as far coronally as possible, completely covering the membrane, and sutured with minimal tension. Care was taken not to compress the flap against the root surface. This same technique was also used to improve esthetics in areas with root caries and failing class V restorations.[42]

Tinti and coworkers[43] modified the technique for space maintenance of the membrane by suturing a pure gold bar to the membrane. The gold bar was shaped to provide proper convexity to the membrane. The bars were ultimately joined, providing a frame that increased the rigidity of the membrane. The gold frames were made to fit the single-tooth, narrow, extra large e-PTFE periodontal membranes.

Titanium-reinforced e-PTFE membranes have been designed and produced commercially (WL Gore, Flagstaff, AZ) to improve the space-making qualities of the membranes. These barriers are used for periodontal defects. The membranes have been evaluated in patients with gingival recession.[44] The new membrane design was reported to facilitate membrane placement and provide greater procedure predictability.

Wound Healing

Gottlow et al[45] and Cortellini et al[46] reported histologic evidence of new connective tissue attachment after treating experimental recession defects with e-PTFE membranes in an animal model. Cortellini and colleagues[47] treated a recession defect in a patient, and after 5 months, the tooth was removed and evaluated histologically. Clinically there was a gain of 4 mm of root coverage and 3 mm of keratinized gingiva. Histologic evaluation revealed 3.66 mm of new connective tissue attachment, 2.48 mm of new cementum, and 1.84 mm of new bone on the facial aspect of the tooth-root complex.

Previous histologic human studies that evaluated various procedures for treatment of recessions have reported healing by a long junctional epithelium with a restricted zone of connective tissue attachment coronal to the crest of bone.[48-50] Preliminary histologic evaluation of recession defects treated by GTR procedures indicate that it is possible to gain new connective tissue attachment for these defects. Further, the treated sites heal with an increased band of keratinized gingiva.

Indications and Contraindications

The esthetic demands of many patients require the development of techniques that predictably cover unesthetic areas of gingival recession. The GTR technique employed to cover isolated root surfaces is indicated for single teeth with wide, deep, localized recessions, 5 mm in width or depth or wider and deeper. The procedure is also indicated for areas of root sensitivity where oral hygiene is impaired and for the repair of recessions associated with failing or unesthetic class V restorations. The technique does not require a secondary donor surgical site, reducing postoperative discomfort. One of the advantages of the procedure is that the new tissue blends evenly with the adjacent tissue, providing a highly esthetic result.

The main limitation of the procedure is that multiple defects cannot be treated at the same surgical session. Another limiting factor is that root coverage is limited by the height of the interproximal bone. A minor disadvantage of the procedure is the necessity for membrane removal 4 to 6 weeks after the initial surgery.

Surgical Procedure

Patient evaluation consists of a determination of the health status and a comprehensive periodontal examination. A full-mouth radiographic survey is used to determine the

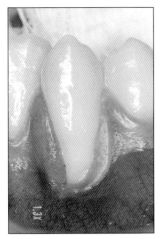

Fig 25-1a A 5-mm-deep facial recession is present on the mandibular left canine. The width of keratinized tissue is less than 1 mm.

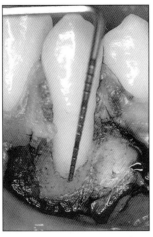

Fig 25-1b A trapezoidal full-partial thickness flap has been raised. Intraoperative measurements reveal 8 mm of attachment loss.

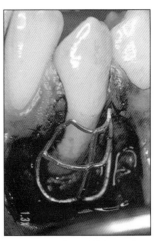

Fig 25-1c The gold frame has been shaped and positioned over the exposed and prepared root to create space for regenerative tissues.

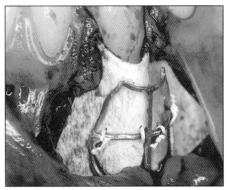

Fig 25-1d An e-PTFE membrane with a gold frame is positioned on the root. The epithelium of the interdental papillae were removed by gingivoplasty. The papillae were then raised at their inner aspects to accommodate the most coronal, lateral portions of the membrane.

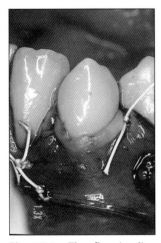

Fig 25-1e The flap is displaced as coronally as possible to fully cover the membrane.

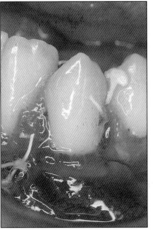

Fig 25-1f Healing after 4 weeks, immediately before membrane removal. No exposure of the membrane has occurred, and there are no clinical signs of inflammation around the sutures.

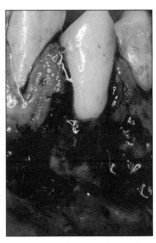

Fig 25-1g The membrane has been removed. Firm, well-attached tissue is present on the root surface. The new tissue almost completely fills the space created by the membrane.

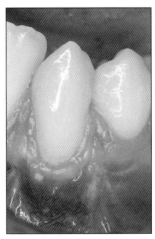

Fig 25-1h Final appearance of tissues at 7 months.

patterns of bone loss; special attention is paid to interproximal bone levels.

After initial therapy, consisting of oral hygiene instructions and scaling and root planing, the areas of recession are evaluated for surgery. Figures 25-1 to 25-3 describe the surgical steps utilizing the gold bar–reinforced membrane and the membrane with the titanium reinforcement.

Flaps are designed for maximum tissue closure. The flap designs are the same for the membrane-reinforced gold and the titanium-reinforced periodontal material. A short horizontal incision is made slightly above the mucogingival junction. This incision is extended to the alveolar bone. Two oblique diverging incisions are made, starting at the ends of the horizontal incision. These oblique incisions are extended beyond the mucogingival junction into the vestibule.

A full-thickness flap is extended from the gingival margin to a level approximately 3 mm apical to the alveolar crest. From this point, a partial-thickness dissection is made and continued apically for approximately 8 to 10 mm into the vestibule. This will allow the flap to be coronally positioned with minimal tension to obtain total membrane coverage. A gingivoplasty is then performed on the interdental

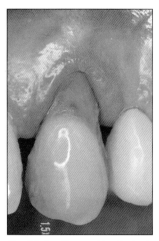

Fig 25-2a Deep-wide gingival recession is present on the maxillary left canine.

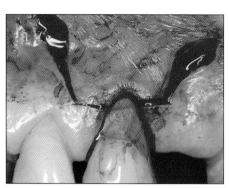

Fig 25-2b A trapezoid-shaped flap is extended into alveolar mucosa. The two diverging incisions create a large apical base.

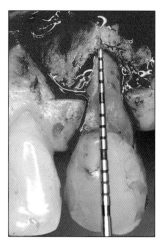

Fig 25-2c A trapezoidal flap has been reflected. There is 7.5 mm of attachment loss.

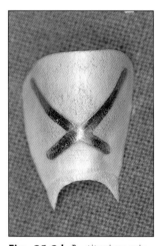

Fig 25-2d A titanium-reinforced membrane has been shaped to the desired convexity.

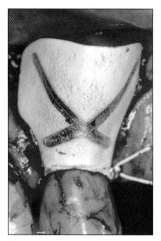

Fig 25-2e The membrane has been positioned and sutured in place at the cementoenamel junction.

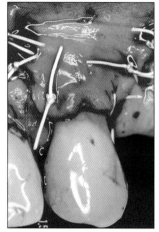

Fig 25-2f The coronally displaced flap, which completely covers the membrane, is secured with e-PTFE sutures.

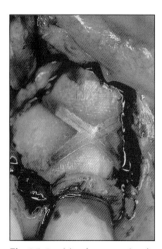

Fig 25-2g Membrane retrieval, 4 weeks after surgery. Flap reflection reveals that the membrane has retained its convex shape, providing space for new tissue ingrowth.

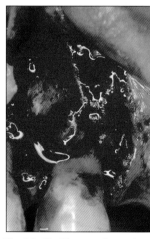

Fig 25-2h The membrane has been removed, exposing the newly formed tissue. The tissue has covered the previously denuded root (compare with Fig 25-2c).

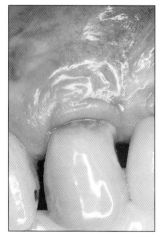

Fig 25-2i Clinical appearance 15 months after treatment.

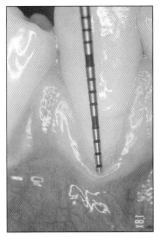

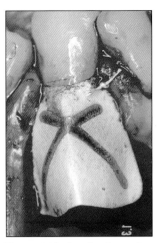

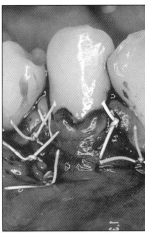

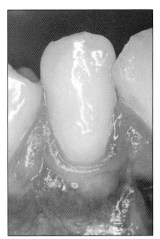

Fig 25-3a A 5-mm-deep facial recession is present on a mandibular right canine.

Fig 25-3b A titanium-reinforced e-PTFE membrane has been shaped to create sufficient space beneath the membrane.

Fig 25-3c The flap is coronally sutured to completely cover the membrane.

Fig 25-3d Clinical appearance 15 months after treatment. Note the complete root coverage and the increased amount of keratinized gingiva.

papillae to remove the outer epithelial layer. The papillae are raised from bone with a small chisel to provide space for the coronal and lateral parts of the membrane.

The root surfaces are planed with either hand or rotary instruments. A single-tooth, narrow e-PTFE membrane (extra large) is trimmed and adapted to cover the exposed root. The material is extended a minimum of 2 mm beyond the buccal bone crests and placed beneath the raised papillae. Once the membrane is positioned, it is necessary to determine the proper membrane curvature that will be necessary to secure adequate space between the membrane and the root. The membrane is then removed, contoured, and replaced for suturing. A sling e-PTFE suture is then made so as to secure the membrane in place at the cementoenamel junction.

The periosteum is severed along the entire base of the flap to allow coronal repositioning with minimal tension and flap compression. The flap is fixed with an e-PTFE sling suture. The lateral borders of the flaps are sutured with mesial and distal periosteal sutures.

To minimize flap compression, periodontal dressings are not applied. The patient should avoid contact with the wound area for approximately 2 weeks. Ice packs are not employed at the surgical area, to avoid unintended compression. Antibiotic therapy is recommended (amoxicillin, 1 g, twice a day for 6 days). Medications for discomfort can be dispensed, depending on the needs of the patient. Chemical plaque control with topical application of chlorhexidine-digluconate gel two times a day for 1 minute is instituted for 14 days. Toothbrushing is discontinued at the surgical site for the first 2 weeks postoperatively. Patients return weekly for plaque control, and the sutures are removed after 1 month.

Membrane Retrieval

The sutures and membrane are removed 4 weeks after the initial surgery. A trapezoidal flap, similar to the one described previously, is made over the membrane, and the membrane-retaining suture is removed. The membrane is then carefully removed from the underlying new tissue. The newly formed tissue that fills the space beneath the membrane must not be injured or manipulated. Flap margins are gently debrided, positioned as coronally as possible to cover the newly formed tissue, and secured with a combination of sling and interrupted sutures. A periodontal dressing is applied, and the topical application of chlorhexidine-digluconate gel is prescribed for 2 weeks. The sutures and dressing are removed after 1 week.

Evaluation of Results

The procedure results in successful root coverage and optimum esthetics with minimal patient discomfort. Tinti et al[41] reported clinical results after deep and wide recession defects were treated with GTR. At 1 year, for patients treated with membrane material shaped with sutures, there was an average of 77.3% root coverage and 73.9% gain in clinical attachment. There was a 75.1% gain in root coverage after the use of gold-reinforced material and an average of 73.6% root coverage after treatment with the titanium-reinforced membranes.[44] Ricci and coworkers[51] compared subepithelial connective tissue grafts with GTR for root coverage. The average gain in root coverage was similar for both groups. The group undergoing subepithelial connective tissue grafting had an average gain of root coverage of 3.83 mm, while the average gain for the group undergoing GTR was 4.61 mm. The mean gain in clinical attachment for the grafted group was 3.1 mm, while the GTR group had an average gain of 5.5 mm. These results documented evidence of the benefits of both procedures and indicated that recession defects treated by GTR procedures will experience gains in both clinical attachment and root coverage.

Conclusion

Guided tissue regeneration can be used in the treatment of deep and wide isolated facial recessions, resulting in improved esthetics and gains in clinical attachment. The provision and maintenance of adequate space to allow formation of a blood clot are critical prerequisites for successful treatment. The protection of the blood clot during the tissue-forming phase and the newly formed tissue during its period of maturation appears to be critical to a successful clinical outcome.

This surgical technique may provide the same extent of root coverage as conventional mucogingival surgery, while enhancing clinical attachment gain, reducing probing depth, and increasing connective tissue attachment on the previously exposed root surface. Results suggest that conventional mucogingival surgery may provide a greater percentage of root coverage in shallow (smaller than 5-mm) facial recessions along with a greater increase in keratinized tissue width. The e-PTFE membrane procedure may provide greater root coverage in the treatment of deep and wide (larger than 5-mm) recessions presenting with a lesser quantity of tissue.

From a clinical point of view, the technique can be improved through the development of more ideal GTR devices and more refined surgical techniques.

References

1. Grupe H, Warren R. Repair of gingival defects by a sliding flap operation. J Periodontol 1956;27:92.

2. Pennel BM, Higgason JD, Towner JD, King KO, Frita BK, Sadler JF. Oblique rotated flap. J Periodontol 1965;36:305.

3. Cohen DW, Ross SE. The double papilla repositioned flap in periodontal therapy. J Periodontol 1968;39:65.

4. Tarnow DP. Semilunar coronally repositioned flap. J Clin Periodontol 1986;13:182.

5. Bjorn H. Free transplantation of gingiva propria. Sven Tandlak Tidskr 1963;22:684.

6. Nabers JM. Extension of the vestibular fornix utilizing a gingival graft. Case history. Periodontics 1966;4:77.

7. Miller PD. Root coverage using a free soft tissue autograft following citric acid application. I. Technique. Int J Periodont Rest Dent 1982;2(1):65.

8. Caffesse RG, Alspach SR, Morrison EC, Burget FG. Lateral sliding flaps with and without citric acid. Int J Periodont Rest Dent 1987;7(6):43–57.

9. Hall WB. Gingival augmentation/mucogingival surgery. In: Nevins M, Becker W, Kornman K (eds). Proceedings of the World Workshop in Clinical Periodontics. Chicago: American Academy of Periodontology, 1989, VII-1–VII-21.

10. Smukler H. Laterally positioned mucoperiosteal pedicle flaps in the treatment of denuded roots. A clinical and statistical study. J Periodontol 1976;47:590–595.

11. Bernimoulin JP, Lüscher B, Mühlemann HR. Coronally repositioned periodontal flap. J Clin Periodontol 1975;2:1–13.

12. Allen EP, Miller PD. Coronal positioning of existing gingiva: Short-term results in the treatment of shallow marginal tissue recession. J Periodontol 1989;60:316–319.

13. Jahnke PV, Sandifer JB, Gher ME, Gray JL, Richardson ACA. Thick free gingival and connective tissue autografts for root coverage. J Periodontol 1993;64:315–322.

14. Nyman S, Lindhe J, Karring T, Rylander H. New attachment following surgical treatment of human periodontal disease. J Clin Periodontol 1982;9:290–296.

15. Gottlow J, Nyman S, Karring T, Lindhe J. New attachment formation as the result of controlled tissue regeneration. J Clin Periodontol 1984;11:494–503.

16. Gottlow J, Nyman S, Lindhe J, Karring T, Wennström J. New attachment formation in the human periodontium by guided tissue regeneration: Case reports. J Clin Periodontol 1986;13:604–616.

17. Becker W, Becker BE, Prichard J, Caffesse R, Rosenberg E. Root isolation for new attachment procedures: A surgical and suturing method: Three case reports. J Periodontol 1987;58:819–826.

18. Becker W, Becker BE, Prichard J, Caffesse R, Rosenberg E. New attachment after treatment with root isolation procedures: Report for treated class II furcations and vertical osseous defects. Int J Periodont Rest Dent 1988;8(3):18–23.

19. Schallhorn R, McClain P. Combined osseous composite grafting, root conditioning, and guided tissue regeneration. Int J Periodont Rest Dent 1988;8(4):8–31.

20. Stahl S, Froum S. Human infrabony lesion responses to debridement, porous hydroxyapatite implants and Teflon barrier membranes. Seven histologic case reports. J Periodontol 1991;62:605–610.

21. Claffey N, Motinnger S, Ambruster J, Egelberg J. Placement of porous membrane underneath the mucoperiosteal flap and its effect on periodontal wound healing in dogs. J Clin Periodontol 1989;16:12–16.

22. Gottlow J, Karring T, Nyman S. Guided tissue regeneration following treatment of recession-type defects in the monkey. J Periodontol 1990;61:680–685.

23. Tonetti MS, Pini Prato GP, Cortellini P. Periodontal regeneration of human intrabony defects. IV. Determinants of healing response. J Periodontol 1993;64:934–940.

24. Dahlin C, Sennerby L, Lekholm U, Linde A, Nyman S. Regeneration of new bone around titanium implants using a membrane technique: An experimental study in rabbits. Int J Oral Maxillofac Implants 1989;4:19–25.

25. Becker W, Becker BE, Handelsman M, et al. Bone formation at dehisced dental implant sites treated with implant augmentation material: A pilot study in dogs. Int J Periodont Rest Dent 1991;10:93–102.

26. Dahlin C, Gottlow J, Lindhe J, Linde A, Nyman S. Healing of maxillary and mandibular bone defects using a membrane technique. An experimental study in monkeys. Scand J Plastic Reconstr Surg 1990;24:13–19.

27. Seibert J, Nyman S. Localized ridge augmentation in dogs: A pilot study using membranes and hydroxyapatite. J Periodontol 1990;61:157–165.

28. Buser D, Bragger U, Lang NP, Nyman S. Regeneration and enlargement of jaw bone using guided tissue regeneration. Clin Oral Implant Res 1990;1:22–32.

29. Dahlin C, Albeerius P, Linde A. Osteopromotion for cranioplasty. An experimental study in rats using a membrane technique. J Neurosurg 1991;74:487–491.

30. Haney JM, Nilveus RE, McMillan PJ, et al. Periodontal repair in dogs: Expanded polytetrafluoroethylene barrier membranes support wound stabilization and enhance bone formation. J Periodontol 1993; 64:883–890.

31. Sigurdsson TJ, Hardwick R, Bogle GC, et al. Periodontal repair in dogs: Space provision by reinforced e-PTFE membranes enhances bone and cementum regeneration in large supra-alveolar defects. J Periodontol 1994;65:350–356.

32. Dahlin C, Andersson L, Linde A. Bone augmentation at fenestrated implants by an osteopromotive membrane technique. A controlled clinical study. Clin Oral Implant Res 1991;2:159–165.

33. Jovanovic SA, Spiekermann H, Richter EJ. Bone regeneration around titanium dental implants in dehisced defect sites: A clinical study. Int J Oral Maxillofac Implants 1992;7:233–245.

34. Lekovic V, Kenney EB, Carranza FA Jr, et al. Treatment of grade II furcation defects using porous HA in conjunction with an e-PTFE membrane. J Periodontol 1990;61:575–579.

35. Cortellini P, Pini Prato G, Baldi C, Clauser G. Guided tissue regeneration with different materials. Int J Periodont Rest Dent 1990; 10:137–151.

36. Trombelli L, Schincaglia GP, Scapoli C, Calura G. Healing response of human buccal gingival recessions treated with e-PTFE membranes. A retrospective report. J Periodontol 1995;66:14–22.

37. Anderegg CR, Mellonig JT, Gher M, et al. Clinical evaluation of the use of decalcified freeze-dried bone allograft with guided tissue regeneration in the treatment of molar furcation invasions. J Periodontol 1991;62:264–268.

38. Kramer G. Surgical alternatives in regenerative therapy of the periodontium. Int J Periodont Rest Dent 1992;12:11–31.

39. Tinti C, Vincenzi G. La rigenerazione guidata dei tessuti con Gore-Tex: Nuove prospettive? Quintessence Int (edizione Italiana) 1990;6:45–49.

40. Tinti C, Vincenzi G. Il trattamento delle recessioni gengivali con la tecnica di "rigenerazione guidata dei tessute" mediante membrane Gore-Tex. Variante clinica. Quintessence Int (edizione Italiana) 1990;6:456–468.

41. Tinti C, Vincenzi G, Cortellini P, Pini Prato GP, Clauser C. Guided tissue regeneration in the treatment of human facial recession. A 12-case report. J Periodontol 1992;63:554–560.

42. Pini Prato GP, Tinti C, Cortellini P, Magnani C, Clauser C. Periodontal regenerative therapy with coverage of previously restored root surfaces. Case reports. Int J Periodont Rest Dent 1992; 12:451–461.

43. Tinti C, Vincenzi G, Cocchetto P. Guided tissue regeneration in mucogingival surgery. J Periodontol 1993;64:1184–1191.

44. Tinti C, Vincenzi GP. Expanded e-PTFE titanium-reinforced membranes for regeneration of mucogingival recession defects: A 12-case report. J Periodontol 1994;65:1088–1094.

45. Gottlow J, Nyman S, Karring T, Lindhe J. Treatment of localized gingival recessions with coronally displaced flaps and citric acid. An experimental study in the dog. J Clin Periodontol 1986;12:57–63.

46. Cortellini P, De Sanctis M, Pini Prato G, Baldi C, Clauser C. Guided tissue regeneration procedure using a fibrin-fibronectin system in surgically induced recessions in dogs. Int J Periodont Rest Dent 1991;11:151–163.

47. Cortellini P, Clauser C, Pini Prato GP. Histologic assessment of new attachment following the treatment of a human buccal recession by means of a guided tissue regeneration procedure. J Periodontol 1993;64:387–391.

48. Sugarman EF. A clinical and histological study of the attachment of grafted tissue to bone and teeth. J Periodontol 1969;40:381–387.

49. Pfeifer JS, Heller R. Histologic evaluation of full and partial thickness lateral repositioned flaps. A pilot study. J Periodontol 1971; 42:331–333.

50. Common J, McFall W. The effects of citric acid on attachment of laterally positioned flaps. J Periodontol 1983;54:9–18.

51. Ricci G, Silvestri M, Tinti C, Vincenzi GP. Subpedicle connective tissue grafts versus GTR for root coverage. A biometrical evaluation. Presented at the European Federation of Periodontology, Europerio 1, Paris, 12–15 May 1994.

CHAPTER 26

Supportive Periodontal Care

Ralph P. Pollack, DMD, MScD

Periodontal recall for maintenance has been described by Cohen[1] as "an extension of periodontal therapy." He further stated that maintenance is important to the survival of the dentition. At the World Workshop in Clinical Periodontics,[2] the maintenance and recall phase of periodontal therapy was renamed *supportive periodontal care* (SPC), or *supportive periodontal therapy* (SPT). The term SPC is a more realistic description of the follow-up periodontal therapies used for the treated patient. This chapter will discuss both the SPC provided when initial phase therapies have been performed (with or without surgery), as well as the "holding program" followed when surgical therapies have not been performed because the patient demonstrates inadequate oral hygiene practices. Patients will be categorized by age cohorts: adolescents to young adults, aged 8 to 25 years; adults, aged 26 to 64 years; and older adults aged 65 years and older.

The problems associated with SPC are first realized when patients do not comply with recommendations. Wilson et al[3] studied 961 patients over an 8-year period. Only 16.4% of the individuals were compliant, while 83% never returned for SPC or were erratic in their return to the office. This group of patients underwent scaling and root planing with or without periodontal surgery. Mucogingival patients were not included in the study. The mean age of the 961 patients was 44.4 years. They noted that more than 57% of all of these patients had only scaling and root planing performed. Ninety-two percent of all the patients were on a 3- to 4-month recall program. Wilson et al[3] and Becker et al[4] further noted that compliance decreases as the number of years after active therapy increases.

Periodontists can expect successful results only if the patient returns to the office for follow-up care. It has been well established that tooth loss is increased in individuals who do not comply with maintenance periodontal therapy.[4–6] Conversely, patients who do comply and who return to the periodontist for SPC retain more of their teeth.[7]

Active Periodontal Therapy

Active periodontal therapy consists of initial phase therapy, followed by either SPC or a surgical phase and subsequent SPC. The initial phase of periodontal therapy is the most important of all therapies. This was referred to as the *initial preparation phase of therapy* by Goldman.[8] He stated that the objectives of initial phase therapy consist of elimination or reduction of local causes and the correction of local environmental influences prior to the rendition of operative procedures devoted to treating marginal lesions and lesions of the attachment apparatus.

Many patients only require an initial preparation phase of therapy.[3] Grant et al[9] described the initial phase therapy as consisting of *(1)* plaque control, *(2)* scaling and root planing, *(3)* occlusal adjustment, *(4)* nightguards, *(5)* splinting, *(6)* periodontal orthodontics, and *(7)* reexamination. It may not be necessary to apply all of the aforementioned procedures, eg, orthodontics.

When required, caries control, endodontics, and extraction of hopeless teeth must also be included in this initial preparation phase. If, following the initial phase of treatment, the local etiology, pockets, and mobility have been controlled, the patient should enter the SPC program. The timing of the SPC program can vary from 3 to 6 months, and the patient should also be sent back to the referring dentist for other evaluations and therapies.

Holding Program

If, after the initial preparation phase has been performed, the patient cannot properly maintain the periodontium, he or she should be placed on a holding program. This holding program is designed to maintain and improve the periodontal status; it is hoped that, with reinforcement and encouragement, the individual can and will perform good oral hygiene habits in the future. If shallow pockets are still evident without osseous defects, the periodontist should prescribe a 2- to 3-month recall schedule for SPC. At this stage, chlorhexidine rinses may also be employed.

If poor plaque control and concomitant osseous defects with deep pockets still exist, bacterial cultures may be taken to assay for prevalence of specific pathogenic organisms, eg, *Porphyromonas gingivalis* in adult disease. Systemic antibiotics or local drug delivery and/or chlorhexidine could be prescribed as adjunctive measures for disease control. Tetracycline can be given systemically or incorporated in a fiber system for placement into pockets. A more stringent 4- to 8-week SPC holding program is necessary under these adverse periodontal conditions. The patient should also see the referring dentist for detection of caries.

Surgery

When the surgical phase is performed, it may consist of gingival grafting (or other plastic surgical procedures), osseous recontouring, or osseous addition grafting procedures. Implant therapy has also become a prominent facet of periodontal therapy and may be included in the overall treatment plan. Supportive periodontal care should be on a 3-month basis during and following this surgical phase.

Records and Documentation

It is imperative to have a complete series of radiographs depicting all of the structures surrounding the teeth. If periapical changes are noted, they must be compared to those in previous radiographs. The radiographic schedule is usually on a 3- to 4-year basis to discern if any periodontal loss of bone has occurred. It is also quite important to document whether bone apposition has increased after periodontal therapy.

A very important aspect of records involves clinical photographs of each section in the oral cavity. The importance of photographs taken before the initial phase of therapy involves the assessment of the color, position, and texture of the soft tissues, as well as the local environmental factors conducive to disease. Following the initial phase therapy, there should be improvement of the quality and form of the soft tissues; this should be well documented in the patient's records.

The areas of progressive gingival recession that are noted at the SPC visit must be documented. Using clinical photographs rather than relying on charting alone is a distinct advantage. The ability to compare the photographs taken after therapy with the 3-year follow-up photographs is important. Initiation of mucogingival procedures, such as gingival grafting, connective tissue grafting, or the sliding pedicle graft procedure, would be necessary to stop further tissue recession. Along with recession of the gingiva, it is also very important to document whether root coverage has been attained or the extent of creeping attachment that has occurred during the follow-up period. Creeping attachment (the progression of the level of the gingival margin in a coronal direction), a phenomenon that has not been satisfactorily explained, has been shown to occur after gingival grafting.[10] Where it does take place, root coverage is augmented.

The SPC Office Visit

The patient's level of compliance with the periodontal program often depends on the attitude of the staff. A friendly atmosphere is always beneficial. A typical visit's duration would be slightly less than 1 hour. The frequency of SPC visits is demonstrated schematically in Figure 26-1. The basic checklist would include:

1. *Review of the patient's medical history.* It should be established whether the patient needs to be premedicated because he or she has a prosthetic heart valve, an organic heart murmur, or certain orthopedic implants. If the patient has forgotten to take the recommended drug in the appropriate dosage, then another appointment should be made. A separate questionnaire page can be used prior to each SPC visit to document the patient's name, the date, any changes in medical history, and new medications being taken (Fig 26-2). This flow sheet, used at every SPC visit, has a different color and is made of stiff, heavy paper. If the patient is taking several types of medication, a separate form is used (Fig 26-3). This form lists the patient's physicians and the medications prescribed. Many individuals take over-the-counter medication or substances secured from friends; this information should also be recorded.

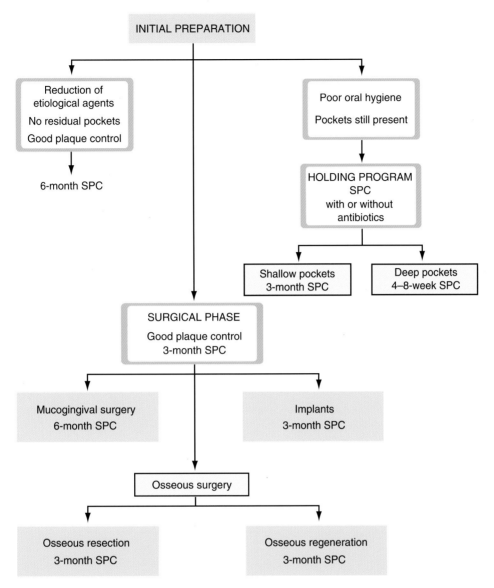

Fig 26-1 Schematic diagram describing treatment flow. Starting with an initial preparation, the timing of the SPC visits are dependent on the treatment performed and the patient's ability to maintain the periodontium.

2. *Review of any dental changes.* Often new restorations have been placed or the patient has undergone recent endodontic therapy or extractions.

3. *Examination for oral cancer.* A common disease in adults is lichen planus. White-laced tissues, with or without redness, are often noted. Any suspicious white lesions should be recorded and followed up with a biopsy. If increased supracrestal bony areas are observed, benign and malignant osseous lesions have to be ruled out.[11]

4. *Facial examination.* In locations where individuals spend a large amount of time in the sun, skin lesions are common; pigmented lesions may be precancerous or malignant, requiring evaluation by a medical specialist. Basal-cell carcinomas may be noted at a routine SPC visit (Fig 26-4); the patient should be referred to a dermatologist.

5. *Periodontal examination.* This consists of probing to determine any changes made in probing depths. If implants are present, the use of a nonmetallic probe is recommended so as not to damage their surfaces. The color, position, and texture of the gingiva should be noted. Areas of bleeding should likewise be recorded.

6. *Application of disclosing solution.* The use of a disclosing solution allows the patient and hygienist to see if plaque has accumulated. The disclosing solution should not be used until after the color of the gingiva and other soft tissues has been established. Plaque control measures are reinforced with various implements. Where furcations exist, the use of a Stimudent (Johnson & Johnson, New Brunswick, NJ) with sodium fluoride paste can be demonstrated (Figs 26-5a and 26-5b) along with proper brushing techniques. Where interproximal spaces exist, the use of interproximal brushes is demonstrated for more efficient plaque control (Fig 26-6).

RECALL

NAME: DATE:

Changes in medical history   [ ] No
                                   [ ] Yes_____

New medications   [ ] No
                                   [ ] Yes_____

Comments:_____

RECALL

NAME: DATE:

Changes in medical history   [ ] No
                                   [ ] Yes_____

New medications   [ ] No
                                   [ ] Yes_____

Comments:_____

RECALL

NAME: DATE:

Changes in medical history   [ ] No
                                   [ ] Yes_____

New medications   [ ] No
                                   [ ] Yes_____

Comments:_____

RECALL

NAME: DATE:

Changes in medical history   [ ] No
                                   [ ] Yes_____

New medications   [ ] No
                                   [ ] Yes_____

Comments:_____

Fig 26-2 Flow sheet on which the hygienist can record the patient's current medical status and any new medications taken since the last SPC visit.

7. *Assessment of changes in mobility.* Increased tooth mobility or displacement should be recorded and compared to previously obtained values.

8. *Assessment of gingival recession.* The position of marginal tissue levels should be compared to those noted in earlier records. A 56-year-old woman initially presented for a periodontal evaluation on May 7, 1984 (Fig 26-7a). During her SPC visit on September 4, 1986, progressive gingival recession was noted on the maxillary right canine (Figs 26-7b and 26-7c). A gingival graft was placed during a follow-up visit.

9. *Scaling and root planing.* Where sulci exist, scaling would be sufficient. Where pockets exist, the teeth need to be root planed. The length of time of this visit varies from patient to patient and depends on the number and location of pockets.

10. *Rescheduling.* When scalings and root planings have been accomplished and the patient can maintain the periodontium until the next SPC visit, the patient is then given an appointment 3 to 6 months in the future. If isolated pockets, periodontal abscesses, or other areas of attachment loss are noted, early treatment should be considered.

Before the patient leaves the office, an appointment is arranged for the next SPC visit. A week before the scheduled appointment, a postcard is sent out as a reminder. The day before the patient's appointment, a personal call is made to confirm the appointment. These procedures reinforce the periodontist's commitment to maintaining the periodontium, as well as the patient's obligation and responsibility to be effectively maintained.

To allow us to better evaluate your periodontal status,
please fill out the following to the best of your knowledge.

Medications prescribed by _____MD

1._____ mg _____times per day
2._____ mg _____times per day
3._____ mg _____times per day
4._____ mg _____times per day

Medications prescribed by _____MD

1._____ mg _____times per day
2._____ mg _____times per day
3._____ mg _____times per day

Medications over the counter (OTC)

1._____ mg _____times per day
2._____ mg _____times per day
3._____ mg _____times per day
4._____ mg _____times per day

Medication from friends

1._____ mg _____times per day
2._____ mg _____times per day

Signed _____

Date _____

Fig 26-3 Questionnaire indicating the patient's medications. Often the older adult takes myriad prescribed and over-the-counter medications. Often these patients take medications obtained from friends. All these should be listed.

Communications With the Referring Dentist

Communication between the periodontist and restorative dentist is imperative. At the SPC visit, the patient is evaluated for oral hygiene status and the periodontal condition. Tooth mobility is also recorded. A note is sent to the referring dentist with a checklist of important aspects of the patient's SPC visit (Fig 26-8). Of importance is the scheduling of future visits between offices.

The communication will inform the dentists of their mutual patient's status and will indicate how both offices, working cooperatively, can help the patient maintain and retain as many teeth as possible, in health, for as long as possible.

Re-treatment

Where increased pocket depth or loss of attachments is recorded, scaling and root planing should be the first re-treatment attempted.[12] The patient should be reinstructed and motivated in oral hygiene at the root planing sessions. Depending on the severity of bleeding and purulence, administration of antibiotics with or without bacterial cultures should be considered. The patient should be reevaluated after 2 weeks to determine the degree of healing that has occurred. The need for surgical treatment can then be assessed.

When younger adults take phenytoin for epilepsy, and gingival overgrowth is noted at the SPC visit,[13] the excess tissue may require surgical removal. In individuals who

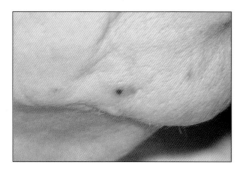

Fig 26-4 Basal-cell carcinoma noted at SPC visit. Referral to a dermatologist was subsequently made and this lesion was successfully treated.

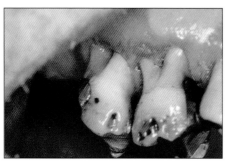

Fig 26-5a Note the severe buccal gingival recession and buccal furcations on the right maxillary first and second molars on this 55-year-old man.

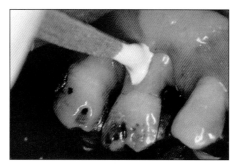

Fig 26-5b Application of sodium fluoride paste via a Stimudent in the buccal furcation. This application is employed to control root caries in the furcation area.

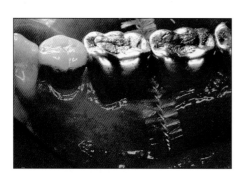

Fig 26-6 Use of an interproximal brush to successfully clean the plaque from a wide embrasure space.

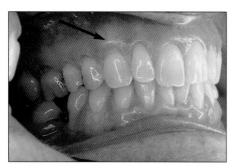

Fig 26-7a Clinical appearance of a 56-year-old woman at the initial office visit.

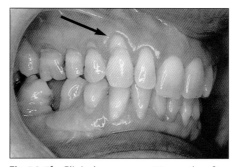

Fig 26-7b Clinical appearance 27 months after her initial visit. Note the progressive gingival recession on the maxillary right canine *(arrow)*. A gingival graft was placed.

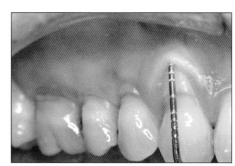

Fig 26-7c Periodontal probe revealing a 5-mm denudation of the root.

Date: _____

To:_____

Regarding:_____

We have recently seen_____for supportive
periodontal care (SPC).

The following conditions were noted:

Oral hygiene:

_____Excellent_____Good_____Fair_____Poor

Periodontal condition:

_____Excellent _____Good_____Fair_____Poor

Teeth with guarded prognosis: _____

Hopeless teeth: Please arrange for removal:

Progressive mobility: _____

Caries: *Please place on your caries recall*

_____

Endodontic lesions: _____

Scheduled SPC, our office: _____

Suggested SPC, your office: _____

Remarks: _____

_____

_____

If at any time you have any questions, please do not hesitate
to contact me.

Sincerely,

Fig 26-8 Communication note. This note allows both the periodontist and referring dentist to evaluate tooth mobility and the status of hard and soft tissues.

have undergone organ transplant surgery and are taking cyclosporine A, similar gingival overgrowth may occur.

Comparable gingival hyperplasia may occur in older adults taking antihypertensives such as nifedipine[13,14] or Cardizem.[15,16] These agents are calcium blockers that inhibit calcium ion transfer into myocardial cells, thereby relieving angina by relaxation and prevention of coronary artery spasm. The gingival overgrowth is due to increased numbers of fibroblasts in the tissue secreting increased amounts of ground substance[17] (Fig 26-9). The re-treatment for patients taking the above-mentioned medications consists of visits for scaling and root planing with reinstitution and remotivation in oral hygiene. When these individuals realize the primary cause of the overgrowth, namely bacterial plaque, they will then frequently become more compliant

patients. When the inflammation has been brought under control and bleeding is essentially absent, the hyperplastic tissue can be removed via gingivectomy. If, however, osseous defects are present, flap procedures and osseous therapies to eliminate the pocketing would be the proper treatment modality.

Chlorhexidine can be used as an adjunctive agent. It has been used in Europe since the 1970s in a concentration of 0.2%; however, the side effects included brown staining of the teeth and a bitter taste. Since 1987, the concentration of 0.12% has been found to be effective, and the taste has been made more palatable with the addition of a mint flavor. Chlorhexidine is an effective supragingival antiplaque agent to control surface bacteria.

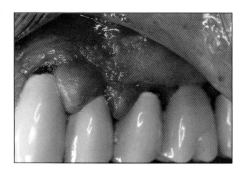

Fig 26-9 Gingival overgrowth in a 66-year-old man who had recently begun taking Procardia, a calcium channel blocker, for his cardiac condition. Note the bulbous nature of the interproximal papillae.

Local Drug Delivery

The use of a local drug delivery system employing antibiotics was first investigated by Goodson et al[18] in 1979. This led to the development of tetracycline-filled hollow fibers, composed of cellulose acetate, which were placed in the inflamed gingival crevice. This treatment changed the microflora and alleviated the clinical signs of periodontal disease. Goodson et al[18] claimed that, with local drug delivery, a 1,000-fold reduction in dose is possible compared to the systemic use of tetracycline hydrochloride; a reduction in the systemic side effects is also evident. With the recent US Food and Drug Administration approval of this form of tetracycline hydrochloride therapy, the fiber is now composed of an extruded ethyl vinyl acetate copolymer loaded with 25% tetracycline.

When Maiden et al[19] studied the effectiveness of the tetracycline fibers via DNA probes, they found that the numbers of periodontal pathogens were greatly reduced compared to those found in the control group in which the antibiotic was not employed. The pathogens they studied were *Actinobacillus actinomycetemcomitans*, *Prevotella intermedia*, *Eikenella corodens*, *Fusobacterium nucleatum*, *Porphyromonas gingivalis*, and *Wolinella recta*.

If a surgical flap procedure was previously performed and continued osseous breakdown is noted at the SPC visit, tetracycline fiber therapy may promote the further reduction of the pathogenic periodontal organisms. A 50-year-old woman had a purulent, recurrent 5-mm pocket in the lingual area of the mandibular central incisors (Fig 26-10a). Tetracycline fibers were applied in the distal and lingual pockets (Fig 26-10b). The fibers were retained in place for 10 days and then removed. Two months after removal of the fibers, purulence was nonexistent, and a residual 3-mm area remained (Fig 26-10c). A careful evaluation of this area

at the SPC visit will reveal the effectiveness of the local drug delivery technique in periodontal therapy.

Noncompliance (Dropout)

In a previously described article, only 16.4% of the patients actually complied with their supportive care.[3] The Ontario Exercise-Heart Collaborative Study studied a group of 678 subjects after myocardial infarctions.[20] More than 46% of these individuals dropped out of the prescribed exercise program. This noncompliant group was studied to determine the reasons for the large number of dropouts. One of the major reasons for dropout was found to be transition, when people moved out of the area; this group constituted about 25% of the dropout group. Psychological reasons accounted for almost 40% of the noncompliance; almost 16% had medical reasons, lacked motivation, or were "too busy." A significant part of this study showed that the blue-collar smokers dropped out at a rate four times higher than white-collar nonsmoking individuals. The continuance of smoking after myocardial infarction was an indication of poor compliance.

In a study of 40 patients who had peripheral vascular disease and who had smoked, only 17% stopped smoking after they were informed that cigarette smoking was associated with their development of peripheral vascular disease.[21] Interestingly, the age group studied was approximately 63 years old. The adult group is also the largest growing cohort in periodontal practices. It should be noted that this study was done in England and not in the United States. It has been well established that smoking is related directly to periodontal bone loss.[22] Cigarette smokers who exhibit good plaque control and who do not have any form of periodontal disease also experience periodontal bone loss.[23]

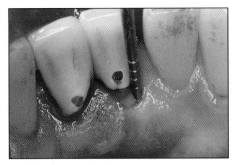

Fig 26-10a Mandibular left central incisor with a 5-mm probing depth. Purulent exudate is visible.

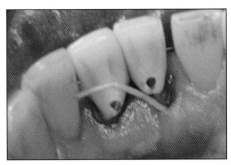

Fig 26-10b Placement of a tetracycline fiber.

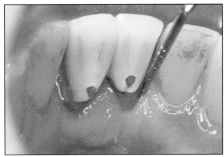

Fig 26-10c Appearance 2 months after removal of the tetracycline fiber. Purulence is nonexistent, and only a 3-mm crevicular depth is recorded. Careful evaluation is needed at the SPC visit.

Implements for Proper Maintenance

Although supportive care is provided, the patient must clean the periodontium on a daily basis. The important "tools" that a patient needs include a soft rounded-end bristle brush, floss (which may have end tufts), and a toothpick with a holder. If spaces are enlarged in the interproximal region after periodontal therapy, the small narrow floss may not be adequate. Interproximal brushes are manufactured by many different companies. These are invaluable aids to proper oral cleanliness. If a patient is arthritic, is physically handicapped, or lacks manual dexterity, an electric toothbrush may be of valuable assistance. Some electric brushes either rotate or oscillate in different directions.

The use of chlorhexidine has been found to be of great benefit for individuals who cannot maintain proper plaque control. Resin composite or silicate restorations will become stained by the germicide and may have to be replaced. The use of chlorhexidine is extremely important in the maintenance of implants. The sulcular-junctional epithelium may be vulnerable to breakdown should inflammation develop in peri-implant tissues.

Tooth Loss

Several studies have discussed tooth loss in treated areas and tooth loss occurring during the maintenance phase in periodontal practices. In a study of 100 patients treated for periodontal disease over a 15-year period, only 9.8% of teeth were lost because of periodontal disease during the maintenance phase and 1.5% were lost because of other causes.[24] The subjects were divided into well-maintained cases, numbering 77; downhill cases, numbering 15; and extremely downhill cases, numbering eight. A total of 2,627 teeth were studied. The population studied included 59 females and 41 males with an average age of 43.8 years.

In Hirschfeld and Wasserman's[25] study of 600 patients, periodontal therapy consisted of selective gingival and subgingival scaling with local anesthesia. The pockets were reduced but not always eradicated. The study revealed a 25% loss of teeth. Only 14 of the 600 patients were 60 to 73 years of age. The other 586 patients ranged from 12 to 59 years old; the average age of all patients was 42 years old.

In a longitudinal study by Pollack[26] over a 13-year period, the average group age was 68.7 years at the start of therapy and 76.8 years at the end of the study. Periodontal therapy consisted of the initial phase of therapy in all individuals. Of the periodontal case types studied (American Academy of Periodontology), 52% were type II, 36% were type III, and 12% were type IV. Twenty-one percent of the individuals only received initial preparation, whereas in 78% initial preparation was followed by surgical procedures, such as gingival grafts, osseous resection or addition procedures, and root resections. Tooth loss throughout the treatment and maintenance phases totaled 4.14%. A total of 950 teeth were present at the start of the study, and only 37 teeth were lost by the end of the study. Of all the studies of periodontal treatment, this study had the greatest number of older patients. These individuals can be successfully treated and maintained.

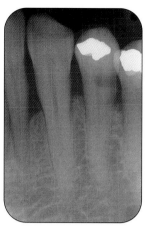

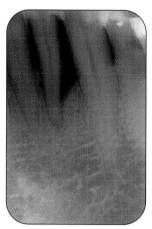

Fig 26-11a Pre–initial preparation radiograph of the area of the mandibular left canine and lateral incisor area (December 1991). Note the 7-mm bone loss distal to the lateral incisor.

Fig 26-11b Radiograph taken in November 1994. After 2.5 years of noncompliance, the patient exhibits progressive bone loss. Bone loss extends to a level of about 3 mm from the apex. The mandibular anterior teeth were stabilized in 1992 with wire mesh and resin composite.

Case Study

A 47-year-old man presented in December 1991 with periodontal probing depths ranging from 4 to 9 mm generally throughout his periodontium. Mobility patterns were in the range of 2 to 3 degrees on the Miller scale of 0 to 3 in the mandibular anterior region. Moderate-to-advanced bone loss was noted in the mandibular incisor canine area (Fig 26-11a). Initial therapy consisted of four visits of scaling and root planing; plaque control measures were demonstrated at each visit. The patient had a history of smoking one and a half packs of cigarettes per day for more than 20 years. It was suggested he stop smoking because of the many systemic and oral hazards of smoking, such as periodontal bone loss.[22,23] The mandibular anterior teeth were stabilized via lingual placement of resin composite and wire mesh. After these areas were splinted in 1992, mandibular anterior surgical procedures were contemplated for pocket elimination. Because of familial problems, the patient did not return for two and a half years.

In 1994, an advanced area of bone loss was noted in the mandibular left canine–lateral incisor region (Fig 26-11b). Progressive bone loss in the rest of the periodontium was also noted and documented. Pockets were now generally even deeper in most of the anterior and posterior regions. The only positive finding was the fact that the mandibular anterior teeth were no longer mobile. This is the history of a patient who was compliant during initial phase therapy. However, the follow-up surgical treatment and SPC were not performed; advanced bone loss ensued. The mode of therapy at this time would be to reinstitute four operative sessions for root planings and then reassess the tissue tone and color. This individual had started taking a calcium channel blocker during the prior year; this could also be a factor in his difficulty in the performance of plaque control.

Longitudinal Studies

The progression of disease in the aforementioned patient paralleled that described by Becker et al,[27] in a longitudinal study of 40 patients with untreated periodontal disease. The patients presented with moderate-to-advanced periodontal disease. The mandibular and maxillary molars had the greatest incidence of tooth loss in the period between the initial and final examinations. They also found that the increase in probing depth was smaller in patients older than 44 years of age. The age of these 30 patients ranged from 25 to 71 years, with a mean of 44.6 years. Sixteen men and fourteen women were in this study. The mean time of study of these patients was 3.72 years. The distolingual and mesiolingual interproximal surface areas had the greatest increase in probing depth, while the lingual and buccal surfaces had the smallest increase in probing depth. This is probably because it is easier for the patient to clean the buccal and lingual surfaces of the teeth than to floss the interproximal regions.

In another longitudinal evaluation of untreated periodontal disease in 1,016 Irish textile workers,[28] 82 patients had never been periodontally treated. This subgroup of 39 males and 43 females, who had an average age of 27 years, was the subject of the study. An average loss of two and a half teeth per individual was observed over a 10-year period. The teeth that were most frequently lost were the maxillary molars. This agrees with the findings of other authors, including Hirschfeld and Wasserman,[25] Becker et al,[27] Marshall-Day et al,[29] and Pollack.[26] Evidence indicates that in older populations periodontal disease progresses steadily from gingivitis to periodontitis.[27] However, younger groups show less rapid deterioration. The findings of Buckley and Crowley[28] suggest that teeth with periodontal disease have a poorer prognosis in younger individuals because of the age involved. One shortcoming of their study is that they did not correlate these findings for untreated periodontal disease with those of a similar group of individuals who were treated for periodontal disease; nor did they describe what types of periodontal services were rendered.[28]

Nabers et al,[6] in their study of tooth loss in 1,535 treated periodontal patients who were recalled over an average period of time of 12.9 years, found that 89% of the individuals did not lose any teeth from periodontal disease. A total of 444 teeth were lost. Surgical procedures were performed in 74% of the patients. At their recall examination, 15.9% of the patients required surgical re-treatment; many of the teeth that were re-treated were of a questionable prognosis. Almost all of the patients in this study were maintained on a 3- to 6-month recall schedule. The recall visits were scheduled according to the patient's periodontal health and oral hygiene effectiveness. The study did not specify the therapy that was performed during recall, other than plaque control procedures.[6]

Goldman et al[30] studied tooth loss in 211 patients who were treated for periodontal disease. Their therapy consisted of oral hygiene instruction and supragingival and subgingival scaling. The only surgical procedures were gingivectomy, gingivoplasty, and, in a few patients, flaps or open curettage. Neither ostectomy nor osteoplasty was performed. Occlusal adjustments were performed for all 211 patients. The patients were maintained for 15 to 34 years on a 3- to 6-month recall schedule; their average age was 42 years. The average time in maintenance was 22 years. Of the 5,761 teeth studied, 771 (13.4%) were lost. The researchers divided the patients into three groups: well-maintained (62%), downhill (28%), and extremely downhill (10%). Approximately 50% of the teeth, excluding the third molars, were lost in the extremely downhill group. In the downhill group, 17.5% of the teeth, excluding the third molars, were lost. Radiographic evidence of furcation bone loss was noted in 636 teeth; however, only five teeth had root amputations during the average 22-year maintenance period. Perhaps if osseous therapies and root resections had been performed, a larger number of teeth would have been retained.

Wilson et al[5] reported that none of the patients who complied with their maintenance schedule lost any teeth. Oliver[31] demonstrated that periodontal disease can be effectively treated and that tooth loss resulting from periodontal disease can be prevented. Over a 5-year period, 442 patients were treated with an average 4.6-month maintenance periodicity. Two of three patients were older than 40 years at the time of treatment. Preventive care consisted of oral hygiene education and prophylaxis only. A total of 11,000 teeth were available for periodontal therapy, and only 178 teeth (just 1.6%) were lost. Oliver[31] did not delineate the type of therapy instituted or the severity of the preexisting periodontal disease.

Adolescent to Young Adult Patients (to 25 Years Old)

This group of individuals, ranging from 8 to 25 years of age, presents several concerns for the periodontist. Common periodontal problems in the adolescent are gingivitis, gingival recession in the mandibular anterior region, and localized juvenile periodontitis. Altered passive eruption is a condition in which the marginal gingiva has not receded to the cementoenamel junction after active eruption of the teeth.[32] The young adult may also have pain and blunting of the gingival papilla. These are signs and symptoms of necrotizing ulcerative gingivitis or, when this progresses further, necrotizing ulcerative periodontitis.

Gingivitis is treated with scalings (initial phase therapy) and oral hygiene instruction; usually SPC visits every 6 months are sufficient. Localized gingival recessions are treated with gingival grafting or other applicable mucogingival surgical procedures. When localized juvenile periodontitis occurs, bacterial studies and antibiotic therapy with or without surgical care are needed. The SPC visits are usually on a 2- to 3-month schedule. When the periodontium has become stable and healthy, a 3- to 6-month SPC regimen would be recommended. The young adult can have signs and symptoms of periodontal disease similar to those found in older cohorts. Smoking, poor oral hygiene, and gingival recession are common complicating and etiologic agents. An initial preparation phase consisting of two to four root planing visits would allow initial healing of the soft tissues. The complications of smoking or chewing tobacco on the periodontium and their relationship to oral cancer should be carefully explained to these individuals. The SPC time schedule depends on the fragility of the periodontium and severity of the periodontal case type.

Young Adult to Middle-Aged Patients (26 to 64 Years Old)

Persons in this age group appear to be susceptible to stress or tension, both at home and in their jobs. Pregnancy can produce enlargement and bleeding of the gingiva; proper SPC visits and education are important to control or prevent this condition. A 2-month interval for SPC programs is common. Individuals in this age group tend to smoke cigarettes. The relationship of smoking to periodontal bone loss should be explained to these patients.

Older Adult Patients (65 Years and Older)

This group of older adults is the fastest growing cohort in the population. People are living longer and having more robust lives. The majority of older adults present with mild-to-moderate periodontal disease; a smaller percentage present with advanced periodontal disease.

Older adults also suffer from many diseases. The most common are arthritis, hypertension, cardiovascular disease, Alzheimer's disease, Parkinson's disease, depression, osteoporosis, and diabetes mellitus.[33] They also may suffer from hearing and visual impairments. At the SPC visit, more time and care must be given for oral hygiene instructions because of these deficiencies or conditions. More time may have to be devoted to these patients. Calcium channel blockers are used to treat blood pressure and other cardiac problems. Medications such as Cardizem[13,14] and nifedipine[14,15] have been reported to cause overgrowth of gingival tissues in patients in whom the bacterial plaque control has been inefficient. The frequency of the SPC visits of any patient is dictated by the patient's ability to control plaque, host resistance factors, the lack of tooth mobility, or displacement of the teeth. The older adult can be successfully treated periodontally and maintained with a common SPC program on a 3-month interval.[26]

Furcation Management

The buccal farcations are the most accessible of all the molar furcations. If a class I or II furcation exists, brushing and use of a toothpick often controls the plaque accumulation. Where similar lingual furcations exist, the same implements can be used.

Where class I or II furcations exist at the mesial or distal areas of the maxillary molars, the concavities are not accessible by flossing. Often brushing alone is inadequate. However, the use of a tapered interproximal brush is very effective in long-term maintenance. The use of a tapered bristle brush in an individual who has maintained the distal furcation without disease progression for 8 years is demonstrated in Figure 26-12. The mesial furcation of the maxillary left second molar is shown in Fig 26-13a. Radiographs taken 19 years apart revealed no progressive bone loss (Figs 26-13b and 26-13c). The region between the molars was well maintained (Fig 26-13d).

Through and through class III furcations on the mandibular molars may be maintained with Superfloss (Oral-B, Redwood City, CA) or an interproximal brush. The usual cause for demise of these molars is caries. Class III furcations on maxillary molars are usually not maintainable. Root resections, endodontics, and possibly increased support via splinted crown-and-bridge prostheses provide a good short-to-long–term prognosis.

Caries

Adult patients become susceptible to root caries especially if increased root surface exposure occurs either following periodontal therapy or in association with gingival recession. The greatly increased exposure of root surfaces in a 61-year-old woman left the teeth potentially vulnerable to root caries (Fig 26-14a). Periodontal surgical procedures included osseous recontouring and gingival grafting. The restored dentition is shown 14 years after periodontal surgery and SPC (Fig 26-14b).

Crown margins must be carefully checked at the SPC visit because caries can readily occur in these area. An 81-year-old woman, whose existing fixed crowns were placed 17 years earlier, is shown in Figure 26-15a. Root caries developed on the buccal surface of the mandibular right lateral incisor. Subsequently, the referring dentist restored this area with a resin composite (Fig 26-15b).

Wallace[34] studied the prevalence of root caries in 603 people aged 60 years and older and reported that 100% of these individuals had gingival recession and 67% had at least one carious root lesion. A study of 375 Swedish individuals studied the effects of oral hygiene on caries and periodontal disease in three age groups.[35] Two subgroups were evaluated for controlled oral hygiene with maintenance every 2 to 3 months over a 6-year period. They found that the well-maintained groups 1 (younger than 35 years), and 2 (36 to 50 years old) had more than 74 times fewer caries than the corresponding nonmaintained groups; group 3 (older than 50 years) had more than 39 times fewer caries than the corresponding nonmaintained group.

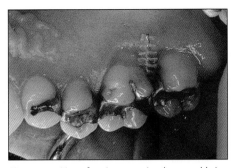

Fig 26-12 Use of an interproximal tapered bristle brush to cleanse the concavities between the roots of each molar.

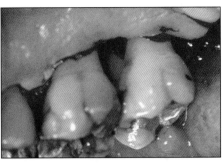

Fig 26-13a Furcation bone loss on the mesial aspect of the maxillary second molar. This patient did not wish any root resections to be performed (1975).

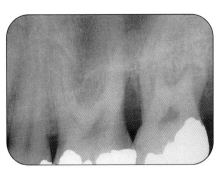

Fig 26-13b Radiograph of the maxillary left molars. Note the distal bone loss on the first molar. The extent of the mesial bone loss on the second molar is not visible.

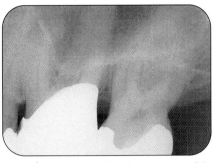

Fig 26-13c Radiograph taken 19 years following the osseous surgery. Bone levels are stable. This patient has faithfully used the tapered interproximal brush. A new crown is present on the first molar.

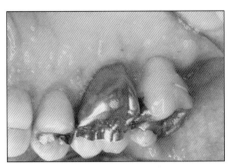

Fig 26-13d Clinical appearance 19 years following the pocket reduction flap surgery. The well-maintained gingival tissues are evident.

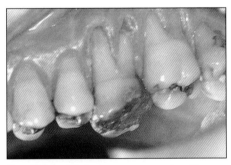

Fig 26-14a Clinical appearance of a 61-year-old woman with severe buccal recession. This exposed root surface is vulnerable to further abrasion and root caries.

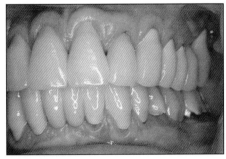

Fig 26-14b Clinical appearance of the same patient 14 years following restorative and periodontal therapies. The first molar was removed.

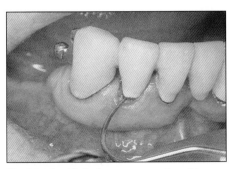

Fig 26-15a Clinical appearance of an 81-year-old woman who presented at her SPC visit. The mandibular reconstruction had been placed 17 years previously. Caries was noted at the buccal crown margin of the mandibular right lateral incisor.

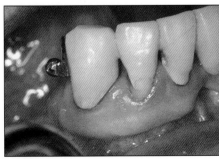

Fig 26-15b Clinical appearance at the patient's next 6-month SPC visit. A resin composite restoration is in place on the lateral incisor.

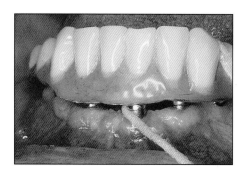

Fig 26-16 Use of Superfloss to cleanse the polished titanium surface of an implant.

Supportive Implant Care

Because the cells of junctional epithelium attach to the surface of titanium via hemidesmosomes with an interposed basement lamina, this junction must be maintained as well as possible. Daily care by the patient is critical to prevent peri-implantitis. Meffert[36] defined an *ailing implant* as one with radiographic bone loss, but no apparent clinical inflammation, at the 3- to 4-month maintenance visit. The *failing implant* is one with radiographic bone loss, signs of inflammation, and steady deterioration observed at the maintenance visit. Mobility is not present. The *failed implant* is one with clinical mobility related to advanced periodontal disease. Meffert[36] further stated that 85% plaque removal may be adequate for proper maintenance.

The patient should apply chlorhexidine on brushes or cotton swabs to the tissue surrounding the implant. Tufted floss, such as Superfloss or Perio-floss (PHB, Inc, Osseo, WI) is effective in areas that a brush cannot reach. Radiographs should be taken every 6 months to evaluate the osseous structures around the implant. Mobility of the superstructure should be recorded, and any loose screws should be tightened. If the implant itself is mobile, it should be removed. A fixed implant case maintained with Superfloss is shown in Figure 26-16.

Halitosis

Patients commonly ask the periodontist or hygienist, "Do I have bad breath?" A family member or friend may mention this to the patient. The origin of halitosis may be local or extraoral. Shklar[37] characterized a fetid odor as an oral sign of acute necrotizing ulcerative gingivitis (ANUG). Otomo[38] listed the local sources of mouth odor as the retention of odoriferous food, ANUG, caries, smokers' breath, and chronic periodontal disease. The extraoral sources may include sinusitis, tonsillitis, lung abscesses, and pulmonary excretion of odors derived from aromatic substances in the bloodstream. Recently, studies show that chemicals are a cause of non–disease-related bad breath.[39] Further investigation is needed to clarify the origin and treatment of halitosis.

Conclusion

The goal of periodontal therapy is to retain the greatest number of teeth for the longest possible time in the healthiest possible functional environment. Well-maintained patients retain more teeth than poorly maintained or non-maintained patients. To allow comparison of the progression of healing after treatment or any distinctive gingival or osseous changes in quality or form, proper initial and post-therapeutic documentation is essential.

References

1. Cohen DW. The maintenance phase. In: Genco RJ, Goldman HM, Cohen DW (eds). Contemporary Periodontics, ed 3. St Louis: Mosby, 1964:878.

2. McFall WT Jr. Supportive treatment. In: Nevins M, Becker W, Kornman K (eds). Proceedings of the World Workshop in Clinical Periodontics. Chicago: American Academy of Periodontology, 1989:IX-1–IX-28.

3. Wilson TG, Glover ME, Schoen J, Baus C, Jacobs T. Compliance with maintenance therapy in a private periodontal practice. J Periodontol 1984;55:468.

4. Becker W, Berg L, Becker BE. The long term evaluation of periodontal treatment and maintenance in 95 patients. Int J Periodont Rest Dent 1984;4(2):55.

5. Wilson TG, Glover ME, Malik AK, Schoen JA, Dorsett D. Tooth loss in maintenance patients in a private periodontal practice. J Periodontol 1987;58:231.

6. Nabers CL, Stalker WH, Esparza D, Naylor B, Canales S. Tooth loss in 1535 treated periodontal patients. J Periodontol 1988;59:297.

7. Lindhe J, Nyman S. Long-term maintenance of patients treated for advanced periodontal disease. J Clin Periodontol 1984;11:504.

8. Goldman HM. Coronal and root surface scaling—Initial preparation. In: Goldman HM, Schluger S, Fox L, Cohen DW (eds). Periodontal Therapy, ed 3. St Louis: Mosby, 1964:347.

9. Grant DA, Stern IB, Everett FG. Treatment plan. In: Grant DA, Stern IB, Everett FG (eds). Periodontics in the Tradition of Orban and Gottlieb, ed 5. St Louis: Mosby, 1979:511.

10. Pollack RP. Periodontal and restorative considerations for the older adult. Periodontal Insights 1994;1:4.

11. Kabani SP, Pollack RP. Osteosarcoma presenting as supracrestal bone formation. J Periodontol 1994;65:93–96.

12. Caffesse RG. Maintenance therapy: Preventing recurrence of periodontal diseases. In: Genco RJ, Goldman HM, Cohen DW (eds). Contemporary Periodontics, ed 6. St Louis: Mosby, 1990:483.

13. Butler RT, Kalkwarf KL, Kaldahl WB. Drug-induced gingival hyperplasia: Phenytoin, cyclosporine, and nifedipine. J Am Dent Assoc 1987;114:56.

14. Barak S, Engleberg IS, Hiss J. Gingival hyperplasia caused by nifedipine. Histopathologic findings. J Periodontol 1987;58:639.

15. Colvard MD, Bishop J, Weissman D, Gargiulo AV. Cardizem induced gingival hyperplasia: Report of two cases. Periodontal Case Reports 1986;8:67.

16. Lederman D, Lumerman H, Reuben S, Freedman P. Gingival hyperplasia associated with nifedipine therapy. Oral Surg Oral Med Oral Pathol 1973;57:620.

17. Lucas RM, Howell LP, Wall BA. Nifedipine-induced gingival hyperplasia: A histochemical and ultrastructural study. J Periodontol 1985;56:211.

18. Goodson JM, Haffajee A, Socransky SS. Periodontal therapy by local delivery of tetracycline. J Clin Periodontol 1979;6:83–92.

19. Maiden MFJ, Tanner A, McArdie S, Najpauer K, Goodson JM. Tetracycline fiber therapy monitored by DNA probe and cultural methods. J Periodont Res 1991;26:452.

20. Oldridge NB, Donner AP, Buck CW, et al. Predictors of dropout from cardiac exercise rehabilitation. Ontario Exercise-Heart Collaborative Study. Am J Cardiol 1983;51:70–74.

21. Clyne CAC, Arch PJ, Carpenter D, Webster JHH, Chant ADB. Smoking, ignorance, and peripheral vascular disease. Arch Surg 1982;117:1062–1065.

22. Bergstrom J, Eliasson S, Preber H. Cigarette smoking and periodontal bone loss. J Periodontol 1991;62:242–246.

23. Haber J, Wattles J, Crowley M, Mandell R, Joshipura K, Kent RL. Evidence for cigarette smoking as a major risk factor for periodontitis. J Periodontol 1993;64:16–23.

24. McFall WT Jr. Tooth loss in 100 treated patients with periodontal disease: A long term study. J Periodontol 1982;53:539–549.

25. Hirschfeld L, Wasserman B. A long term survey of tooth loss in 600 treated periodontal patients. J Periodontol 1978;49:225–237.

26. Pollack RP. An analysis of periodontal therapy for the 65 year old and older: A longitudinal study of 42 patients in a 13 year old periodontal practice. Gerodontics 1986;2:135–137.

27. Becker W, Berg L, Becker BE. Untreated periodontal disease: A longitudinal study. J Periodontol 1979;50:234–244.

28. Buckley LA, Crowley MJ. A longitudinal study of untreated periodontal disease. J Clin Periodontol 1984;11:523–530.

29. Marshall-Day CD, Stephens RG, Quigley LF Jr. Periodontal disease: Prevalence and incidence. J Periodontol 1982;53:539–549.

30. Goldman MJ, Ross IF, Goteiner D. Effect of periodontal therapy on patients maintained for fifteen years or longer: A retrospective study. J Periodontol 1986;57:346–353.

31. Oliver RC. Tooth loss with or without periodontal therapy. Periodont Abstr 1969;17:8–9.

32. Goldman HM, Ruben MP, Everett FG. The normal periodontium. In: Baer PN, Benjamin SD (eds). Periodontal Disease in Children and Adolescents. Philadelphia: Lippincott, 1974:31.

33. Rose ST. Periodontal Care for the Older Adult: An Informational Report. Chicago: American Academy of Periodontology, 1994:3.

34. Wallace M. More root caries for senior class. Dent Today 1987;6:1.

35. Axelsson P, Lindhe J. Effect of controlled oral hygiene procedures on caries and periodontal disease in adults. J Clin Periodontol 1981;8:239–248.

36. Meffert RM. How to treat ailing and failing implants. Implant Dent 1992;1:25–33.

37. Shklar G. Periodontal pathology. In: Carranza FA (ed). Clinical Periodontology, ed 6. Philadelphia: Saunders, 1984:148.

38. Otomo JA. Diagnosis. In: Carranza FA (ed). Clinical Periodontology, ed 6. Philadelphia: Saunders, 1984:497.

39. Kleinberg I, Westbay G. Oral malodor. Crit Rev Oral Biol Med 1990;1:247.

INDEX

G

R